Lecture Notes in Electrical Engineering

Volume 746

The book series *Lecture Notes in Electrical Engineering* (LNEE) publishes the latest developments in Electrical Engineering - quickly, informally and in high quality. While original research reported in proceedings and monographs has traditionally formed the core of LNEE, we also encourage authors to submit books devoted to supporting student education and professional training in the various fields and applications areas of electrical engineering. The series cover classical and emerging topics concerning:

- Communication Engineering, Information Theory and Networks
- Electronics Engineering and Microelectronics
- Signal, Image and Speech Processing
- Wireless and Mobile Communication
- Circuits and Systems
- Energy Systems, Power Electronics and Electrical Machines
- Electro-optical Engineering
- Instrumentation Engineering
- Avionics Engineering
- Control Systems
- Internet-of-Things and Cybersecurity
- Biomedical Devices, MEMS and NEMS

For general information about this book series, comments or suggestions, please contact leontina.dicecco@springer.com.

To submit a proposal or request further information, please contact the Publishing Editor in your country:

China

Jasmine Dou, Editor (jasmine.dou@springer.com)

India, Japan, Rest of Asia

Swati Meherishi, Editorial Director (Swati.Meherishi@springer.com)

Southeast Asia, Australia, New Zealand

Ramesh Nath Premnath, Editor (ramesh.premnath@springernature.com)

USA, Canada:

Michael Luby, Senior Editor (michael.luby@springer.com)

All other Countries:

Leontina Di Cecco, Senior Editor (leontina.dicecco@springer.com)

**** This series is indexed by EI Compendex and Scopus databases. ****

More information about this series at http://www.springer.com/series/7818

Triwiyanto · Hanung Adi Nugroho ·
Achmad Rizal · Wahyu Caesarendra
Editors

Proceedings of the 1st International Conference on Electronics, Biomedical Engineering, and Health Informatics

ICEBEHI 2020, 8–9 October, Surabaya, Indonesia

Springer

Editors
Triwiyanto
Department of Electromedical Engineering
Poltekkes Kemenkes
Surabaya, Indonesia

Hanung Adi Nugroho
Department of Electrical and Information Engineering
Gadjah Mada University
Yogyakarta, Indonesia

Achmad Rizal
Faculty of Electrical and Communication Engineering
Telkom University
Bandung, Jawa Barat, Indonesia

Wahyu Caesarendra
Faculty of Integrated Technologies
Universiti Brunei Darussalam
Gadong, Brunei Darussalam

ISSN 1876-1100 ISSN 1876-1119 (electronic)
Lecture Notes in Electrical Engineering
ISBN 978-981-33-6925-2 ISBN 978-981-33-6926-9 (eBook)
https://doi.org/10.1007/978-981-33-6926-9

This Springer imprint is published by the registered company Springer Nature Singapore Pte Ltd.
The registered company address is: 152 Beach Road, #21-01/04 Gateway East, Singapore 189721, Singapore

Organization

General Chair

Triwiyanto, Poltekkes Kemenkes Surabaya, Indonesia

Conference Chair

M. Ridha Mak'ruf, Poltekkes Kemenkes Surabaya, Indonesia

Program Chair

Endro Yulianto, Poltekkes Kemenkes Surabaya, Indonesia

Local Program Committee

Achmad Rizal, Telkom University, Indonesia
Alfian Pramudita Putra, Universitas Airlangga, Indonesia
Alfin Hikmaturokhman, Institut Teknologi Telkom Purwokerto, Indonesia
Anggun Fitrian Isnanti, Institut Teknologi Telkom Purwokerto, Indonesia
Anita Miftahul Maghfiroh, Poltekkes Kemenkes Surabaya, Indonesia
Bambang Guruh Irianto, Poltekkes Kemenkes Surabaya, Indonesia
Bedjo Utomo, Poltekkes Kemenkes Surabaya, Indonesia
Eka Legya Franita, Universitas Gadjah Mada, Indonesia
Endro Yulianto, Poltekkes Kemenkes Surabaya, Indonesia
Hanifah Rahmi Fajrin, Universitas Muhammadiyah Yogyakarta, Indonesia

Hendra Ari Winarno, Universitas Muhammadiyah Gresik, Indonesia
Herri Trilaksana, Universitas Airlangga, Indonesia
Husneni Mukhtar, Telkom University, Indonesia
I Dewa Gede HW, Poltekkes Kemenkes Surabaya, Indonesia
Inung Wijayanto, Telkom University, Indonesia
Iswanto Iswanto, Universitas Muhammadiyah Yogyakarta, Indonesia
Khusnul Ain, Universitas Airlangga, Indonesia
Latifah Listyalina, Universitas Respati, Indonesia
Made Rahmawaty, Politeknik Caltex Riau, Indonesia
Mochammad Prastawa ATP, Poltekkes Kemenkes Surabaya, Indonesia
Muzni Sahar, Politeknik Caltex Riau, Indonesia
Nada Fitriyatul Hikmah, Institut Teknologi Sepuluh Nopember, Indonesia
Osmalina Rahma, Universitas Airlangga, Indonesia
Priyambada Cahya Nugraha, Poltekkes Kemenkes Surabaya, Indonesia
Ratna Lestari Budiani Buana, Universitas Gadjah Mada, Indonesia
Ridha Mak'Ruf, Poltekkes Kemenkes Surabaya, Indonesia
Riky Tri Yunardi, Universtias Airlangga, Indonesia
Sari Luthfiyah, Poltekkes Kemenkes Surabaya, Indonesia
Syahri Muharom, Institut Teknologi Adhi Tama, Surabaya, Indonesia
Syaifudin, Poltekkes Kemenkes Surabaya, Indonesia
Syevana Dita Musvika, Poltekkes Kemenkes Surabaya, Indonesia
Tenia Wahyuningrum, Institut Teknologi Telkom Purwokerto, Indonesia
Tianur Tianur, Politeknik Caltex Riau, Indonesia
Triana Rahmawati, Poltekkes Kemenkes Surabaya, Indonesia
Triwiyanto, Poltekkes Kemenkes Surabaya, Indonesia
Wahyu Pamungkas, Institut Teknologi Telkom Purwokerto, Indonesia
Wisnu Kartika, Universitas Muhammadiyah Yogyakarta, Indonesia
Yuli Triyani, Politeknik Caltex Riau, Indonesia

International Program Committee

Ejay Nsugbe, Cranfield University, Cranfield, UK
Eko Supriyanto, Universiti Teknology Malaysia, Malaysia
Kharudin Ali, University College TATI, Malaysia
Marwan Nafea Minjal, University of Nottingham, Malaysia
Nehru Nehruk, Institute of Aeronautical Engineering, India
Nirmalya Thakur, University of Cincinnaty, USA
Peter Anto Johnson, University of Alberta, Canada
Pringgo Widyo, Gifu University, Japan
Raja Siti Nur Adiimah Raja Aris, University College TATI, Malaysia
Rezwanul Ahsan, Daffodil International University, Bangladesh
Sidharth Pancholi, Indian Institute of Technology Delhi, India
Suzanna Ridzuan Aw, University College TATI, Malaysia

Preface

ICEBEHI-2020, the International Conference on Electronics, Biomedical Engineering, and Health Informatics, took place during 8–9 October 2020 on virtual platforms (Zoom app). The conference was organized by the Department of Electromedical Engineering, Poltekkes Kemenkes Surabaya, Indonesia, and co-organized by Universiti Colege TATI Malaysia, Universitas Muhammadiyah Yogyakarta, Indonesia, Institut Teknologi TELKOM Purwokerto, Indonesia, with aims of bringing together as family all leading scientists, academicians, educationist, young scientist, research scholars and students to present, discuss and exchange their experiences, innovation ideas and recent development in the field of electronics, biomedical engineering and health informatics.

Taking into account the COVID-19 pandemic, the ICEBEHI-2020 conference was held virtually as agencies around the world are now issuing restrictions on travel, gatherings and meetings in an effort to limit and slow the spread of this pandemic. The health and safety of our participants and members of our research community is of top priority to the Organizing Committee. Therefore, the ICEBEHI-2020 conference was held online through Zoom software. More than 100 participants (presenter and non-presenter) attended the conference; they were from Albania, Canada, China, Columbia, Indonesia, Libya, Malaysia and Russia. The scientific program of this conference included many topics related to electronics and biomedical engineering as well as those in related fields. In this conference, two distinguished keynote speakers and two invited speakers had delivered their research works in the area of biomedical engineering. Each keynote speech lasted 50 min.

ICEBEHI-2020 Conference collects the latest research results and applications on electronics, biomedical engineering and health informatics. It includes a selection of 63 papers from 152 papers submitted to the conference from universities all over the world. All of the accepted papers were subjected to strict peer reviewing by 2–3 expert referees. All the articles have gone through a plagiarism check. The papers have been selected for this volume because of quality and relevance to the conference.

We are very grateful to the Committee which contributed to the success of this conference. Also, we are thankful to the authors who submitted the papers; it was quality of their presentations and communication with the other participants that really made this web conference fruitful. Last but not least, we are thankful to the Lecture Note in Electrical Engineering (Springer) Publishing for their support; it was not only the support but also an inspiration for the organizers. We hope this conference can be held every year to make it an ideal platform for people to share views and experiences in electronics, biomedical engineering, health informatics and related areas. We are expecting you and more experts and scholars around the globe to join this international event next year.

Surabaya, Indonesia

Dr. Triwiyanto
triwi@poltekkesdepkes-sby.ac.id

Contents

Porat^{Rank} to Improve Performance Recommendation System

Sri Lestari, Rio Kurniawan, and Deppi Linda

Abstract The e-commerce recommendation system has experienced tremendous progress and has caused an explosion of information, making it difficult for users to choose items that fit their preferences and take a long time. One way to overcome this condition is to use a collaborative filtering approach. Collaborative filtering generally uses similarity measurements and ranking predictions to produce recommendations. However, the recommendations presented are less reliable when data conditions are sparse. This condition encourages the development of ranking-based collaborative filtering. Some ranking-based methods are Copeland and Borda, which carry out an aggregation process to produce product ratings that are recommended to users. Both of these methods use limited ranking data at the user preference profile stage and do not involve re-ranking data during the aggregation process. This process causes the resulting recommendations to decrease in quality. Therefore, this paper proposes the Porat^{Rank} method. The basic idea of this method is to optimize the utilization of ranking data to produce product ratings that are more in line with user preferences. Ranking data is used as an additional factor in determining product points. Determination of product points not only looks at the ranking value but also considers the same number of ratings, and the position of the product in its appearance. It also sees the effect of the ranking value using the minus function. Optimizing ranking data in the aggregation process can improve the recommendation results, as shown by the average value (NDCG) of the Porat^{Rank} method, which is higher than the Borda and Copeland methods. The Porat^{Rank} method is faster than the Copeland method and manages to overcome the problem

S. Lestari (✉) · R. Kurniawan · D. Linda
Faculty of Computer Science, Institut Informatika dan Bisnis Darmajaya, Bandar Lampung, Indonesia
e-mail: srilestari@darmajaya.ac.id

R. Kurniawan
e-mail: riokurniawan@darmajaya.ac.id

D. Linda
e-mail: deppilinda@darmajaya.ac.id

H. Triwiyanto et al. (eds.), *Proceedings of the 1st International Conference on Electronics, Biomedical Engineering, and Health Informatics*, Lecture Notes in Electrical Engineering 746, https://doi.org/10.1007/978-981-33-6926-9_1

of sparsity and scalability, which is a major problem in the collaborative filtering approach, so the Porat^{Rank} method is feasible to be used in improving performance recommendations system.

Keywords Collaborative filtering · Ranking-based · Porat-Rank

1 Introduction

E-Commerce was introduced around the 1990s and has experienced an unexpected rate of development [1]. The number of companies that leveraged E-Commerce as the primary means of business. The use of E-Commerce for marketing various items from various manufacturers. As E-Commerce developed, there were many manufacturers joined [1] so that there is intense competition. These conditions must be supported by E-Commerce with quick and accurate service in providing item recommendations personally [2, 3]. Item recommendations are based on known users' preferences so that the users can get items quickly and accurately based on their needs.

In general, the E-Commerce recommendation system uses a collaborative filtering approach to provide item recommendations. This approach works by analyzing the rating data pattern to predict user preferences based on similarities with other users [4]. Collaborative filtering consists of two types, namely, user-based [5] and item-based [6, 7]. User-based collaborative filtering observes the similarity of the target user through the rating given by the previous user. The similarity value is used as a reference for providing item recommendations [8].

Meanwhile, item-based collaborative filtering uses the similarity between items to predict user preferences by looking at the similarity between users. As an illustration, an item is similar if there are two items favored by the same user. This thing showed that the user has the same interest in the items purchased [8].

Rating data that is similar to other users and other items in practice is rarely found due to the sparsity of data rating conditions. Sparsity is a condition where the data are not fully completed [9]. One cause of sparsity is the presence of new items that are less desired by the user or the lack of information; thus, the users cannot rate the item. Besides, it can be caused by the presence of new users, who do not like the item or leave the item without giving a rating. If the rating data is rare, it is difficult to determine the similarities between users; therefore, it creates poor recommendations quality [10]. Apart from the sparsity problem, the recommendation system also has scalability problems that require a reliable method. Several approaches have been taken to overcome this problem, such as BordaRank. BordaRank consists of two steps. The first is to fill in the sparsity data using Collaborative Filtering (CF). The second step is to do the aggregation process to produce the product ranking using the Borda Count method [11]. The method can improve precision and recall, but the coverage value is lower than collaborative filtering items. Another research used the Copeland Score aggregation method [12].

The use of this method was to rate the types of products because it can work productively and stably. Also, the Copeland Score method is simple to use for analyzing a portion of an extensive collection of products.

Copeland and Borda method utilizes limited rating data for the user preference profiles stage and does not re-involve rating data during the aggregation process. This process causes the recommendations produced to be of poor quality. Therefore, this study proposed a novel method, namely Porat^{Rank}. The basic idea of the Porat^{Rank} method is to try to optimize the utilization of rating data to produce a better product ranking that is according to user preferences. Rating data is not only for creating a user preference profile; besides that, the use of rating data as an additional factor in determining product points. Determination of the point of the initial product is adjusted to the position of the product in the list of preferences (user preference profiles), i.e., the product in the first position will get n points (n = number of products), and products with the last position get 1 point. So in the research proposed, three conditions determine the product points, namely the rating value, the same number of ratings, and the position of the product according to its appearance. Furthermore, it also looked at the effect of the rating value by using a minus function for products with a rating value <4. Optimizing rating data in the aggregation process of the Porat^{Rank} method has succeeded in improving the quality of recommendations. Porat^{Rank} also managed to overcome the problem of sparsity and scalability. This was happened because Porat^{Rank} can produce recommendations well despite the sparse data conditions, and without having to fill in un-rated data. Besides, the Porat^{Rank} method can solve scalability problems as indicated by running time, which is almost constant even though there is an increase in the amount of input data.

This organization of this paper as follows; Sect. 2 describes the research method, which is Porat^{Rank}. Section 3 describes the experiments conducted from preparing the dataset, basic algorithm as a comparison, and evaluation method used. Section 4 explains the results of the experiments, and Sect. 5 mentions the conclusions.

2 Research Method

2.1 Material

The material used in this research is dataset widely applied in collaborative filtering [13–18]. The MovieLens 100 k dataset has approximately 1682 movies, used by 943 users, and with 100,000 ratings. The rating of the user was on a scale of 1–5, which showed the direction of the user valuation of the item. It means the greater the rating value that was given by the user to an item, the higher the user's interest on the item, and vice versa.

2.2 Proposed Method

The Porat^{Rank} method was proposed in this study to produce more appropriate recommendations by user interests. The Porat^{Rank} method works by optimizing the utilization of rating data. Based on rating data, the same rating is calculated, product points are determined and see the effect of rating values using the minus functions as the results to correct the Copeland and Borda methods. Both of these methods use a data rating limited to user preference profiles. That is sort products by way of decreasing. Products with a high rating will be in a higher position compared to products that have a smaller rating. Also, Copeland and Borda methods in the aggregation process do not involve rating data again. These methods have an impact on the decline in the quality of recommendations produced by the methods of Copeland and Borda. Therefore Porat^{Rank} method is a solution to solve this problem. Porat^{Rank} will produce a better product ranking as a reference to be recommended to users.

Porat^{Rank} method has the following work stages:

(1) Calculate the same number of ratings.

$$S_{(u_g,p_h)} = \sum_{k=1}^{n} SR\left(R_{(u_g,p_h)}, R_{(k,p_h)}\right) \tag{1}$$

$$SR\left(R_{(u_g,p_h)}, R_{(k,p_h)}\right) = \begin{cases} 1, & \textit{if } R_{(u_g,p_h)} = R_{(k,p_h)} \\ 0, & \textit{if } R_{(u_g,p_h)} = 0 \\ 0, & \textit{otherwise} \end{cases} \tag{2}$$

The user is represented as $U = \{u_1, u_2, \ldots, u_g, \ldots u_{l-1}, u_l\}$ and the product is denoted as $P = \{p_1, p_2, \ldots, p_h, \ldots p_{m-1}, p_m\}$. R., for example, denotes the rating given by the user to the product; the user to-g gives the product rating to-h then it is written with $R_{(u_g,p_h)}$.

Eq. 1 states that the same number of ratings $S_{(u_g,p_h)}$ is obtained by calculating the same number of ratings in each SR product $SR\left(R_{(u_g,p_h)}, R_{(k,p_h)}\right)$. The same rating will be given the value of 1. Otherwise, it is 0, as shown in Eq. (2).

(2) Determine product ranking points

$$P_{(u_g,p_h)} = 1 + \sum_{k=1}^{m} PR(u_g, p_h, k) \tag{3}$$

$$PR(u_g, p_h, k) = \begin{cases} 1, & \textit{if } R_{(u_g,p_h)} > R_{(u_g,k)}, \\ 1, & \textit{if } R_{(u_g,p_h)} = R_{(u_g,k)}, S_{(u_g,p_h)} > S_{(u_g,k)}, \\ 1, & \textit{if } R_{(u_g,p_h)} = R_{(u_g,k)}, S_{(u_g,p_h)} > S_{(u_g,k)}, \\ 0, & \textit{Otherwise} \end{cases} \tag{4}$$

Equation 3 determined the product ranking $\left(P_{(u_g,p_h)}\right)$ obtained from value 1 plus the result of the sum of the points that meet the requirements in Eq. 4. The product point is given the value of 1 if:

a. $\left(R_{(u_g,p_h)}\right)$ product rating to-*h* is greater than the product rating to-$k\left(R_{(u_g,k)}\right)$.
b. $\left(R_{(u_g,p_h)}\right)$ product rating to-*h* is equal to the product rating to-$k\left(R_{(u_g,k)}\right)$ and the same number of ratings on the product to-$h\left(S_{(u_g,p_h)}\right)$ is greater than the same number of ratings on the product to-$k\left(S_{(u_g,k)}\right)$.
c. The product rating to-*h* is the same as the product rating to-*k* and the same rating number on the $\left(S_{(u_g,p_h)}\right)$ product to-*h* is the same as the same rating on the product to-$k\left(S_{(u_g,k)}\right)$ and the *h* product index is smaller than the *k* product index.
d. Otherwise, the value of 0 is given.

(3) Calculate Porat

$$Porat_{(u_g,p_h)} = \begin{cases} \left(\left(R_{u_g,p_h}\right) \times \left(S_{u_g,p_h}\right) \times \left(P_{u_g,p_h}\right) \times -1\right) & if \left(R_{u_g,p_h}\right) < 4 \\ \left(\left(R_{u_g,p_h}\right) \times \left(S_{u_g,p_h}\right) \times \left(P_{u_g,p_h}\right)\right) & Otherwise \end{cases} \quad (5)$$

Equation 5 is the $Porat_{(u_g,p_h)}$ calculation process, which is obtained from the product rating process $\left(R_{u_g,p_h}\right)$ multiplication process with the same product rating $\left(S_{u_g,p_h}\right)$ and product ranking point $\left(P_{u_g,p_h}\right)$. If the product rating is smaller than 4 then the value is multiplied by −1.

(4) Calculate Porat^{Rank}

$$Porat - Rank_{(p_h)} = \sum_{k=1}^{n} PR_{(k,p_h)} \quad (6)$$

Equation 6 states that Porat^{Rank} $\left(Porat - Rank_{(p_h)}\right)$ is obtained by summing the rating points for each product $\left(Porat_{(k,p_h)}\right)$.
The output from Porat^{Rank} is a score for each product, which will then be sorted from the highest score to the lowest score and taken by Top-K products.

This study was conducted in two steps; the first step was calculating user similarity by using Cosine similarity [15, 19, 20] (Eq. (7)). Furthermore, based on the following similarity values, Top N users were taken. The next step was to carry out the aggregation process using the proposed Porat^{Rank} method.

$$\text{Cosine } similarity\,(u,v) = \frac{\sum_{j=1}^{n}(r_{u,i})(r_{v,i})}{\sqrt{\sum_{j=1}^{n}(r_{u,i})^2}\sqrt{\sum_{j=1}^{n}(r_{v,i})^2}} \tag{7}$$

The rating of users u and user v for item i is denoted by $(r_{u,\ i})$ and $(r_{v,\ i})$, then for the number of items commonly rated by two users it is denoted by n.

3 Experiment

A series of experiments were conducted to evaluate the Porat^{Rank} method. The experimental protocol and ranking quality analysis were explained in detail as follows.

3.1 Evaluation Methodology

The evaluation was done by measuring the effectiveness of the proposed method in various conditions of user-profiles and the number of ratings from users. Similar to Shams and Haratizadeh's study [21], each user took several T ratings randomly, and they were placed as a training set, and the rest become as a test set. This evaluation involved T = 20, 30, 40, and 50 items. Every T was guaranteed to get a minimum of 10 ratings from each user. This study generated five variants of the 100 k dataset through a random sample.

3.2 Basic Algorithm

Porat^{Rank} implementation was done by combining rating-based and ranking-based collaborative filtering. A combination of similarity (Cosine similarity) approaches with Porat^{Rank} to produce product recommendations. This study compares the performance of the proposed method with the primary ranking-based method, namely Copeland and Borda.

- Copeland Score [22–24] is an aggregation method that works by calculating the frequency of wins, which is then reduced by the results of calculating the frequency of defeat. The frequency of wins and frequency of defeat were obtained from a pairwise contest process between a product with the entire product.
- Borda [11, 24–26] is an aggregation method that is carried out by calculating the points of each product. Points are obtained from the product position in the

preference list. N point is given to the product in the first position, the $n-1$ point was given to the product in the second position, and so on to 1 point for the product in the last position.

3.3 Matric Evaluation

The product ranking, which was the algorithm output, was evaluated using normalized discounted cumulative gain (NDCG). This evaluation was widely used in ranking-based collaborative filtering [21, 27–29]. NDCG@p is calculated using Eqs. (8) and (9).

$$DCG@p = \sum_{i=1}^{p} \frac{2^{rel_i} - 1}{\log_2(i+1)} \tag{8}$$

$$NDCG@p = \frac{DCG@p}{IDCG@P} \tag{9}$$

With i was the range of positions in the recommendation list, and $\mathrm{rel_i}$ showed the item preferences by the user. The $\mathrm{rel_i}$ was sorted in descending order and then calculated using Eq. (8) to obtain the IDCG. NDCG (Eq. (9)) was obtained by dividing DCG with IDCG. Our experiments calculated NDCG@1, NDCG@3, NDCG@5, and NDCG@10 for all algorithms.

3.4 Running Time Evaluation

This study also analyzes the performance of the recommendation system by calculating the running time of the algorithm. The running time evaluation is very dependent on the environment in which the application is running and the complexity of the system being constructed. The running time and the application must be based on the same system environment. This experiment used a Processor Intel Core i7, Hard Disk 1 TB, 8 GB RAM, and MATLAB R2014 software to evaluations all the observed methods. Some researchers conducted running time evaluations such as Da Silva et al. [30] and Chen et al. [31].

3.5 Scalability Evaluation

Scalability is essential as a collaborative filtering recommendation system manages millions of users or goods [32]. Data on a large scale require a lot of resources and reliable computing. In addition to the hardware specifications, the algorithm or method used also plays a role in improving the performance of the system recommendations. Thus, the scalability evaluation was done to analyze how the algorithm ran when the data were on a large scale. Scalability issues were evaluated by Shams and Haratizadeh [21], Shou-Qiang [33] and Tikk [31].

4 Result

The results showed that the performance of the Porat^{Rank} method was superior to the Borda and Copeland methods, as shown in Figs. 1, 2, 3, 4.

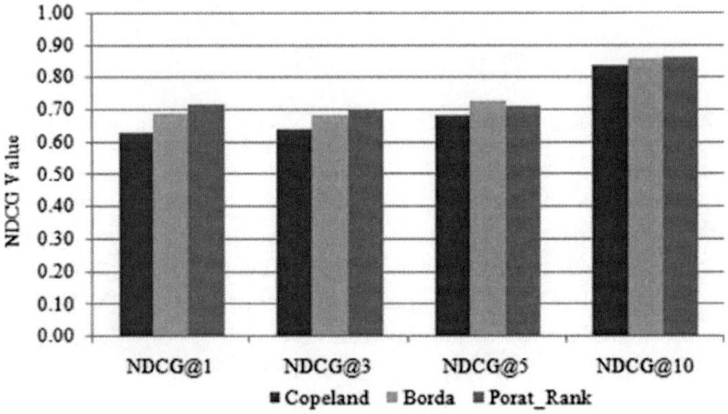

Fig. 1 Performance comparison (NDCG) of algorithms with T = 20

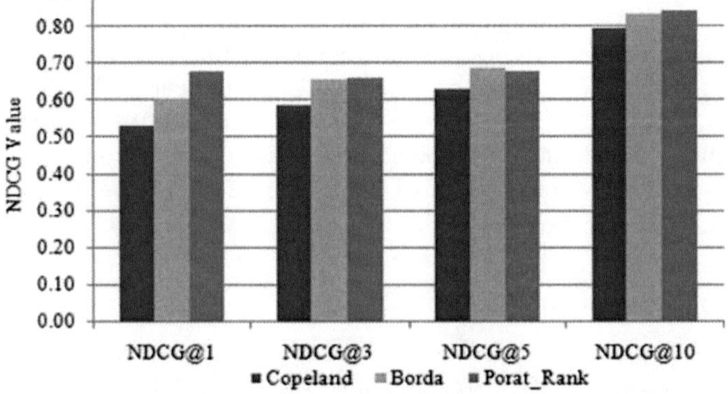

Fig. 2 Performance comparison (NDCG) of algorithms with T = 30

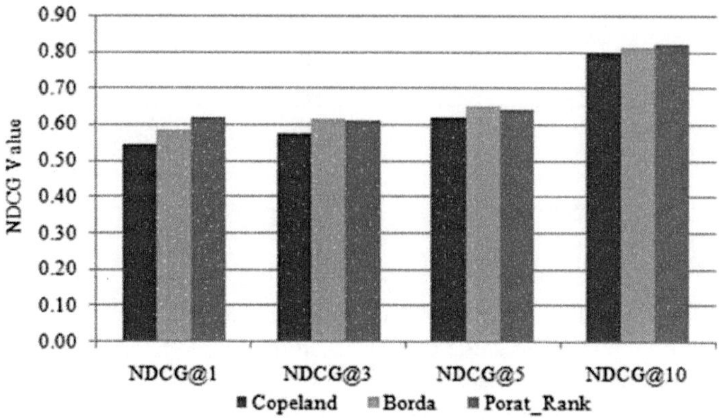

Fig. 3 Performance comparison (NDCG) of algorithms with T = 40

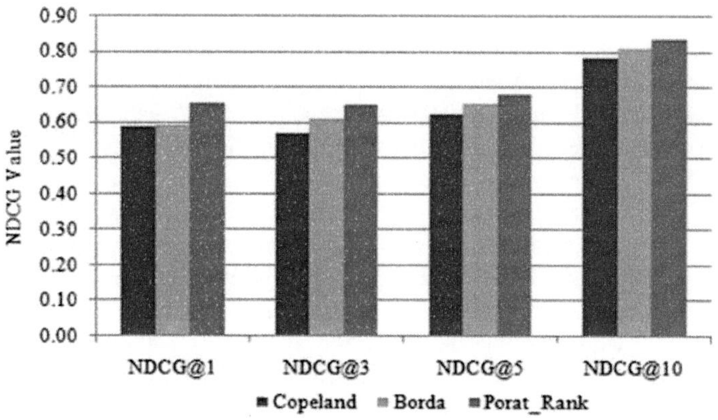

Fig. 4 Performance comparison (NDCG) of algorithms with T = 50

Figures 1 and 2 displayed the performance of the methods when T = 20 and T = 30. At NDCG@1, NDCG@3, and NDCG@10, the Porat^{Rank} method had a higher value than Copeland and Borda methods. Meanwhile, at NDCG@5, the Borda method was better than the Porat^{Rank} and Copeland methods.

Figure 3 shows the performance of the methods when T = 40. At NDCG@1 and NDCG@10, the Porat^{Rank} method had a higher value than Copeland and Borda methods. Meanwhile, at NDCG@3 and NDCG@5, the most significant value was obtained by the Borda method.

Figure 4 shows the performance of the methods when T = 50. The PoratRank method was better than the Copeland and Borda methods in all NDCG.

Table 1 Running Time

Methods	T = 20	T = 30	T = 40	T = 50	Average
	Seconds				
Copeland	158.91	154.64	155.73	153.50	155.69
Porat_Rank	0.21	0.21	0.21	0.20	0.21
Borda	0.01	0.01	0.01	0.01	0.01

The Porat^{Rank} method succeeded increased the relevance of recommendations. As indicated by the average value of NDCG on the Porat^{Rank} method was supreme than Borda and Copeland methods.

Besides, the Porat^{Rank} method overcame sparsity problems since it was able to work well, even in sparse data conditions. This was obtained by utilizing the existing rating data directly (data in the rare state) and not doing a rating prediction process to fill sparse data as commonly done by the traditional collaborative filtering.

The next evaluation was calculating the running time of Borda, Porat^{Rank}, and Copeland methods. Table 1 showed the average running time of Borda, Porat^{Rank}, and Copeland methods, namely 0.01, 0.21, and 155.69 s, respectively.

There were two steps of scalability evaluation. First, evaluate the effect of the number of users on the running time, and then the impact of the number of items on the running time was assessed. The way to experiment was by taking user and item data randomly from the dataset. The first evaluation was done by adding the number of users, from 100, 200, 300, 400, and 500 users with a fixed amount of 100 items (Fig. 5). The same thing happened in the second evaluation by increasing the number of items while the number of users was fixed at 100 users.

The results of the scalability evaluation are shown in Figs. 5 and 6, which show that the time to run the Porat^{Rank} and Borda methods is almost constant.

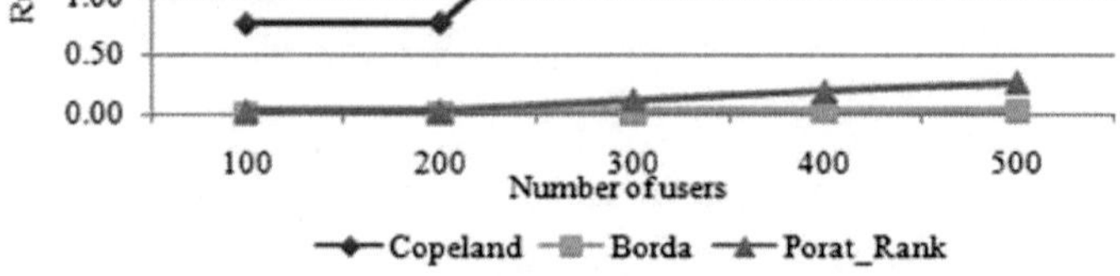

Fig. 5 Scalability analysis of Porat^{Rank} in terms of the number of users

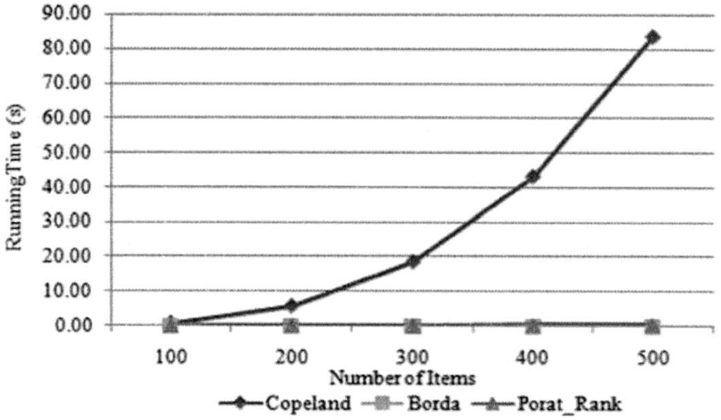

Fig. 6 Scalability analysis of Porat^{Rank} in terms of the number of items

The increase in input data did not significantly affect the running time of both methods. This can be seen from the existing charts, for the Porat^{Rank} and Borda methods, under 0.50 s. While in the Copeland method there is a significant increase in running time, where the addition of the number of users or the number of products greatly affects the processing time, namely the addition of the number of users 500 takes more than 3.50 s and when adding the number of products 500 the time needed is close to 90.00 s. These results indicate that the Porat^{Rank} and Borda methods are able to overcome scalability problems that occur in collaborative filtering.

5 Discussion

This study proposes the Porat^{Rank} method, which functions to rank products according to user preference. The method was then compared with the Copeland, and Borda methods evaluated using NDCG, Running Time, and scalability tests. The test results show that the average value of NDCG in the Porat^{Rank} method is higher than the Borda and Copeland methods. This result means that the product ranking recommended by the Porat^{Rank} method was more relevant to the user interest. This showed that optimizing the use of rating data in the Porat^{Rank} method has succeeded in improving the quality of recommendations. Optimization of rating data consists of adding factors as a condition to determine product points, namely the value of the rating, the same number of ratings, and the position of the product according to its appearance. This results in products with a larger rating, having the same amount of ratings more, and products with an earlier presentation (smaller index) will be in a higher position. It was followed by a minus process for products with a rating <4 so that it will produce a better product ranking.

Furthermore, the evaluation of the running time of the Porat^{Rank} method is faster compared to the Copeland method, but slower 0.2 s than the Borda method. The longest-running time was obtained by Copeland's method because it used a pair-wise comparison process by comparing one product to the entire product for each user, which requires lengthy processing time. Whilst the scalability evaluation shows that the Porat^{Rank} and Borda methods are more stable in processing time (constant) despite an increase in the number of users or the number of products. While the Copeland method, an increase in the number of users or the number of products has a very significant effect on increasing processing time.

6 Conclusion

This paper proposed a new method called Porat^{Rank}, which is a ranking-based method that can overcome the problem of sparsity and scalability in collaborative filtering. Moreover, the Porat^{Rank} method was developed to overcome the weaknesses of Copeland and Borda methods that use rating data only to process user preference profiles and do not involve rating data again in an aggregation process for obtaining the ranking of the items. This condition generates a poor recommendation quality produced. The Porat^{Rank} method optimizes the use of rating data in the aggregation process to produce more qualified recommendations according to user preferences.

The results show that the average value NDCG of the Porat^{Rank} method was superior to the Borda and Copeland methods with the NDCG difference of 0.02 and 0.06, respectively. Meanwhile, the results of the running time evaluation show that the Porat^{Rank} method was faster by 155.49 s than the Copeland method, but it was 0.2 s slower than the Borda method. Moreover, the Porat^{Rank} and Borda methods were able to solve scalability problems. The results were indicated by the fact that the running time of both methods was almost constant. Increasing input data did not significantly increase the running time. Meanwhile, the Copeland method's running time approached quadratic as the input data increased then significantly increase the running time.

For future work, combining with other methods and improving the capabilities of the Porat^{Rank} method so that the recommendations generated an increase in quality.

References

1. Huseynov F, Huseynov SY (2016) The influence of knowledge-based e-commerce product recommender agents on online consumer. Inf Dev 32(1):81–90
2. Xiao B, Benbasat I (2015) Designing warning messages for detecting biased online product recommendations: an empirical investigation. Inf Syst Res 26(4):793–811

3. Heimbach I, Gottschlich J, Hinz O (2015) The value of user' s Facebook profile data for product recommendation generation. Electron Mark 25(2):125–138
4. Adomavicius G, Zhang J (2015) Improving stability of recommender systems: a meta-algorithmic approach. IEEE Trans Knowl Data Eng 27(6):1573–1587
5. Koohi H, Kiani K (2016) User based collaborative filtering using fuzzy C-means. Measurement 91:134–139
6. Naveen N, Kumar SG (2018) Efficient mining and recommendation of extensive data through collaborative filtering in e-commerce: a survey. Int J Eng Technol 7:331–335
7. Kumar NP, Fan Z (2015) Hybrid user-item based collaborative filtering. Procedia Comput Sci 60(1):1453–1461
8. Putra AA, Mahendra R, Budi I, Munajat Q (2017) Two-steps graph-based collaborative filtering using user and item similarities : case study of e-commerce recommender systems. Int Conf Data Softw Eng
9. Venugopal S, Nagraj G (2018) A proficient web recommender system using hybrid possibilistic fuzzy clustering and bayesian model approach. Int J Intell Eng. Syst 11(6): 190–198
10. Sharma S (2017) Suggestive approaches to create a recommender system for GitHub. Int J Inf Technol Comput Sci 9(8):48–55
11. Tang Y, Tong Q (2016) BordaRank: a ranking aggregation based approach to collaborative filtering. In: 2016 IEEE/ACIS 15th international conference on computer and information science ICIS—proceedings
12. Al-Sharrah G (2010) Ranking using the copeland score: a comparison with the Hasse diagram. J Chem Inf Model 50(5):785–791
13. Gupta J, Gadge J (2015) Performance analysis of recommendation system based on collaborative filtering and demographics. In: 2015 International conference on computing and communications technologies, pp 1–6
14. Seo Y, Kim Y, Lee E, Seol K, Baik D (2018) An enhanced aggregation method considering deviations for a group recommendation. Expert Syst Appl 93:299–312
15. Huang BH, Dai BR (2015) A weighted distance similarity model to improve the accuracy of collaborative recommender system. In: Proceedings—IEEE international conference on mobile data management, vol 2, pp 104–109
16. Braida F, Mello CE, Pasinato MB, Zimbrão G (2015) Transforming collaborative filtering into supervised learning. Expert Syst Appl 42(10):4733–4742
17. Polatidis N, Georgiadis CK (2016) A multi-level collaborative filtering method that improves recommendations. Expert Syst Appl 48:100–110
18. Shams B, Haratizadeh S (2017) Graph-based collaborative ranking. Expert Syst Appl 67: 59–70
19. Yu Z, Xu H, Yang Z, Guo B (2016) Personalized travel package with multi-point-of-interest recommendation based on crowdsourced user footprints. IEEE Trans Human-Mach Syst 46 (1):151–158
20. Pereira R, Lopes H, Breitman K, Mundim V, Peixoto W (2014) Cloud based real-time collaborative filtering for item-item recommendations. Comput Ind 65(2):279–290
21. Shams B, Haratizadeh S (2017) Graph-based collaborative ranking. Expert Syst Appl 67: 59–70
22. Zuhairi E, Hartati S, Wardoyo R, Harjoko A (2013) Development of copeland score methods for determine group decisions. Int J Adv Comput Sci Appl 4(6):240–242
23. Dey P, Misra N, Narahari Y (2016) Kernelization complexity of possible winner and coalitional manipulation problems in voting. Theor Comput Sci 616:111–125
24. Lestari S, Adji TB, Permanasari AE (2018) Performance comparison of rank aggregation using borda and copeland in recommender system. In: 2018 International workshop on big data and information security, pp 69–74
25. Wu H, Hua Y, Li B, Pei Y (2013) Personalized recommendation via rank aggregation in social tagging systems. In: Proceedings 10th international conference on fuzzy systems and knowledge discovery 2010, pp 888–892

26. Das J, Mukherjee P, Majumder S, Gupta P (2014) Clustering-based recommender system using principles of voting theory. In: Proceedings 2014 international conference on contemporary computing and informatics, IC3I 2014, pp 230–235
27. Shams B, Haratizadeh S (2017) IteRank: An iterative network-oriented approach to neighbor-based collaborative ranking. Knowl-Based Syst 128:102–114
28. Guo Y, Wang X, Xu C (2016) CroRank: cross domain personalized transfer ranking for collaborative filtering. In: Proceedings—15th IEEE international conference on data mining workshop ICDMW 2015, pp 1204–1212
29. Luo D, Yuan NJ (2017) Representation learning with pair-wise constraints for collaborative ranking. In: Tenth ACM international conference web search data mining, pp 567–575
30. Da Silva EQ, Camilo-Junior CG, Pascoal LML, Rosa TC (2016) An evolutionary approach for combining results of recommender systems techniques based on collaborative filtering. Expert Syst Appl 53:204–218
31. Chen J, Wang H, Yan Z (2018) Evolutionary heterogeneous clustering for rating prediction based on user collaborative filtering. Swarm Evol Comput 38(April 2017):35–41
32. Tikk D (2009) Scalable collaborative filtering approaches for large recommender systems. J Mach Learn Res 10:623–656
33. Shou-qiang L (2016) Research and design of hybrid collaborative filtering algorithm scalability reform based on genetic algorithm optimization. In: International conference on digital home research, vol 6

Design and Implementation of a Registration System with Mobile Application at Public Health Center Based on IoT Using a RESTful API

Sugondo Hadiyoso, Akhmad Alfaruq, Yuli Sun Hariyani, Achmad Rizal, and Tengku Ahmad Riza

Abstract In the health service center, many people often meet in a queue and tend to be chaotic, causing uncomfortable conditions and time inefficiency. From these problems, it was thought that technology was needed to make it easier for users to register and monitor queues. In previous studies, we have successfully implemented a digital queue system using a mini PC as the main control. This system has been implemented at the public health center "Puskesmas" Bojong Soang, Bandung. However, the mechanism of queuing, registration, or ticketing and monitoring could not be done online in an application. Therefore, in this study, an Android-based application was developed to register and monitor queues online and in real-time. The main purpose of this study is to build an integrated system between existing queuing machines and mobile applications so that the queuing mechanism can be done online. The proposed system consisted of three main components, namely the digital queue machine, server-cloud, and client application in the user's smartphone. All modules were connected via the cloud with the developed protocol. This application was called "Q-Puskesmas", which could run on the Android mobile platform with a minimum version of 5.0. The proposed system is able to display location identity, the latest queue number, and a menu for registering. From the test results, the application can update the queue number in real-time according to the existing conditions with a delay of <150 ms and also print a virtual registration number. This developed application was expected to facilitate the public in using health facilities/services.

Keywords Queue · Public health center · Online · Android

S. Hadiyoso (✉) · A. Alfaruq · Y. S. Hariyani · T. A. Riza
School of Applied Science, Telkom University, Bandung, Indonesia
e-mail: sugondo@telkomuniversity.ac.id

A. Rizal
School of Electrical Engineering, Telkom University, Bandung, Indonesia

H. Triwiyanto et al. (eds.), *Proceedings of the 1st International Conference on Electronics, Biomedical Engineering, and Health Informatics*, Lecture Notes in Electrical Engineering 746, https://doi.org/10.1007/978-981-33-6926-9_2

1 Introduction

Technology in information and communication fields is very closely related and is part of the concept of information communication technology (ICT). This can be in the form of media to facilitate and improve the quality of services for the community and services at public service centers in Indonesia. The use of digital queuing system applications using computers is one of technology that is very useful to facilitate and improve the quality of service for the community [1, 2].

One of the public services that use a queue ticket system is a health service center/ clinic or in Indonesia called the Puskesmas. In real conditions, crowds and sometimes tend to be chaotic become one of the problems, especially during rush hour [3]. In the Covid-19 pandemic, where people's activities are restricted, and the crowd had to be avoided, the queue become a problem to be solved [4–7]. One other aspect that needs attention is patient service satisfaction [8]. The patient wants an orderly queue, and the provider provides updated and open information about the queue number. Managing and controlling the queue is one method that can be applied.

Some studies had proposed a digital queuing system including online ticketing, and other studies conduct analyzes then simulate solutions based on queuing theory. Anbuselvan et al. [9] proposed an IoT based application that generates token and senses the position of the queue. A similar study by Dhiman and CK Raina [10] proposed an online ticket checking application. Queue Machine using web applications had also been developed in the study [11, 12]. In other terms, it can be called a paperless ticketing system, which was developed in a study [3, 13, 14]. Several studies conducted simulations based on queuing theory analysis, as reported in [1, 15–17].

From the literature studies, there was still a research gap on how to build an integrated online queuing system with existing conventional digital queue machines. The aim was to build a queuing system that is flexible and can provide convenience to the whole community. Therefore, in this study, we designed an online registration system that is integrated with the existing digital queuing machine at a public health service (Puskesmas) in Bandung, Indonesia. Patients could register, queue, and monitor through the application. Meanwhile, the existing queuing machine could still be used and synchronized with the online application. The proposed system consists of three main components, including digital queue machine, server-cloud, and client application. All components are connected via the cloud with the real-time protocol using RESTful API. Interface. The application that was built was based on Android mobile, and it is called "Q-Puskesmas". The implementation of this system was expected to increase patient convenience and satisfaction, be a value-added service for providers, and support the implementation of health protocols in Indonesia during the Covid-19 pandemic.

As a reminder, the paper is organized as follows: Sect. 2 describes the material and design of the proposed system. Section 3 presents the implementation, testing, analysis, and discussion. Meanwhile, the conclusions of the study and future work are presented in Sect. 4.

2 Material and System Design

This section describes the components or modules used in developing the proposed system, followed by an explanation of system design and workflow diagrams.

2.1 Material Used in the Proposed System

In this study, there were two main sub-systems which are integrated into a compact system. They were digital queuing machines that were installed in Puskesmas and online queuing sub-systems. In the digital queue sub-system, there were the following main components:

1	Mini Computer (PC)	As the central controller to receive input data and provide output such as push buttons, print tickets, displays, and voice call functions. In this study, the Latte panda board is used as the central control. This computer was chosen because it has a compact size and is supported by the digital I/O, which meets the system design requirements. Latte panda uses the Windows operating system so that it can facilitate the development of applications. Also, the Latte Panda has been integrated with the Arduino microcontroller board. This Mini PC is capable of running Linux and Windows 10 operating systems that already exist in Visual Studio, NodeJS, Java, Processing, and others
2	Printing machine	It was used to print the numbers or queue tickets in Puskesmas. We used a commercial thermal printer with a USB interface for communication with Latte Panda
3	Display monitor	As a medium to display the queue numbers and counters. In this study, we used LCD TV as a monitor
4	Speaker	As the loudspeaker in calling the queue number

Meanwhile, the designed online queue sub-system performed the function of registering and monitoring the queue number. These two functions were performed on an android-based application called "Q-Puskesmas". In carrying out this function, there were two main components, namely the server and the user's smartphone, which were then connected through a cloud database with the developed protocol.

2.2 Proposed System Architecture

In this study, a digital queue system equipped with an application user interface for registration and monitor of the queue number was implemented using a Latte panda, thermal printing machine, monitor, and an Android smartphone to perform

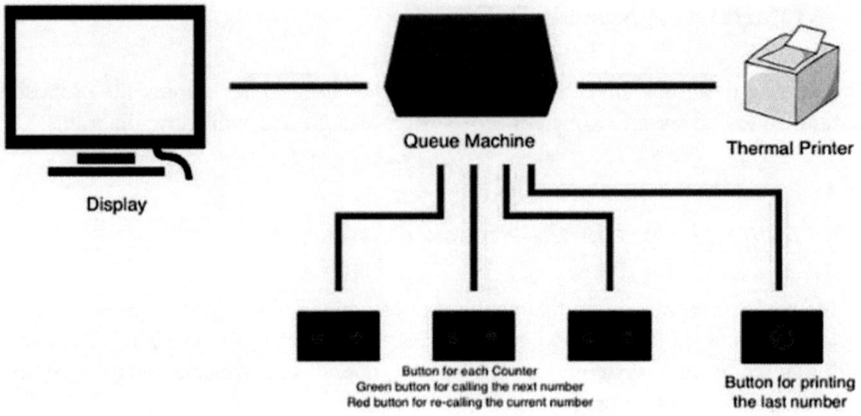

Fig. 1 Queue machine architecture

Fig. 2 Architecture of the proposed online queue registration system

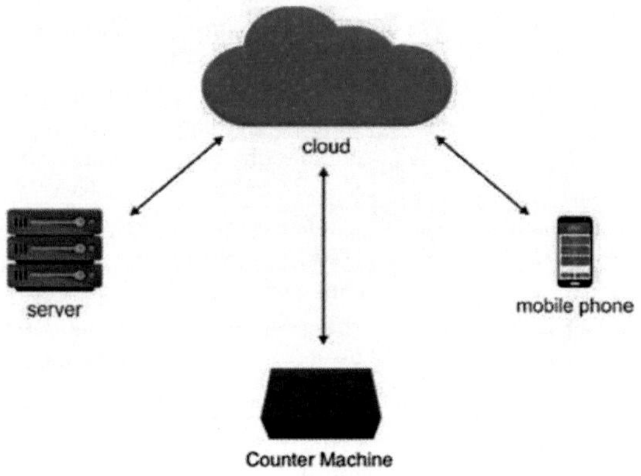

online registration and monitoring functions. Figure 1 displays the system architecture designed in this study. Meanwhile, the design of a queue registration and monitoring system through the internet network is shown in Fig. 2.

Based on Fig. 1, the developed queuing system has the main components, as already explained, namely mini PCs, printing machines, speakers, and displays. In this study, additional features were in the form of a monitoring application designed using the Android platform installed on a smartphone so that it can see the status of the queue in real-time and online. To support the application, the mini-computer was connected to the WiFi Router as a gateway to the internet network. Queue data would be sent to the server so that it could be accessed online through the internet network.

2.3 *Hardware Queue Machine and Desktop Applications Implementation*

Figure 1 shows the hardware design of the queuing system at the Public Health Center. The central control was carried out by a mini personal computer based on the Windows operating system with QT-Creator as the basis for developing desktop applications. This desktop application performed: reading input from buttons, printing queue ticket numbers, performing digital display the queue status, and calling functions. The workflow of the proposed system can be seen in Fig. 3.

When the queue number button was pressed, the device would retrieve the latest queue number data from the server, and then the printer would print the ticket number. The queue number was obtained from the last queue number +1 in decimal

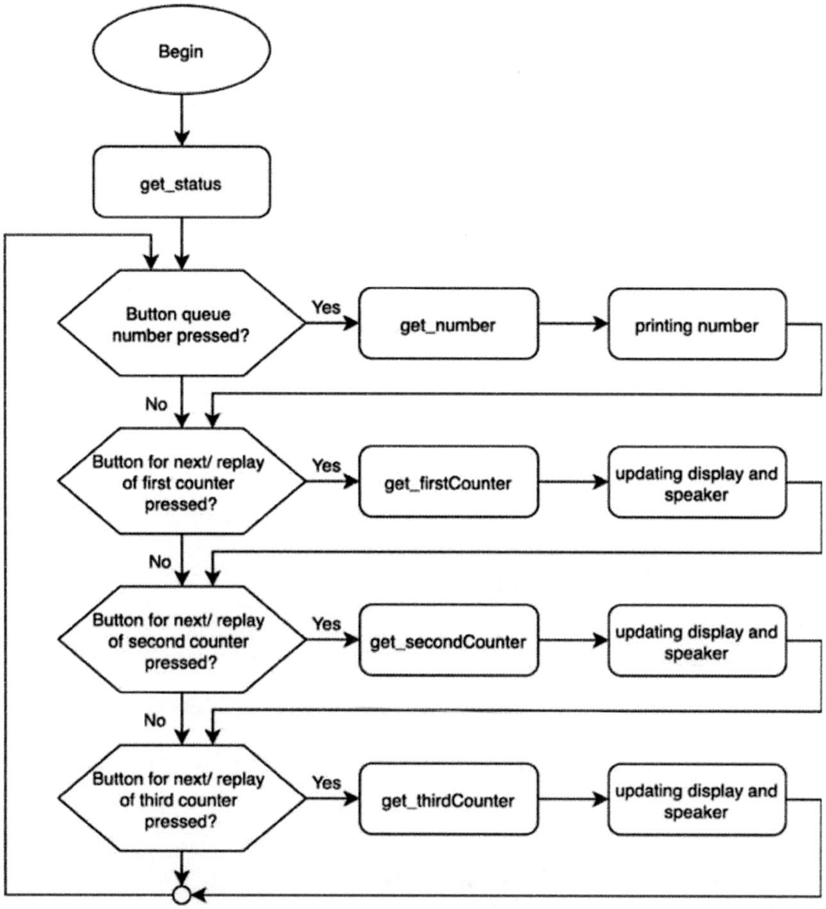

Fig. 3 The workflow of the hardware queue machine

value. If the clerk pressed the call button (either counter 1, counter 2, or counter 3), the device would retrieve the counter number data from the server, then showed it on display and sound the speaker to call the queue number. The counter number was obtained by finding the highest value from counter-1, counter-2, and counter-3, which then +1 in decimal value.

The desktop application was designed to display queue numbers and counters according to the administrator registration instructions. The system implemented in this study supports calling and displaying queue numbers up to three counters.

2.4 Database Design on Cloud Servers

The database is one of the main functions that is run on the server application to store and update the condition of the queue number in accordance with the conditions at the health center. The database was developed using SQL with a structure, as shown in Table 1.

In order to make the queuing machines and applications could access existing data on the server, then we created the RESTful API interface, as in Table 2.

Table 1 The function of database component

No.	Name	Function
1	id_device	Queue machine identity (Id). Id is unique and different on each device. Data accessed refers to this id
2	counter1	Save queue position on counter-1
3	counter2	Save queue position on counter-2
4	counter3	Save queue position on counter-3
5	total	Save the last queue number

Table 2 The interface of the queue machine with the server

No.	API name	Annotation
1	get_counter	Used to get the last number of the queue on the counter Parameter: id_device: the identity of each queue machine id_counter: the identity of the counter Type: used to select the type of calling (next or repeat)
2	get_number	Used to get a queue number position Parameter: id_device: the identity of each queue machine
3	get_status	Used to get the position of each counter Parameter: id_device: the identity of each queue machine

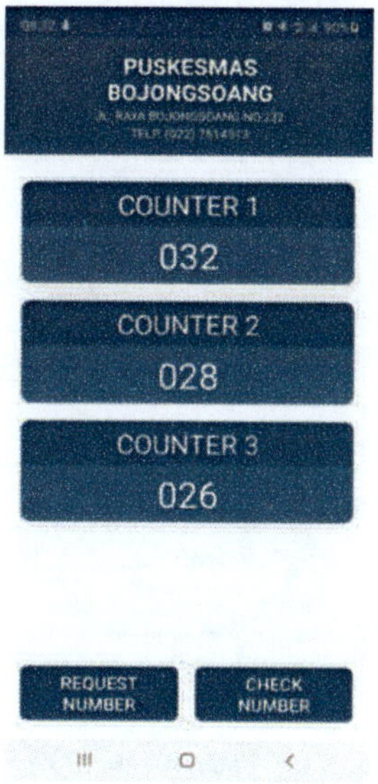

Fig. 4 The user interface of the Q-Puskesmas application

2.5 Design of Q-Puskesmas Applications

The Q-Puskesmas application was developed to be able to run on the Android operating system. The primary function of this application is registration, print tickets, and monitor queue numbers online. The user interface of this application consisted of the identity of the health center, the counter queue number, and a menu list. The Q-Puskesmas application interface is shown in Fig. 4. This application was connected to the server and the queuing machine at the Puskesmas through cloud services. By this system, the queue number position would always be updated according to the last number called. The number of counters displayed on the application could be adjusted to the needs or existing conditions at the health center. In the application, there was a queue number position information for each counter and a button for queue number registration. Registered numbers can be seen in the number view menu. Users could re-register the queue number if the registered queue number were missed. The workflow of Q-Puskesmas is shown in Fig. 5.

3 Results and Discussion

The implementation of the digital queue system at the health center is shown in Fig. 6. The implemented system worked well, including printing tickets, displaying and calling queue numbers. From the overall queuing machine functionality test on

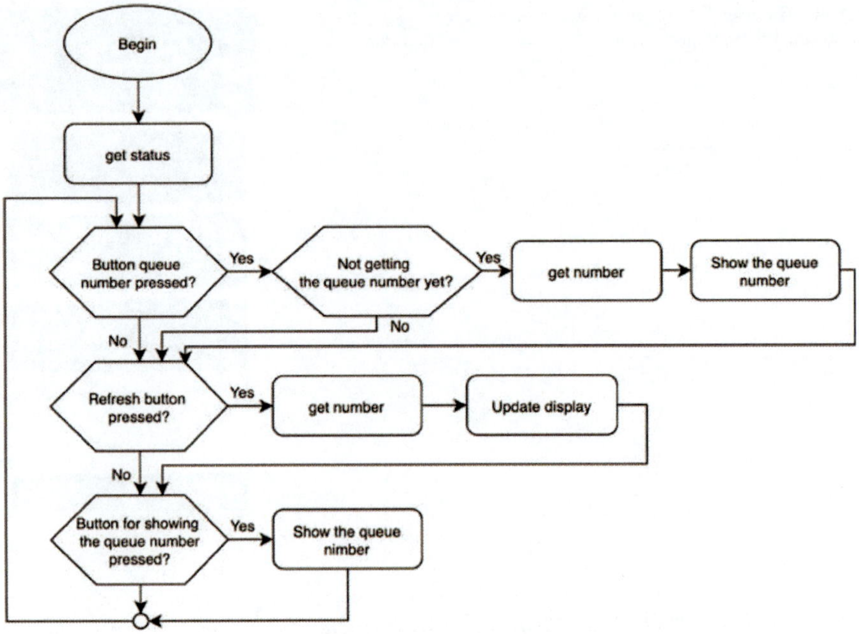

Fig. 5 The workflow of Q-Puskesmas

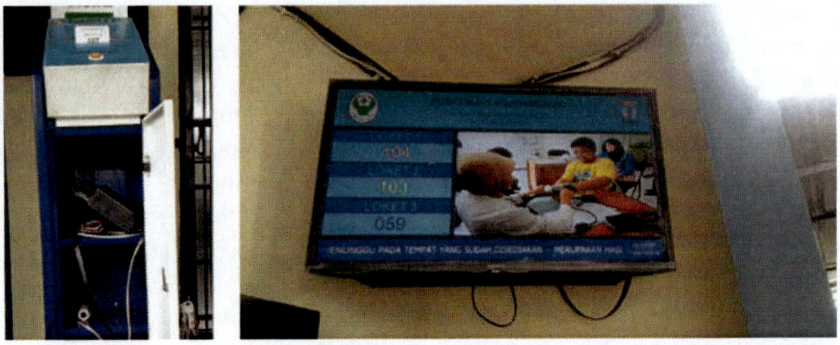

Fig. 6 Digital queuing machine implemented at the health center

the side of the health center showed performance by the design specification. All integrated components performed functions synchronously, which were controlled by a computer.

Testing functionality was then focused on the application of Q-Puskesmas. Testing network parameters was also carried out to determine the quality of service. Several test scenarios were carried out to be discussed and analyzed. Testing the functional performance of Q-Puskesmas applications that are integrated with digital

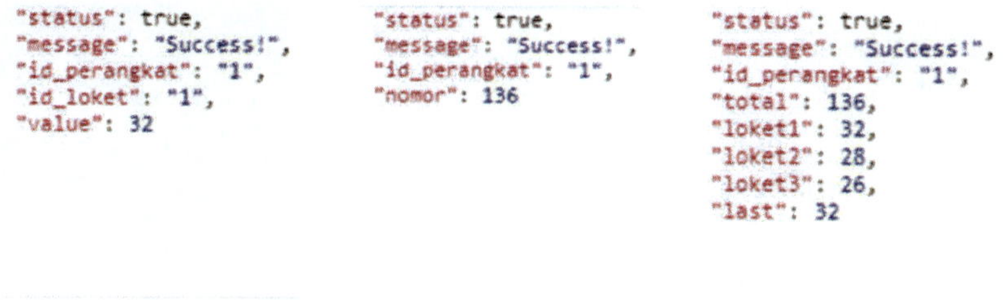

(a) (b) (c)

Fig. 7 Testing of query **a** get_counter **b** get_number **c** get_status

queuing machines is done through visual observations displayed both on desktop and mobile applications. Validation of new registrations and online monitoring of queue numbers is done by observing database queries. Figure 7 below is an example query for each function presented in Table 2, including get_counter, get_number, and get_status.

From this test, it could be concluded that the RESTful API interface as a database connection on a server with Q-Puskesmas could work well according to design specifications. This was indicated by the status of "success". That means each request generated by the user could be responded to by the server. The following Fig. 8 is an example of a request to see the registration ticket number. Meanwhile, Fig. 9 shows the response system when a user requests a number but has previously created a ticket number request. Under the specifications of the designed algorithm, the user could re-register when the registered number had been called by the admin counter.

Fig. 8 Display in the application to view the registration number (e-ticket)

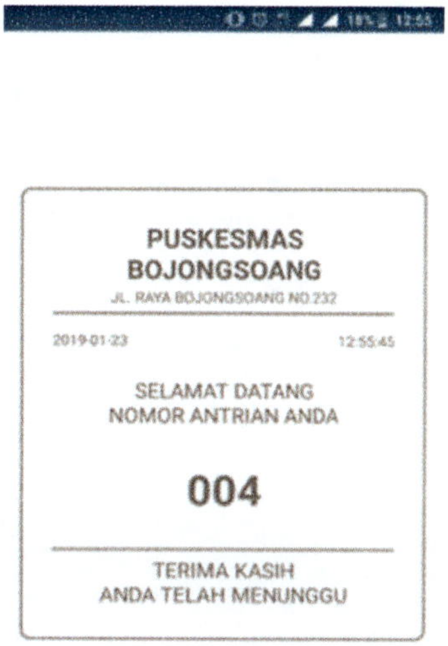

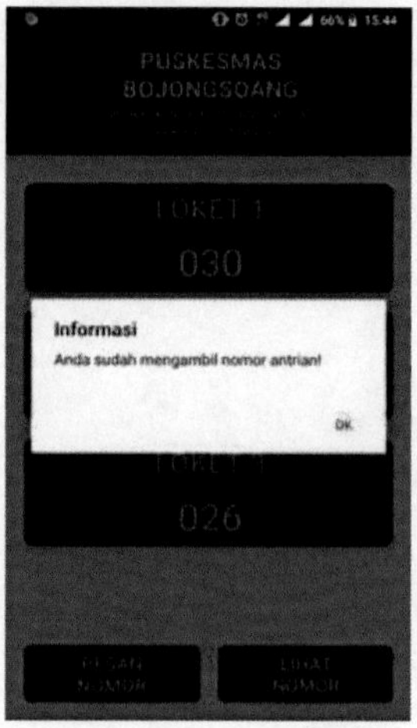

Fig. 9 Application response when the user requests a queue number more than once

Since the proposed system supports online registration using Q-Puskesmas, network quality testing was also carried out on the cloud server. It aimed to determine the performance of the system in providing real-time services, especially in the mobile application sub-system. Tests carried out include delays and web server loads. Performance parameters were then compared with the ITU-T standard. Delay testing was done when the client requests the status or position of the latest queue number through the mobile application. From 10 tests that were carried out, the processing delay was obtained, as shown in Table 3. The average delay generated by the system was 67.8 ms with a standard deviation of 12.47 ms, referring to the ITU-T standard where the delay <150 ms, the proposed system complies the real-time communication standard.

Since the application is designed to serve many users, a server load test is also performed to determine system performance if the server is flooded by simultaneous user requests. In this test, Load Impact is used as a tool that generates virtual users and virtual request activities. Users are generated from 10 to 350 to access the

Table 3 Delay test results with 10 times measurement

Test	Delay (ms)	Average, Std. Dev (ms)
1	61.31	67.8 ± 12.47
2	75.94	
3	65.19	
4	78.32	
5	50.99	
6	63.89	
7	80.87	
8	88.55	
9	59.63	
10	53.33	

Table 4 Request waiting time on server load test

Number of users	Req_waiting_time (ms)
10	6.08
25	6.14
50	5.94
75	6.76
100	9.87
150	8.76
200	9.14
250	10.48
300	14.92
350	632.11

server simultaneously, then response time is observed. Table 4 shows the results of the server load test referring to the number of virtual users served. Based on these tests, the average waiting time request for 10–350 users is 6.02 ms and 632.11 ms, respectively. There was an increase in waiting time, however, it was not significant (<1 s) so that the server performance remained stable in serving many users who access it simultaneously.

From all the test scenarios that have been carried out, it can be concluded that the proposed system is able to run well in accordance with the design specifications. However, there are limitations of this system including the minimum Android version of 5.0 so that the Q-Puskesmas application can be run on a mobile phone. In addition, this system has not been able to provide reminding the upcoming patients that their turns are nearly arriving as implemented in the study [3, 18]. However, the system which was implemented in this research outperformed to the system that proposed in the study [3]. Its advantages include easy registration via mobile applications, real-time monitoring and integrated with the existing queuing machine. Finally, the public can choose which mechanism they consider easier and more efficient.

4 Conclusion

This research has successfully developed and implemented an integrated online registration system at Public Health Center, Bandung. The created system consists of a digital queue machine and an online registration application through a mobile application. The queue machine can print ticket numbers, call and display queue number positions. This machine consists of a mini-computer as the main control, thermal printer, buttons and LED monitors to display the queue number. This device supports calling queue numbers for up to three counters. The mobile application can be used for online registration and monitoring. This developed application is then called Q-Puskesmas which can work on Android-based smart phones. Testing of network service quality is also carried out to determine the performance of the system in providing real-time services to users. Quality of service tests performed include delay and server load. The average delay generated when user requests an update queue number is 67.8 ms which complies with the delay standard in real-time communication. The results of load tests on the server show that the developed system is capable of serving 350 users simultaneously with low waiting times. The proposed system is expected to improve the quality of services to the community and support social distancing during the Covid-19 pandemic. Future research, this system can be equipped with a reminder and notification feature if the upcoming patients that they turn are nearly arriving.

References

1. Uddin MN et al (2016) Automated queue management system. Glob J Manag Bus Res An Adm Manag 16(1):1–9
2. Ghazal M et al (2016) A smart mobile system for the real-time tracking and management of service queues. Int J Comput Digit Syst 5(4):305–313
3. Jidin AZ, Yusof NM, Sutikno T (2016) Arduino based paperless queue management system. Telkomnika (Telecommun Comput Electron Control 14(3):839–845
4. Mattioli AV, Ballerini Puviani M, Nasi M, Farinetti A (2020) COVID-19 pandemic: the effects of quarantine on cardiovascular risk. Eur J Clin Nutr May:1–4
5. Remuzzi A, Remuzzi G (2020) COVID-19 and Italy: what next? Lancet 395(10231): 1225–1228
6. Saadat S, Rawtani D, Hussain CM (2020) Environmental perspective of COVID-19. Sci Total Environ 728:1–23
7. Nicola M et al (2020) The socio-economic implications of the coronavirus and COVID-19 pandemic: a review. Int J Surg April
8. Xiao H, Zhang G (2010) The queuing theory application in bank service optimization. In: 2010 International conference on logistics systems and intelligent management, ICLSIM 2010, vol 2, pp 1097–1100
9. Anbuselvan J, Citharthan D, Varatharaj M (2017) IoT based solution to reduce queue in the banking sector. Int J Eng Sci Comput 7(3):5973–5975
10. Dhiman K, CK Raina ER (2017) IoT based ticket checking system. Int J Adv Res Comput Commun Eng 6(3):916–919
11. Istoko AD, Rifa'i AF (2018) Web-based queue machine development using raspberry and ESP8266. IJID Int J Inf Dev 7(1):4
12. Warlina L, Noersidik SM (2018) Designing web-based food ordering information system in restaurant. IOP Conf Ser Mater Sci Eng 407(1)
13. Lin CY, Jhu GY, Siao S (2019) An innovative queue management system based on bluetooth beacon technology. In: Proceedings—22nd IEEE international conference on computational science and engineering and 17th IEEE international conference on embedded and ubiquitous computing, CSE/EUC 2019, pp 427–430
14. Putra RO, Musoffa SF, Nurhasanah S, Anggadjaja E, Santoso H (2018) QBLE-theme park queueing system using wearable device. In: 2017 IEEE 3rd international conference on engineering technologies and social sciences, ICETSS 2017, 2018, vol 2018-Janua, pp 1–6
15. Pankratova E, Moiseeva S (2014) Queueing system MAP/M/∞ with n types of customers. Commun Comput Inf Sci 487(1):356–366

16. Nair AN, Jacob MJ (2015) An (s, S) production inventory controlled self-service queuing system. J Probab Stat 2015:1–8
17. Obinwanne E, Darlingtina A (2015) On application of queuing models to customers management in banking system. Am Res Bio Sci 1(2):14–20
18. Dyatmika D, Sudana O, Putri GAA (2019) Untethering the queue based on multi channel access (MCA) technology at hospital radiology section. J Inf Syst Eng Bus Intell 5(2):146

Fuel Truck Tracking for Real-Time Monitoring System Using GPS and Raspberry-Pi

Rohmat Tulloh, Dadan Nur Ramadan, Sugondo Hadiyoso, Rohmattullah, and Zikra Rahmana

Abstract Trucks are the main transportation in fuel distribution from the dispatch center to the gas station. The lack of a security system of fuel shipments from the dispatch center to the gas station is an opportunity for theft by illegally moving fuel from trucks. Therefore, an application is needed to support the security system on the truck. In this study, we designed a fuel truck monitoring system by combining a global positioning system (GPS) module and a mini-computer. The purpose of this study is to implement an integrated which perform the function of tracking the position of the truck and to ensure the truck arrives at the gasoline station. The limit sensor on the tap will detect if the valve is open. This function is to ensure that the tap is only opened at locations with predetermined coordinates. Monitoring is done through online and real-time websites. The website will display a database of GPS where the coordinates of the fuel truck are located. If a theft is detected, the system will display a warning with the coordinates of its location. From the test results obtained tracking accuracy of 100%. The average difference in the coordinates of GPS tagging with GPS tracking of 5.48 m. The averaged of one-way delay and response time of the proposed system are 4.95 s and 160 ms respectively, it has good criteria according to the ITU-T G10.10 standard for real-time application. This designed system is expected to be implemented on existing fuel trucks for security reasons.

Keywords Fuel truck · Global positioning system · Website · Real-time

1 Introduction

Fuel oils are one of the most important commodities and are needed by the community. However, Indonesia's oil production cannot cover domestic fuel consumption needs. The condition is exacerbated by the presence of fuel oil theft

R. Tulloh (✉) · D. N. Ramadan · S. Hadiyoso · Rohmattullah · Z. Rahmana
School of Applied Science, Telkom University, Bandung, Indonesia
e-mail: rohmatth@telkomuniversity.ac.id

H. Triwiyanto et al. (eds.), *Proceedings of the 1st International Conference on Electronics, Biomedical Engineering, and Health Informatics*, Lecture Notes in Electrical Engineering 746, https://doi.org/10.1007/978-981-33-6926-9_3

activities. This can be done by illegally removing fuel oil from the transport truck. This theft modus is usually done by opening the fuel truck tank and taking fuel using a hose pipe through the mouth of the tank. To deal with it, the Global Positioning System (GPS) technology in real-time monitoring applications can be applied in this case.

The use of GPS as a tracking system has been commonly used in various fields of life including vehicle tracking [1–3], tracking people's positions both indoors and outdoors [4], tracking the location of hospitals [5], tracking wild animals for purposes nature conservation [6–8]. Web Progressive Apps (WPA) as a user interface monitoring provides several advantages in terms of cost, ease of access and ease in building applications [9–11]. Website usage is commonly used for project monitoring user interface [12, 13], energy system monitoring [14], vehicle monitoring [15], Mobilize Community monitoring [16].

GPS has been widely applied, especially in supporting low-cost monitoring systems but has a high benefit if it can be applied to fuel truck monitors. Therefore, this research aims to realize a prototype fuel truck monitoring and fuel security system with a combination of GPS and WPA as a user interface monitoring system.

2 Methodology

2.1 Global Positioning System

The Global Positioning System (GPS) is a global navigation system using satellite radio [17]. This system was first launched in 1978 by the United States (U.S.) Department of Defense [18]. Until now, GPS has become an important tool for navigation, land surveying and cartography [18]. GPS satellites can be accessed free of charge. GPS covers all areas of the earth including ground, sea, air and space [1]. GPS provides accurate information about position, speed and time. The position of the GPS receiver is calculated by measuring the distance with four or more GPS satellites [19]. GPS receivers are constantly receiving and then analyzing radio signals from satellites, so that distances can be measured. GPS has now been widely applied to commercial and research uses. GPS applications such as logistics, plantations/forests, farming, tracking, area mapping, disaster, sports and some health applications. In this study, GPS is used to track the fuel trucks. The GPS module used in this study is Ublox NEO-6 M as shown in Fig. 1. This module is a family of GPS receivers that stand alone with size 16 × 12.2 × 2.4 mm. Modules are ideal for applications with low power and high mobility. The capabilities of this module include: horizontal position accuracy is 2.5 m with a maximum Altitude of 50,000 m and a maximum Velocity of 500 m/s. This module supports UART and SPI serial communication as an interface. In this study, UART communication is used as an interface with Raspberry-Pi.

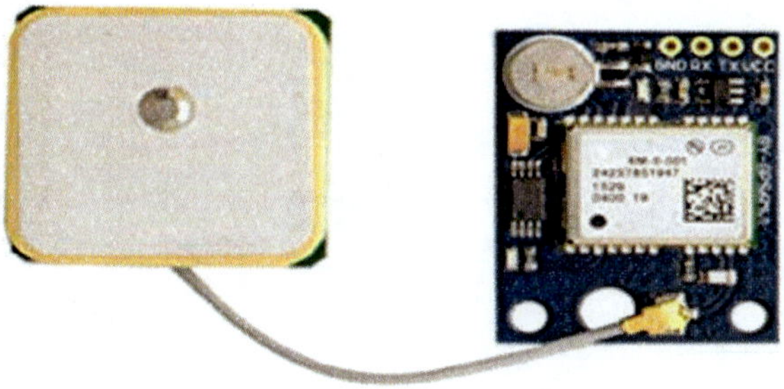

Fig. 1 GPS Module used in the proposed system

The following Eq. 1 is used to calculate the distance from point to point. This calculation is used to calculate the distance and accuracy of the coordinates that are read on Google Maps with reference points.

$$\begin{aligned} S = &6371 \times \cos^{-1}[\cos(90^\circ - y2) \times \cos(90^\circ - y1) + \sin(90^\circ - y2) \\ &\times \sin(90^\circ - y1) \times \cos(x1 - x2)] \times 1000 \end{aligned} \quad (1)$$

where

s: Distance,
x1: Latitude first node,
y1: Longitude first node,
x2: Latitude second node,
y2: Longitude second node.

2.2 *Fuel Truck*

Fuel Truck is a vehicle used to distribute fuel oil. Fuel Truck capacity that exists in Indonesia consists of 8000, 16,000, 24,000, 32,000 and 40,000 L. Fuel Truck can be filled with various types of fuel oil. In one tank car can load diesel, gasoline, and Pertamax at once, depending on the capacity of the tank car. Figure 2 shows a fuel truck with a capacity of 16,000 L. Has two holes on it. These tank compartment holes are called Menholes, where each hole contains 8000 L each. This storage container is called a tank compartment with a divider or boundary.

In Fig. 2, at the bottom left-hand side of the truck, there is a box where the fuel is received when the truck is about to issue contents at the fuel station. In the box the liquid delivery pipes (dismantling pipes) are connected to each of the compartments. There is a lever or a button on/off the wind valve as mentioned earlier. The end of the unloading pipe is wrapped with Bottom Loading, which is a water tap with a lever to open the pipe hole. Before the process of receiving fuel oils at the Fuel station, the bottom loading was still closed by the sealed API Dust Cap. The

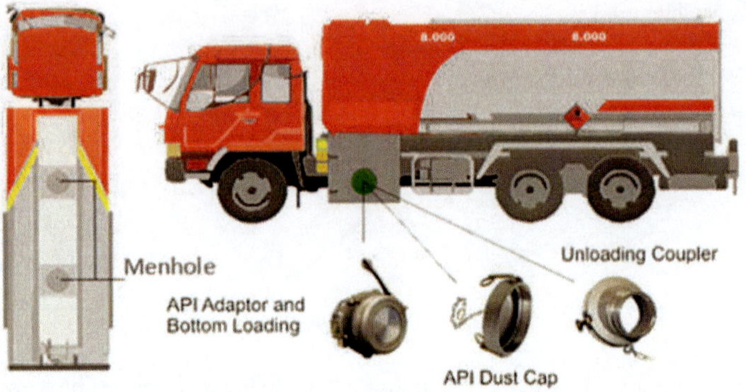

Fig. 2 The standard component of fuel truck in Indonesia

Dust Cap API will be opened and installed Unloading Coupler or commonly known as pigtail. To simulate these parts, in this study a prototype of the fuel oil receipt box which was given a sensor switch that detected the condition of the box being opened or closed.

2.3 System Architecture

The proposed system consists of Raspberry-Pi 3 as main control, Ublox Neo 6 m GPS Sensor which functions to send the coordinates of the truck's position, limit switch as a box position detection sensor (open or closed), fuel tap and LCD 16 × 2 as a component to display status on system device (Fig. 3). To connect to the internet using an external modem. All of these devices are mounted on fuel trucks. The power supply uses 4000 mAh batteries.

On the website-based monitoring software application consists of a website in which there are fuel station coordinates (Latitude and longitude) and truck driver data database. The website functions to control, display valve condition notifications, display maps, vehicle tracking, departure hours, arrival hours and truck license plates. The database in this system uses the Firebase application connected to the Raspberry-Pi. GPS plays the role of tracking the whereabouts of the coordinates of trucks that are distributing fuel to fuel stations to be displayed on the website in real time. When a truck releases fuel not at the destination fuel station, a notification will appear on the website in the form of a warning message for administrators. Conversely, if the fuel is released at the appropriate fuel station, the open status will be recorded in the system and an open sign will be displayed.

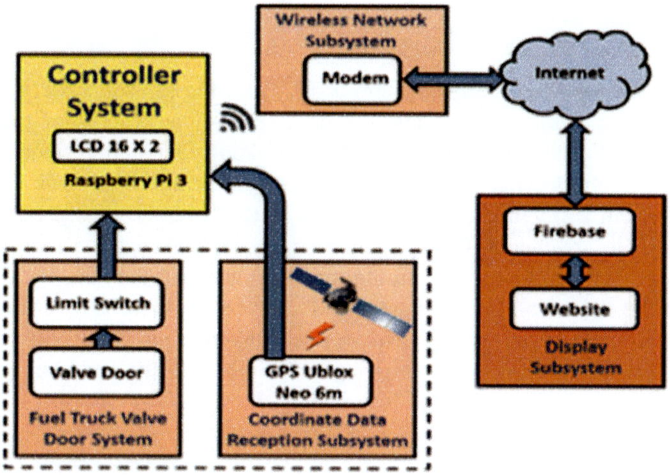

Fig. 3 Proposed system architecture

2.4 Wiring System

Figure 4 explains that all components are connected directly to the Raspberry-Pi Pin 3. The Ublox Neo 6 m GPS module has 4 pins namely Vcc, Rx, Tx and ground. The GPS module gets a 5v supply for Rx and Tx using the Raspberry-Pi UART pin. The GPS module is connected to Raspberry using, Pin GPIO 6 for Vcc, GPIO 4 for Rx, GPIO 8 for Tx and GIPO 10 for Ground. The pins that are connected to process positioning data are in the form of Latitude and Longitude that will be sent to the database. For sensors get a 3.3 V supply. On the LCD 16 × 2 display connected to the I2C pin on the Raspberry-Pi.

Fig. 4 Wiring diagram

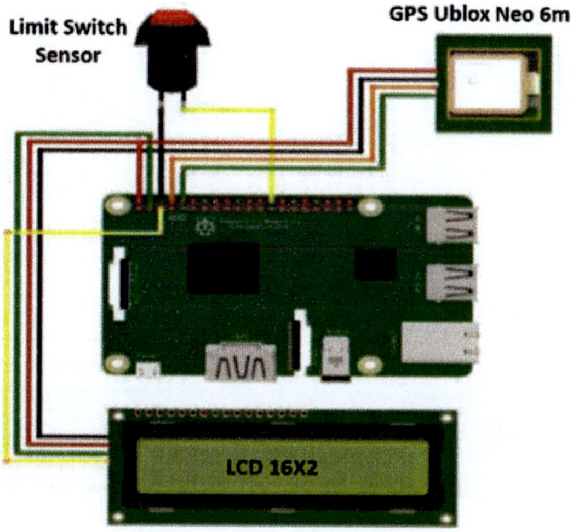

2.5 System Workflow

The workflow of the monitoring system is shown in Fig. 5. The system starts with fuel truck filling. After being filled, the next step is the process of tracking the position by GPS. The truck departs to the destination fuel station. During the trip the system will check whether the tank valve is open or not. If the tank tap valve is open, the system will validate the current coordinates with the inputted coordinates. If the results do not match, the system will provide a notification message in the form of a warning to the admin through the website, then the data will be sent to firebase. If the validation tracking process is appropriate, there is a notification that the truck has arrived at the destination fuel station, then data will be sent to Firebase. Finally the process of removing the contents of the tank can be done.

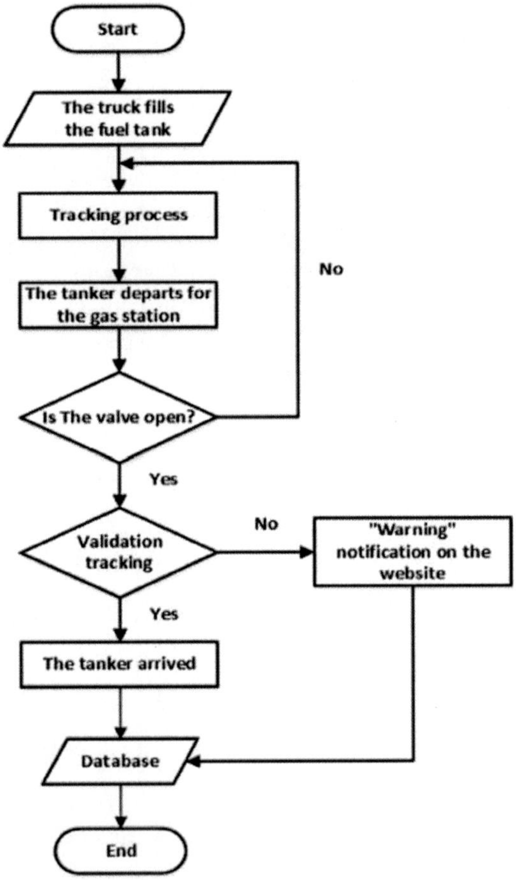

Fig. 5 Workflow system

2.6 API Interface for Maps Display

API (Application Programming Interface) is used so that Google maps can be displayed on the website. The first stage is create the API code from the Google Maps account. After that, the following stages are performed to display the Google Maps map on the website.

- Insert the Google Map library inside the <head> tag or inside <body>.

```
<script
src="http://maps.googleapis.com/maps/api/js"></script>
```

- Create the initialize function () to prepare the map.

```
Function initialize(){…}
```

- Create properties on the map.

```
Var propertiMap ={
    Center:new google.maps.LatLng(-
    8.5830695,116.3202515),
    zoom:9,
    mapTypeId:google.maps.MapTypeId.ROADMAP
};
```

- This property is written in the initialize function ().

```
Google.maps.event.addDomlistener(window,'load',initiali
ze);
```

- Add the initialize function () to the window load event so that it is called when the web is opened.

```
<div id="googleMap"
style="width:100%;height:380px;"></div>
```

3 Result and Discussion

3.1 Hardware Implementation

The prototype implementation that was designed consisted of two sub-systems that were placed in the casing box. The first box is the GPS Tracking system and the second box is a receiver that is installed on the fuel truck. The first box functions as a controller system that contains a Raspberry-Pi, GPS Module and LCD as shown in Fig. 6.

The second box functions as a fuel valve sensor that has a limit switch along with reception coordinates. Then connected using a DC connector. Two prototype boxes as shown in Fig. 6. Inside the box are fluid delivery pipes (dismantling pipes) that are connected to each of the compartments. Mechanical design using a PVC box with dimensions of 18.5 × 11.5 × 6.5 cm.

3.2 Testing System Functionality

Tests carried out with several scenarios to prove that the system made is in accordance with the initial design. Figure 7 shows the first scenario. In this scenario, the truck goes to the fuel station without any process to open the valve on the truck so there is no notification. The GPS bottom view can map the movement of trucks in real-time. On the website appearance, data such as the name of the driver, time of updating, destination of the fuel station, vehicle license plate, time of departure, time of arrival and notification can be displayed properly.

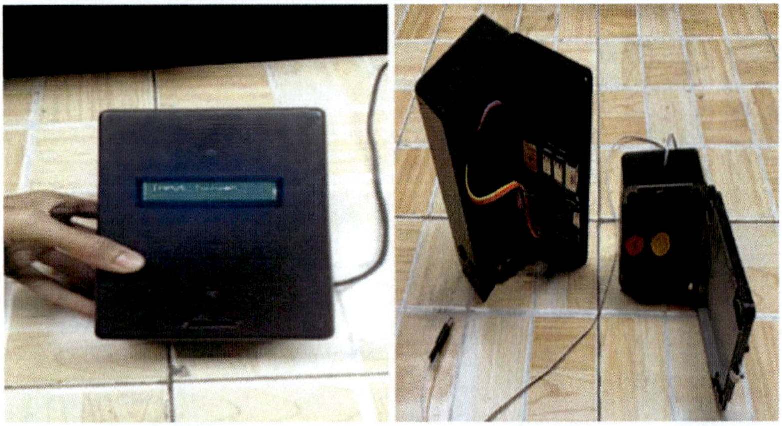

Fig. 6 Tracking system hardware

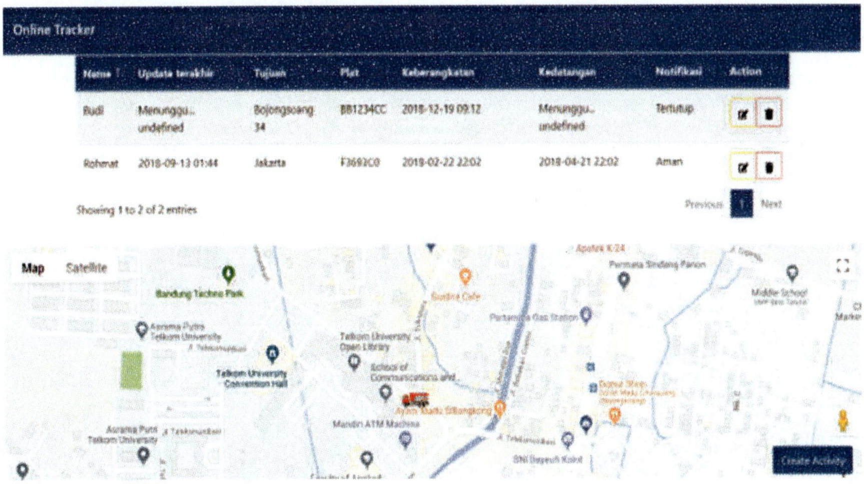

Fig. 7 The monitoring system results on the website

In the second scenario the system testing is done by opening the fuel filling valve not at the specified coordinates or not at the specified fuel station. Figure 8 shows the notification “WARNING!!” on the website and arrival status is still undefined.

Figure 9 shows the results of the third scenario: the valve opens when the truck’s tank is less than one meter from the radius at the destination gas station. In this condition the notification “Open” appears on the website. For this test it can be said to be successful because there is an influence of distance tolerance between GPS coordinates with coordinates on google map of 1–6 m.

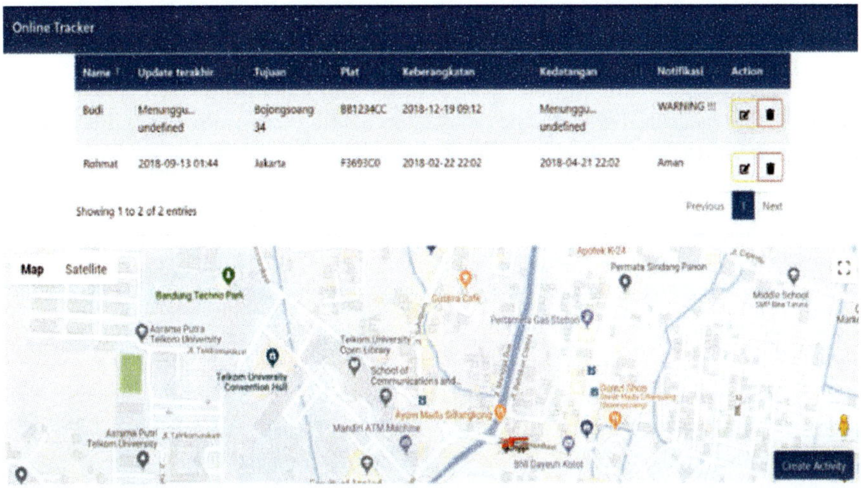

Fig. 8 Monitoring results when the valve is open is not at the destination gas station

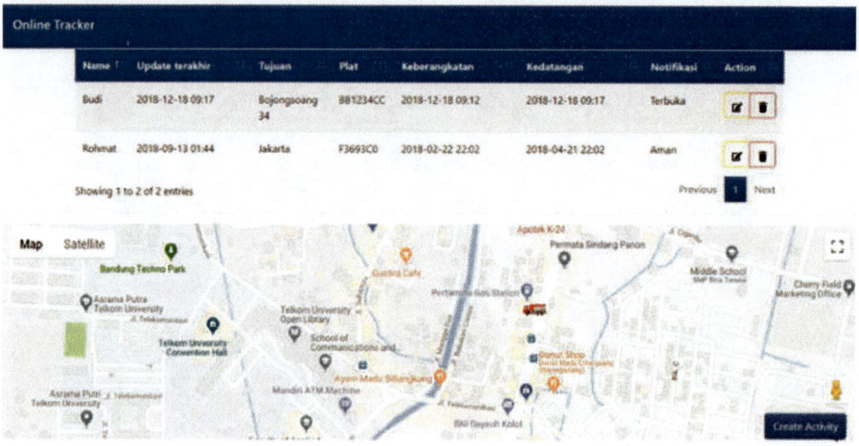

Fig. 9 Monitoring results when the valve is not open at the destination fuel station

3.3 Coordinate Reading Error Testing

Testing the accuracy of the location coordinates carried out 10 times. The test is done by comparing the results of reading the Ublox 6 m GPS module coordinates with a reference device, the Garmin GPS etrex 10 (Fig. 10). From the two coordinates, the distance difference is then calculated to determine the fault tolerance. The calculation uses Eq. 1. The test results as in Fig. 11 are referred to as GPS location error data. The average error testing for GPS coordinates reading is 5.48 m.

3.4 Measurement of Delay

Delay measurements are carried out 10 times and calculated the average delay obtained. The measured delay is the delay from reading the Ublox 6 m GPS module to Firebase until it is displayed on the website.

Fig. 10 Testing the coordinates

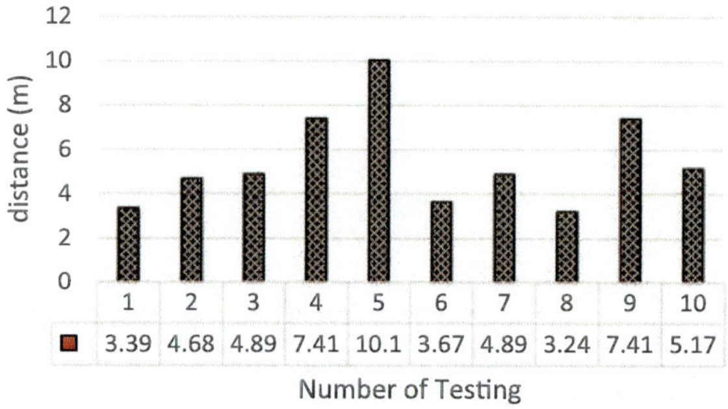

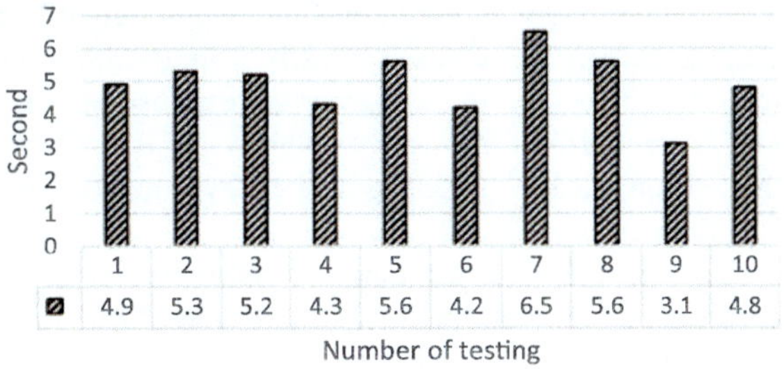

Fig. 11 One-way delay measurement results

From the measurement results shown in Fig. 11, it appears that the average delay of 10 attempts was 4.95 s. The amount of delay obtained is included in the good category in accordance with ITU-T standard G.1010 [20] about one way delay for data transfer preferred <15 s. The delay value obtained depends very much on the speed of the Internet, the processor on Raspberry-Pi 3 and the ability of the web server to process data.

3.5 Testing Website Performance

This test is carried out using Load Impact software. Load Impact is a cloud service to load tests of the performance of websites, apps and APIs. Load impact verify the stability and reliability of the API under extreme conditions. The test scenario simulates as many as 50 clients who access the website at the same time with a duration of 10 min with the results shown in Fig. 12.

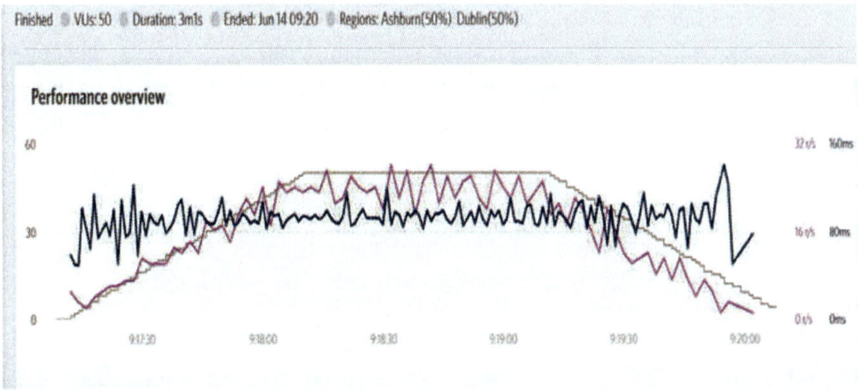

Fig. 12 Website performance measurement results (Blue line: Response time website, Purple line: Request rate per second, Gray line: Active visitors browsing the website)

Based on the web server testing results obtained stable quality. The number of users accessing is increased linearly from 0 to 50 users. Based on website response time, it can be seen that the average response time is still below 160 ms. Based on ITU-T standard for one-way web browsing delay less than 2 s [20]. This means that the response time in this proposed system conform to the standard criteria for real-time communication.

On a website, performance is an important part of the user experience. This performance is often measured by response time to visualize or interact with some information. The two main factors that influence user experience response time are frontend and backend. Frontend performance focuses on browser metrics such as rendering time, interactive time, load time. Whereas Backend Performance, on the other hand, mostly focuses on server response time and the number of errors returned. Because the website is connected to the IoT system, the influence of network connections and devices is also very influential.

4 Conclusion

In this study, a security system for fuel trucks has been designed and implemented in terms of monitoring and fraud detection applications. The system which implemented can work well according to the initial design. This proposed system consists of GPS, Raspberry-Pi, sensor, and a real-time database. The system can perform tracking the position of the truck, display the departure time, arrival time, and license plates in real-time so that it can help the information system. The sensor which is installed on the tank pipe can detect the condition of valve. The application can display valve notifications in 3 conditions, namely Closed, Warning (The valve is opened not at the destination fuel station), and Open (the valve is opened at the destination fuel station). From the tests that have been carried out on the proposed system is obtained: (1) the average difference in the coordinates of GPS tagging with GPS tracking of 5.48 m, (2) the average of one-way system delay of 4.95 s, (3) the average response time with a value of less than 160 ms. The delay generated by the system meets the criteria for real-time communication based on ITU-T G10.10 standards. In the future it is hoped that the proposed system can be applied to existing fuel trucks for security purposes.

References

1. Choi E, Chang S (2017) A consumer tracking estimator for vehicles in GPS-free environments. IEEE Trans Consum Electron 63(4):450–458
2. Gao C, Yang D, Hong X, Xu Y, Wang B, Zhu Y (2018) Experimental results about traffic flow detection by using GPS reflected signals. IEEE J Sel Top Appl Earth Obs Remote Sens 11(12):5076–5087

3. Singla L, Bhatia P (2016) GPS based bus tracking system. In: IEEE international conference on computer, communication and control, IC4 2015
4. Hutabarat DP et al (2017) Human tracking in certain indoor and outdoor area by combining the use of RFID and GPS. In: APWiMob 2016—IEEE Asia Pacific conference on wireless and mobile 2016, conference proceedings, pp 59–62
5. Samah KAFA, Ibrahim S, Ghazali N, Suffian M, Mansor M, Latif WA (2020) Mapping a hospital using openstreetmap and graphhopper: a navigation system. Bull Electr Eng Inf 9 (2):661–668
6. Patel A, Stocks B, Fisher C, Nicolls F, Boje E (2017) Tracking the cheetah tail using animal-borne cameras GPS, and an IMU. IEEE Sens Lett 1(4):1–4
7. Gaspar T, Oliveira P, Silvestre C (2015) Model-based filters for 3-D positioning of marine mammals using AHRS- and GPS-equipped UAVs. IEEE Trans Aerosp Electron Syst 51 (4):3307–3320
8. Roeleke M, Blohm T, Kramer-Schadt S, Yovel Y, Voigt CC (2016) Habitat use of bats in relation to wind turbines revealed by GPS tracking. Sci Rep
9. Turner-McGrievy GM et al (2017) Choosing between responsive-design websites versus mobile apps for your mobile behavioral intervention: presenting four case studies. Transl Behav Med 7(2):224–232
10. Papadopoulos EP, Diamantaris M, Papadopoulos P, Petsas T, Ioannidis S, Markatos EP (2017) The long-standing privacy debate: Mobile websites vs mobile apps. In: Proceedings of the 26th international conference on world wide web WWW 2017, pp 153–162
11. Tandel SJA (2018) Impact of progressive web apps on web app development. Int J Innov Res Sci Eng Technol
12. Hambali A, Pratama RM, Negara RM, Ramdhani M, Fadhilah A, Tulloh R (2017) Controlling and monitoring project based on Android application for fiber optic infrastructure. In: ICCEREC 2016—international conference on control, electronics, renewable energy and communications, Proceedings, 28, pp 17–22
13. Landicho JA (2016) A web-based geographical project monitoring and information system for the road and highways. J Electr Syst Inf Technol 5(2):252–261
14. Hamzah A, Chaniago B, Suwitno S, Rosma IH, Gussyafri H, Kurniawan I (2018) Web based wind energy conversion system monitoring. In: Proceedings—2018 2nd international conference on electrical engineering and informatics (ICon EEI) 2018, Oct, pp 179–182
15. Moushi OM, Kamal M, Haque M, Ahsan MS (2019) Design and development of an online bus monitoring system. In: ICECE 2018—10th International conference on electrical and computer engineering, pp 69–72
16. Tulloh R, Negara RM, Prasetya YEY, Saputra S (2019) HERO: maximizing student potential to mobilize community empowerment activities around campus. In: Proceeding—2019 international conference of artificial intelligence and information technology ICAIIT 2019, pp 431–436
17. Abulede FO, Akinnusotu A, Adeyemi A (2015) Global positioning system and it's wide application. Cont J Inf Technol 9(1):22–32
18. Maddison R, Ni Mhurchu C (2009) Global positioning system: a new opportunity in physical activity measurement. Int J Behav Nutr Phys Act 6(73):1–8
19. Scott MTU, Scott TJ, Kelly VG (2016) The validity and reliability of global positioning systems in team sport: a brief review. J Strength Cond Res 8:1249–1254
20. International Telecommunication Union, ITU-T (2001) Recommendation G. 1010: End-user multimedia QoS categories (Quality of service and performance). Int Telecommun Union

Room Searching Robot Based on Door Detection and Room Number Recognition for Automatic Target Shooter Robot Application

Syahri Muharom, Ilmiatul Masfufiah, Djoko Purwanto, Ronny Mardiyanto, Budi Prasetyo, and Saiful Asnawi

Abstract Parameters of room are the presence of a door and room number, where to detected room need a system that can detected part of room. From it the researcher created a robot that can detected room target based on door and room number recognition. The way robot in finding a room is by tracing the corridor of the room by using the PID control method, PID value $K_p = 5$, $K_i = 2$ and $K_d = 0.4$, from it, the robot movement is stable with value is 55 RPM. To find room target the robot's way of detecting a room is by recognizing the door frame, which is first processed using the Hough-transform method, where the results of it will be eventually processed as a parameter of a room door. After it the system will match the corresponding image to the existing image storage using template matching. After the door detection, the system will capture the image of the room, and process using OCR method and template matching. The experiment of robots in recognizing room doors has a success rate of 81.8%, while the success rate of robots in detecting room numbers is 84.6%, this result is due to the change of illumination level in the corridor of a room, and the size of the room number that affects the robot's recognition. The result of experiment that has been done, the robot has a 88.8% success rate in finding the room, and has a time of 43–65 s from the robot's starting point. From result, the researcher expected to be applied to the shooter robot application.

Keywords Shooter robot · Door detection · Number recognition · Hough transform · OCR · Template matching · PID

S. Muharom (✉) · I. Masfufiah · B. Prasetyo · S. Asnawi
Department Electrical Engineering, Institut Teknologi Adhi Tama Surabaya, Surabaya, Indonesia
e-mail: syahrimuharom@itats.ac.id

D. Purwanto · R. Mardiyanto
Department Electrical Engineering, Institut Teknologi Sepuluh Nopember Surabaya, Surabaya, Indonesia

H. Triwiyanto et al. (eds.), *Proceedings of the 1st International Conference on Electronics, Biomedical Engineering, and Health Informatics*, Lecture Notes in Electrical Engineering 746, https://doi.org/10.1007/978-981-33-6926-9_4

1 Introduction

Robot is becoming an increasingly popular technology to help and ease human for doing hard work such as underwater and space exploration, or any other field in the industrial world application [1]. The development of this has entered to a larger scope such as weaponry [2] where the robot can shoot targets automatically controlled remotely, human daily life [3] where it can help to ease the household chores such as dish washing robot, dust cleaning robot, and helping people with physical limitations, etc. The main advantage of having robot is to help human activity [4]. The initial interest of robot development was to have a system work in each specific area [5].

The use of a control system on the robot's navigation is to speed up the movement in reaching the target [6]. The application of navigation systems in robots uses several types of sensors, as well as cameras to become the main system in robot navigation [7]. Cameras are often used to track down moving objects in the field of vision, this explains the design and development of cameras used in a robot [8]. In addition to some of the advantages they has, Continuous camera-based tracking and recognition can recognize and capture moving objects without calibration [9]. by having image from the target area that will be a robot reference in term of recognizing those areas directly [10]. In mapping area, the navigation robot is influenced by various factors such as detection of a Doors and public objects in the environment [11], and it present a new approach to detecting areas based on doors in the room [12]. The system needs an image to process using Hough-Line Transform method [13].

Since the computer vision is a breakthrough method [14] used by the system, the room system must be structured so the robot is able to recognize the area [13, 15]. The process of recognizing a room need to have a room address, a room number through optical character recognition (OCR) method [16]. Sensing Mobile Robot is able to navigate in an indoor environment, which is a method approach for door verification based on vision systems [17]. However, all of researcher result has not been integrated into a robot system. From it, the researcher makes a robot that can searching room based on door detection and room number recognition, this system reveals full potential to be used for automatic target shooter robot application.

2 Methodology

The design of the room searcher robot based on the door and room number can be made a block diagram, where in the robot work system block diagram, there is the initial process of the robot in moving up to the room detection process. Below are parts of the robot system.

2.1 Diagram Block System

Making this room searcher robot system, there are several parts that become the main parameters in making robots, where the parameters of the parts of the robot that are built is the camera, where the camera on the robot functions as a sensor to detect the presence of doors and room numbers, then the personal computer (PC) which has the function to process the image captured by the camera, the image processing on the PC includes the process detection of door frames to the introduction of the number of the environment, the results of image processing are then sent via Bluetooth to the microcontroller Atmega128. Atmega128 Microcontroller processes commands given by PC, where the data processing on Atmega128 Microcontroller is to convert commands from a PC into an output signal, the converted signal is sent to the L298 motor driver, where the driver will move the robot to move forward, backward, turn left or left turn right. The movement of this robot is influenced by reading and detecting images from the camera in detecting targets.

2.2 Navigation System

In the design of this room searcher robot, a system diagram block was created to control the movement of the robot, the robot's navigation system was built using the application of the PID method, this method was designed to accelerate the robot's response in moving forward, backward, turning right or turning left, more clearly in This robotic navigation system can be seen in Fig. 1.

The design of this robot based on navigation system aims to accelerate the response of robot movements, where the robot's movement is influenced from the target's position, where the target's position can be near or far from the robot's starting point. In the robot's navigation system has two feedbacks where the first is the rotary encoder, and the second is the target coordinate position based on the robot's angle, the rotary encoder functions as a robot speed sensor in moving, where every robot's movement is monitored by this sensor, position and distance

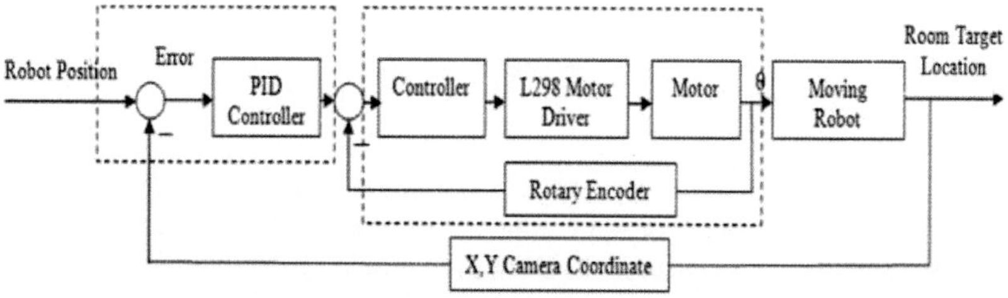

Fig. 1 Block diagram robot controller

the target becomes a parameter to regulate the speed of the robot, the farther the target the faster the robot's speed. As for the target position, the PID serves to make the robot be in the coordinates of the X, Y point of view on the specified camera.

2.3 Flowchart System

The design of the work system on the robot that is made can be seen in the flowchart, the robot work system can be seen by providing initial parameters for the robot in finding the existence of the room, the parameters given to the robot is to enter the room number of the room. After the target is entered the robot will walk with the navigation settings using the PID method, the robot will walk through the corridor of the room to find the door frame, on the left or right side of the robot. After the door frame is detected, the robot will process the door frame image using Hough transform, the result of the door line image processing is matched with the parameters of the door that have been prepared using template matching, this matching aims to identify the image and ensure the detected image is the same as the parameter has been set, if the parameters match, the robot has found the door to the room. This robot working system can be seen in Fig. 2.

The next process is to identify the room number, the camera will detect from the room number based on the shape, where the room number design in this study, is marked with a box shape and there are letters or numbers in the box, the shape of this box will be detected using shape detection. After the target box is found, OCR will work to convert the image of the room in the box to ASCII using tesseract, where the tesseract master is number 0–9 and alphabet a to z, the results of this processing will be processed again using template matching. Template matching will identify the image of the room number whether it matches the template image that has been prepared, if it is not the same, the robot will walk through the corridor of the room to find the door frame, or the robot will be given an order to find a new room number. If the matching results from the door and the room number match the input command given, the robot succeeded in finding the room.

3 Result and Discussion

3.1 Result Door Frame Detection

Figure 3 shows the position of the target room door in the right side of the robot, as shown in the figure, the robot is placed as far as 4.25 m from door, this experiment is done to get the robot's detection response to the door of the room based on the robot's perspective.

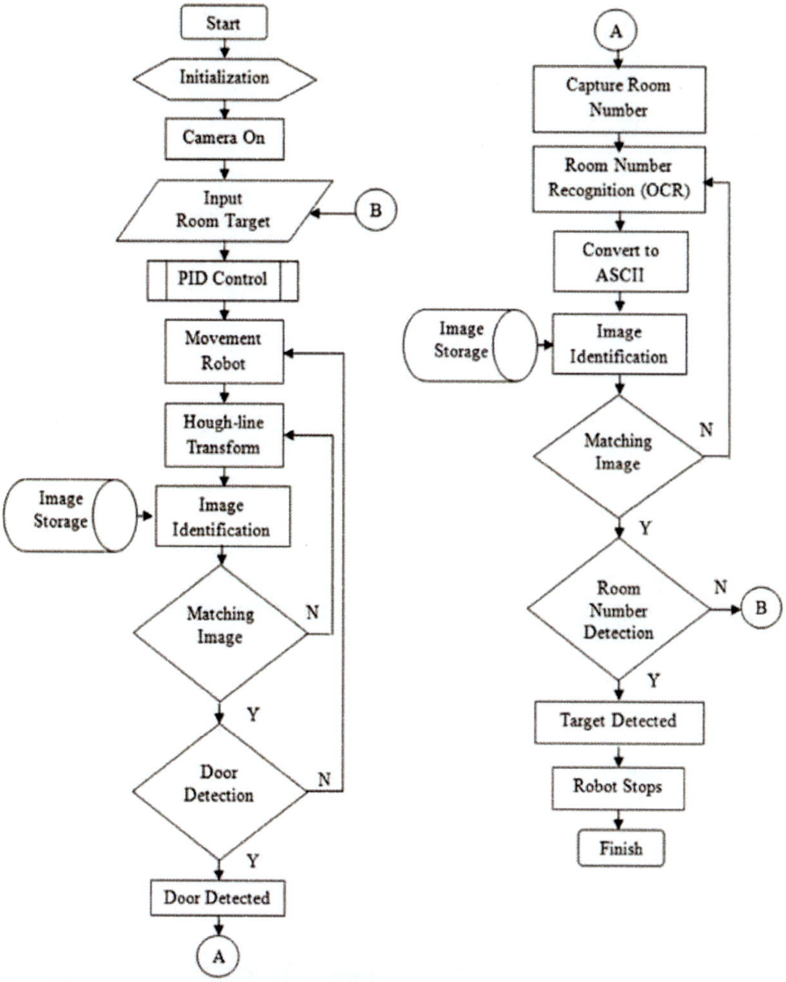

Fig. 2 Flowchart robot

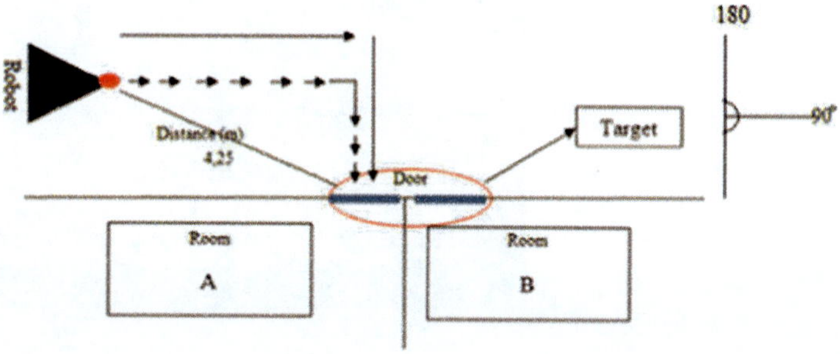

Fig. 3 Robot's position in detecting door

Table 1 Door frame detection based on distance and robot's point of view

No	Distance (Meter)	Angle robot (Degree)	Door frame position (Degree)	Light illumination (Lux)	Explanation
1	4.25	90	80	128	Detected
2	4.25	90	80	122	Detected
3	4.25	90	80	126	Detected
4	4.25	90	80	122	Detected
5	4.25	90	75	125	Detected
6	4.25	90	75	127	Detected
7	4.25	90	75	122	Detected
8	4.25	90	60	123	Detected
9	4.25	90	60	122	Detected
10	4.25	90	45	120	Fail
11	4.25	90	45	127	Fail

This study conducted 11 attempts by changing the robot's perspective of the target angle from 45 to 90°. These attempts are done by adjusting the lighting with a range of light luminance values between 120 and 130 lx. This study is summarized in Table 1.

The percentage of this study is 81.8% as it obtained several different results, those are influenced by the target angle and lighting luminance value. Those have been successfully conducted 9 times out of 11 experiments, with angle between 60 and 80°. The system gets 2 times failed when the target angle is reduced to 45°, this failure is caused by the small target angle so it cannot be detected by the camera. From the testing of the detection of the door frame in this room. The process of detecting room door frames is shown in Fig. 4.

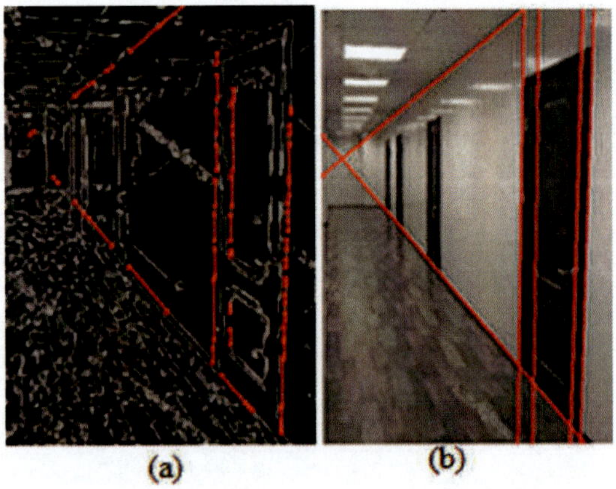

Fig. 4 Door frame detection results with hough transform and template matching, **a** hough transform, **b** matching with template result

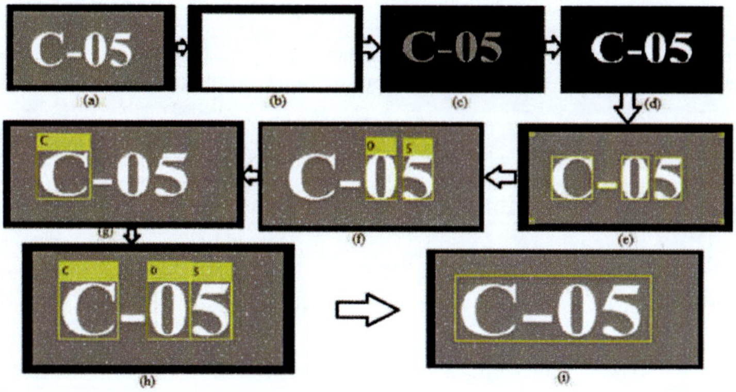

Fig. 5 OCR system process and template matching, **a** convert image to gray, **b** blob analysis, **c** eroded, **d** diladed, **e** Roi, **f** OCR number, **g** OCR alphabet, **h** OCR result, **i** template matching result

3.2 OCR System Testing Result

Figure 5 shows the process of detecting the room number. It is done to see the optimum result of robot in detecting a room number, the room number used is in a box shape as the initial marker of the system in recognizing the room number. The system will detect the shape using shape detection, then the OCR system and template matching will work to detect the room number.

The process of this study begins with the box shape detection in the room number, the image will then be converted to gray level and processed through blob detection. After the blob detection is finished, the next step is Erosion and dilation process, the results of this process will be then processed in the Roi process to limit the detection of white images only. The next step is the OCR process for numbers, and for letters. The result of combining OCR numbers and letters is matched with parameters using template matching. The results of this room number detection test can be seen in Table 2.

The successful rate is linearly decreasing as the light luminance decreases. The results show OCR reading is 101 for the detection of room number B-01 when detection process using a 76 of light luminance value so that the template matching cannot match the parameters that have been set. While the experiment with a light luminance value of 120–130 show OCR systems and template matching can detect and recognize room numbers. Thus, we can conclude that the successful rate of changing this light luminance value is 84.6%.

Table 2 Room number detection

No	Room number	OCR number	OCR alphabet	Matching template result	Light illumination (Lux)	Explanation
1	A-01	A	01	A01	128	Detected
2	A-22	A	22	A22	122	Detected
3	B-01	–	101	–	76	Fail
4	C-A2	CA	2	CA2	122	Detected
5	C-01	C	01	C01	125	Detected
6	C-05	C	05	C05	98	Detected
7	C-12	C	12	C12	122	Detected
8	D-02	D	02	D12	123	Detected
9	D-11	D	11	D11	122	Detected
10	E-01	E	01	E01	120	Detected
11	E-11	E	11	E11	127	Detected
12	E-AA	AA	1	–	80	Fail
13	E-0A	EA	0	E0A	128	Detected

3.3 *Robot Control Result*

The aim of this study is to know the robot speed movement response toward the detected target by placing the robot in a corridor of the room with the determined distance. The illustration of the robot's navigation system can be seen in Fig. 6.

Figure 7 explains the coordinates of the camera pixel is 0–640 with the midpoint is 320 pixels, it shows the target room is in coordinates 0 or 360 pixels, where the target is on the left or right of the robot. Y target and Y set pin is door position at pixel camera capture. This experiment was carried out to obtain the most optimal PID value setting in the robot navigation system, where the test results can be seen in Table 3.

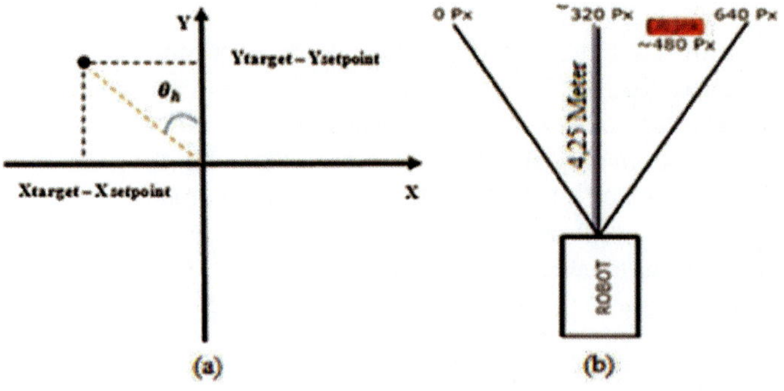

Fig. 6 The illustration robot against the position the detected door frame target, **a** position of target point, **b** capture area camera

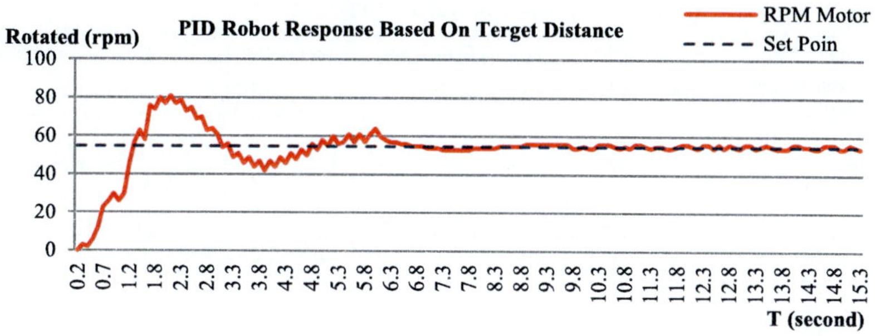

Fig. 7 Robot system PID response

The process to find the most optimal PID value is by placing the robot from the target with a distance of 4.25 m. The initial setting of the given K_p values is = 2, K_i = 2 and K_d = 0.7, while a rise time result is 0.3, with peak time of 0.8 and settling time of 2.8 s. This value indicates that the robot moves too fast, and become unstable so the detection of the room is remain constrained. After several attempts, the new value is obtained by setting K_p = 5, K_i = 2 and K_p = 0.4. While the rise time to 1.4 and peak time 2.2, with a settling time of 4.8 s, this value is chosen because the robot can stably run and detect the target room. The response image from PID can be seen in Fig. 7.

3.4 *Result of Robot System*

The main purpose of this overall experiment is to find space based on the door and the room number and to speed up the movement in reaching the target. In this study, robot-target distance is made constant at 5.5 m, while the target room to be located is on the right side of the robot, this study is done by setting a light luminance value of 120–130 lx. Result of this overall experiment can be summarized in Table 4.

This study is done by providing command input in the form of room number, then robot will walk through the corridor of the room to detect the target. the process of detecting the first target is to detect the door frame of the room, after the results match the template matching parameters that have been provided then it is concluded that the robot has successfully detect the room door. The next step is to detect the room number using OCR and template matching, if the results of OCR and template matching are in accordance with the input robot commands given, then the robot has concluded to have successfully found a room.

There were 2 failures out of 18 attempts of experiment, it is influenced by the inability of robot in detecting the presence of the door frame for room B10. The first failure is the robot keeps moving forward until it hit the corridor of the room, while the second failure is the lack of exposure resulting in the inability of OCR system to

Table 3 Robot movement response based on value of PID

No	Distance robot with target (m)	PID value			PID response (second)				RPM robot target
		K_p	K_i	K_d	Rise time	Peak time	Settling time	Error steady state	
1	4.25	2	2	0.7	0.3	0.8	2.8	3.8	55
2	4.25	3	2	0.7	0.3	0.5	3.2	4.1	55
3	4.25	4	2	0.7	0.4	0.6	2.6	3.7	55
4	4.25	5	2	0.7	0.5	0.8	2.6	3.9	55
5	4.25	5	2	0.6	0.6	0.9	2.4	4.2	55
6	4.25	5	2	0.5	0.9	1.2	3.2	5.8	55
7	4.25	5	2	0.4	1.4	2.2	4.8	6.3	55
8	4.25	5	2	0.3	1.6	2.8	6.8	8.3	55

Table 4 Robot system testing result

No	Input target	Distance (m)	Door detected	Room number detected	Room detected	Time (s)	Explanation
1	A01	5.5	Detected	A01	Detected	44.2	Target detected
2	A01	5.5	Detected	A01	Detected	47.9	Target detected
3	A01	5.5	Detected	A01	Detected	43.6	Target detected
4	A01	5.5	Detected	A01	Detected	44.5	Target detected
5	A01	5.5	Detected	A01	Detected	59.7	Target detected
6	C05	5.5	Detected	C05	Detected	43.2	Target detected
7	C05	5.5	Detected	C05	Detected	49.7	Target detected
8	C05	5.5	Detected	C05	Detected	63.8	Target detected
9	C05	5.5	Detected	C05	Detected	44.5	Target detected
10	C05	5.5	Detected	C05	Detected	43.9	Target detected
11	D02	5.5	Detected	D05	Detected	43.2	Target detected
12	D11	5.5	Detected	D11	Detected	43.4	Target detected
13	D10	5.5	Detected	D10	Detected	48.5	Target detected
14	E01	5.5	Detected	E01	Detected	44.8	Target detected
15	E11	5.5	Detected	E11	Detected	65.8	Target detected
16	E10	5.5	Detected	E10	Detected	58.3	Target detected
17	B01	5.5	–	–	Fail	–	Can't find room target
18	B01	5.5	Detected	101	Detected	132.5	Wrong target

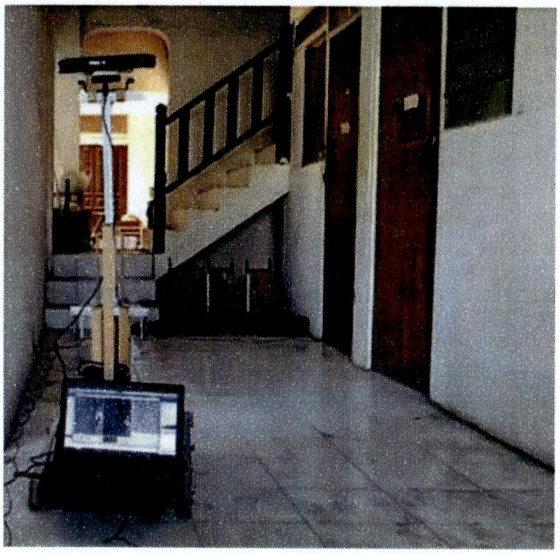

Fig. 8 Room searching robot process

translate the room number, B01 command OCR translates 101, it leads robot to misidentify the target room. Thus, the success rate was 88.8% with an average time for the robot to find the target was 49.3 s, respectively. The process of finding a room based on the door and room number is shown in Fig. 8.

From the result of robot system, it has advantages over previous studies, where the detection process is carried out automatically using robot system, and has an time average is 49.3. The robot system having limitation process, where this robot only works in a predetermined area, this is because the parameters of room corridor, the type of door and room number models are different.

4 Conclusion

Robot based on navigation system is proposed and investigated for finding the target room based on the door and the room number. The detection of the room door frame uses Hough-transformation and template matching, and by setting the light luminance value of 120–130 lx. The system has a success rate of 81.8% in door room detection at robot point of view of as large as 60–80°. Furthermore, the process of detecting the number of rooms is using OCR and template matching. The system can recognize the target room number with a success rate of 84.6%, with a light luminance value of 120–130 lx. The PID setting on the robot's navigation system is, $K_p = 5$, $K_i = 2$, and $K_d = 0.4$, hence, the system can achieve steady state error with a time of 8.3 s. The robot system has a success rate of 88.8%, and, requires an average time of 49.3 s. Thus, This Robot provides considerable advantages in detecting target, such as the value of success rate, low-cost fabrication, ease in handling and reliable measurement results. And the researcher expected to be applied to the shooter robot application.

References

1. Hawari K, Finawan A, Kamal M (2016) Rancang bangun robot sebagai alat bantu penjelajah bawah air. Jurnal LITEK 13(2):91–96
2. Herdiana B, Pratama YB (2017) Sistem deteksi dan penembak target pada robot tank pengendali nirkabel. Jurnal TELEKONTRAN 5(1)
3. Widodo B, Santoso A, Purwanto D, Jazidie A (2011) A method for path planning strategy and navigation of service robot. Paladyn 2(2):100–108
4. Muharom S, Odinanto T, Fahmiah S, Siwi DPP (2019) Design of design of wheelchairs robot based on ATmega128 to people with physical disability. ICATECH, IOP Conf Ser Mater Sci Eng 462(1):012016
5. Fuad M, Purwanto D (2014) Wall-following using a Kinect sensor for corridor coverage navigation. J Theor Appl Inf Technol 70(1)
6. Muharom S (2018) Tukadi, control of wheelchair robot movement using flex sensor Glove. Jurnal INFORM 3(2):84–89
7. Mir-Nasiri N (2006) Camera—based 3D object tracking and following mobile robot. School of Engineering Swinburne University of Technology
8. Chen Z (2011) Visual detection of lintel-occluded doors by integrating multiple cues using a data-driven Markov chain Monte Carlo process. Electrical and Computer Engineering Department, Clemson University, Clemson, SC 29634, United States Robotics and Autonomous Systems p 59
9. Majumdar J (2012) Intelligent vision system for door sensing mobile robot. Department of Research and Development Nirtte Meenakshi Institute of Technology
10. Deepu R, Honnaraju B, Muradi S (2015) Path generation for robot navigation using single camera. ICICT, Procedia Comput Sci 46
11. Fernandez C, Moreno V, Curto B, Rodriguez JF, Serrano FJ (2014) A real-time door detection system for domestic robotic navigation. JIRS 76(1):119–136
12. Uroidhi A, Mardiyanto R, Purwanto D (2016) Automatic navigation for a mobile robot with real time depth Kinect sensor and map database. Jurnal JAVA 14(1)
13. Muharom S (2017) Penerapan Metode Hough Line Transform Untuk Mendeteksi Pintu Ruangan Menggunakan Kamera. Jurnal IPTEK 21(1):79–86
14. Budiharto W, Jazidie A, Purwanto D (2010) Indoor navigation using adaptive neuro fuzzy controller for servant robot. ICCEA, IEEE pp 582–586
15. Firmansyah RA, Pambudi WS, Suheta T, Zuliari EA, Muharom S, Hidayatullah MBS (2018) Implementation of artificial neural networks for localization system on rescue robot. EECIS, IEEE, pp 305–309
16. OZ-Salinas RM, Hernandez A (2005) Door-detection using computer vision and fuzzy logic. Department of Computer Science and Artificial Intelligence University of Granada
17. Muharom S (2019) Pengenalan Nomor Ruangan Menggunakan Kamera Berbasis OCR Dan Template Matching. Jurnal INFORM 4(1)

A Comparative Evaluation of Acceleration and Jerk in Human Activity Recognition Using Machine Learning Techniques

Nurul Retno Nurwulan and Gjergji Selamaj

Abstract Acceleration data have been widely used to study human activity recognition. However, the acceleration data collected from the accelerometer do not consider the force of gravity. Thus, it has a difficulty in discriminating closely similar activities. Jerk, the derivative of acceleration, is able to describe the changes of body accelerations correctly and mutually exclusive from the sensor orientation. This study aimed to compare the performance of jerk compared to acceleration data. The dataset used to do the comparison was collected from a triaxial accelerometer built-in Samsung smartphone with a sampling frequency of 50 Hz attached to the waist of thirty subjects. The subjects performed walking on a flat surface, walking upstairs, walking downstairs, sitting, standing, and lying down. The feature data were then grouped into three categories: acceleration features, jerk features, and combined features of acceleration and jerk. The evaluation was done using k-Nearest neighbors (KNN), linear discriminant analysis (LDA), support vector machine (SVM), and random forest (RF). The results showed that jerk features performed worse than the acceleration features. However, the combined acceleration and jerk features yielded the highest accuracy with above 87% for all classifiers. The present findings show that acceleration is still better than jerk in recognizing the pattern in human activity. The present study is, therefore, increasing the understanding of acceleration data and its derivative in human activity recognition.

Keywords Human activity recognition · Accelerometer · Acceleration · Jerk · Pattern recognition

N. R. Nurwulan (✉)
Sampoerna University, Jakarta 12780, Indonesia
e-mail: nurul.nurwulan@sampoernauniversity.ac.id

G. Selamaj
Universiteti Ismail Qemali, Vlorë 9401, Albania
e-mail: gjergji.selamaj147@gmail.com

H. Triwiyanto et al. (eds.), *Proceedings of the 1st International Conference on Electronics, Biomedical Engineering, and Health Informatics*, Lecture Notes in Electrical Engineering 746, https://doi.org/10.1007/978-981-33-6926-9_5

1 Introduction

Human activity recognition has been proven for its benefits in various fields such as healthcare [1–3]. Human activity recognition is often used to help the physicians to make a correct diagnosis for patients. Accelerometers are a common device in human activity recognition due to its ability to provide an objective, non-intrusive measure of activity and the high resolution of data acquisition [1]. Triaxial accelerometers in smartphones are the practical and cost-effective choice for human daily activity recognition [4].

Various studies evaluating human daily activity using the acceleration data by extracting its features either the time or frequency-domain features. High accuracy results with more than 90% accuracy have been reported in past studies [5–7]. However, the high accuracy results are only possible when the activities are simple, well-separated, and performed carefully based on researchers' instructions. If the activities are more complex, closely similar to each other, and performed in a more natural manner, human activity recognition becomes a challenging problem since there is no clear way to relate the signal data to a specific activity.

Past studies reported promising results obtained from using jerk-based features for activity recognition in animals [8]. Jerk was used because it is not possible to direct the animals with specific instructions to perform the tasks. Further, jerk could describe the sensor orientation although the sensor is loosely attached and frequently shifted [8]. Motivated by the promising results in animals, the aim of the present study was to evaluate the performance of jerk compared to the acceleration in recognizing human daily activities. This study examined whether jerk, the derivative of acceleration, could overcome the low sensitivity of acceleration data in discriminating complex and closely similar human daily activities. Machine learning techniques were used for the evaluation due to their robustness [9].

This paper is organized as follows. Section 2 describes the materials and method in obtaining the dataset and a brief description of the theoretical background behind acceleration and jerk, feature extraction, and machine learning classifiers. Section 3 presents results and discussion. Finally, the conclusion is presented in Sect. 4.

2 Materials and Method

The dataset used to evaluate the performance of acceleration and jerk was taken from the study by Anguita et al. [4]. The data was collected using the triaxial accelerometer built-in Samsung smartphone from thirty subjects aged between nineteen and forty-eight. The smartphone was attached to the waist with the sampling frequency rate was set to 50 Hz. Each subject performed walking, walking upstairs, walking downstairs, sitting, standing, and lying down. The dataset was pre-processed with a fifty percent overlapping window of 2.56 s. Then, time- and frequency-domain features from acceleration and jerk data were extracted.

The extracted features were then analyzed using supervised machine learning techniques, namely K-Nearest neighbors (KNN), Fisher's linear discriminant analysis (LDA), support vector machine (SVM), and random forest (RF). Ten-fold cross-validation using Weka environment was done to evaluate the performance of acceleration and jerk datasets.

2.1 *Acceleration and Jerk*

Acceleration is the rate of change of velocity in terms of speed and/or direction. The acceleration is commonly used in human activity recognition researches. However, acceleration data exclude the force of gravity and thus it is just a consequence of static load [10]. Jerk is the derivative of acceleration and it is felt like the change of accelerations. The magnitude of jerk describes the changes of accelerations independently from the sensor orientation [8]. Thus, jerk can overcome the problem of unknown sensor orientation that might happen when the smartphone on the subjects' pocket moves its position.

2.2 *Feature Extraction*

There are two modes of features in human physiological data: time-domain features that refer to the variation of the amplitude of the signal with time; and frequency-domain features that are more robust and need signal pre-processing such as the Fast Fourier Transform (FFT) [11]. In this study, the features are mean, standard deviation, mean absolute deviation, maximum, minimum, signal magnitude area, energy, interquartile range, and spectral entropy in both the time- and frequency-domain modes.

2.3 *Classifiers*

In this study, we evaluated the performance of acceleration and jerk data using supervised classifiers: K-Nearest neighbors (KNN), Fisher's linear discriminant analysis (LDA), support vector machine (SVM), and random forest (RF). Weka environment was used for the machine learning analyses. The KNN is a fast and simple supervised classifier [9]. The classification is done by determining the similarity between the training set and new observation that is assigned to the most similar class based on the most votes [12]. Despite its simplicity, KNN is an effective classifier for human activity recognition [13].

The LDA is capable of ensuring the projections of samples from different classes to a line are well-separated. It can separate the classes with an obvious distance between mean values and small variances [14]. Whereas, the SVM can distinctly classify the patterns of the data points into different classes. The difference between the SVM and LDA is that the SVM selects the hyperplane with maximum margin distance [15]. The RF constructs a large number of uncorrelated decision trees as an ensemble at training time with the output is the classification of individual trees [16]. Each individual tree has a class prediction and the class with the most votes will become the model prediction. Past studies reported high accuracy using the RF as a classifier [9, 16, 17].

3 Results

This study evaluated the performance of both acceleration and jerk in order to see whether jerk could really recognize human activity better than acceleration. The evaluation was conducted for three different groups: acceleration, jerk, and combination of both acceleration and jerk. Then, these groups were evaluated using KNN, LDA, SVM, and RF. Ten-fold cross-validation with 90% of the data used for training was selected in this study. The dataset was divided into ten folds with the same class distribution as the original dataset. Each fold was used once to test the performance of the classifier from the combined data of the remaining nine folds. As can be seen in Table 1, the RF outperformed the other classifiers in all groups with the highest accuracy is 88.30% in the combination of acceleration and jerk group.

Since the RF outperformed the other classifiers, we focus on the RF to compare the performance of acceleration and jerk. Tables 2, 3, and 4 show the confusion matrices of the RF for acceleration, jerk, and combination of acceleration and jerk, respectively. The standing, sitting, and lying are misclassified with one another. However, acceleration and combination groups classified better than jerk.

4 Discussion

We used ten-fold cross-validation because it has a low variance than a single hold-out set estimator. For the dataset in this study, the test set is very small if the single hold-out set is used because 90% of the data are used for training, and 10%

Table 1 Performance evaluation of the classifiers

Attribute	KNN (%)	LDA (%)	SVM (%)	RF (%)
Acceleration	85.06	85.84	85.79	87.15
Jerk	81.24	83.82	83.45	83.52
Combined	87.27	87.31	87.42	88.30

Table 2 Confusion matrix of RF for acceleration

Labeled	Recognized results					
	Standing	Sitting	Lying	Walking	Downstairs	Upstairs
Standing	323	174	171	0	0	0
Sitting	231	218	174	0	0	0
Lying	200	151	328	0	1	1
Walking	0	0	0	508	14	81
Downstairs	0	0	0	25	431	37
Upstairs	0	0	1	106	24	410

Table 3 Confusion matrix of RF for jerk

Labeled	Recognized results					
	Standing	Sitting	Lying	Walking	Downstairs	Upstairs
Standing	240	197	231	0	0	0
Sitting	226	198	199	0	0	0
Lying	218	196	265	0	0	2
Walking	0	0	0	369	146	88
Downstairs	0	0	0	114	329	50
Upstairs	0	0	1	96	20	424

Table 4 Confusion matrix of RF for the combination of acceleration and jerk

Labeled	Recognized results					
	Standing	Sitting	Lying	Walking	Downstairs	Upstairs
Standing	353	156	159	0	0	0
Sitting	235	224	164	0	0	0
Lying	165	126	388	0	0	2
Walking	0	0	0	572	5	26
Downstairs	0	0	0	12	431	50
Upstairs	0	0	0	31	25	485

used for testing. The findings of this study showed that RF yielded the highest accuracy. RF is an effective method to rank the importance of variables. Unlike the other decision tree classifiers, each tree in RF can only select a random subset of features that makes it possible to increase the variation among the trees in the model. Thus, the classification will result in higher accuracy considering the low correlation across trees [9, 17].

The performance of a combination of both acceleration and jerk yielded in the highest accuracy. However, when the acceleration and jerk were evaluated as individual groups, acceleration resulted in higher accuracy than jerk. The logic behind using jerk-based features is because jerk is the derivative of acceleration.

Thus, it is supposed to be able to detect slight changes in closely similar activities [8]. However, it is not the case in this current study. This could be caused by the fact that the past study [8] used jerk to evaluate the activity recognition in animals with less-to-none instructions from the researchers. On the contrary, the dataset in this study was taken from human subjects with detailed instructions for each activity. Therefore, in contrast to the past study [8], jerk did not perform well in recognizing human activities. This might happen because there were little changes in forces in human signal data during standing, sitting, and lying. Jerk is felt when there is an obvious change in force [10].

As for walking on a flat surface, walking downstairs, and walking upstairs, jerk is also the worst in classifying the activities correctly. Both acceleration and combined groups are able to distinguish the walking activities. This might also happen because the subjects in this study were young adults with good postural control [18]. They could compensate with both increasing and decreasing forces that happened during walking downstairs and upstairs. Based on the results in this study, it can be said that jerk does not perform better than acceleration in human activity recognition when the change of force in the activities is minimum. This finding increases the understanding of the usage of acceleration data and its derivative in human activity recognition. Further studies with more variation of activities including activities with an obvious change of force, to evaluate the performance of jerk and other derivatives of acceleration are needed. In addition, future studies should also evaluate the performance of jerk in other age brackets such as older adults since the other age brackets might not have a good postural control like the young adults.

5 Conclusion and Future Work

This paper has presented the performance evaluation of jerk compared to acceleration using machine learning techniques, namely the k-Nearest neighbors (KNN), Fisher's linear discriminant analysis (LDA), support vector machine (SVM), and random forest (RF). Based on the evaluation results, it can be concluded that the RF outperformed the other machine learning techniques in terms of accuracy and jerk did not perform better than acceleration in recognizing human activities. This could happen because there were only slight force changes in acceleration in the activities being evaluated. The results of the current study increase the understanding of the usage of acceleration data and its derivative in human activity recognition. Further studies evaluating activities with an obvious change of force are important to confirm whether jerk is more sensitive than acceleration in activities with a bigger change of force.

References

1. Nurwulan NR, Jiang BC (2016) Possibility of using entropy method to evaluate the distracting effect of mobile phones on pedestrian. Entropy 18:390
2. Ogbuabor G, Labs R (2018) Human activity recognition for healthcare using smartphones. In: Proceedings of the 10th international conference on machine learning and computing, Macau, pp 41–46
3. Yan W, Shuang C, Yu H (2019) A survey on wearable sensor modality centred human activity recognition in health care. Expert Syst Appl 137:167–190
4. Anguita D, Ghio A, Oneto L, Parra X, Reyes-Ortiz JL (2013) A public domain dataset for human activity recognition using smartphones. In: Proceedings of the 21th European symposium on artificial neural networks, computational intelligence and machine learning, ESANN, Bruges, Belgium
5. Walse KH, Dharaskar RV, Thakare VM (2016) PCA based optimal ANN classifiers for human activity recognition using mobile sensors data. In: Proceedings of 1st international conference on information and communication technology for intelligent systems, Ahmedabad, India, pp 429–436
6. Fullerton E, Heller B, Munoz-Organero M (2017) Recognizing human activity in free-living using body-worn accelerometers. IEEE Sens J 17(16):5290–5297
7. Pavey TG, Gilson ND, Gomersall SJ, Clark B, Trost SG (2017) Field evaluation of random forest activity classifier for wrist-worn accelerometer data. J Sci Med Sport 20(1):75–80
8. Hämäläinen W, Järvinen M, Martiskainen P, Mononen J (2011) Jerk-based feature extraction for robust activity recognition from acceleration data. In: Proceedings of the 11th international conference on intelligent systems design and applications (ISDA 2011). IEEE computer society, pp 831–836
9. Nurwulan NR (2020) Performance evaluation of decomposition methods in perturbed walking. Revue d'Intelligence Artificielle 34(1):45–50
10. Eager D, Pendrill AM, Reistad N (2016) Beyond velocity and acceleration: jerk, snap and higher derivatives. Eur J Phys 37:065008
11. Nurwulan N, Jiang BC (2020) Window selection impact in human activity recognition. Int J Innovative Technol Interdisc Sci 3(1):381–394
12. Suto J, Oniga S, Pop Sitar P (2016) Feature analysis to human activity recognition. Int J Comput Commun Control 12(1):116–130
13. Subasi A, Radhwan M, Kurdi R, Khateeb K (2018) IoT based mobile healthcare system for human activity recognition. In: Proceedings of 15th learning and technology conference, Jeddah, Saudi Arabia
14. Hassan MM, Uddin MZ, Mohamed A, Almogren A (2018) A robust human activity recognition system using smartphone sensors and deep learning. Future Gener Comput Syst 81:307–313
15. Zeng H, Li K, Tian X, Wei N, Song R, Zhou L (2018) Classification of hand motions using linear discriminant analysis and support vector machine. Chinese Autom Congr, Jinan, China
16. Nunes UM, Faria DR, Peixoto P (2017) A human activity recognition framework using max-min features and key poses with differential evolution random forests classifier. Pattern Recogn Lett 99:21–31
17. Mehrang S, Pietila J, Korhonen I (2018) An activity recognition framework deploying the random forest classifier and a single optical heart rate monitoring and triaxial accelerometer wrist-band. Sensors 18(2):613
18. Selamaj G (2020) Impacts of mobile phone distractions on walking performance. Indonesian J Comput Eng Design 2(1):32–37

Rapid Thermal Modelling of Power MOSFET Using Bump Test Method to Evaluate Performance of Low Cost Heatsink

Dista Yoel Tadeus, Heru Winarno, and Priyo Sasmoko

Abstract Heat dissipator or heatsink is crucial for the reliability of MOSFET-based converters and inverters. Currently, products such as To-220 are low cost passive aluminium heatsink that fit to a single discrete MOSFET package did not followed by proper documentation about its thermal model and performance. Thermal modelling has been used widely for thermal studies, but the methods were often time consuming, complex setup, and require sophisticated equipments. This study proposed a different method in thermal modelling that is specifically applied to evaluate the performance of low cost heatsink through the Bump Test experiment. It emphasizes on rapid, simple setup and calculations. The experiment were finished in less than 1000 s in order to obtain dataset that were used to develop case to ambient thermal model of IRF840 n-channel MOSFET that was constructed by third order transfer function. Also, it was converted to Cauer equivalent RCs circuit to obtain physical meaning of heatsink block layers. The conducted experiments were applied to two different low cost heatsinks shapes; heatsink A resulted in a dissipation of MOSFET's power limit to 4.21 W, while the attached heatsink B produced 5.38 W. In other words, heatsink B has 27.79% higher dissipated power handling, or 13.06% higher continuous Drain current utilization, than heatsink A. These values represented quantitative measure of heatsink performance. This study can be used as a technical reference for MOSFET based electronic circuit board fabricator in order to obtain rapid measure of low cost heatsink performance.

Keywords Power MOSFET · Thermal model · Low cost heatsink

D. Y. Tadeus (✉) · H. Winarno · P. Sasmoko
Electrical Engineering, Department of Industrial Technology, Vocational School, Diponegoro University, Semarang, Indonesia
e-mail: distayoel@gmail.com

H. Triwiyanto et al. (eds.), *Proceedings of the 1st International Conference on Electronics, Biomedical Engineering, and Health Informatics*, Lecture Notes in Electrical Engineering 746, https://doi.org/10.1007/978-981-33-6926-9_6

1 Introduction

Power electronics have a major role in switch mode converters and inverters. The applications are widely applied in various fields such as household electronic appliances, offices, telecommunications, transportation, medical, military, and power plants. Semiconductor technology that is constantly developing and available today offers various types of power electronic components with their own characteristics. Power Metal Oxide Semiconductor Field Effect Transistor (MOSFET) is one of power electronic components that have advantage in switching speed and small On-resistance. Its low voltage handling characteristic, making it suitable for small and medium power applications. Thermal management is a critical concern since it is easy to damage due to excessive heat generated as a result of poor performance of heatsinks. There are available on market low cost passive aluminium heatsinks in various shapes that fit to a single discrete MOSFET package such as To-220. Its low price, easy to install design, and high availability making it excellent choice for small and home industries to be applied as MOSFET heatsink for wide electronic circuit applications as shown on Fig. 1. But unfortunately, these low cost heatsinks does not have any technical information about its thermal characteristic and performance measure. So it was hard for electronic manufacturers to put limit on MOSFET's power utilization according to its applied heatsink. Thermal modelling was widely used to obtain object's thermal characteristic and model, but the methods were often time consuming, require complex setup and sophisticated equipments [1, 2, 3, 4, 5]. This study proposed a different method that is specifically applied to evaluate the performance of low cost heatsink through the Bump Test experiment. It was usually applied to tune PID controller [6, 7]. It emphasizes on rapid, simple setup and calculations also does not require sophisticated equipments. Dataset obtained from rapid experiment were used in Matlab System Identification Toolbox to develop case to ambient thermal model of IRF840 n-channel MOSFET. This software-based computation was commonly used as a tool to study thermal characteristic [1, 2, 8, 9]. The mathematical model was constructed as third order transfer function and converted to Cauer equivalent RCs circuit to obtain physical meaning of heatsink block layers [3, 10]. Static gain from developed model then used in calculation to evaluate performance of low cost heatsinks in terms of its effect to limit MOSFETS's power handling capability and Drain current utilization.

2 Research Method

N-channel power MOSFET IRF840 with TO-220 package was used as an example here because it is easy to find in the market and suitable for general purpose applications. Dallas D18B20 temperature sensor was used with any general purpose microcontroller based data logger device with time sampling of 1 s to aquire

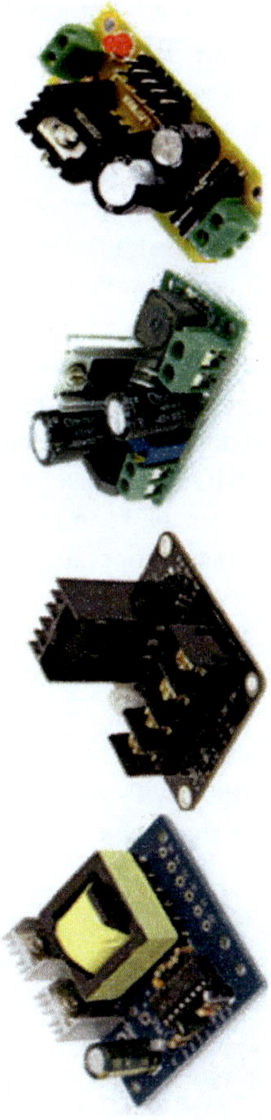

Fig. 1 Examples of low cost heatsinks applied to commercially available small electronic power converters

MOSFET case realtime temperature and input signal in the Bump Test procedure. 100 W 8 O resistor is used as load. The Bump Test was conducted as a simple open loop system [11] as shown by Fig. 2. The recorded measurement data from data logger are extracted and arranged to form graph as shown by Fig. 6.

Electric power as step input signal was supplied to system to obtain its heating characteristic until steady state condition was reached. Circuit schematic for experiment is shown by Fig. 3, microcontroller outputs High logic (5 V) as voltage trigger to activate MOSFET and drive it to its saturation region with 8 V Drain-Source voltage and generated 1.3 A continuous Drain current. IRF840 has typical 0.85 O Drain-Source On-State Resistance, so the calculated dissipated power used to perform Bump Test was 1.44 W.

This study takes two examples of common low cost commercially available aluminium heatsink. Its shape is shown by Fig. 4. The A shape is lighter and has smaller surface area than B shape. Both of them was sticked to MOSFETs case with silicone thermal pad in Fig. 5 to increase surface contact area between material while providing electrical insulation and secured with bolt. Temperature sensor was mounted on MOSFET's case with skun lug.

There were three rapid conducted Bump Tests that were done in period of 1000 s to obtain three thermal output responses according to different setup: MOSFET without heatsink attached, with heatsink shape A attached, and with heatsink shape B attached. Figure 6 shows plots of MOSFET case temperature transient and steady state from each Bump Test setup. It can be seen that by heatsink attachment there was significant effect to steady state case temperature, for heatsink A it was reduced to around 12 °C and for heatsink B it was reduced to around 20 °C where the ambient temperature was around 28 °C. Thermal instability at steady state condition seems to occure easily on No-Heatsink attached, it can be noticed from Fig. 7 after around 650 s there were several small temperature ramp-ups that pushed steady state temperature to higher point. This behaviour is probably caused by low thermal mass characteristic of MOSFET with no heatsink attached, since there was not enough 'inertia' to 'suppress' disturbance caused by fluctuation in load-loop

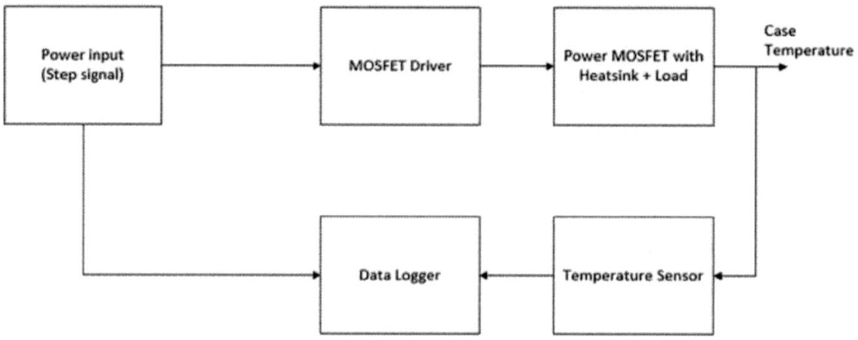

Fig. 2 Block diagram of bump test step response experiment

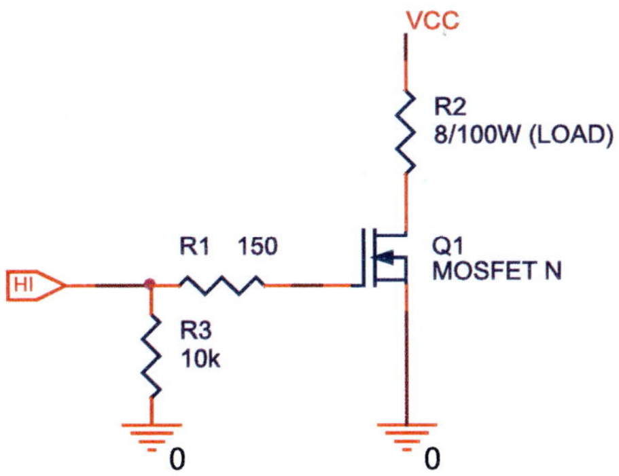

Fig. 3 MOSFET's circuit setup for conducted experiment, two resistors were used as simple driver

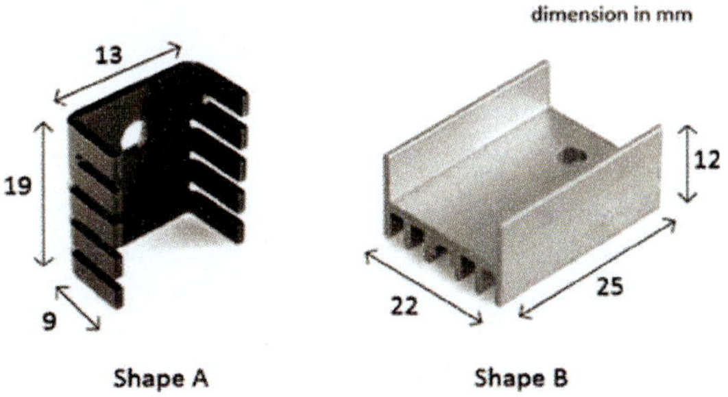

Fig. 4 These two kind of low cost heatsinks in different shape were so popular and easily got from market

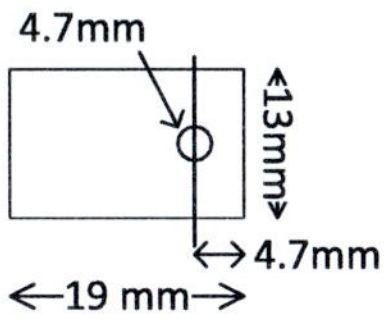

Fig. 5 Common low cost silicon based thermal pad

circuit total resistance that was arised from dependency character of resistance with temperature.

System Identification Toolbox Matlab was used to estimate model of unknown Black Box system using input-output data obtained from Bump Tests with heatsink attached. Ambient temperature was removed in the process in order to meet zero initial condition requirement from the Toolbox.

Thermal model was constructed by third order strictly proper transfer function where:

$$H(s) = \frac{B(s)}{A(s)},\ {}^{\circ}(B(s)) = 2 < {}^{\circ}(A(s)) = 3 \tag{1}$$

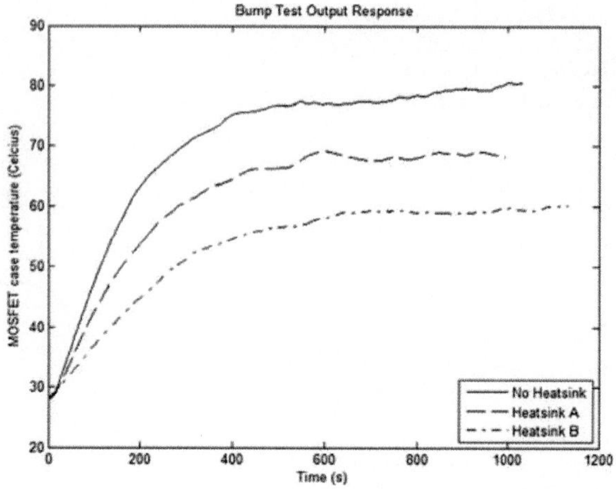

Fig. 6 Output responses from bump tests

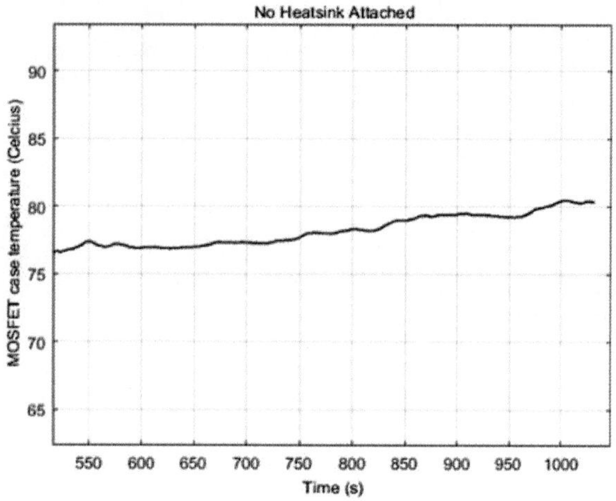

Fig. 7 Small ramp-up heating at steady state condition

The number of numerator and denumerator were choosen according to the structure of Cauer impedance transfer function in Eq. (4). Figure 8 shows normalized zero initial temperature responses from estimated model and actual data generated from Toolbox. For heatsink A setup there was 96.24 best fits and 96.53 best fits for heatsink B setup. These values represent the 'goodness' of estimated model, it can be seen that estimated model can captured transient and steady state dynamic very well.

Equations (2) and (3) show transfer function of MOSFET's case to ambient thermal estimated model for heatsink A setup and heatsink B setup respectively,

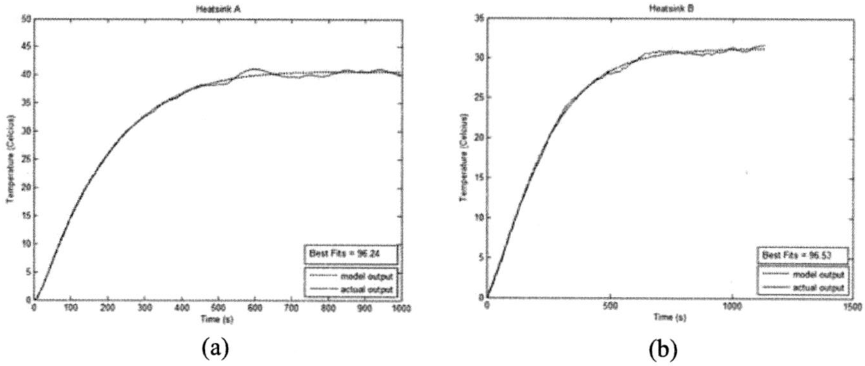

Fig. 8 Normalized zero initial temperature responses from estimated model and actual data, **a** heatsink A setup, **b** heatsink B setup

$$H_A = \frac{13647.59s^2 + 4855.83s + 27.97}{457665.9s^3 + 38297.48s^2 + 347.46s + 1} \tag{2}$$

$$H_B = \frac{-402.21s^2 + 784.49s + 21.65}{851.78s^3 + 17155.02s^2 + 266.78s + 1} \tag{3}$$

Cauer third order equivalent thermal network was realized in order to obtain physical meaning of MOSFET's case to ambient thermal estimated model. It was used to get the structure of decomposition model: case to silicon pad, silicon pad to heatsink, heatsink to ambient. The general recursive definition of Cauer impedance in Laplace-transformed [12]:

$$Z_{\text{neq}} = \frac{1}{sC_n + \frac{1}{R_n + Z_{n-1}}} \tag{4}$$

Symbolic computations was performed to obtain explicit equation for third order system, this leads to:

$$Z_{3\text{eq}} = \frac{b_2 s^2 + b_1 s + b_0}{a_3 s^3 + a_2 s^2 + a_1 s + a_0} \tag{5}$$

$$\mathrm{b}_2 = \mathrm{C}_1\mathrm{C}_2\mathrm{R}_1\mathrm{R}_2\mathrm{R}_3 \tag{6}$$

$$\mathrm{b}_1 = \mathrm{C}_1\mathrm{R}_1\mathrm{R}_2 + \mathrm{C}_1\mathrm{R}_1\mathrm{R}_3 + \mathrm{C}_2\mathrm{R}_1\mathrm{R}_3 + \mathrm{C}_2\mathrm{R}_2\mathrm{R}_3 \tag{7}$$

$$\mathrm{b}_0 = \mathrm{R}_1 + \mathrm{R}_2 + \mathrm{R}_3 \tag{8}$$

$$a_3 = C_1C_2C_3R_1R_2R_3 \tag{9}$$

$$a_2 = C_1C_2R_1R_2 + C_1C_3R_1R_2 + C_1C_3R_1R_3 + C_2C_3R_1R_3 + C_2C_3R_2R_3 \tag{10}$$

$$a_1 = C_1R_1 + C_2R_1 + C_2R_2 + C_3R_1 + C_3R_2 + C_3R_3 \tag{11}$$

$$a_0 = 1 \tag{12}$$

where,

Z_{3eq} Cauer third order equivalent thermal impedance
R_1, R_2, R_3 Cauer resistance 1, 2, 3
C_1, C_2, C_3 Cauer capacitance 1, 2, 3

Equating all coefficients in Eqs. (2) and (3) respectively to Eq. (5) and solved it numerically, resulted Cauer equivalent RCs value as shown on Table 1.

3 Results and Discussion

In Table 1, there were negative values in both of models. Since there were no absolute negative values of resistance and capacitance in physical world and in the thermal domain there is not an equivalent to negative charges [2], so this decomposition model was loosing it's physical meaning and did not gave insight of MOSFET's physical layer, although it was mathematically valid. Figure 9 shows realization of Cauer circuit as represented by Eq. (5). Actually, from MOSFET's junction to case, there were thermal dynamics that can be characterized by the same procedure explained earlier, but this was not easy to achieved especially for practical purposes. It requires case temperature to be independent of junction temperature. This is very difficult to achieve experimentally so thermal information from manufacturer's datasheet usually preferred for practical purposes.

To evaluate performance of heatsink, b_0 coefficient from Eqs. (2) and (3) need to be extracted from transfer function model. This is known as model's static gain or steady state gain [11], for step signal input it has general form defined by:

$$K = \frac{\text{output value at steady state} - \text{output value at initial condition}}{\text{input value at steady state} - \text{input value at initial condition}} \tag{13}$$

Table 1 Cauer equivalent resistances and capacitances value

	R_1	R_2	R_3	C_1	C_2	C_3
Heatsink A model	−6.29	34.38	−0.10	−22	−26	33.53
Heatsink B model	25.57	−3.9	−0.02	−7.93	23.78	−2.11

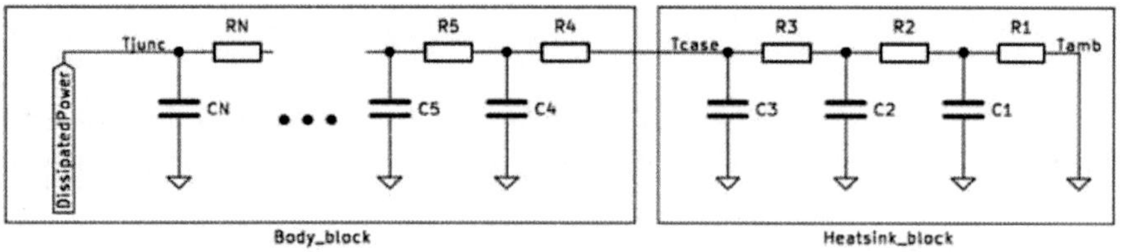

Fig. 9 RC Cauer realization circuit, body block's dynamic was ignored and replaced by data from manufacturer's datasheet

K value can be directly calculated using Bump Test step response data experiments, [13] this is useful in the case there is no access to Matlab or other software based computation. Model's static gain reflects direct relationship between dissipated power occurred in MOSFET and steady state case temperature. It also enables simple rapid calculation to estimate maximum allowed dissipated power on MOSFET's according to heatsink attachment, example as follows for heatsink A setup: From datasheet, IRF840 has 1 °C/W maximum junction to case thermal resistance $\left(R_{\mathrm{jc}}\right)$, 150 °C maximum junction temperature $\left(T_{\mathrm{j}_{\max}}\right)$, model's static gain (K) 27.97, then maximum allowed dissipated power $((\mathrm{P}_{\mathrm{d}_{\max}})$:

$$\mathrm{P}_{\mathrm{d}_{\max}} = \frac{T_{\mathrm{j}_{\max}} - T_{\mathrm{amb}}}{R_{\mathrm{jc}} + K} \tag{14}$$

$$\mathrm{P}_{\mathrm{d}_{\max}} = \frac{150 - 28}{1 + 27.97}$$

$$\mathrm{P}_{\mathrm{d}_{\max}} = 4.21 \text{ W}$$

For continues Drain current operation, this limits maximum Drain current to 2.22 A. In switch mode operation, this value needs to be reduced since dissipated power from switching operation also contributing. In the case of heatsink B setup, same procedure was applied, resulted a $\mathrm{P}_{\mathrm{d}_{\max}} = 5.38$ W with maximum Drain current to 2.51 A. It can be said that heatsink B is 27.79% more effective than heatsink A in term of handling dissipated power and 13.06% more effective in term of maximizing drain current utilization. Comparing model's static gain obtained from Bump Test experiment also usefull to obtain immediate performance of heatsinks. The smallest model's static gain value giving qualitative sense indicating good performance of heatsink.

4 Conclusion

Case to ambient thermal model of Power MOSFET was successfully developed on this study. It successfully captured the transient and steady state dynamic responses of black box system, simply by using input and output data from Bump Test. The equivalent Cauer RC circuit was also developed to obtain physical meaning of layer structure from case to ambient, but unfortunately it generated negative values of resistance and capacitance, so it only can be existed mathematicaly. Model's static gain combined with information from manufacturer's datasheet was very useful to evaluate performance of low cost heatsink and also enabled simple calculation to set limitation on maximum MOSFET's Drain current according to the type of low cost heatsink applied so junction temperature can be maintained below maximum limit. This will increase realibility of MOSFET applications. The method described in this study was rapid, simple, and practically easy to be conducted, there were no sophisticated equipments needed, and even if there was no access to software based computation such as Matlab, the work still can be done by manual calculations. From calculations it can be shown that heatsink A set MOSFET's power dissipation limit to 4.21 W, and 5.38 W for heatsink B. This means that heatsink B has 27.79% higher dissipated power handling, or 13.06% higher continuous Drain current utilization, than heatsink A. These values represented quantitative measure of heatsink performance, it can be used further as a basis to improve or optimize power density of circuit boards. Finally, this study can be used as a technical reference to small and home industries as fabricator of MOSFET based electronic circuit board in order to obtain rapid measure of low cost heatsink performance.

References

1. Hernandez-Perez JG, Carrillo JG, Bassam A, Flota-Banuelos M, Patino-Lopez LD (2020) A new passive PV heatsink design to reduce efficiency losses: a computational and experimental evaluation. Renew Energy 147:1209–1220
2. Sun L, Zhu J, Wong H (2016) Simulation and evaluation of the peak temperature in LED light bulb heatsink. Microelectron Reliab 61:140–144
3. Mitterhuber L et al (2018) Thermal transient measurement and modelling of a power cycled flip-chip LED module. Microelectron Reliab 81:373–380
4. Yoon Y, Kim DR, Lee KS (2020) Cooling performance and space efficiency improvement based on heat sink arrangement for power conversion electronics. Appl Therm Eng 164:114458
5. Lin SC, Tsai R, Chiu CP, Liu LK (2019) A simple approach for system level thermal transient prediction. Therm Sci Eng Prog 9:177–184
6. Bahavarnia M, Tavazoei MS (2013) A new view to Ziegler–Nichols step response tuning method: analytic non-fragility justification. J Process Control 23(1):23–33
7. Amoura K, Mansouri R, Bettayeb M, Al-Saggaf UM (2016) Closed-loop step response for tuning PID-fractional-order-filter controllers. ISA Trans 64:247–257

8. Rahmani MA et al (2014) Thermal management and design optimization of heatsink for cooling performance improvement during transient heat generation. Energy Procedia 61:1665–1668
9. Hu J, Huang M, Liu Y, Zha X (2018) Transient junction temperature estimation of IGBT using improved thermal model. Microelectron Reliab 88–90:1146–1150
10. Kim T, Funaki T (2016) Thermal measurement and analysis of packaged SiC MOSFETs. Thermochim Acta 633:31–36
11. McIntosh AR, Mahalec V (1991) Calculation of steady-state gains for multivariable systems from closed-loop steady-state data. J Process Control 1(4):178–186
12. Gerstenmaier YC, Kiffe W, Wachutka G (2009) Combination of thermal subsystems by use of rapid circuit transformation and extended two-port theory. Microelectron J 40(1):26–34
13. Özdemir N, Townley S (2003) Integral control by variable sampling based on steady-state data. Automatica 39(1):135–140

Facial Skin Type Classification Based on Microscopic Images Using Convolutional Neural Network (CNN)

Sofia Saidah, Yunendah Nur Fuadah, Fenty Alia, Nur Ibrahim, Rita Magdalena, and Syamsul Rizal

Abstract Skin is part of the human body that has a function as a barrier from the external environment and gives a physical appearance to an individual. In general, human skin types are classified into normal, dry, oily and combination skin. These skin types affected by the amount and change in facial sebum secretion and hydration ability. Determination of the type of facial skin is needed to determine skin care products and cosmetics in accordance with the type of facial skin they have. In this research, a system design for digital-based facial skin types using Convolutional Neural Network (CNN) method which has advantages to produce features and characteristics from the microscopic images dataset. The primary datasets taken directly using microscopic cameras and have been validated by a dermatologist. The CNN proposed model in this study consists of 3 hidden layers that use 3 × 3 size filters with output channels 8, 16 and 32 respectively, fully connected layer and softmax activation. The proposed model was able to classify the skin types into normal, dry, oily skin conditions and the combination with the best accuracy of 99.5% from 1200 training images and 400 test images used, meanwhile the parameters of recall precision and f-1 score produce values close to 1, which means that it is almost perfect or it can be said that the error is small.

Keywords CNN · Microscopic images · Skin types

1 Introduction

The skin functions as physical arid chemical barrier from external environment and gives physical appearance to an individual [1]. Generally facial skin types are classified into normal, dry, oily, and the combination skin type. These types are affected by the change and amount of facial hydration status and sebum secretion [2, 3]. The factors that regulate normal skin are an act of stratum corneum (SC), normal

S. Saidah (✉) · Y. N. Fuadah · F. Alia · N. Ibrahim · R. Magdalena · S. Rizal
School of Electrical Engineering, Telkom University, Bandung, Indonesia
e-mail: sofiasaidahsfi@telkomuniversity.ac.id

H. Triwiyanto et al. (eds.), *Proceedings of the 1st International Conference on Electronics, Biomedical Engineering, and Health Informatics*, Lecture Notes in Electrical Engineering 746, https://doi.org/10.1007/978-981-33-6926-9_7

level of SC lipids, balanced sebum secretion, normal levels of natural moisturizing factor (NMF) and hyaluronic acid (HA), normal aquaporin (AQP3) expression. Dry skin has low sebum secretion and skin hydration, and can be identified from rough texture, dull grey-white colour, and elevated number of ridges, leaving a tightness sensation and dry looks at the skin. Oily skin comes with excessive sebum secretion, giving the oily appearance [3, 4]. The combination skin type is when an individual has regional differences in skin type. Both U-zone (both cheeks) and T-zone (chin, nose, and forehead sites) face have different skin types, and the individual can feel the symptoms and signs of dry skin type or oily skin type together [2, 3]. Sebum secretion throughout lifetime affected by internal factor such as aging, and also external factors such as seasonal change and application of moisturisers [2]. Therefore, there must be a continuous skin type determination while using skin care and cosmetic products.

Nowadays, there are a noticeable growing in nonmedical skin care and cosmetic use of over-the-counter products. The need in understanding variations of skin types and appropriate measurement tools is important in order to choose the suitable cosmetics and skin care products for specific skin types [4]. Regarding the sebum level as the key of facial skin types classification, various techniques have been used to measure its level, including visual grading that is done by experts, absorbent paper or tape, gravimetry absorption, and the widely used quantitative measurement device Sebumeter® with photometric techniques [5].

Some studies on the classification of facial skin types based on digital images have been conducted. In previous studies, Support Vector Machine (SVM) is used for classification method and also Discrete Wavelet Transform (DWT) and Local Binary Pattern (LBP) is used for feature extraction method to classify facial skin types for oily, normal, dry and combination types, with resulted accuracy of 91.6% [6], while the dataset of an overall face image taken using a camera. In research [7] by using K-Nearest Neighbor (K-NN) and statistical characteristics of order 1 and 2, an accuracy of 92.85% was obtained to classify 3 types of facial skin, namely oily skin, normal to oily skin, and normal to dry skin. Research [8] classified oily and non-oily facial skin using Haar Wavelet and K-Nearest Neighbor methods to obtain an accuracy of 90%. Research [9] classified men's facial skin types based on texture with Support Vector Machine (SVM) method and Gray Level Co-occurance Matrix (GLCM) method and it given an accuracy of 88.89% for 2 classes of skin types namely dry and oily skin. Some of these studies require several process that must be passed to produce the best accuracy. Several studies have shown that Convolutional Neural Networks (CNN) are suitable for processing microscopic images. In the study [10] CNN was used to classify 2D-Hela microscopic images and PAP-smear datasets with an accuracy of 92.57% for 2D-Hela and 92.63% for PAP-Smear. Meanwhile, in the research [11] it can be seen that the CNN method showed a significant improvement in the F1-score value compared to other methods used to detect microscopic images of cells. In addition, a researcher from NHK Broadcasting Science Research Laboratories, Tokyo, Japan named Kunihiko Fukushima developed CNN under the name NoeCognitron for the first time [12]. Then Yann LeChun, a researcher from AT&T Bell Laboratories in Holmdel, New

Jersey, USA, developed the concept and successfully applied the CNN model named LeNet in his research on number and handwriting recognition [13].

In this study, classification of facial skin types will be carried out using Convolutional Neural Network (CNN) in terms of microscopic images. The CNN proposed model design in this study uses 3 hidden layers, max pooling, RelU activation, fully connected layer and softmax activation.

2 Method

In this study, a system was designed to classify normal, dry, oily and combined facial skin types using the CNN method. The CNN model used consists of 3 hidden layers where in the three hidden layers 3 × 3 size filters are used with output channels 8, 16 and 32 respectively, fully connected layer and softmax activation. Generally, Fig. 1 show the CNN model proposed in this study.

2.1 Dataset

This study used primary datasets taken directly using microscopic cameras. The primary dataset taken consists of normal, oily, dry skin, and a combination skin

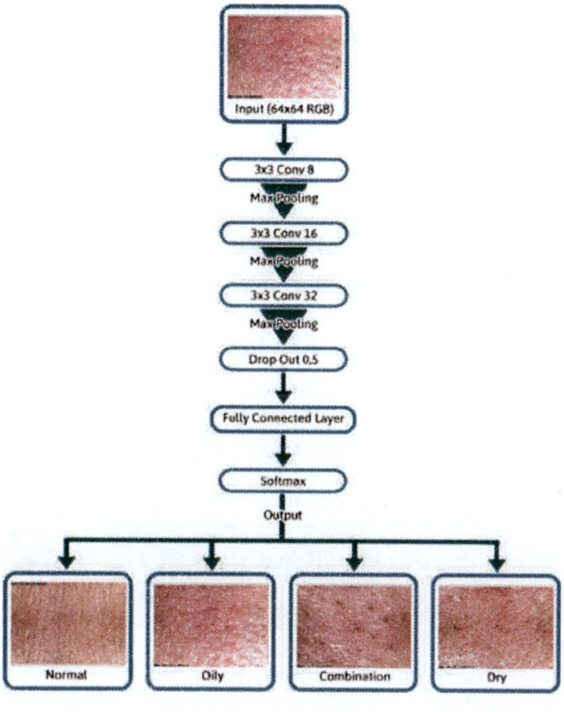

Fig. 1 Proposed system model of facial skin types classification using CNN

conditions that has been validated by a dermatologist. Total data used are 1600 data, each skin condition consisting of 400 skin images. The division of training data and validation data in this study were 1200 training data and 400 validation data. The validation data used consists of 100 data for each skin condition.

2.2 *Convolutional Neural Network*

Convolutional Neural Network (CNN) is a development of the Multilayer Perceptron (MLP) which is designed to process two-dimensional data in the form of images. CNN is a part of Deep Learning methods that can be used to detect and recognize an object on a digital image. Deep Learning is an implementation of the basic concepts of Machine Learning that implements Artificial Neural Network (ANN) algorithms with more layers. The MLP method is not suitable for image classification because MLP does not store spatial information from the data of an image and considers each pixel to be an independent feature resulting in unfavorable results. The way CNN works is the same as in MLP, but on CNN each neuron is presented in two dimensions, different from MLP that presented in one-dimensional for each neuron. On CNN, both weight parameters and linear operation are different because of the data propagated are in two-dimensional form.

The first layer in CNN model is Convolutional Layer, where the linear operations is proceed through convolution that have four dimensions of weights form, which are a collection of convolution kernels. The weight dimensions on CNN are:

$$\text{weight dimension} = \text{input neurons} \times \text{output neurons} \times \text{height} \times \text{weight} \quad (1)$$

Due to the nature of the convolution process, CNN can only be used on data that has a two-dimensional structure such as an image. The purpose of convolution in the image data is to extract features from the input image. Convolution will produce a linear transformation of the input data according to special information in the data. The weight of the layer specifies the convolution kernel used, so that the convolution kernel can be trained based on input on CNN. Feature extraction layer consists of convolutional layers and pooling layers. The convolution process is carried out to change the image to produce a convolved feature which is a unique character of the original image. The convolution process is shown in Fig. 2 [14].

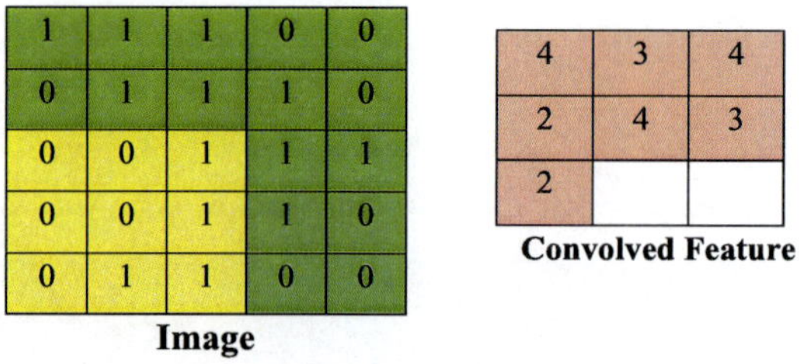

Fig. 2 Convolution process of CNN

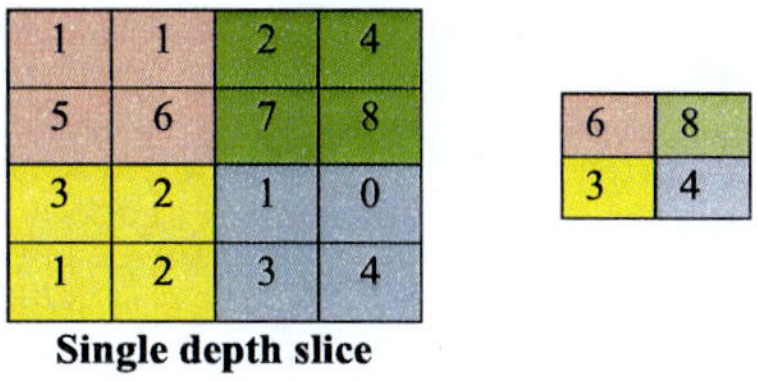

Fig. 3 Max pooling with 2 × 2 filters and stride 2

After the convolution layer, then there is the pooling layer. Pooling is a reduction in the size of the matrix by using the pooling operation. Basically, the Pooling layer consists of a filter of a certain size and stride that will alternately shift throughout the feature map area. The shape of the pooling layer generally uses a 2 × 2 filter which is applied in two steps and operates on each slice of the input. Figure 3 below is an example of a max-pooling operation image [15].

The use of the pooling layer on CNN are reduce the size of the image so that it can be easily replaced with a convolutional layer with the same stride as the corresponding pooling layer, and for looking the image in the big picture.

Dropout is a technique used to reduce overfitting in neural networks by preventing complex adaptations to training data. In this research 0.5 dropout was used, meaning that 50% of the unit will be dropped from the neural network.

The Fully Connected Layer is a layer in which all the activation neurons from the previous layer are all connected to the neurons in the next layer just like an ordinary neural network. Basically, this layer is usually used in MLP which has the purpose of transforming data dimensions to be classified linearly.

The activation function used in the CNN model proposed in this study are RelU in the hidden layer and softmax for the output layer. The Softmax function calculates the probability of each target class for all possible target classes and will help to determine the target class for a given input. The main advantage of using

Table 1 Detail of CNN proposed model

Layer	Filter size	Output shape
Input image	–	64,64,3
Convolution2D	3 × 3, padding	64,64,8
RelU	–	64,64,8
Max pooling	2 × 2, stride 2	32,32,8
Convolution2D	3 × 3, padding	32,32,16
RelU	–	32,32,16
Max poolling	2 × 2, stride 2	16,16,16
Convolution2D	3 × 3, padding	16,16,32
RelU	–	16,16,32
Max pooling	2 × 2, stride 2	8,8,32
Dropout	–	8,8,32
Flatten	–	2048
Dense	–	4
Softmax	–	4

Softmax is the range of output probabilities with values from 0 to 1, and the sum of all probabilities will be equal to one. The softmax function can be used for multi-classification models. The softmax function is defined as follows:

$$F(X_i) = \frac{\text{Exp}(X_i)}{\sum_{j=0}^{k} \text{Exp}(X_i)}, \text{ dimana } i = 0, 1, 2, \ldots k \tag{2}$$

The following Table 1 is a table of the CNN models proposed in this study along with the output of each layer.

3 System Performance

The parameters used to measure the performance system for classifying facial skin types are include accuracy, recall, precision and F1-score. Confusion matrix is used to present the results of system testing in classifying dry, normal, oily and combination facial skin types. Here are the equations for measuring those parameters:

$$\text{Accuracy} = \frac{TP + TN}{TP + FP + TN + FN} \tag{3}$$

$$\text{Recall} = \frac{TP}{TP + FN} \tag{4}$$

$$\text{Precision} = \frac{TP}{TP + FP} \tag{5}$$

$$F1 - \text{Score} = 2 \times \frac{\text{recall} \times \text{precision}}{\text{recall} + \text{precision}} \tag{6}$$

TP (True Positive) shows positive data that is predicted to be true (positive), TN (True Negative) is negative data that is predicted to be true (negative). FP (False Positive) is negative data but is predicted as positive data. FN (False Negative) is positive data but predicted as negative data.

4 Result and Discussion

The skin condition classification system designed in this study can classify skin conditions into normal, oily, dry and combination skin conditions. The data used in this study are private datasets that have been validated by dermatologists. Total data used amounted to 1600 data, each skin condition consisting of 400 skin images. In testing the system performance, training has been carried out using the proposed

CNN model for 1200 training data and 400 test data. The test data used consisted of 100 data for each skin condition. The proposed CNN model uses Adam optimizer with a learning rate of 0.001 and uses the loss categorical cross entropy equation. System performance in classifying the four skin conditions is evaluated using the performance of accuracy, precision, recall and F1-score. Based on the results of the proposed model training using 100 times iteration (epoch 100) the accuracy and loss results for each iteration are shown in Figs. 4 and 5 respectively.

The CNN model used in the skin condition classification system that was designed in this study did not experience overfitting, meaning that both the training stage and the model testing were able to recognize each skin condition, this is based on Fig. 4 which shows an increase in accuracy in each iteration and the results of training data accuracy and the test data obtained are not much different. Likewise with the loss performance shown in Fig. 5, it can be seen that the loss value for both training data and test data has decreased for each iteration and the error value is very minimum. The best performance of the system obtained an accuracy of 99.50% and a loss value of 0.0216.

Fig. 4 Accuracy of the proposed model

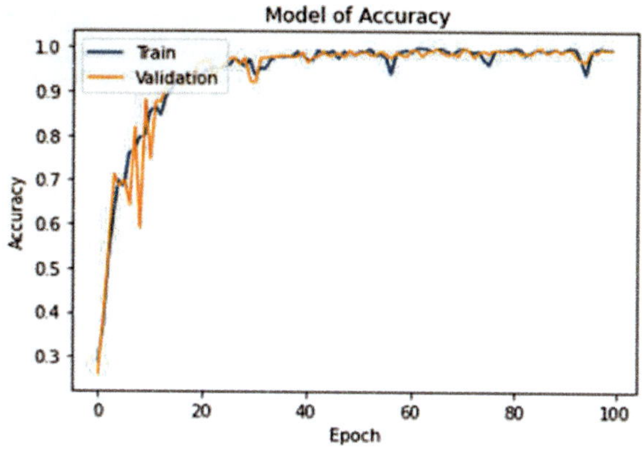

Fig. 5 Loss of the proposed model

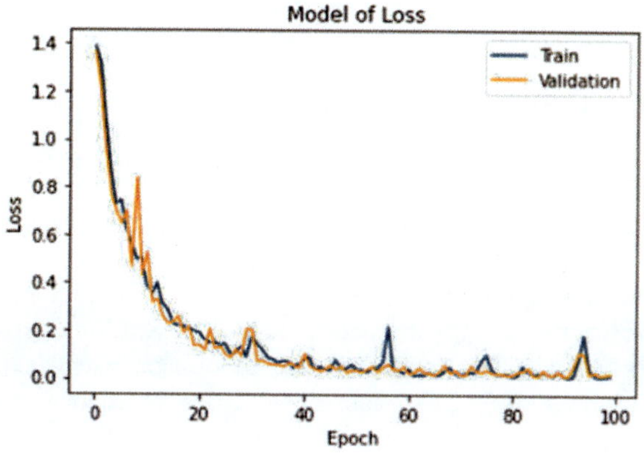

Table 2 System performance of CNN proposed model

Class	Precision	Recall	F-1 score	Number of image
Oily	0.98	1	0.99	116
Normal	1	1	1	92
Dry	1	1	1	88
Combination	1	0.98	0.99	104
Total	0.995	0.995	0.995	400

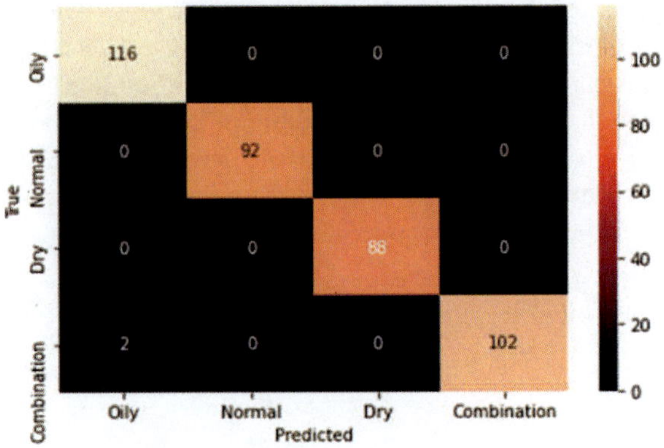

Fig. 6 Confusion matrix of validation data

The performance of the system is show in Table 2 below.

Figure 6 is a Confusion Matrix system test results, based on the results obtained can be seen that from the 400 test data used, almost all test data can be classified according to skin conditions both for normal, oily, dry and combination conditions. There are only two oily skin data detected as a combination condition. In addition, in Table 2 it can be seen that other performance parameters such as precision, recall and f1 score get an average value close to 1 (almost perfect). This shows that the CNN model proposed in this study has a very accurate and promising performance as a tool to diagnose skin conditions.

5 Conclusion

In this study, a system was designed to classify dry, normal, oily and combination facial skin types. The dataset used is a primary dataset total 1600 data that has been validated by a dermatologist. The CNN model used in this study consists of 3 hidden layers, with a filter size of 3 × 3 with output channels 8, 16 and 32 respectively, fully connected layer and SoftMax activation. Based on testing, the proposed CNN model is able to classify facial skin image data with the best accuracy of 99.5%, a loss of 0.0216, a precision value of 0.995, a recall of 0.995

and an average f1-score of 0.995. In subsequent studies this method can be used for a classification system for facial skin types and provide alternative types of treatment suitable for each skin type.

References

1. Chu DH (2012) Structure and development of the skin. in fitzpatrick's dermatology in general medicine, 8th edn. In: Goldsmith LA, Katz SI, Gilchrest BA, Paller AS, Leffell DJ, Wolff K (eds) The McGraw-Hill Companies, Inc. pp 58–75
2. Youn SW (2015) Cosmetic facial skin types. In: P. H. et al (ed) Measuring the skin. Springer International Publishing Switzerland, pp 1–6
3. Choi CW, Choi JW, Youn SW (2013) Subjective facial skin type, based on the sebum related symptoms, can reflect the objective casual sebum level in acne patients. Ski Res Technol 19 (2):176–182
4. Baumann L (2015) Baumann skin type indicator—a novel approach to understanding skin type. In: Maibach H (ed) Handbook of cosmetic science and technology, pp 29–39
5. Crowther JM (2016) Method for quantification of oils and sebum levels on skin using the Sebumeter®. Int J Cosmet Sci 38(2):210–216
6. Indriyani I, Sudarma M (2020) Classification of facial skin type using discrete wavelet transform, contrast, local binary pattern and support vector machine. J Theor Appl Inf Technol 98(5):768–779
7. Neighbor DMK, Tritoasmoro II, Susatio E (2012) Klasifikasi Jenis Kulit Wajah Berdasarkan Analisis Tekstur Dengan Metode K-Nearest Neighbor, pp 0–6
8. Farhan MR, Widodo AW, Rahman MA (2019) Ekstraksi Ciri Pada Klasifikasi Tipe Kulit Wajah Menggunakan Metode Haar Wavelet. J Pengemb Teknol Inf dan Ilmu Komput 3 (3):2903–2909
9. Firaz T, Nusantara B, Atmaja RD, Elektro FT, Telkom U (2018) Klasifikasi Jenis Kulit Wajah Pria Berdasarkan Tekstur Menggunakan Metode Gray Level Co-Occurrence Matrix (Glcm) Dan Support Vector Machine (Svm) Classification of Men' S Face Skin Types Based the Texture Using Gray Level Co-Occurrence Matrix Glcm 5(2):2130–2137
10. Nguyen LD, Lin D, Lin Z, Cao J (2018) Deep CNNs for microscopic image classification by exploiting transfer learning and feature concatenation. In: Proceedings of IEEE International Symposium on Circuits Systems 2018 May
11. Xue Y, Ray N (2018) Cell detection in microscopy images with deep convolutional neural network and compressed sensing, pp 1–29
12. Fukushima K (1980) Neocognitron: a self-organizing neural network model for a mechanism of pattern recognition unaffected by shift in position. Biol Cybern 36(4):193–202
13. Carruthers A, Carruthers J (2013) Handwritten digit recognition with a back-propagation network. Dermatol Surg 39(1 Pt 2):149
14. Unsupervised feature learning and deep learning tutorial. http://ufldl.stanford.edu/tutorial/supervised/ExerciseConvolutionAndPooling/. Accessed on 15 Jun 2020
15. Kegunaan Layar Pooling Pada Penerapan Deep Learning menggunakan Convolutional Neural Network. https://medium.com/@mukhlishatunnada02/kegunaan-layar-pooling-pada-penerapan-deep-learning-menggunakan-convolutional-neural-network-140146078f28. Accessed on 15 Jun 2020

Electrodermal Activity-Based Stress Measurement Using Continuous Deconvolution Analysis Method

Yang Sa'ada Kamila Ariyansah Putri, Osmalina Nur Rahma, Nuzula Dwi Fajriaty, Alfian Pramudita Putra, Akif Rahmatillah, and Khusnul Ain

Abstract Stress is a psychological response that must be handled properly, or it can affect psychology and trigger other complicated diseases. Nowadays, stress measured by filling out stress-related forms or interviews with a psychologist. This method still requires a willingness from the patient to consult their condition, which is often not giving the best result due to late treatment. Therefore, we need a system to monitor a person's stress level conditions independently so they could be threatened quickly if their state gets worsen. One of the non-invasive methods that can be used to measure stress is an Electrodermal Activity (EDA) sensor. EDA is known to be associated with sweat gland activity regulated by SudoMotor Nerve Activity (SMNA), which response to a stressor. However, the SMNA need to decompose into the Skin Conductance Response (SCR) before it could represent stress condition. Hence, the decomposition stage is essential in measuring the quality of the stress condition. In this study, the EDA sensor placed in the palm to obtain the skin conductivity signal. Then, the skin conductivity signals were deconvolved using the Continuous Deconvolution Analysis (CDA) method to capture the SCR. CDA was chosen because it could produce a zero-based line SCR driver and could separate two overlapping peaks in SCR. The result, CDA is adequate to extract SCR, which is shown by the zero baseline of the SCR driver line with a clear peak. The clear SCR peaks are essential for identifying the responses related to the stimulus (stressor).

Keywords CDA · EDA · SCR · SMNA · Stress

Y. S. K. A. Putri · O. N. Rahma · N. D. Fajriaty · A. P. Putra · A. Rahmatillah · K. Ain (✉)
Biomedical Engineering Study Program, Department of Physics, Faculty of Science and Technology, Universitas Airlangga, Surabaya 60115, Indonesia
e-mail: k_ain@fst.unair.ac.id

O. N. Rahma · A. P. Putra · A. Rahmatillah · K. Ain
Biomedical Signals and Systems Research Group, Faculty of Science and Technology, Universitas Airlangga, Surabaya 60115, Indonesia

H. Triwiyanto et al. (eds.), *Proceedings of the 1st International Conference on Electronics, Biomedical Engineering, and Health Informatics*, Lecture Notes in Electrical Engineering 746, https://doi.org/10.1007/978-981-33-6926-9_8

1 Introduction

According to data from the World Health Organization (WHO) in 2016, approximately 800,000 people die every day from suicide [1]. The leading cause of high suicide rates is poorly managed on severe stress. Stress is a psychological response from threats or demands of the task that are felt and marked by certain emotions [2]. It can also trigger mental health disorders, such as depression and anxiety disorders, which can lead to suicide. Not only effect on psychologically, but stress can also interfere with other diseases, such as increases the risk of heart disease and stroke [3].

Given that stress can affect the body's psychology and trigger various diseases, a monitoring system is needed to measure stress level conditions. Stress usually measures by filling out forms, such as the State-Trait Anxiety Inventory Test [4] or interviews with a psychologist. However, this method still requires intervention from humans because not all sufferers consult their condition to the doctor, which leads to inappropriately handled due to the late treatment. This method also takes a long time (up to 10–20 min in filling the form) and requires the professional to identify.

Therefore, it is essential to develop an alternative method for stress measurement, which is non-invasive and could independently be done by the patient. Previously, stress measured by using various physiological signals, namely Electrocardiogram (ECG), Electrodermal Activity (EDA), Electromyogram (EMG), and Reaction Time (RT), which were then classified using Support Vector Machine (SVM) and obtained an accuracy of 88.5% [5]. A review from "*Towards an Automatic Early Stress Recognition System for Office Environments Based on Multimodal Measurements*" concluded that the ECG and EDA are the most accurate physiological signals in detecting stress [6]. EDA is one of the best methods used for real-time measurement and linearly related to arousal, which has been widely used in stress and emotion detection. Besides, EDA can also be used as a direct examination index to find out the effects of stress on bodily functions [7].

EDA measures the conductivity of the skin, which is usually measured in units of micro siemens and changes due to the sweat excretion [8]. However, the results of the measurement signal from EDA in the form of raw data Skin Conductivity (SC) cannot be directly extracted. The SC signal obtained is a combination of two components, tonic and phasic components. The tonic component is known as Skin Conductance Level (SCL), while the phasic component is Skin Conductance Response (SCR). The SCL changes based on many factors, including the focus level, but it will continue to exist even though no stimulus is given. Biologically, SCL arises due to the diffusion of ions from the sweat glands to the outermost epidermis (stratum corneum), although the epidermis prevents ion diffusion from being impermeable to water.

On the other hand, SCR as a phasic component only exists in a certain period because SCR arises when the sympathetic nervous system reacts to certain stimuli [9]. If the original SC signals are not separated, there will be overlapping SCRs, which cause less precise information when feature extracted [10]. Hence, it is essential to separate the SCR and SCL signals by deconvoluting the SC signal [11]. In this study, the deconvolution obtained using the Continuous Deconvolution Analysis (CDA) method. This method was chosen because it is faster and more efficient compared to Discrete Non-Negative Deconvolution Analysis [12]. This deconvolution process aims to obtain a clear SCR with no overlapping and get the zero baseline SCR driver. The clear SCR peaks are essential for identifying the responses related to the stimulus (stressor). In the future, the SCR could be processed further to become a feature for the stress level classification system.

2 Deconvolution of Skin Conductivity

Separation of SC into SCL and SCR was done using the Continuous Deconvolution Analysis (CDA) decomposition technique [12]. This method is based on the pharmacokinetic model of the incidence of sweat glands as the first compartment to sweat into the stratum corneum (which is the second compartment) depicted in Fig. 1. These models show how the concentration of sweat changes due to diffusion, and because the area of the stratum corneum is much larger than the gland, it can be considered as restricted diffusion [13].

The mathematical equation of the relationship of two compartments is a two coupled first-order differential equation that is shown by Eq. 1 for the sweat gland compartment and Eq. 2 for the stratum corneum compartment.

$$\frac{dC_1}{dt} = -\frac{C_1}{\tau_1} \tag{1}$$

$$\frac{dC_2}{dt} = \frac{C_1}{\tau_1} - \frac{C_2}{\tau_2} \tag{2}$$

The solution of these two coupled first-order differential equations is the Impulse Response Function (IRF), which is also known as the Bateman Function, as in Eq. 3, assuming that the concentration of sweat only changes through diffusion.

$$\text{IRF}\,(t) = C.\left(e^{-\frac{t}{\tau 1}} - e^{-\frac{t}{\tau 2}}\right) \tag{3}$$

This Bateman function is known from the form of onset that rises steeply and returns slowly where tau (τ_1 and τ_2) are constants that determine how steep

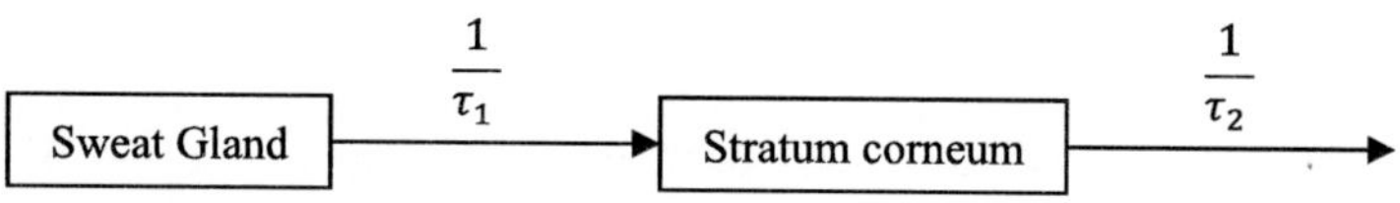

Fig. 1 Pharmacokinetic modeling on sweating process

the function will rise and fall again, and criterion (*C*) is the gain or the Bateman area [14].

Furthermore, the skin conductivity or SC is modeled as a convolution process between SudoMotor Nerve Activity (SMNA), part of the sympathetic nervous system, with IRF shown in Eq. 4.

$$SC = SMNA*IRF \tag{4}$$

SMNA in Eq. 4 is the sum of SCR driver with SCL driver [12]. SC will be deconvolved with IRF to get the SMNA. This SMNA is the key to predict the SCL model and getting the SCR separated. The tau value in IRF will be optimized using criterion (*C*) in Eq. 5 until it approaches zero or reach the minimum value to get a better result. *Indist* in criterion equation is indicators of differentiation between hills formed in the SCR by redefining the threshold for negative values (5% of the SCR peak), this *indist*, also known as discreteness error. Then *neg* is the negative proportion of SCR driver which is shown by Eq. 6 and *alpha* (α) is a constant equal to $6\, s^2/(s\mu S)$. The average is calculated using the gradient descent method to reach the minimum value of criterion.

$$c = indist + neg.\alpha \tag{5}$$

$$ERROR_{neg} = \sqrt{\frac{\sum (DRIVER_{phasic-neg})^2}{n}} \tag{6}$$

The detailed process of this deconvolution will be explained step by step further in the next Sect. 3.2.

3 Experimental Setup

3.1 Data Collection Setup

The subjects in this research are taken from Biomedical Engineering students of Airlangga University, which consisted of eight males and ten females (18–22 years old), each in good health (no mental disorder or depression), enough sleep, not taking drugs and in relax condition before measurement started. We prepare the equipment by connecting the Ag-AgCl electrode to the EDA sensor by BITalino then to the microcontroller connected to the laptop via Bluetooth. The electrodes were placed on the subject's palm to obtain the skin conductivity signal. Before collecting the data, subjects were asked to wash their hands first, then sat comfortably in front of the laptop and wore the provided headphones. The headphones became the source of the audio stimulus, while the laptop became the visual stimulus.

We played 12 min of relaxing songs before the test began to make the subject relaxed. Furthermore, the subjects were asked to answer 100 Stroop tests provided in Bahasa with six color variants: red, blue, green, yellow, purple, and brown. Stroop test is a cognitive test to choose the color according to the font color of the writing, not according to the reading of the writing. Then the subjects were given a variety of stimuli that become stressors in the form of sounds and videos that are frightening and terrifying, like Pocong (Indonesian ghost), hollow hand, and maggot, as shown in Fig. 2. From that figure, the subject was required to choose yellow or "kuning". If the subject chooses the wrong color, there would be a buzzer sound, and a red cross appears. Stimuli that were given here belongs to the emotional stressors. The emotional stressors were chosen because this stress represents human fear and could be measured well by EDA [15].

3.2 Signal Pre-processing and Deconvolution Process

The signal is processed using the continuous deconvolution analysis (CDA) method that is in the Ledapy, one of the python libraries. This method separates the phasic or SCR components from the SC, as raw data obtained from the recording.

At first, the SC was imported into the program. Then we pre-processed the signal by downsampling and smoothing it to eliminate ripples on the signal. After that, IRF or Bateman function according to Eq. 3 was formulated. The IRF is formulated by defining the initialization of τ_1 at 2, τ_2 at 40, and the gain is 1/sampling rate (sr = 100 Hz). The visualization of IRF is shown in Fig. 3. Based on this IRF, we could deconvolute the SC that has been carried out after the pre-processing to get SMNA (SudoMotor Nerve Activity) according to Eq. 4.

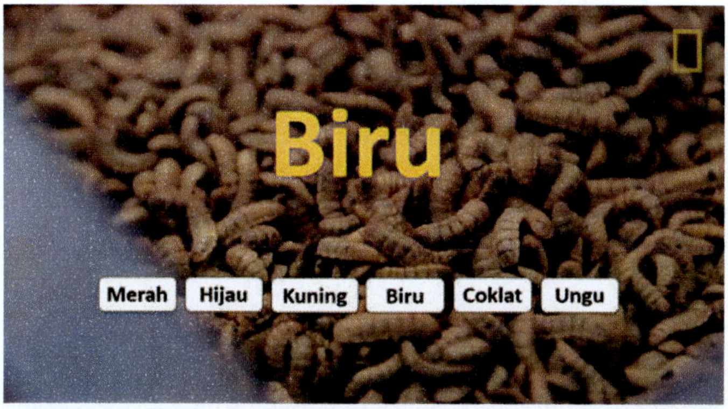

Fig. 2 Stroop test with maggot stimuli as the stressor, the main center text is 'Biru' (en: Blue), three six options are 'Merah' (en: Red), 'Green' (en: Green), 'Kuning' (en: Yellow), 'Coklat' (en: Brown), 'Ungu' (en: Purple)

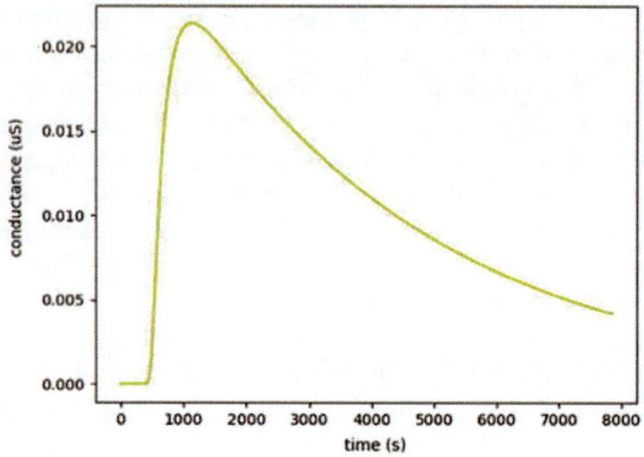

Fig. 3 IRF with $\tau_1 = 2$ and $\tau_2 = 40$

3.3 SCL Estimation

SCL can be observed in the absence of any SCR activity. The SMNA that has been obtained from the previous process is then smoothed with a 200 ms-wide Gauss window. Smoothing is done to eliminate ripples if they arise during the deconvolution process. Then the peak detection is conducted at the 0.2 μS threshold. Peaks that are more than 0.2 μS will be considered as SCR, while other peaks will be flattened into interpolation points to arrange SCL drivers. The SCL driver can then be calculated by interpolating all points below the threshold with the cubic spline fitting method. Results from the interpolating process will be deconvolved with IRF to obtain SCL.

3.4 SCR Estimation

SCR driver can be calculated by subtracting the SMNA with SCL driver. Drivers are then smoothed to get better results. Then, the SCR is obtained by subtracting the raw data SC with the SCL, remember the sum of SCR and SCL will become the original SC. Finally, we compute error *indist* (discreteness) and negativity errors that already described in Sect. 2 with Eqs. 6 to get the value of criterion in Eq. 5.

3.5 Optimization

This optimization stage must be conducted for optimizing the value of tau that will affect the performance of the IRF parameter set. First of all, several sets are prepared for various levels of optimization. After that, optimization is done by calculating criterion (c) according to Eq. 5, which is a function of error *indist* and negativity errors that have been calculated previously. Then the minimum value of criterion was found by calculating the average using the gradient descent method so that the tau with the smallest error is obtained. After the optimization process, the signal is recomposed with new parameters, and better signals will be obtained with zero baseline SCR driver, and two SCR peak, which is overlapping, can be distinguished as two different peaks.

4 Result

EDA raw data recorded from eighteen subjects with details of eight males and ten females in the age range 18–22 years with the criteria mentioned in Sect. 3.1. Data retrieval of the subject was done in a sitting position. Then the EDA sensor placed on the subject's palm is connected to the microcontroller on channel A3. Then, the microcontroller will send data to the laptop via Bluetooth transmission. The hardware installation process from EDA to this laptop is documented in Fig. 4.

Recordings began with listening to relaxation songs for 12 min, and the subject will take the Stroop test with various stimuli, as explained in Sect. 3.1. During the session, the subject will be recorded to see the situation and the real condition of the subjects. The data collection process can be seen in Fig. 5.

The signal (see Fig. 6) was obtained using Open Signals software. This signal shows the combination of tonic and phasic components, which indicated by the fluctuated signal and the peaks that change rapidly over time. The recordings were then stored in an H5 file extension, which then processed further using python.

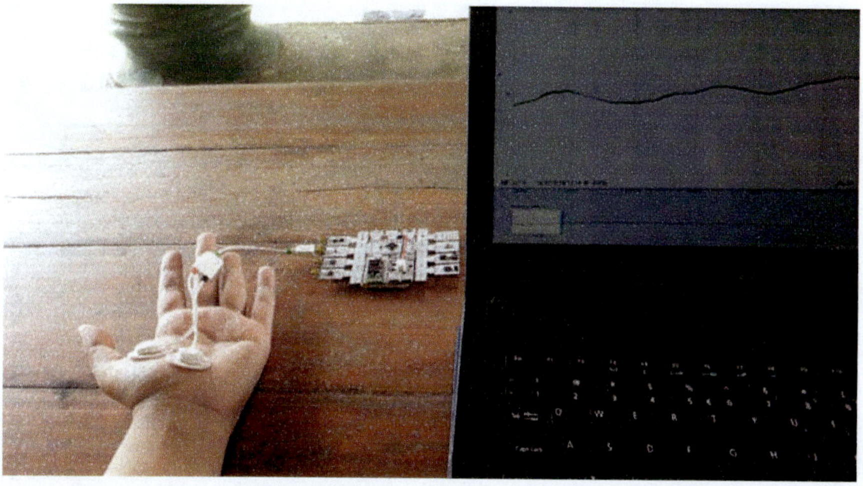

Fig. 4 The hardware installation of EDA Recordings

The recorded signal then deconvoluted using CDA to retrieve the SCR signal. The SCR is representing the subject's stress response to the stressor. In the Ledapy module, a series of processes occurs from pre-processing, followed by deconvolution, estimate the SCL, SCR, and optimization, as explained in Sect. 3. The best results of the SCR are then plotted to see a difference when compared to the original SC. Figure 7 shows the results of a comparison of SC with SCR driver and the SCR itself.

From Fig. 7, we can see that a zero baseline SCR driver is obtained, which is shown by the value of 0 on the Y-axis, and there is no driver with a negative value. Similarly, overlapping SCRs can also be separated, which is proven at around 75–105 s, showing two different SCRs that were not previously seen on the original SC. These two different signals showed that the CDA method was able to separate SCR from original SC raw data accurately.

The SCR obtained was further analyzed to find out whether the SCR were arising due to a given stimulus or not. SCR Analysis from subjects while doing the Stroop test with a variety of emotional stressors is shown in Table 1. Based on Table 1, it can be seen that various kinds of emotional stressors related to the body response (sign by the peak occurred). Some stressors produce significant peaks, while others not. The stimulus that produced small peaks was the horror night atmosphere sound and when the subject answers the Stroop test incorrectly. The small SCR peak occurred because the subject already made a mistake before, or the subject experience the repeating stressor, so the subject was not afraid of the sound anymore. This assumption following the post-experimental questionnaire, which stated so. Hence, stress quickly falls back during the adapted situation. Nevertheless, the stimuli were considered as a stressor by the body. Moreover, for

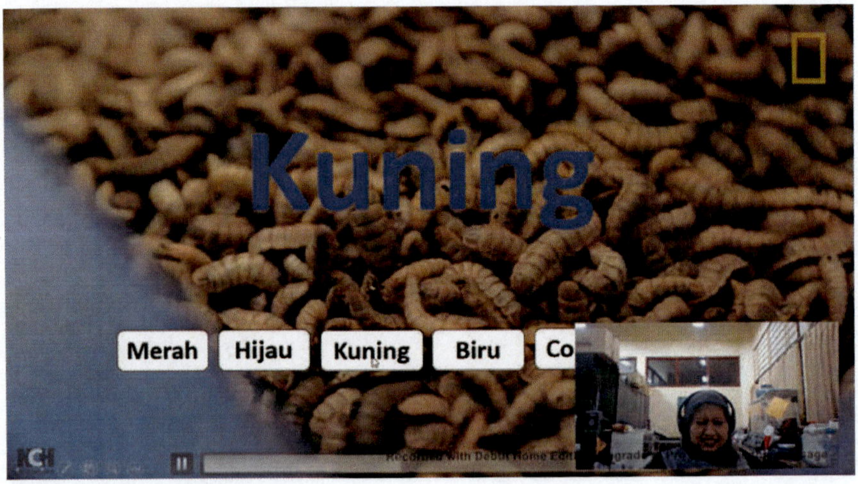

Fig. 5 Stroop test experiments

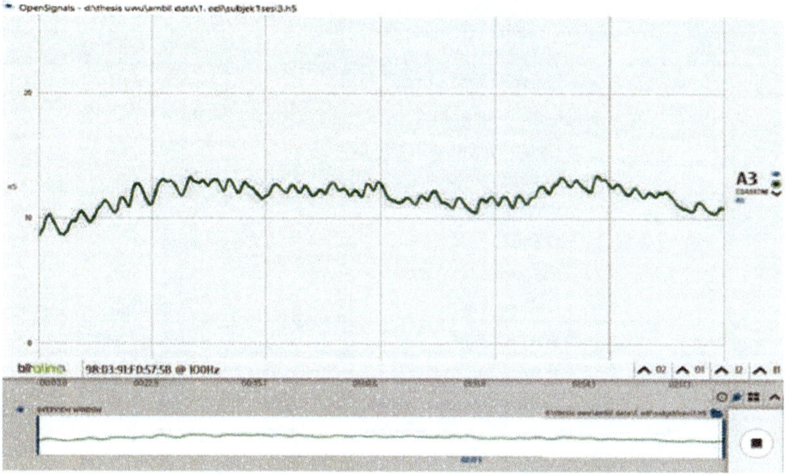

Fig. 6 EDA recordings in open signal interface

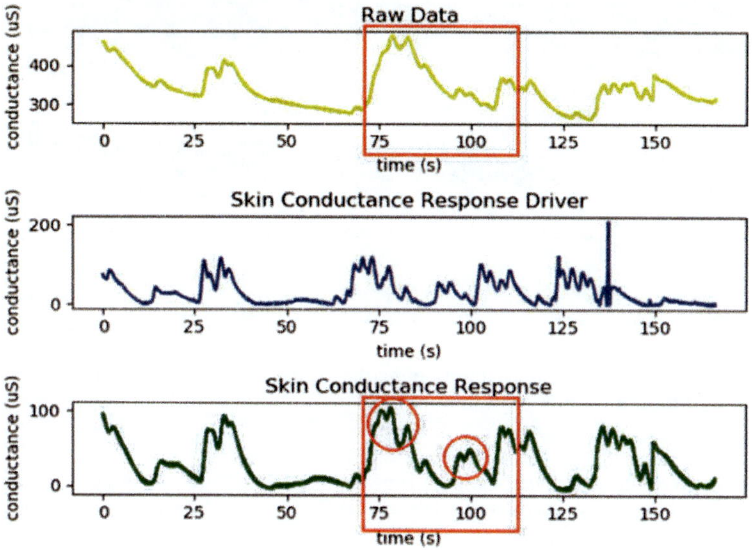

Fig. 7 The comparison between original skin conductivity signal (upper row), with skin conductance response driver (middle row) and estimated skin conductance response (lower row)

stimuli such as Pocong (Indonesian ghost), grinder, maggot, and hollow hands become a stimulus that provides a significant rise. The very high peak occurred because of the stress that made by the fear and surprise feelings at something new that had never been felt before. The subject responds by covered her eyes or looks

Table 1 SCR peak amplitude corresponds to given stressor

Time (seconds)	Given stressor	Peak amplitude
30	Horror night atmosphere	Very high
41	Lightning sound	Low
51	Horror night atmosphere	Very low
75	Pocong (Indonesian ghost)	Very high
87	Wrong answer	Low
98	Grinder	High
111	Maggot	Very high
130	Hollow hand	Very high
135	Wrong answer	Low
145	Wrong answer	Low
155	Hollow hand stopped	High

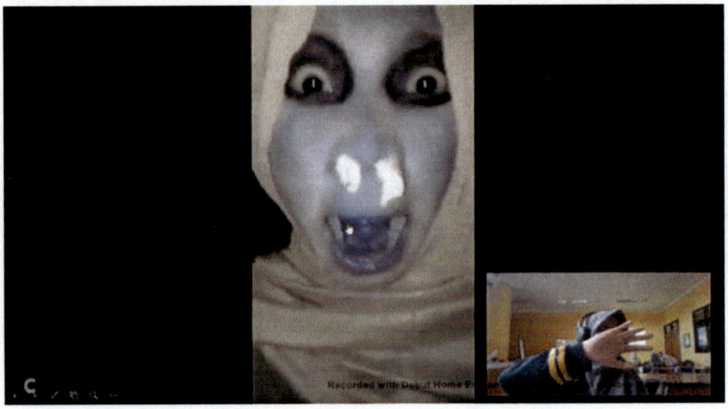

Fig. 8 The fear response from a subject during the Stroop test (she covered her eyes and then looked away from the monitor)

away from the monitors, as seen in Fig. 8. The results of the post-experimental questionnaire also showed that the subject did feel scared when they saw Pocong, maggot, and hollow hands.

5 Conclusion

As a sum up, there are four main stages in the CDA method: pre-processing and deconvoluting SC raw data, tonic estimation (Skin Conductance Level/SCL), phasic estimation (Skin Conductance Response/SCR), and optimizing the value of tau to get the lowest criterion to obtain the best estimation of SCR. Separation of the SCR from the Skin Conductivity data performed using the Continuous Deconvolution Analysis (CDA) method produces a pretty good SCR signal with the characteristics of a zero baseline SCR driver and the overlapping SCR signals that can be distinguished well as two different SCR peaks. Besides, the peaks in SCR are the result of some stimulus that represents the emotional stressors given in this study. This method could be used as the fundamental analysis to find the essential feature for classifying the level of stress.

References

1. World Health Organization. Suicide Data. https://www.who.int/mental_health/prevention/suicide/suicideprevent/en. Last Accessed on 29 June 2020
2. Lumban Gaol NT (2016) Teori stres: Stimulus, Respons, dan Transaksional. Bul Psikol 24(1):1
3. Noerhadi M (2008) Hipertensi dan Pengaruh Terhadap Organ-Organ Tubuh, pp 1–18
4. Beckler K (2010) State-trait anxiety inventory for adults—manual, instrument and scoring guide. Psychol Press Inc Mind Gard Inc 0–78
5. Zhang B (2017) Stress recognition from heterogeneous data. University of Lorraine
6. Alberdi A, Aztiria A, Basarab A (2016) Towards an automatic early stress recognition system for office environments based on multimodal measurements: a review. J Biomed Inform 59:49–75
7. Critchley H, Nagai Y (2013) Electrodermal activity (EDA). In: Gellman MD, dan Turner JR (eds) Encyclopedia of behavioral medicine. Springer New York, NY, pp 666–669
8. Jones R, Rowe M (2013) A guide for analysing electrodermal activity (EDA) and skin conductance responses (SCRs) for psychological experiments. pp 1–42
9. Hernando-Gallego F, Luengo D, Artes-Rodriguez A (2018) Feature extraction of galvanic skin responses by nonnegative sparse deconvolution. IEEE J Biomed Heal Inf 22(5):1385–1394
10. Alexander DM, Trengove C, Johnston P, Cooper T, August JP, Gordon E (2008) Separating individual skin conductance responses in a short interstimulus-interval paradigm. J Neurosci Methods 146(1):116–123
11. Cho D, Ham J, Oh J, Park J, Kim S, Lee NK, Lee B (2017) Detection of stress levels from biosignals measured in virtual reality environments using a kernel-based extreme learning machine. Sensors Switzerland 17:10
12. Benedek M, Kaernbach C (2010) A continuous measure of phasic electrodermal activity. J Neurosci Methods 190(1):80–91
13. Greco A, Valenza G, Scilingo EP (2016) Advances in electrodermal activity processing with applications for mental health
14. Garrett ER (1994) The Bateman function revisited: a critical reevaluation of the quantitative expressions to characterise concentrations in the one compartment body model as a function of time with first-order invasion and first-order elimination. J Pharmacokinet Biopharm 22(2):103–128
15. Birjandtalab J, Cogan D, Pouyan MB, Nourani M (2016) A non-EEG biosignals dataset for assessment and visualization of neurological status. IEEE Int Work Signal Process Syst 110–114

Monitoring Stress Level Through EDA by Using Convex Optimization

Nuzula Dwi Fajriaty, Osmalina Nur Rahma, Yang Sa'ada Kamila Ariyansah Putri, Alfian Pramudita Putra, Akif Rahmatillah, and Khusnul Ain

Abstract This study designed an effective system for monitoring stress levels based on Electrodermal Activity (EDA) sensors by knowing the signal patterns and characteristics using convex optimization decomposition. The EDA sensor considered accurate and sensitive for identifying stress by analyzing the skin conductivity (SC) due to the changes in sympathetic nerve activity. However, the SC signal consists of phasic and tonic components, which needed to decompose to analyze stress levels. The SC signals also followed by the white Gaussian noise, which represents the error value. Hence, deconvolution is a crucial stage for the further process because the quality of the measurement depends on this result. This study aims to deconvolve the SC signal using the convex optimization method (cvxEDA). This model is physiology inspired by EDA based on Bayesian statistics, convex mathematical optimization, and sparsity. This research conducted with 18 subjects through three sessions of measurement. The given stimuli arise in each session to increase the level of stress. The results showed that this method could separate and identify SC. The Phasic component shows an increase in the stimulus of each session, as seen from the number of peaks. In contrast, there were no significant differences in the tonic component. This study shows that the phasic component is closely related to changes in sudomotor nerve activity (SMNA) and response to a stressor, which could be useful to classify stress levels in the future study.

Keywords Convex optimization · EDA · Phasic · SC · SMNA · Stress · Tonic

N. D. Fajriaty · O. N. Rahma · Y. S. K. A. Putri · A. P. Putra · A. Rahmatillah · K. Ain (✉)
Biomedical Engineering Study Program, Department of Physics, Faculty of Science and Technology, Universitas Airlangga, Surabaya 60115, Indonesia
e-mail: k_ain@fst.unair.ac.id

O. N. Rahma · A. P. Putra · A. Rahmatillah · K. Ain
Biomedical Signals and Systems Research Group, Faculty of Science and Technology, Universitas Airlangga, Surabaya 60115, Indonesia

H. Triwiyanto et al. (eds.), *Proceedings of the 1st International Conference on Electronics, Biomedical Engineering, and Health Informatics*, Lecture Notes in Electrical Engineering 746, https://doi.org/10.1007/978-981-33-6926-9_9

1 Introduction

Recently, there are many cases of suicide caused by mental health, such as stress and anxiety. According to the World Health Organization (WHO), human deaths due to suicide almost reach 800,000 people per day. In 2016 the number of suicides at a productive age reached 50,000 people, and it is estimated that by 2020 mental health disorders due to depression will be rampant to the level of HIV/AIDS or heart disease [1].

Generally, stress is measure with filling in forms containing several questions such as those conducted by Cohen et al. in 1983 [2] or by consulting with a psychologist. However, this method is entirely ineffective in preventing suicide due to late treatment. Not all of the stress sufferers are willing to fill in the form or consult their condition. Hence, it is essential to develop an alternative method for stress measurement, which is non-invasive and could independently be done by the patient. So they will know when they need to be threatened before it goes worse. One of the promising methods, which has been widely used in detecting stress and emotion, is EDA. EDA is said to be one of the best methods used for real-time measurement and linearly related to arousal [3].

EDA sensor measures the changes of the skin conductance (SC), which represents the activity of the sudomotor nerves while the sweat gland secretes the sweat [4]. Although sweating is a mechanism of the thermos-regulation, sweat glands located on the surface, such as in the palmar and plantar, are more responsive to psychological stimuli that related to stress. Hence, the EDA sensor for measure the stress condition is usually placed in the palm.

The SC signal consists of tonic and phasic components, which have a different characteristic in time scales and peaks in any given stimuli. The tonic component reflects the baseline of the skin conductance level (SCL) and spontaneous fluctuations (SF), which differ in each people [5]. The phasic component reflects the short-time response to the stimulus, called skin conductance response (SCR). The typical shape of the SCR indicates a rapid rise from the SCL, followed by an asymptotic exponential decay back to the baseline. Hence, the decomposition of the SC into its phasic and tonic components is essential in the EDA measurement for analyzing the stress characteristic. However, the overlapped issue still became a limitation in the decomposition process. The SCRs could be overlapped if the gap between stimuli is shorter than the decay of the previous response. This overlap makes the SCR peaks unclear and lessens the accuracy of identifying the stress through the stressors.

Previous studies have been developed to decompose the phasic signal into individual SCRs associated with each stimulus. Barry et al. [6] subtracted each SCR from an extension of the preceding SCR to correct the baseline using graphical tools, which required visual observation to select the best model. Alexander et al. [7] estimated the sudomotor nerve activity (SMNA) using the Linear time-invariant (LTI) model, where the SC is the result of a convolution between the SMNA, and the skin conductance Impulse Response Function (IRF) assumed a priori and time-invariant.

Benedek and Kaernbach proposed a new LTI model by modified the assumption to calculate the variability in SCR shape. This new model is known as continuous deconvolution analysis (CDA) [8]. The CDA deconvolved the SMNA into two components; one was describing the phasic activity and the other representing EDA variations of different origins by the Bateman function. Although noise was not mathematically calculated in any of these models [7, 8], all three assume its existence.

This study tried to analyze the SCR activity from the EDA related to stress using a convex optimization approach (cvxEDA), called a Convex Optimization Approach to Electrodermal Activity Processing (cvxEDA) by Greco et al. [5]. The cvxEDA also modeled based on the Bateman function, similar to the CDA model, but added three main concepts: maximum a posteriori probability, convex optimization, and sparsity. The cvxEDA modeled the phasic component, as an infinite impulse response (IIR) function utilizing an ARMA model. The phasic component then could be separated from the SC signal and analyzed the pattern through the given stressor for monitoring the stress level. The stress was only limited to the cognitive stress, which is considered as a psychological stress, not neurological stress. The cognitive stress could create nervous or tense for the unpleasant feeling, and alert or excited for the pleasant feeling. We tried to observe the trend on EDA related to different level of stressor given on the subjects.

2 Deconvolution of Skin Conductivity

2.1 Convex Optimization

The deconvolution of SC signals was obtained using the cvxEDA model, proposed by Greco et al. [5], which decomposed the SC signals (y) into phasic (r), tonic (t), and a noise component (∈).

$$y = r + t + \in \tag{1}$$

The single phasic response (r) is modeled using a biexponential impulse response function, called the Bateman function:

$$h(\tau) = \left(e^{-\frac{\tau}{\tau_0}} - e^{-\frac{\tau}{\tau_1}}\right)u(\tau) \tag{2}$$

where τ_0 and τ_1 represent the time constant and $u(\tau)$ is a unit step function. By utilizing ARMA model of Eq. 1 into ARMA cascade,

$$q = A^{-1}p, \quad r = Mq \tag{3}$$

$$r = MA^{-1}p \tag{4}$$

where p represents the SMNA and M and A are tridiagonal matrix. Tonic component (t) is represented as the cubic B-spline basis function

$$t = B\lambda + C \tag{5}$$

where B is a matrix for cubic B-spline basis function, λ is the vector of spline coefficients, C is a N × 2 matrix with $C_{i,1} = 1$ and $C_{i,2} = i/N$, d is a 2 × 1 vector with the offset and slope coefficients for the linear trend.

The observation model could be written by substituting Eqs. (4) and (5) into Eq. (1). The goal is to find the maximum posteriori spike of p and t for measured the EDA signals.

By substituting these terms into

$$P[q, \lambda, d|y] \propto P[y|q, \lambda, d]P[q]P[\lambda]P[d] \tag{6}$$

and taking the algorithm of Eq. (6), the convex optimization that representing cvxEDA is

$$\begin{aligned} &\text{minimize } \tfrac{1}{2} \parallel Mq + B\lambda + Cd - y \parallel_2^2 + \alpha \parallel Aq \parallel_1 + \tfrac{\gamma}{2} \parallel \lambda \parallel_2^2 \\ &\text{Subj. to } Aq(x) \geq 0 \end{aligned} \tag{7}$$

3 Method

3.1 Experimental Setup

In this experiment, 18 healthy subjects (18–22 years old; ten females and eight males) were asked to answer Stroop test in three sessions with assume the level of difficulty increased in each session by the increment of the given stimulus. The stimulus is given from the very beginning of recording, which is started with the Stroop test for about 3 min, then continued with session 2 and session 3 for about 4 min, respectively. In the session 2 and session 3, the subjects were asked to do the Stroop test while interrupted with noisy or scary sound and annoying or terrifying video to add to the difficulty and stress in answering the question. The number of questions in session 2 and 3 also increased, from 75 questions in session 1–100 in session 2 and 3. The time for answering the strop test also shortened and the buzzer would on if the subject wrong in answering the question.

The Stroop test consist of text with color. During the test, subjects were asked to choose the answer according to the font color, not the written text. The first session

Table 1 Audio stimuli given in the session 2

Time (s)	Given stressor	Duration (s)
14	Sound of Cats fight	20
36	Squall (baby's cry)	27
80	Sound of horror night atmosphere	7
100	Lightning sound	22

Table 2 Audio and Visual stimuli given in the session 3

Time (s)	Given stressor	Duration (s)
25	Sound of horror night atmosphere	7
33	Lightning sound	22
52	Sound of horror night atmosphere	7
54	Lightning sound	22
70	Pocong (Indonesian ghost) video	2
80	Sound of the grinder	30
95	Maggot (video)	13
120	Picture of hollow hand	15

had three color variants without any interferences, while in the second session had five color variants interrupted with noisy or shocking sound, as seen in Table 1. The last session had six color variants interrupted with terrifying or shocking sound and videos, as seen in Table 2. The Stimuli in this experiment belong to the cognitive and emotional stressor because it represents human fear which indicates stress [9] and the given stressor also multiplied, assuming session 1 is the lowest level of tress.

Before the test began, we set up the equipment by the electrodes are placed on the subjects' palm, connecting the electrode to the EDA sensor BITalino (fs = 100 Hz) which connected to the microcontroller and laptop via Bluetooth. The subject must wash their hand to prevent the dirt on the palm which could disturb the recording. The subjects also wore the headphone for the audio stimulus, and sit relaxed in front of the laptop.

3.2 EDA Processing

The cvxEDA separated the phasic component from the raw SC signal described in Sect. 2. The fast time constant $\tau 1 = 0.7$ s was used for all subjects, the optimal slow time constant $\tau 0$ was determined on a per-subject basis as the value $\tau 0 \in [2.0, 4.0]$ s that minimized the λ^2—norm of the residual after fitting the cvxEDA model. Fixed values $\alpha = 0.0008$ and $\gamma = 0.01$ were chosen during previous exploratory tests on previous studies and implemented throughout this analysis.

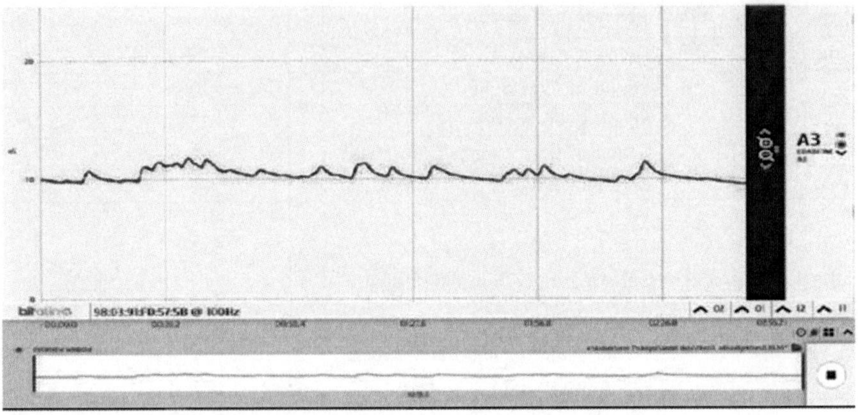

Fig. 1 EDA recordings in Open Signal Interface (the raw SC Signal)

4 Result and Discussion

The recording data process is obtained using Open Signals software, as seen in Fig. 1. The signal shows the combination of tonic and phasic components that indicated with the fluctuated peaks that change at a particular time. The recordings are then stored in an H5 file extension, which will then be input for signal processing using python.

The cvxEDA model produced the expected result (see Figs. 2, 3 and 4): the raw SC data, z-score normalized was decomposed into two signals, tonic component (*t*), parametrized by a cubic B-spline and phasic component (*r*) that is the convolution of the sudomotor nerve activity with a Bateman IRF.

We deconvolved the raw signal or the Skin Conductance (SC) to observe the SCR or the phasic component, which will change when the stressors are given to the subjects, while the tonic will relatively unchanged or changes slowly. Before the deconvolution process, we could not see the peak obviously, especially when the time for the consecutive stimulus are short. Therefore, we need to deconvolve the signal to see the real phasic driver that related to the stimulus. After the SC signal deconvolved, the overlapped peak could be calculated separately in the phasic driver figures, as seen in the box located in Figs. 2c, 3c, and 4c.

From Figs. 2, 3 and 4, we can also see whether stress level was increasing in each session or not from the number of peaks. Besides, we can see phasic component were arising by peak amplitude corresponds to a given stimulus when doing the Stroop test. In Table 3, It can be seen that phasic component in first session produced 9 peaks with peak amplitude 1 very high, 0 high, 4 low dan 4 very low. The second session produced 16 peaks with peak amplitude 2 very high, 7 high, 3 low, 4 very low, and in the last session produced 23 peaks with peak amplitude 3 very high, 8 high, 12 low and 0 very low. Some stressors produced significant

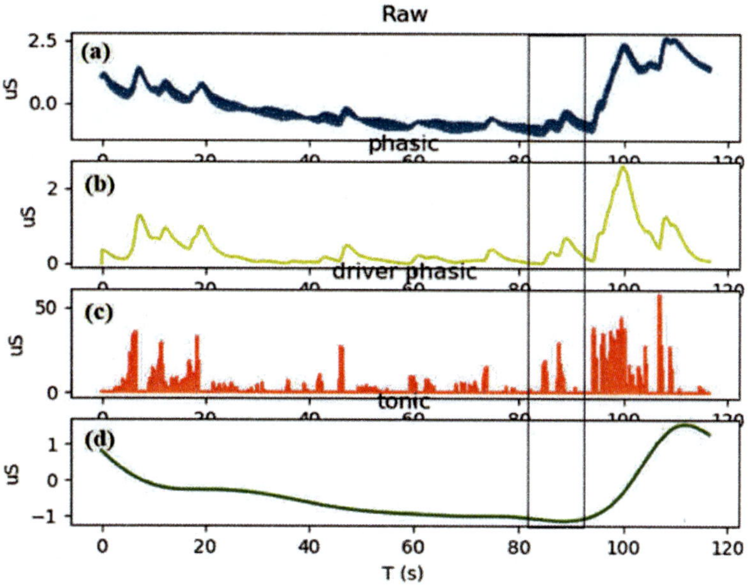

Fig. 2 Example of application of the cvxEDA decomposition SC signal in first session: **a** raw SC signal, z-score normalized, **b** phasic component r, **c** driver phasic component p, **d** tonic component t

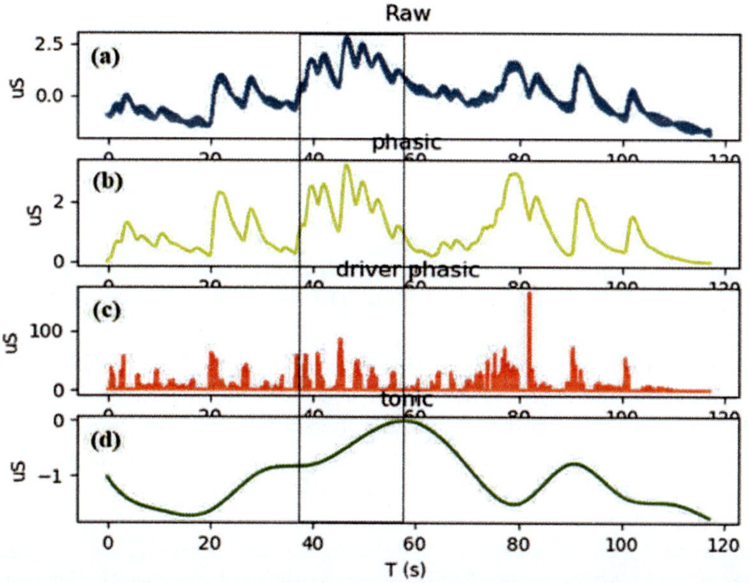

Fig. 3 Example of application of the cvxEDA decomposition SC signal in second session: **a** raw SC signal, z-score normalized, **b** phasic component r, **c** driver phasic component p, **d** tonic component t

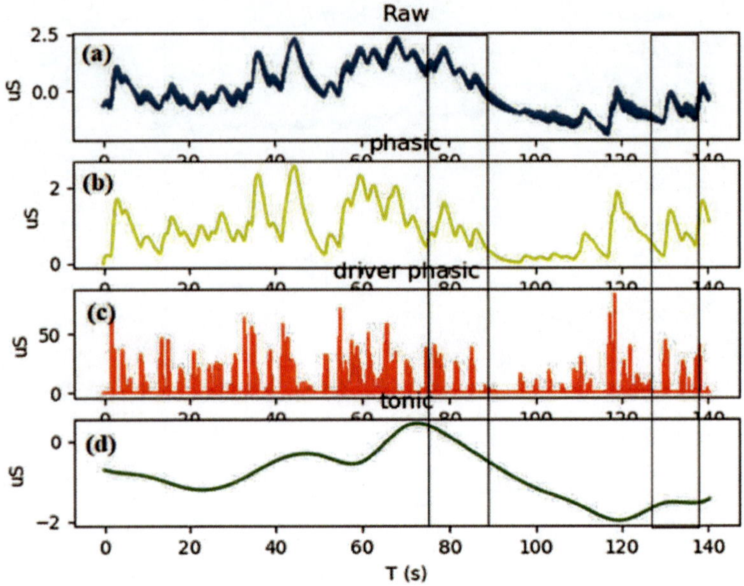

Fig. 4 Example of application of the cvxEDA decomposition SC signal in third session: **a** raw SC signal, z-score normalized, **b** phasic component r, **c** driver phasic component p, **d** tonic component t

Table 3 Phasic number of peak and peak amplitude in each session

Session	Number of Peak	Peak Amplitude
1	9 Peaks	1 Very high; 0 High; 4 Low; 4 Very low
2	16 Peaks	2 Very high; 7 High; 3 Low; 4 Very low
3	23 Peaks	3 Very high; 8 High; 12 Low; 0 Very low

peaks, and some did not. The stressor which is not giving the significant peaks could be caused by the subject's reactions. The amplitude of this peak depends on how the subject responds to a variety of the stimulus, whilst repeated stimuli resulted smaller reaction that leads to lower amplitudes. This phenomenon called habituation [10]. This phenomenon explained the reduced peak or the decreased amplitude in the phasic component while the repeated stressor given, such as in session 3 at the seconds 25 and 52 when the sound of horror night atmosphere and the lighting sound repeated in seconds 33 and 54.

There is no standard unit for stress level, usually only based on scoring on the questioners that leads to the mild, moderate and severe stress. However, based on the previous studies there is correlation between EDA and stress level and the standard unit for EDA signal is micro Siemens (μS). The peaks show the changes of the phasic component while receiving the stimuli. Even though each subject has different values of amplitudes and peaks, but all of them giving the similar trend which shows the more frequent of the stimulus given, the higher SCR (phasic component) produced. The increased number of peaks in the phasic component also showed that the level of stress increases in each session. The results showed that increasing from the given stimuli in each session, related with increase the level of stress.

5 Conclusions

This paper confirms that the cvxEDA model based on convex optimization could produce decomposition of the EDA. Even though each subject has different values of amplitudes and peaks, but all of them giving the similar trend which shows the more frequent of the stimulus given, the higher SCR (phasic component) produced. The Phasic component was able to show an increase in the stimulus of each session, as seen from the number of peaks that represent the cognitive and emotional stressor given in this study.

References

1. World Health Organization. Suicide Data, https://www.who.int/mental_health/preven-tion/suicide/suicideprevent/en. Accessed 2020/06/29
2. Cohen S, Kamarck T, Mermelstein R (1983) A global measure of perceived stress. J Health Soc Behav, 385–396
3. Alberdi A, Aztiria A, Basarab A (2016) Towards an automatic early stress recognition system for office environments based on multimodal measurements: a review. J Biomed Inf 59:49–75
4. Fowles D et al (1981) Publication recommendations for electrodermal measurements. Psychophysiology 18(3):232–239
5. Greco A, Valenza G, dan Scilingo EP (2016) Advances in Electrodermal Activity Processing with Applications for Mental Health
6. Barry RJ et al (1993) Elicitation and habituation of the electrodermal orienting response in a short interstimulus interval paradigm. Int J Psychophysiol 15(3):247–253
7. Alexander DM, Trengove C, Johnston P, Cooper T, August JP, dan Gordon E (2005) Separating individual skin conductance responses in a short interstimulus-interval paradigm. J Neurosci Methods 146(1):116–123
8. Benedek M, dan Kaernbach C (2010) A continuous measure of phasic electrodermal activity. J Neurosci Methods 190(1):80–91
9. Birjandtalab J, Cogan D, Pouyan MB, dan Nourani M (2016) A non-EEG biosignals dataset for assessment and visualization of neurological status. IEEE Int Work Signal Process Syst, 110–114
10. Sarchiapone M et al (2018) The association between electrodermal activity (EDA), depression and suicidal behaviour: a systematic review and narrative synthesis. BMC Psychiatry 18(1):1–27

Design of Banana Ripeness Classification Device Based on Alcohol Level and Color Using a Hybrid Adaptive Neuro-Fuzzy Inference System Method

M. R. E. Ariono, F. Budiman, and D. K. Silalahi

Abstract The ripeness classification device of banana-based on Internet of Things (IoT) was designed utilizing the Adaptive Neural Fuzzy Inference (ANFIS) method is presented. The ripeness of banana was identified from its color and alcohol level, utilizing MQ-3 gas sensor and TCS34725 color sensor. The built device has consisted of Arduino Mega, ANFIS for classification tool, and NodeMCU as the IoT Gateway. Google Firebase was used as an IoT platform and a database for the classification result. The inputs for the classification process were obtained from the alcohol level and RGB values from the sensors. The results showed that the device was successfully classified the ripeness level with an accuracy of 99.07%, that categorized into unripe, ripe, or rotten conditions. The final tuning of ANFIS classifier was using: 960 datasets and divided into 864 training data and 96 test data, Pi-shaped MF as input MF type, Linear MF as output MF type, (3-2-2-2) structure as the structure of MFs and Hybrid Algorithm as the optimizer. The average required time for predicting the ripeness level was 3.57 s. It is expected this device could be implemented for advanced applications such to classify other types of fruits and/or vegetables.

Keywords Adaptive Neuro-Fuzzy inference system · Banana ripeness classification · Internet of things

M. R. E. Ariono · F. Budiman (✉) · D. K. Silalahi
School of Electrical Engineering, Telkom University, Jl. Telekomunikasi no. 1, Bandung 40257, West Java, Indonesia
e-mail: faisalbudiman@telkomuniversity.ac.id

M. R. E. Ariono
e-mail: esarizki5@gmail.com

D. K. Silalahi
e-mail: desrikristina@telkomuniversity.ac.id

H. Triwiyanto et al. (eds.), *Proceedings of the 1st International Conference on Electronics, Biomedical Engineering, and Health Informatics*, Lecture Notes in Electrical Engineering 746, https://doi.org/10.1007/978-981-33-6926-9_10

1 Introduction

1.1 Background

Banana is one of the most popular fruits consumed by people due to its nutritions and contains carbohydrates. A ripe banana has quite high calories [1], therefore, often consumed by people before/after exercising. Banana is also often processed into various kinds of products, for example in the form of smoothies, fruit salad, and banana chips. For merchants and industries who use of banana as raw materials, the quality (i.e. ripeness) of the banana determines the sales potential level.

Generally, the quality of the banana could be determined through its ripeness level, particularly through its mass, color, fragrance, and texture [2]. Ethylene substance is mostly found in climacteric fruits, such as in banana fruit [3]. The ethylene substance indicates the acceleration of respiration pace, chlorophyll degradation, and essence starch conversion into glucose processes [4]. This means that the ripeness of climacteric fruits can easily be detected by the alcohol level. Moreover, the fruit color is also changed when ripening, due to the effect of chlorophyll degradation: the green color of the fruits will be fading [4]. Presently, the ripeness level of fruits mostly is detected manually by human senses [5]. Therefore, the obtained accuracy will be diversed and may decrease the banana-based product sales. To overcome such issues, requires a device that able to collect the banana ripeness data accurately and automatically classifying the ripeness condition. One solution, the device requires to be trained by using an Artificial Intelligence (AI) method.

Some researchers have been worked on different fruit ripeness classification devices. Ajizi et al. reported a banana ripeness classification device based on its mass and color, utilizing Naïve Bayes as a classifier method, and the obtained accuracy of classification was up to 90% [6]. Simamora et al. worked on durian ripeness classification devices based on alcohol level using the Naïve Bayes method and reported 100% accuracy of prediction [7], but using the Naïve Bayes method its conditional probability is non-zero otherwise, it will not classify the subject [8]. Tomato ripeness classification device was also investigated by Villasenor-Aguilar et al. through computer vision utilizing the Fuzzy Inference System (FIS) and reported 99.9% accuracy [9], but, FIS method is difficult to be implemented when the dataset is too large and cannot be trained automatically [10]. In terms of banana case, Ariono et al. designed a device to detect the ripeness of banana-based on color and alcohol level utilizing the Artificial Neural Network (ANN) method with the classification accuracy up to 93.3% [11], but, if the measurements were done under noise conditions from the outside, the output will not predict as the expectation [12]. Therefore, a method that could adapt to the problem is required. Here, a combination of the fuzzy method and ANN was selected for classifications since it is more noise resistant and provides a wider range of input [13–15]. It is expected to combine ANN with a fuzzy method while using a database to store the collected dataset and retrained the classification method could make the system to classify more accurately [16].

In this present work, a banana ripeness classification device based on the Internet of Things (IoT) was designed utilizing the Adaptive Neuro-Fuzzy Inference System (ANFIS) method. The ripeness of banana was identified from its color and alcohol level, utilizing MQ-3 gas sensor and TCS34725 color sensor. The built device consisted of Arduino Mega, ANFIS method was used for classification tool, and NodeMCU as the IoT Gateway. Google Firebase was used as an IoT platform and a database for the classification result. The classification was done utilizing a combination of ANN and FIS method. Having this device will help the users to predict the ripeness of the banana, or even the remains day before it turns to rot and in other words, it could classify the quality of the banana. It is also expected this device could be implemented for advanced applications such to classify other types of fruits and/or vegetables.

2 Materials and Methods

2.1 System Design

The banana object that studied here was "*Musa Acuminata*" species [17]. The ripeness level was investigated utilizing MQ-3 alcohol sensor and TCS34725 color sensor, that connected to Arduino Mega as the main controller. The ANFIS classifier was employed as a feature for classification processes. The classification results were displayed on an LCD (16 × 2). Here, NodeMCU was used as IoT Gateway and sent the given results to Google Firebase as IoT platform and database, with domain in https://banana-3c9e5.firebaseio.com/. This ANFIS classification device is consisted of 2 box: sensor box (a.k.a. box for acquiring data) and controller box (a.k.a box for configuring the device), as shown in Fig. 1a. In this classification method the sensors box attached to a conveyor to automatically classify the ripeness of each banana that enters from the right side through to the left side of the conveyor as shown in Fig. 1b. The diagram block in this research is shown in Fig. 2.

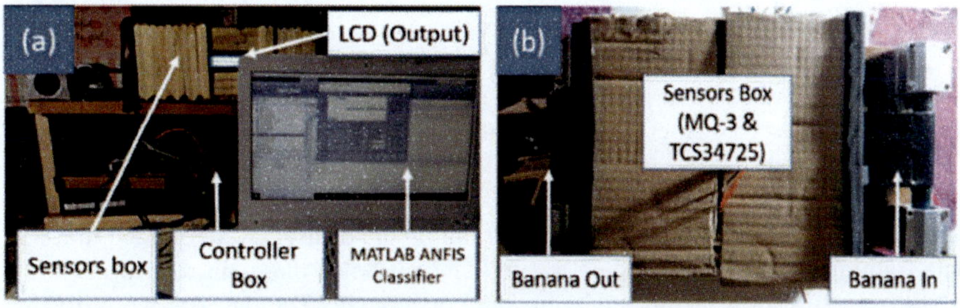

Fig. 1 **a** Front shoot of the built device. **b** Above shoot of the built device

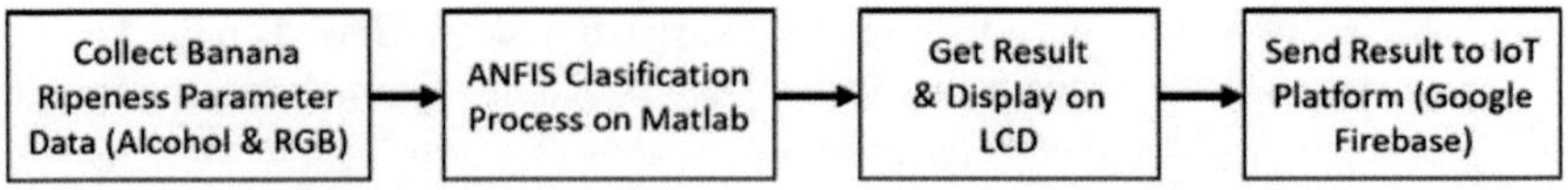

Fig. 2 Block diagram of the system

2.2 Sensor Calibration

The MQ-3 sensor and TCS34725 sensor were calibrated before used. For MQ-3 sensor, the calibration was performed by heating the sensor for 2 days, based on the datasheet instruction. Conversion of analog data into mg/L unit for the alcohol level followed the predefined equation from the datasheet (Eq. 1). The alcohol sensor values were compared by the detected mg/L from an alcohol sensor model "Breathanalyzer AT6000", while the RGB values from TCS34725 were compared by RGB output from mobile apps "RGB color detector version 1.1.4". The ripeness experiments were performed by recording the alcohol level and color of the banana as well, for 3 min, for each sensor, for six days. The above experiments purposes to monitor the characteristic of banana ripeness from unripe to rot condition.

$$Alcohol(\mathrm{mg/L}) = 0.39(Analog\,Input/2275\,\mathrm{K})^{-1{,}49} \tag{1}$$

2.3 Sensor Calibration

ANFIS is one of the AI Hybrid methods that consists of the combination of ANN and Sugeno's FIS method [13, 14]. The topology consists of 5 layers: the input layer, fuzzification layer, rule layer, defuzzification layer, and output layer. Similar to neural network characteristics, the ANFIS classification method requires an optimization process, to attain high accuracy prediction level.

Tuning Parameters and Training process of ANFIS Classification Method. When designing an ANFIS classifier system, several parameters are necessary to be tuned: type of input membership function (MF), type of output MF, the structure of input MF and optimizer [18]. Tuning process is required, since it will shows the optimum condition for faster classification, with more accurate results. A smaller value of testing error will give a better parameter for classification. The average testing error was calculated using Root-Mean-Square-Error, as shown in (Eq. 2) The target for the ripeness condition was set to 0.25, 0,50 and 0,75 for unripe, ripe and rotten respectively as the ANFIS output [15]. Here, the list of the parameters tuned is summarized in Table 1. During training, the datasets were divided first into data training and the rest for data testing, since it holds the main role to make the ANFIS classification method to train more accurately. The datasets were divided using a scenario of X:Y ratio, with X is for training, while Y is for testing the

Table 1 List of parameters in ANFIS classification tuning process

Tuning	Parameter studied
Input Type MF	Triangular; Generalized bell-shaped; Gaussian combination; Gaussian; Trapezoidal; Sigmoidal
Structure of Input MF	**3 MF** for each/some features of inputs; **2 MF** for each/some features of inputs; **More than 3 MF** for each/some features of inputs
Output Type MF	Linear; constant
Optimizer	**Backpropagation** (BP); **Hybrid** (BP + Least Squares Estimation (LSE)

trained classification method [18]. The most popular dividing dataset scenario is the 90:10 ratio [18].

$$RMSE = \left(\frac{\sum \text{Target}_i - ANFISOutput_i}{n} \right)^{0.5} \tag{2}$$

3 Result and Discussion

3.1 Banana Ripeness Profile

The banana ripeness profile was obtained by recording the alcohol level (Fig. 3a) and RGB values (Fig. 3b) of a banana for 6 days, from unripe condition to rot condition. It can be seen that the alcohol level gradually increases every day during the ripening process, especially from unripe to ripe conditions. The alcohol level rises very sharply when the banana entered the rot condition. The alcohol level for unripe, ripe, and rotten banana was recorded at 0.30, 0.99, and 2.01 mg/L, respectively, after 3 min of recording for each experiment. Moreover, the tendency

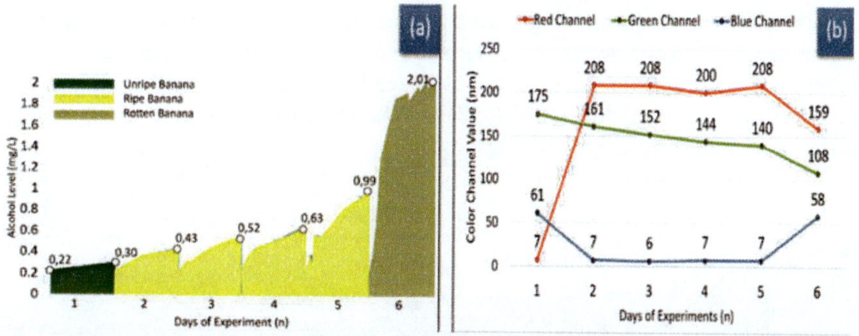

Fig. 3 **a** Banana ripeness profile based on alcohol gas level. **b** Banana ripeness profile based on RGB color changes

of each color channel during ripeness banana was different. The red channel value from unripe condition (1st day) to ripe condition (2nd day) increased from 7 to 208 nm, then almost constant at 200 nm from the 2nd day to 5th day. When entering the rot condition (6th day), the value decreased from 208 to 159 nm. In the case of the green channel, the value decreases gradually on each day started from 175, 160–140, and 108 nm for unripe, ripe, and rotten conditions, respectively. Moreover, the blue channel has a reverse tendency compared with the red channel. From the unripe (1st day) to ripe condition (2nd day), the value decreased from 61 to 7 nm and has a constant value at below 10 nm from 2nd to 5th day. From ripe (5th day) to rot condition (6th day), the value rises again to 51 nm. Based on the results, the region of RGB value on each ripeness can be divided into 2 regions: above the average value or below the average value. The average value here represents as the average of the collected data on each color channels measurements result. The total collected ripeness dataset of this banana was 960 data, with (162, 636, 162) as data of unripe, ripe and rot banana, respectively.

3.2 *Tuning Process of ANFIS Classification Method*

The tuning process of the ANFIS classification method purposes on optimizing the accuracy level as well as the time for classification. The tested parameters were: (1) types of input MF with (Trapezoidal, Gaussian, Pi Shaped), (2) types of output MF with (Constant, Linear), (3) structure of input MFs (3-3-3-3, 3-2-2-2, 3-4-4-4) and (4) optimizer that compared (BP, Hybrid). After testing and comparing all parameters, the selected criteria from each parameter were used for the final process, based on the lowest value of average testing error. The collected data from the banana ripeness profile was divided to 90:10 ratio, which means that 864 data as to train the ANFIS classification method and 94 data for testing the performance of the ANFIS classification method, after trained. The number of dataset training was 147, 571, and 146 data for unripe, ripe, and rot banana, respectively, while the data testing is the remains data, as seen in Table 2.

Table 3 shows the comparison of average errors on the ANFIS classification tuning process using Trapezoidal, Gaussian, and Pi-shaped as the selected type of input MF. According to the results, Pi- Shaped input MF has the lowest average error testing value, which is 0.05786. Therefore, the Pi-Shaped input MF was used as the next parameter for the tuning process.

Table 2 Divided datasets with 90:10 ratio

Condition	No. of Training Dataset	No. of Testing Dataset
Unripe	147	15
Ripe	571	65
Rot	146	16

Table 3 Comparison of each selected types of Input MF

Types of Input MF	Average Training Error	Average Testing Error
Trapezoidal MF	0.026081	0.05809
Gaussian MF	0.040031	0.10593
Pi-shaped MF	0.024372	**0.05786**

Table 4 Comparison of each selected type of output MF

Output MF Type	Input MF Type	Average Training Error	Average Testing Error
Constant	Pi-shaped MF	0.026491	0.06246
Linear	Pi-shaped MF	0.024372	**0.05786**

Table 5 Comparison of each structure combination of inputs MF

Structure of inputs MF	Number of Nodes	Number of Fuzzy Rules	Number of Linear Parameters	Number of Non-Linear Parameters	Average Training Error	Average Testing Error
3-3-3-3	193	81	405	48	0.0243	0.057
3-2-2-2	73	24	120	36	0.0386	**0.044**
3-4-4-4	421	192	960	60	0.0253	0.062

The comparison of an average error on the ANFIS classification tuning process utilizing constant and linear as selected output MF with selected input MF from earlier tuning process is shown in Table 4. Based on the tuning results, the lowest average testing was had by Linear MF at 0.05786. Hence, the linear output MF was used for the next parameter of the tuning process.

Table 5 shows the comparison of average errors of ANFIS classification tuning process using 3 values of MFs referring as fuzzified input on each alcohol level and RGB inputs or called as (3-3-3-3) input MF structure; 3 total values on alcohol MFs and 2 total values on each RGB MFs a referred as (3-2-2-2) input MF structure; and (3-4-4-4) input MF structure as for 3 total values on alcohol MF and 4 total values on each RGB MFs. The total nodes, fuzzy rules, linear parameters, and non-linear parameters of ANFIS topology were generated accordingly to the inputs MF structure. The number of nodes generated was proportional to the required time for training or testing the ANFIS classification method. The (3-2-2-2) input MF structure was considered as the optimum selection for this device, since the total values of alcohol input MFs was 3 values and that referring to the 3-banana ripeness condition (unripe, ripe and rot). Meanwhile, the total values on each RGB MF were 2, according to the divided region of RGB values on banana ripeness that as explained in Sect. 3.1 in Chap. 3.

Table 6 presents the comparison of average errors on the ANFIS classification tuning process using BP and Hybrid optimizer, with selected input-output MF type and (3-2-2-2) input MF structure from the previous tuning process. Usage of hybrid

Table 6 Comparison of each selected optimizer

Structure of inputs MF	Optimizer	Classifying Duration (sec)	Average Training Error	Average Testing Error
3-2-2-2	BP	0.55	0.0386	0.044
	Hybrid	**1.23**	6.53e-06	**0.0093**

algorithm gave the lowest average testing error, which was 0.0093 and 1.23 s of classification time, while BP algorithm had the shortest time of classification which is 0.55 s but has a larger average error, 0.044. Since the main purpose of this device was mostly required an accurate classifier system and despite the classification time, as long as it still under 5 s. Therefore, the Hybrid algorithm was used as the optimizer.

The optimum parameters for classification were summarized in Table 7. The topology of ANFIS generated based on the tuning has (73, 24, 120, 36) of nodes, fuzzy rules, linear and non-linear parameters, respectively. The accuracy of this device utilizing ANFIS as a classifier using 10% of the dataset (96 data) as the tested data up to 99.07% using (Eq. 3). In our previous work, research on banana ripeness using ANN method based on alcohol and color as parameters has only 93.3% accuracy [11], while the ANFIS method's accuracy up to 99.07%. Moreover, the required time for the classification process using this device was also conducted by using a digital stopwatch and the timespan from Arduino IDEs serial monitor for 15 times of experiments (exclude from the tested dataset), and the results are shown in Table 8. It was obtained that the average duration of the prediction process of this device was 3.57 s.

Table 7 Final tuning of the ANFIS classification method

Tuning		Result on Tested Data			Result of Trained Data	
		Average Testing Error	Prediction Time	Testing Accuracy (%)	Average Training Error	Training Accuracy (%)
Data used for training	864	**0.0093**	**1.23**	**99.07**	**6.53e-06**	**100**
Data used for testing	96					
Inputs MF Structure	(3-2-2-2)					
MF Input Type	Pi-shaped					
MF Output Type	Linear					
Optimizer	Hybrid					

Table 8 Duration of the device classification process

Average Duration (s)					
Transfer data Arduino to PC	ANFIS Classification Method Process	Transfer data PC to Arduino	Transfer data Arduino to NodeMCU	Upload Data to Firebase	Total
0.5	1.23	0.65	0.5	0.69	3.57

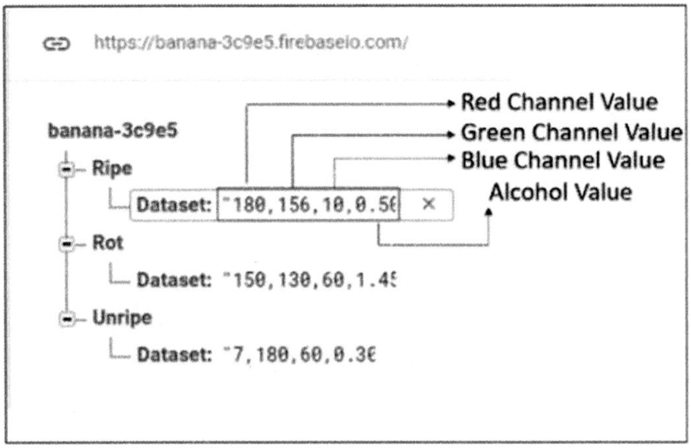

Fig. 4 Display of Firebase Realtime Database

$$Accuracy = (1 - AverageTestingErrors) * 100\% \tag{3}$$

3.3 *Display of Firebase Realtime Database*

The display of Firebase real-time database platform is shown in Fig. 4. There are 3 data existed on the database, which are: "unripe", "ripe", and "rot" for each ripeness dataset list of each classified banana. The dataset itself consists of 4 features which are R, G, B value, and alcohol level, respectively, and was delimited by commas.

4 Conclusion

We have shown how to design the banana ripeness classification device based on alcohol level and color using ANFIS as a classifier system. The inputs for the classification process were obtained from the alcohol level and RGB values from

MQ-3 alcohol sensor and TCS34725 color sensor. The output targets of the ANFIS classifier were set to 0.25, 0.5, and 0.75 for unripe, ripe, and rotten conditions, respectively. ANFIS classifier has several parameters that need tuning processes such as: selecting Input-Output MF type, the structure of input MF, and its optimizer. The final tuning of the ANFIS classifier was using: 864 training data and 96 test data, Pi-shaped MF as input MF type, Linear MF as output MF type, (3-2-2-2) structure as the structure of MFs and Hybrid algorithm as the optimizer. The accuracy of this device after the tuning process was 99.07%. The average required time for classification was 1.23 s. This device could be developed further to increase the accuracy by using the collected dataset on Google Firebase and also possible to classify other fruits as long the type of fruits is climacteric and the parameters are the same.

References

1. Hapsari L, Lestari DA (2016) Fruit characteristic and nutrient values of four Indonesian banana cultivars (Musa.spp) at different genomic groups. AGRIVITA J Agric Sci, 303–311. Author F, Author S. Title of a proceedings paper. In: Editor F, Editor S (eds.) Conference 2016, vol 9999. LNCS. Springer, Heidelberg, pp 1–13
2. Prayogi S, Fitmawati, Sofiyanti N (2016) Karakteristik Morfologi dan Uji Kandungan Nutrisi Pisang Batu (Musa Balbisiana Colla) di Kabupaten Kuantan Singingi. Biologi Papua. 8 (2):97–110. Author F. Contribution title. In: 9th international proceedings on proceedings, pp 1–2 (2010)
3. Tripathi K (2016) Fruit ripening of climacteric and non-climacteric fruit. J Environ Appl Biores
4. Winarno FG (1997) Kimia Pangan dan Gizi. Gramedia Pustaka Utama, Jakarta
5. Hameed K, Chai D, Rassau A (2018) A comprehensive review of fruit and vegetable classification techniques. Image Vis Comput 80. https://doi.org/10.1016/j.imavis.2018.09.016
6. Ajizi MF, Syauqy D, Ichsan MH (2019) Klasifikasi Kematangan Buah Pisang Berbasis Sensor Warna dan Sensor Load Cell Menggunakan Metode Naive Bayes. Pengembangan Teknologi Informasi dan Ilmu Komputer, pp 2472–2479
7. Simamora J (2019) Rancang Bangun Alat Pendeteksi Tingkat Kematangan Buah Durian dengan M etode Naïve Bayes. (Malang). Artikel ilmiah Teknik Elektro. 01(2):87–95
8. Kaviani P, Dhotre S (2017) Short survey on Naive Bayes algorithm. Int J Adv Res Comput Sci Manage 04
9. Villasenor-Aguilar MJ et al (2019) Fuzzy classification of the maturity of the tomato using a vision system. J Sens 2019:12. Article ID 3175848
10. Guth MAS (1989) Some uses and limitations of fuzzy logic in artificial intelligence reasoning for reactor control. Nucl Eng Des 113(1):99–109
11. Ariono MRE, Lestari I, Silalahi KD, Budiman F (2020) Proceeding FisTEK 2020. Perkumpulan Robot Edukasi Indonesia (PREI), pp 29–35
12. Ennet CM, Frizet M (1998) Investigation into the strength and limitations of artificial neural network: an application to an adult ICU patient database. University of Ottawa, S.I.T.E., 161 Lous Pasteur, Ottawa
13. Afroozeh M, Sohrabi MR, Davallo M, Mimezami SY, Motlee F, Khosravi M (2018) Application of artificial neural network, fuzzy inference system and adaptive neuro-fuzzy inference system to predict the removal of Pb(II) ions from aqueous solution by using magnetic graphene/nylon 6. Chem Sci J 9(2):1–7

14. Dewi VC, Amrizal V, Agustin FEM (2015) Penggunaan Metode ANFIS (Adaptive neuro fuzzy inference system) Pada Aplikasi Prediksi Usia Kertas. Jurnal Teknik Informatika 8(2)
15. Naik S, Patel B (2017) Machine vision based fruit classification and grading—a review. Int J Comput Appl (0975–8887) 170(9):22–34
16. Khedkar S, Thube S (2017) Real time databases for applications. Int Res J Eng Technol (IRJET) 4:20178–2082
17. D'Hont A, Denoeud F, Aury J et al (2012) The banana (Musa acuminata) genome and the evolution of monocotyledonous plants. Nature 488:213–217
18. Elif Ü, Ahmet K (2019) Design and simulation of ANFIS controller for increasing the accuracy of leaf spring test bench. Procedia Comput Sci 158:169–176

Design of Electrical Energy Storage System Produced by Thermoelectric Generator

Rizky Septiawan, Mohamad Ramdhani, and Wahmisari Priharti

Abstract Many home appliances can generate waste heat that are released to the surrounding. This waste heat can be utilized by converting it directly into electrical energy using a Thermoelectric Generator (TEG). However, the electrical energy produced by TEG from waste heat is quite low, hence a proper energy storage is essential to enable its use. This study aims to design an electrical energy storage system for TEG and assess its performance and capabilities. Six TEG module TEC1-12706 connected in series were utilized to harness the waste heat energy. A refrigerator compressor was used as the waste heat producer and a 3.7 V 400 mAh Li-Po battery was used as the electrical energy storage. A boost converter CE8301 was utilized to increase and stabilize the output voltage to extend the battery life. The storage system proposed in this study was successfully increased 27,3% of the battery capacity during 120 min of charging.

Keywords Boost converter · Li-Po battery · Thermoelectric generator

1 Introduction

Please Electrical energy is a source of energy that is most needed for humans today. The high demand for electricity triggers the development of alternative energy in various sectors. According to the data from the Ministry of Energy and Mineral

R. Septiawan (✉) · M. Ramdhani · W. Priharti
Teknik Elektro, Fakultas Teknik Elektro, Telkom University, Jl. Telekomunikasi no. 01, Bandung, Indonesia 40257
e-mail: rseptiawan19@gmail.com

M. Ramdhani
e-mail: mohamadramdhani@telkomuniversity.ac.id

W. Priharti
e-mail: wpriharti@telkomuniversity.ac.id

H. Triwiyanto et al. (eds.), *Proceedings of the 1st International Conference on Electronics, Biomedical Engineering, and Health Informatics*, Lecture Notes in Electrical Engineering 746, https://doi.org/10.1007/978-981-33-6926-9_11

Resources (ESDM), Indonesia's electricity consumption in 2018 reached 1064 kWh per capita [1]. It is estimated that electricity consumption will increase for the next few years.

Many renewable energy sources such as solar, wind or hydro energy has been widely explored as an alternative electricity generator. However, there is an important energy source that is often overlooked such as heat or thermal energy. Apart from the sun, heat energy can also be generated as the waste or byproduct of industrial processes, machines, electrical and domestic appliances [2].

According to Bertoldi et al. [3], in the European Union (EU-27), the number of domestic appliances such as heating systems/electric boilers, refrigerator, oven, washing machine, dishwasher and many others is continuously growing and the same tendency may also be observed for their frequency of use and the duration of their duty cycles. Heating systems/electric boilers contribute to 19.1%, of the residential electricity consumption at European level. Refrigerators and freezers give the second most relevant contribution for almost 14.5%. While, electric ovens, washing machines/dryers and dishwashers contribute on electricity consumption for 6.6%, 7.2% and 3% respectively [3]. Therefore, the possibility of recovering and reusing their waste heat, is becoming more relevant.

According to Bansal et al., the potential energy savings from waste heat recovery can be up to 25% [4]. Especially for refrigerator that are used continuously (up to 24 h a day), the wasted energy reaches 2000Wh/24 h with a constant temperature of 50–70 °C at the condenser [2]. The recovery of waste heat can generate a used heat by using an adsorption refrigerator with a combined mass and heat recovery system as proposed by Lu and Bansal et al. [5, 6]. The recovery of waste heat can also generate an electrical energy by using a device that can directly convert heat into electrical energy called Thermoelectric Generator (TEG).

TEG is a device that consists of an array of p and n semiconductors, connected electrically in series and thermally in parallel as shown in Fig. 1. These conductors are connected electrically in series to increase the operating voltage and connected thermally in parallel to increase the thermal conductivity [7].

TEG working principle are based on an effect called the Seebeck effect, which was first discovered in 1821 by Thomas Johann Seebeck. The Seebeck effect occurs when the two conductors with different temperatures connected at its end, creating a flow of electric current and a potential difference. The difference in potential or voltage produced is proportional to the temperature difference between two

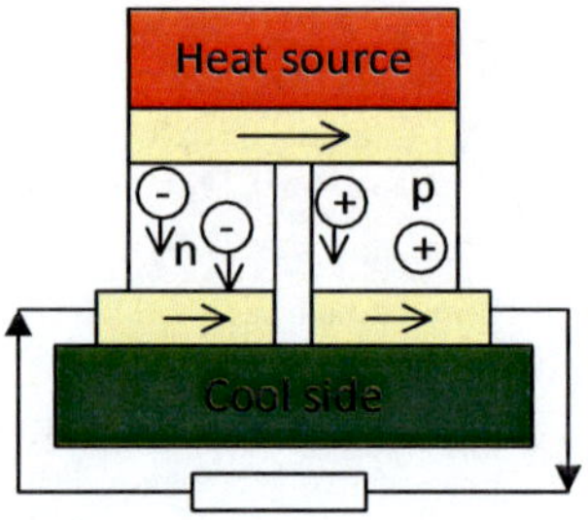

Fig. 1 Semiconductor arrangement on TEG

intersections between the two conductors. This potential difference does not depend on the temperature distribution along the conductors. This effect is the basis of thermocouples, which are often used for temperature measurements [8].

Seebeck coefficient equation can be described as follows [9].

$$\alpha = (V_h - V_c)/(T_h - T_c) = \Delta V/\Delta T \quad (1)$$

where:
α = Seebeck coefficient
V_h = voltage of hot junction (V)
V_c = voltage of cold junction (V)
T_h = temperature of hot junction (°C)
T_c = temperature of cold junction (°C)
ΔV = Voltage difference
ΔT = Temperature difference

In addition, the voltage acquired from the Seebeck effect can be written as follows.

$$E = \alpha(T_h - T_c) \quad (2)$$

where:
E = electromotive force (V)
α = Seebeck coefficient (V/°C)
T_h = temperature of hot junction (°C)
T_c = temperature of cold junction (°C)

There are three parameters that must be considered in using the TEG, namely Q is the heat load to be transferred (Watt), T_h is the hot side temperature of the TEG (°C), T_c is the cold side temperature of the TEG (°C). Heat load is the total amount of heat that must be transferred by the TEG from the object or to be cooled/taken heat into the environment [10].

The electrical energy produced by TEG from waste heat is quite low, hence a proper energy storage is essential to enable its use [4]. An electrical energy storage device such as battery can be used, however, due to the unstable output of the voltage produced by TEG, a current or voltage stabilizer and a boost converter are needed in order to stabilize the current or voltage and increase the voltage value that will be stored in the storage device. The voltage stabilizer is also intended to extend the life of the electrical energy storage device.

The purpose of this research is to design a storage of electrical energy converted from heat by a TEG. A 3.7 V400 mAh Li-Po battery was utilized as the energy storage device. A boost converter was also design to boost the output voltage in order to match the operating voltage of the battery. An assessment was conducted to measure the capability of Li-Po battery to stored electrical energy produced by TEG.

2 Methodology

2.1 Selection of Materials

Thermoelectric generator. In this study, six TEG module TEC1-12706 connected in series were utilized to harness the waste heat energy and convert it into the electrical energy. The specification of the TEC1-12706 are as follows: T_h 27 °C (at dry air condition), ΔT_{max} 70 °C, V_{max} 16.0 V and I_{max} 6.1 A. The dimension of TEG is $40 \times 40 \times 3.8$ mm^3 with 10% tolerance for thermal and electricity parameters.

Battery. The battery is a device that can store electrical energy by converting chemical energy into electricity. The ability of the battery is called an electrochemical reaction. The battery itself is divided into 2 types, primary batteries and secondary batteries. The primary batteries can only be used once since the chemical reaction cycle in the primary battery is unidirectional. While secondary batteries are rechargeable batteries that can be used more than once [11].

In order to charge a battery, voltage and current are required. Voltage is the potential difference between two points (nodes) in an electrical circuit. The electric voltage value can be read due to the current flowing in a closed circuit and a certain load like a resistor. Therefore, the value of the voltage that occurs is the amount of current flowing multiplied by the amount of resistance it passes. Here is the general equation for potential difference [11].

$$V = I \cdot R \tag{3}$$

where:
V = Potential Difference (Volt)
I = Electric Current (Ampere)
R = Resistance (Ohm/Ω)

This system uses a Li-Po 3.7 V 400 mAh battery as storage to store the electrical energy produced by TEG. The battery has 4.1 V over charging and 3.0 V over discharging, so it can be stated that the capacity of the battery is 0% at 3.0 V and 100% or full charge at 4.1 V.

Boost Converter. Boost Converter or Step-up Converter is able to increase the voltage using a switch. Boost Converter consists of several components, namely the inductor (L), diodes (D), resistor (R), capacitor (C), and a switch (S). Switch or Switching can be a thyristor, MOSFET, IGBT, and others [12]. The diagram of the boost converter is shown in Fig. 2.

The Boost Converter works in two states, namely when the switch opens (Fig. 3a) and when the switch closes (Fig. 3b). To find out when the MOSFET should open and when to close the current flow, a control circuit is needed. When the MOSFET closes (ON) at t = 0, the current in the inductor increases and flows through the MOSFET (switch). So that the energy that was stored in the inductor will increase. When the MOSFET is open (OFF) at t = t1, the current in the inductor will flow through the capacitor, diode, and load [12].

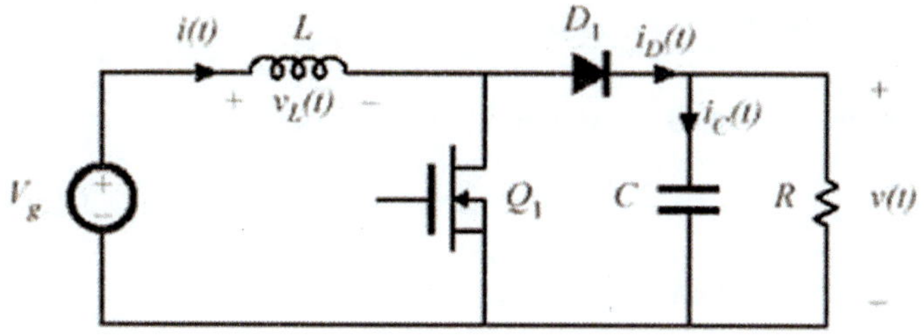

Fig. 2 Boost converter circuit

Fig. 3 Boost converter in: (**a**) open state (**b**) closed state

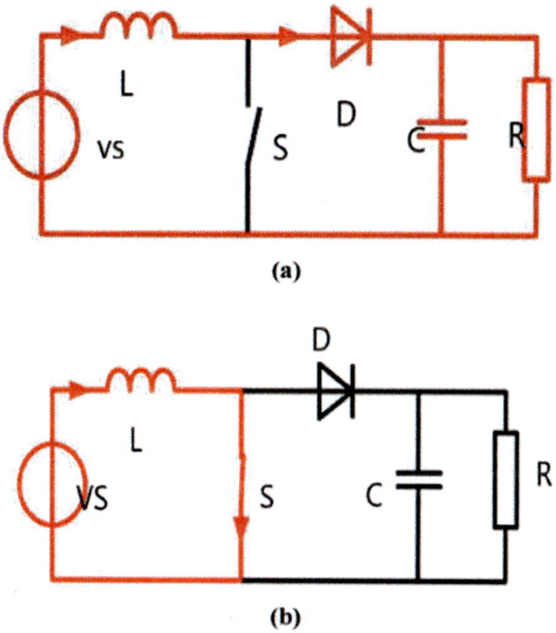

IC CE8301 was chosen as the boost converter since this IC has a PFM feature that can control the duty ratio automatically, so it has a small ripple and a stable output voltage. There is an LED as an indicator when the circuit works at a voltage of 0.9–5 V. the Boost Module above has the following features:

- Input DC voltage 0.9–5 V.
- Output booster using the USB Port feature.
- Has an indicator light as a warning that the booster is on or not.
- Maximum transfer efficiency of 85%.
- Portable and stable booster performance.

2.2 System Design

This research was intended to design a storage system for electrical energy converted from waste heat by a TEG. The waste heat was obtained from the refrigerator compressor whereas the Li-Po 3.7 V 400 mAh battery was utilized as the energy storage. The system also consists of boost converter to increase the output voltage, microcontroller Arduino Uno to control the converter and LCD and LED as battery capacity display and indicator. The block diagram and flow chart that shown the connection of all apparatus and processes are shown in Figs. 4 and 5 respectively.

The details of the design of storage system are as follows:

1. Electrical energy was generated from the conversion of heat energy into electrical energy by the Thermoelectric Generator. In this process, the hot side of TEG was attached to a refrigerator compressor while the cold side of TEG was attached to a heat sink and aluminum water block to reduce excess heat. The setup of the apparatus is shown in Fig. 5.
2. The produced voltage was increased and stabilized using a boost converter type CE8301 0.9–5 V in order to match the operating voltage of the Li-Po battery.
3. The stabilized voltage and current flows into the Li-Po 3.7 V 400mAh battery.
4. The capacity of the battery was monitored from the flow of current in the battery obtained by current sensor INA219.

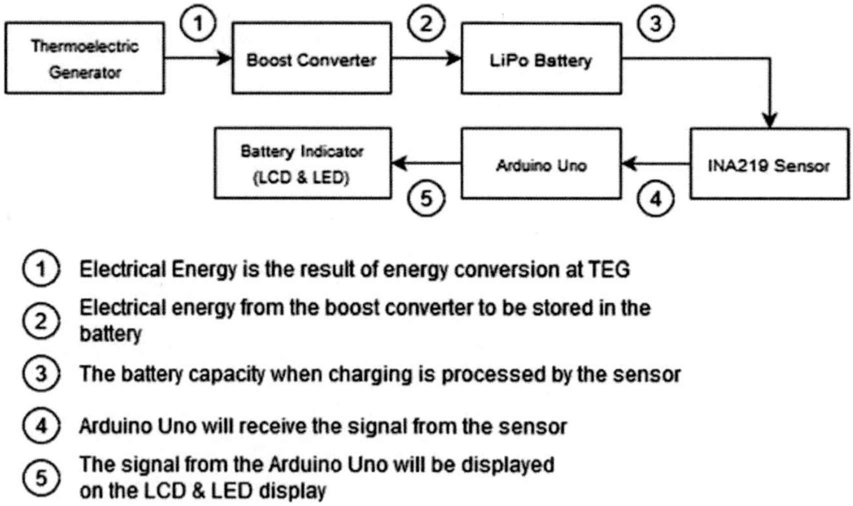

Fig. 4 Block diagram system

Fig. 5 Flowchart diagram

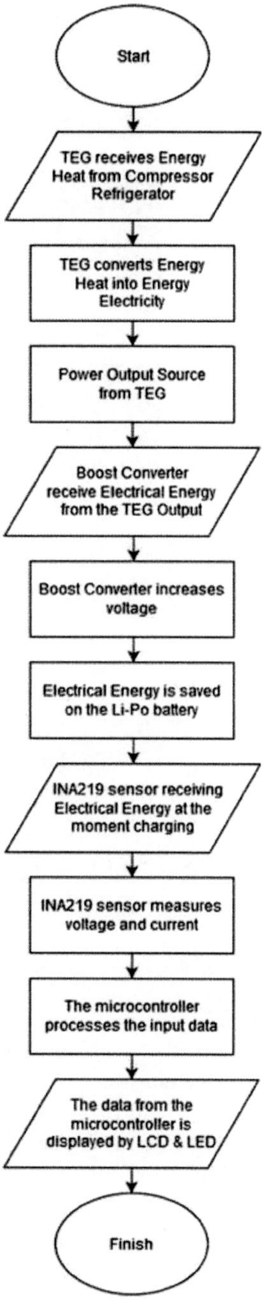

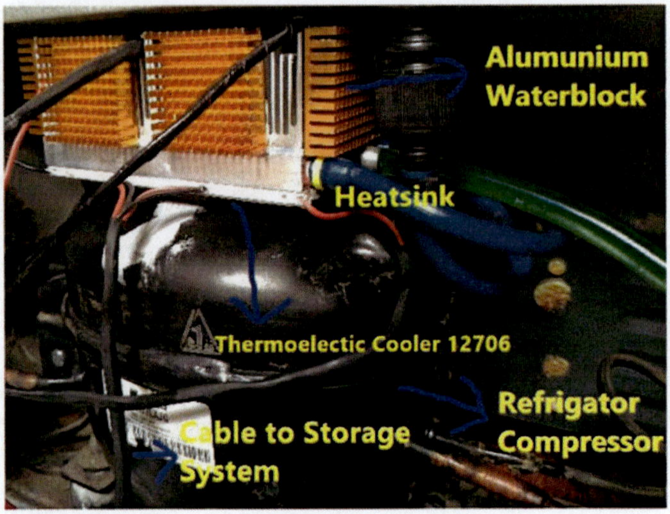

Fig. 6 Heat to electrical energy conversion system by TEC-12706

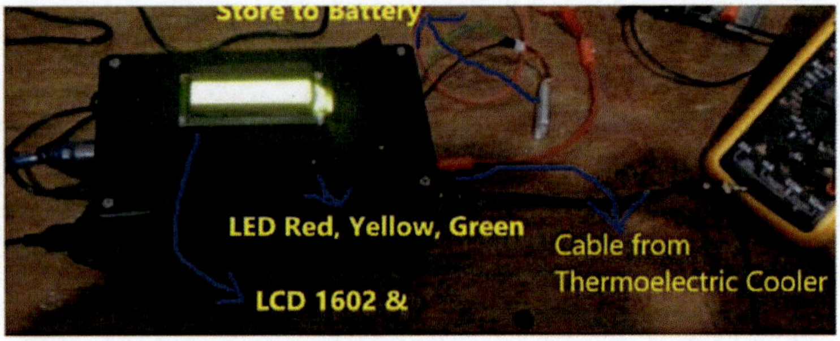

Fig. 7 Storage system with LED indicator and LCD display

5. The data was sent to the Arduino Uno microcontroller to activate the auto cut-off mechanism.
6. LCD and LED are used to display the capacity of the Li-Po battery as shown in Figs. 6 and 7. Red, yellow and green LED indicated the condition of 0%, 50% and 100% of the battery capacity.

2.3 System Assessment

Several assessments were carried out in order to measure the performance and capability of the storage system. The first assessment was to check the capability of the boost converter in increasing and stabilizing the output voltage of TEG. The purpose of this assessment is to ensure that the boost converter can increase the output voltage of the TEG to 5 V to ensure the output stability. The assessment was carried out by attaching the hot side of TEG to the refrigerator compressor while the cold side of the TEG was attached to a heatsink and aluminum water block to reduce excess heat. The TEG was connected to the boost converter. The boost converter was connected to current sensor INA219 that was also connected to the Arduino Uno board. The voltage and current flows through the boost converter was observed using the Arduino IDE serial monitor.

The second assessment was to ensure the capability of the system to charge or store electrical energy in the battery. The purpose of this assessment was to measure the duration needed to charge 3.7 V Li-Po battery using the energy produced by thermoelectric generator. The measurement was carried out by connecting the TEG to a boost converter and a Li-Po battery. The voltage sensor which has been connected to the Arduino Uno board was connected to the battery to observe the battery capacity. The measurement was only carried out for 120 min and can be done longer if possible.

3 Result and Discussion

3.1 Boost Converter Performance

Figure 8 shown the performance of boost converter in increasing and stabilizing the output voltage of TEG. During 60 min of measurement, it was found that the boost converter can immediately increased the output voltage to 4.84 V and was stable from the 1st to the 60th minute. The minimum output voltage produced by TEG was 1.45 V and the maximum voltage was 2.72 V. The average output voltage was 1.5 V. This result indicated that the boost converter was able to operate properly even though the output of the TEG conversion was unstable. The boost converter was fully activated and able to increased and stabilized the voltage throughout the measurement provided that the output voltage was not less than 0.3 V.

3.2 Battery Charging Performance

The battery charging performance was measured for 120 min and the stored voltage was recorded as shown in Fig. 9. In the measurement, the initial voltage was 3.6 V

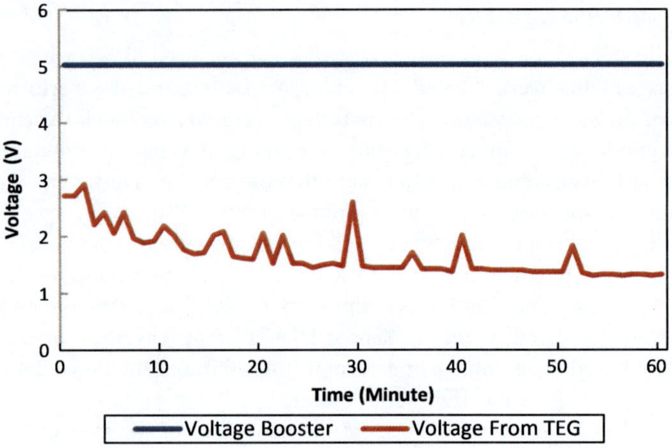

Fig. 8 Boost converter performance

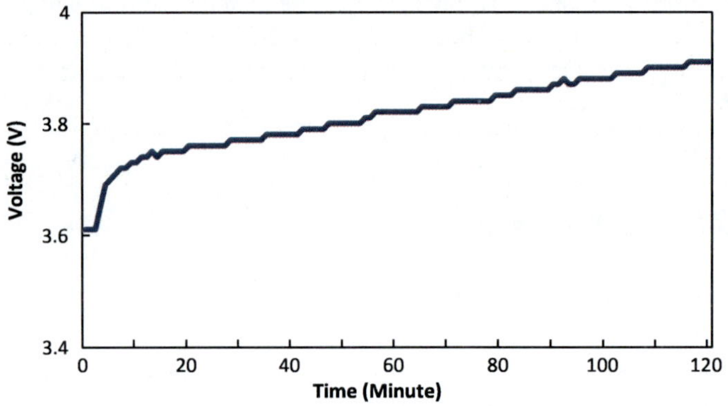

Fig. 9 Battery charging performance

and continued to increase to 3.9 V after 120 min. It is indicated that the Li-Po battery can store 0.30 V during 120 min of charging.

The battery capacity percentage was calculated using the equation below:

$$\frac{Measurable\ Voltage - Min\ Voltage}{Max\ Voltage - Min\ Voltage} \times 100\% \qquad (4)$$

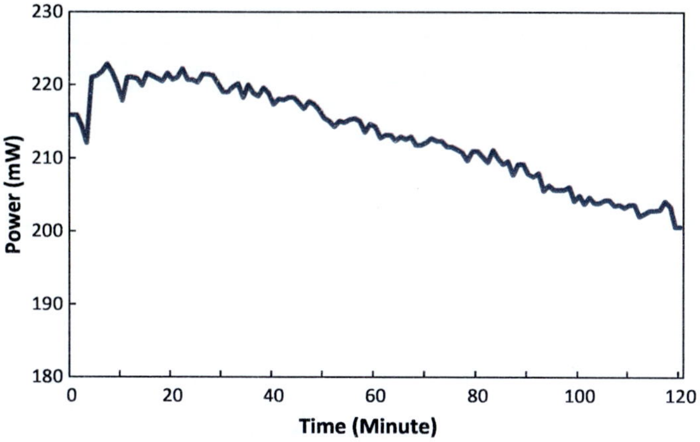

Fig. 10 The power stored during battery charging

If the initial voltage on the battery:

$$\frac{3.61 - 3.0}{4.1 - 3.0} \times 100\% = 55,4\% \quad (5)$$

and the voltage after 120 min of charging:

$$\frac{3.91 - 3.0}{4.1 - 3.0} \times 100\% = 82,7\% \quad (6)$$

Therefore, the increase in battery capacity,

$$\Delta\% = 82.7\% - 55.4\% = 27.3\% \quad (7)$$

The flow of current into the battery decreased over time during the charging process. From the measurement, it was recorded that the maximum current during charging is at 60 mA and ends at 51 mA. During 120 min of charging, the average flow of current was 0.056 A or 56 mA. The decreased flow of current resulted in the decreased amount of power stored in the battery as shown in Fig. 10. The maximum power was recorded at 20th minute (220.71 mW) and the minimum power at the end of the charging process at 120th minute (200.58 mW).

4 Conclusion

This study proposed a design of electrical energy storage system produced by thermoelectric generator. Li-Po 3.7 V 400 mAh battery equipped with boost converter CE8301 0.9–5 V was utilized as the storage. The boost converter was able to maintain a stable output TEG voltage at 5 V in order to be stored in the battery. Using this converter, the battery capacity was successfully increased 27.3% during 120 min of charging. Therefore, it can be concluded that the storage system proposed in this study has a good performance and can be used to store electrical energy produced by TEG.

References

1. Liputan6.com. https://www.liputan6.com/bisnis/read/3863789/konsumsi-listrik-terus-meningkat-ri-menuju-negara-maju. Last accessed on 20 January 2020
2. Simone AZ, Garcia-Polanco N, Capablo J, Doyle JP, Barbato MC (2014) Household appliances wasted heat storage by means of a Packed bed TES with Encapsulated PCM. In: 13th International Conference on Sustainable Energy tech
3. Bertoldi P, Hirl B, Labanca N (2012) Energy efficiency Status Report 2012. JRC—Joint Research Centre, s.l.
4. Bansal P, Vineyard E, Abdelaziz O (2011) Advances in household appliances—A review. Appl Therm Eng 31:3748–3760
5. Lu Z, Wang L, Wang, R (2011) Experimental analysis of an adsorption refrigerator with mass and heat-pipe and heat recovery process. Energy Convers Manag 53:291–297
6. Bansal Azzouz K, Leducq D, Gobin D (2009) Enhancing the performance of household refrigerators with latent heat storage: An experimental investigation. Int J Refrig 32:1634–1644
7. Priharti W, Ramdhani M, Putra FRJ, Khansalya A (2020) Feasibility Study of Thermoelectric Generator Configuration in Electricity Generation. In: Proceedings of the 2nd Faculty of Industrial Technology International Congress
8. Alfiyyah K (2019) Konversi Energi Panas Menjadi Energi Listrik Menggunakan Termoelektrik Generator. Skripsi. Teknik Elektro. FTE-Universitas Telkom, Bandung
9. Anwar S, Sari SP (2013) Generator Mini dengan Prinsip Termoelektrik dari Uap Panas Kondensor pada Sistem Pendingin. Universitas Gunadarma, Jakarta
10. Hidayat A, Putra P (2006) Pengembangan Alat Uji Kualitas dan Karakteristik Elemen Peltier, Seminar Nasional Tahunan Teknik Mesin V. Rizki, Amelia Septiani. (2018). Perancangan Sistem Kendali Untuk Kestabilan Pendulum Terbalik Menggunakan Metode Logika *Fuzzy*. Bandung. pp 9–12
11. Firmanda R (2019) Penyimpanan Energi Listrik Dari Konversi Energi Panas Menjadi Energi Listrik Menggunakan Thermoelectric Generator. Skripsi. Teknik Elektro. FTE-Universitas Telkom, Bandung
12. Subramani S, Babu NR (2017) A modified high step-up non-isolated DC-DC converter for PV application. Proc J Appl Res Technol 15(3):242–249

Performance Comparison of Three Thermoelectric Generator Types for Waste Heat Recovery

Adhitia Rachman, Wahmisari Priharti, and Mohamad Ramdhani

Abstract Waste heat recovery using thermoelectric generator (TEG) is believed to be promising solution to the needs of the community's electrical energy sources. TEG can produce electrical energy when there is a temperature difference between two different semi-conductor materials hence creating a voltage difference and a current flow. There are several types of TEG commercially available at the market with different specification and capabilities. This research was conducted to compare the power generation capability (Watt/m^2) and the power production cost (Rp/Watt) of three TEG module i.e. TEC1-12706, TEC1-12710 and TEC1-12715. The test was conducted with and without the cooling system for the TEG module. The results showed that TEC1-12706 provide the best performance with 3800 W/m^2 and 12 $/Watt with heatsink and 475 W/m^2 and 97 $/Watt without heatsink.

Keywords Thermoelectric generator · Seebeck effect · Waste heat

1 Introduction

The need of electricity consumption has been gradually increased in in the last few years. In order to meet that need, several sources of renewable energy such as solar, wind, biomass or hydro energy has been widely explored to generate electricity in a large scale. Moreover, lower level electricity generation using different physics phenomenon has also been studied such as using pressure [1], vibration [2], radio frequency (RF) [3] and thermal energy [4].

A. Rachman (✉) · W. Priharti · M. Ramdhani
Telkom University, Jl. Telekomunikasi no. 01, Bandung, Indonesia 40257
e-mail: adhitiarachman.student@telkomuniversity.ac.id

W. Priharti
e-mail: wpriharti@telkomuniversity.ac.id

M. Ramdhani
e-mail: mohamadramdhani@telkomuniversity.ac.id

H. Triwiyanto et al. (eds.), *Proceedings of the 1st International Conference on Electronics, Biomedical Engineering, and Health Informatics*, Lecture Notes in Electrical Engineering 746, https://doi.org/10.1007/978-981-33-6926-9_12

Thermal energy is an abundant source of energy that are also easy to obtain from the environment. Moreover, thermal energy can also be generated as the byproduct of industrial processes, machines, electrical and domestic appliances in the form of waste heat [5]. There many types of domestic appliances that can provide a low temperature waste heat such as refrigerator, water heater/boiler, dishwasher and many others. Therefore, the possibility of recovering their waste heat is becoming more relevant.

The low temperature waste heat recovery can be carried out using a thermoelectric generator (TEG). TEG is a device that capable of directly converts heat energy into electrical energy and vice versa using a principle known as the Seebeck effect [6]. This effect occurs when there are two different materials connected in a closed circuit and the two connections are maintained at different temperatures, hence creating a flow of electric current in the circuit. When one of the wires is disconnected and then connected with a galvanometer, the difference in voltage will be obtained from the two the tip [7].

TEG consists of p-type and n-type semiconductors that are connected in series as shown in Fig. 1. When heat is applied to a TEG surface, electrons in the n-type semiconductor and holes in the p-type semiconductor will move away from the heat source. This movement of electrons and holes creates an electric current, the direction of the current is opposite to the movement of electrons, and in the direction of the movement of holes. By creating an appropriate electricity connection, the thermoelectric generator current flows in a closed loop through p-type and n-type semiconductors and external loads. A pair of n-type and p-type semiconductors form a thermocouple. Thermoelectric generators can consist of several thermocouples connected in series, which increase the output voltage, and parallel by increasing the output current [8].

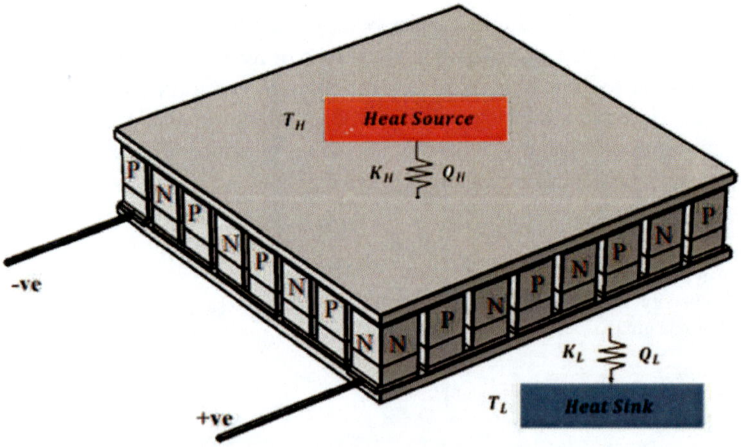

Fig. 1 Semiconductor arrangement on Thermoelectric

Electrical energy output obtained from TEG can be stored in electrical energy storage devices such as batteries, superconductors and many others. However, before being stored in a storage device, TEG output must be increased or stabilized using a boost converter and volt/ampere stabilizer. The use of boost converter and volt/ampere stabilizer can also maintain the quality and extend the life of the storage device.

Nowadays, there many types of TEG modules commercially available at the market. Each of the TEG has different specification, capabilities and price according to the manufacturer. In order to create an optimum waste heat recovery system, the optimum performance of TEG must be selected.

Rana et al. in Australia, have conducted an experiment to carefully select the most suitable TEG for waste heat recovery system. The selection of TEG was compared based on the power generation capabilities and power production cost. However, the same TEG that available at their market maybe quite different from ours. Hence in this study, we perform a comparison of three different TEG commercially available in Indonesia, namely TEC-12706, TEC-12710 and TEC-12715. The purpose of this study is to select the most suitable TEG that can be used for waste heat recovery system that will be conducted in the future.

2 Method

2.1 Materials

Thermoelectric Generator. Thermoelectric generator use the principle of the Seebeck effect that was first discovered in 1821 by Thomas Johan Seebeck. In the experiment, he connected copper and iron in a series and placed a compass needle between the two metals. When the metal side is heated, the needle turns to move. This happens because the flow of electricity that occurs in metals creates a magnetic field, this magnetic field is what drives the compass needle. This phenomenon is then known as the Seebeck effect [9]. The power generated by TEG is very dependent on the difference in temperature obtained, all of this is also related to the efficiency of the thermoelectric itself [10].

If the temperature difference is greater then the output power will also be greater to the maximum efficiency of the Peltier. So it's possible even though the temperature difference is very large but the power produced is smaller. The efficiency value of the thermoelectric module can be increased by giving the use of a heatsink, fan, or water bath on the cold side of the module to maintain the temperature difference from the hot side. Seebeck coefficient equation can be described as follows.

$$a = (V_h - V_c)/(T_h - T_c) = \Delta V/\Delta T \quad (1)$$

where:
α = Seebeck coefficient
V_h = voltage of hot junction (V)
V_c = voltage of cold junction (V)
T_h = temperature of hot junction (°C)
T_c = temperature of cold junction (°C)
ΔV = Voltage difference
ΔT = Temperature difference

Heat sink. A heat sink is designed to increase the surface area of contact with the surrounding fluid, such as air. Air velocity in the surrounding environment, material selection, fin design (or other forms) and surface treatment are some of the factors that influence the thermal resistance of a heat sink. Thermal adhesive (also known as thermal grease) is added to the bottom surface of the heat sink so that no air is trapped between the heat sink and the part that will be absorbed by heat.

An optimal heat sink will increase the coefficient of performance of the electronic system. This can be done by maximizing surface area or using heat absorbers which have large heat storage capacities so that heat can be attenuated at low temperatures [11].

Thermocouple Temperature Sensor. Temperature sensor is a component that can change the amount of heat into electrical quantities so that it can detect changes in temperature on certain objects [12]. Thermocouples are temperature measuring sensors using thermoelectric working principles. This thermocouple is composed of two non-homogeneous conductors which are connected at one point of the steel and copper connections. One end of the thermocouple as a heat signal receiver, while the other side as a reference or low temperature.

Voltage Sensor. The voltage divider is used to express the voltage across one of the two series resistors, expressed as the voltage across the combination. The voltage that arises across one of the series resistors is the total voltage multiplied by the ratio of the total resistance and resistance. The distribution of stress and the combination of the resistors can be used [13].

Current Sensor. Using the principle of the transfer function, which compares the output value with the input value, the current sensor slightly differs from the transfer function is the correlation between the physical measured value of the sensor and the ADC (Analog to Digital Converter) value that reads it [14].

Data Logger. The automatic process of collecting and recording data from sensors for archiving or analytical purposes. The sensor is used to convert physical quantities into electrical signals that can be measured automatically and finally sent to a computer or microprocessor/microcontroller for processing [14].

2.2 Selection of Thermoelectric Generator

Based on market research results, three different types of low-performance thermoelectric modules were selected as shown in Fig. 2. These three thermoelectric modules are thermoelectric peltier cooling types, which in this study will be used as electricity generator based on the Seebeck effect. Basic data such as dimension and price were provided by the manufacturer as presented in Table 1.

Several experiments have been carried out using the thermoelectric generator test settings shown in Fig. 3. an experiment has been carried out for the same temperature operating conditions as heat using an aluminum heater plate with temperature T_h = 80–100 °C as a simulation temperature for the utilization of low temperature waste heat.

2.3 System Design

The main idea of this study was to design a system capable to convert heat energy into electrical energy using a thermoelectric generator with the principle of the

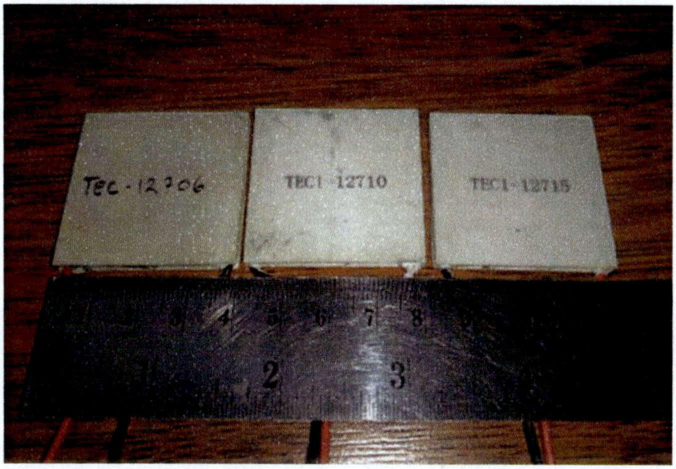

Fig. 2 Selected thermoelectric generator module, TEC1-12706, TEC1-12710, TEC1-12715

Table 1 TEG dimensions and price (Exchange rate IDR14.500/$1 USD)

TEG Type	Dimension (mm)	Price ($)
Peltier TEC-12706 Thermoelectric 12 V 6A	40 × 40 × 0.4	1.86
Peltier TEC-12710 Thermoelectric 12 V 10A	40 × 40 × 0.4	3.37
Peltier TEC-12715 Thermoelectric 12 V 15A	40 × 40 × 0.4	4.47

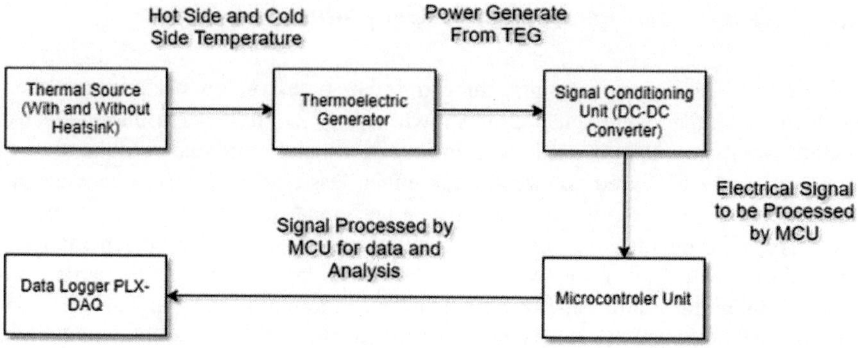

Fig. 3 Heat conversion system block diagram

Seebeck effect. The peltier modules of type TEC-12706, TEC-12710, TEC-12715 was us as the generator using 80–100°C heating plates as the heat source.

A heatsink was used as the passive cooling system to reduce excess heat. The generated voltage was measured using the voltage sensor while the temperature on both sides of the thermoelectric generator was measured using the temperature sensor. All sensor data were sent to the Arduino microcontroller to convert analog to digital data. Data retrieval was done using PLX-DAQ data logger acquisition software with Microsoft Excel for Arduino. The block diagram of this system design is shown in Fig. 3.

2.4 System Testing

The purpose of the test in this study was to measure the power generation capability ($Watt/m^2$) of each type of TEG i.e. TEC1-12706, TEC1-12710, TEC1-12715. The test were conducted in two conditions, namely (1) without and (2) with the cooling system for the TEG module. In this test, the passive type cooling system using heatsink was utilized. The cooling system was intended to reduce excess heat and maintain the temperature difference (ΔT) between the hot and cold sides of TEG module. Each of the test was conducted for 30 min.

The first condition of the test was carried out by installing a heating plates as heat waste simulation on the hot side of TEG and allows the cold side of TEG to be directly exposed to the environment. The second condition was done in the same manner as the first test, but the cold side of TEG was attached to a heatsink. Voltage and temperature sensor connected to a microcontroller was attached to each module during testing to record the output power (P) generated by TEG modules. The detail setup of the testing is shown by Fig. 4.

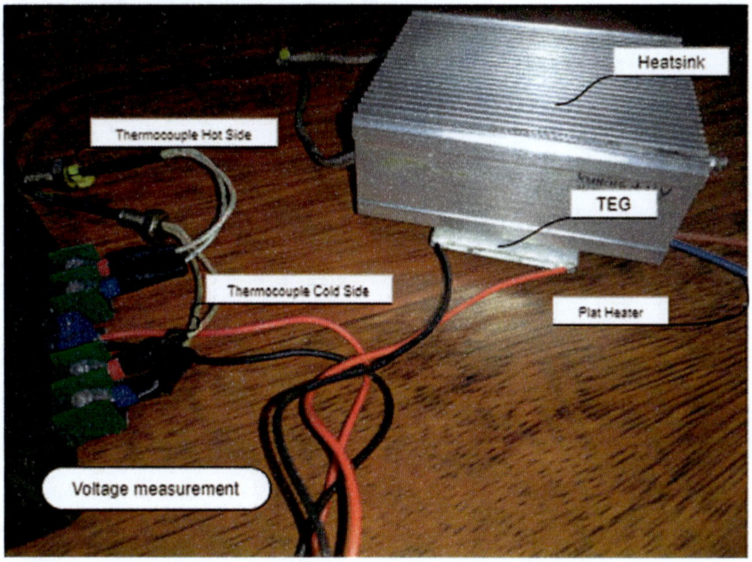

Fig. 4 Thermoelectric generator test setup

3 Result and Discussion

Several tests have been conducted to measure the output of the Thermoelectric Generator. The purpose of these test is to compare the power generation capability (Watt/m^2) and the power production cost ($/Watt) of three TEG module i.e. TEC1-12706, TEC1-12710 and TEC1-12715. The test were conducted in two conditions, namely (1) without and (2) with the cooling system for the TEG module. In this test, the passive cooling system using heatsink was utilized. The temperature difference (ΔT) and generated power (P) for each type of TEG recorded for 30 min were shown in Fig. 5, for both testing condition. The average value of ΔT and P collected from the test summarized in Table 2.

From the results presented in Table 2, it is found that, in the first condition of testing without heatsink as the cooling system, TEC1-12706 obtained the highest value of the temperature difference i.e. 11.32 °C with the generated power of 0.019 W. The order of the highest temperature difference was followed by TEC-12710 and TEC-12715 respectively. However, there are no change in the value of generated power for all types.

In the second condition, where a heatsink is attached to TEG, TEC1-12706 still recorded the highest temperature difference value of 38.63 °C with the generated power of 0.152 W. The temperature difference and generated power were tend to decrease when the TEG type TEC-12710 and TEC-12715 were utilized.

It can be seen that the power generated from TEG modules attached to a heatsink was greater than the one that did not use a heatsink. This is because heatsink can act

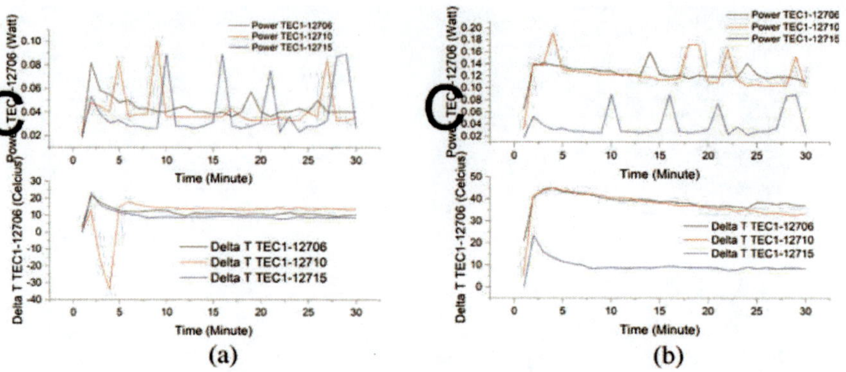

Fig. 5 TEG module testing: (**a**) without and (**b**) with heatsink

Table 2 TEG module testing data without and with heatsink

Testing Condition	TEG Type	Temperature difference (°C)	Voltage (V)	Current (A)	Power (Watt)
Without heatsink	TEC-12706	11.32	0.441	0.044	0.019
	TEC-12710	11.04	0.415	0.415	0.017
	TEC-12715	9.46	0.387	0.038	0.014
With heatsink	TEC-12706	38.63	1.237	0.123	0.152
	TEC-12710	37.08	1.235	0.123	0.152
	TEC-12715	29.72	0.907	0.097	0.082

as a cooling material can reduce the heat on the cold side of TEG and flow it into the environment through the process of heat convection. This phenomenon maintain the higher temperature difference between the hot and cold side of the TEG and therefore increase the output power generated by TEG.

According to the yielded data, it can also be observed that at the start of the test, the power obtained is relatively small since the temperature difference is also small. As the operation of the system lengthens, the difference in the temperature between the sides of the TEG increases due to the increase in temperature on the hot side of the module. The cold side of the module also experiences a small increase in temperature. It can be observed that the output voltage is directly proportional to the temperature difference between the hot side and the cold side of the TEG module.

From the data yielded from the test, the power generation capability (Watt/m^2) of three types of TEG was then calculated from the value of generated power (presented in Table 2) divided to the area of TEG module (presented in Table 1). While the power production cost ($/Watt) was calculated from the price of TEG module divided to the value of generated power. The summarize of these results is presented in Table 3.

Table 3 Comparison of power generation capability and power production cost for three types of TEG

Testing conditon	TEG type	Power generation capability (Watt/m^2)	Power production cost ($/Watt)
Without heatsink	**TEC1-12706**	**475**	**97**
	TEC1-12710	425	198
	TEC1-12715	350	319
With heatsink	**TEC1-12706**	**3800**	**12**
	TEC1-12710	3800	22
	TEC1-12715	2080	54

From the data presented in Table 3, it is clearly seen that TEG type TEC1-12706 and TEC1-12710 generally have better performance among other modules in term of power generation capability for both testing conditions. However, in terms of power production cost, TEC1-12706 was clearly superior with the lowest value of the cost compared to both TEC1-12710 and TEC1-12715. Hence it can be concluded that the TEC1-12706 is the most suitable TEG since it provides the best power generation capability with the minimum production cost. This result can become the basis for the selection of TEG in the next step of TEG experimentation for waste heat recovery system.

4 Conclusions

Three commercially available TEG modules have been tested to select the most suitable TEG for waste heat recovery system. The selection was made by measuring and calculating the power generation capability (*Watt/m^2*) and power production cost (*$/Watt*) for each TEG. Each TEG was tested for 30 min under two different conditions i.e. with and without heatsink. Among other modules, TEC1-12706 module was found to have the highest generation power capability of 475 W/*m^2* with the lowest power production cost of 97 *$/Watt*. Hence it can be concluded that TEC1-12706 is the most suitable TEG that can be used for waste heat recovery system conducted in the future.

References

1. Liu H, Zhong C, Lee SW Lin L (2018) A Comprehensive Review on Piezoelectric Energy Harvesting Technology: Materials, Mechanisms, and Applications. Appl Phys Rev
2. Wei C, Jing X (2017) A Comprehensive Review on Vibration Energy Harvesting: Modelling and Realization. Renew Sustain Energy Rev 74:1–18

3. Aparicio MP, Bakkali A, Sebastian T, Sogorb V, Bou A (2016) Radio Frequency Energy Harvesting—Sources and Techniques, 155–169
4. Moreno RJ, Grbovic D, Pollman, A (2016) Harvesting Waste Thermal Energy From Military Systems. In: Proc of the ASME 2018 Power and Energy Conference, 1–6, June
5. Simone A, Garcia-Polanco Z, Capablo J, Doyle JP, Barbato MC (2014) Household Appliances Wasted Heat Storage by means of a Packed bed TES with Encapsulated PCM. In: 13th International Conference on Sustainable Energy technologies
6. Setiawan A, Ayub T (2012) Perancangan, Pembuatan dan Pengujian Prototipe Generator Termoelektrik Berbahan Bakar Gas. Universitas Kristen Satya Wacana Jalan Diponegoro 52–60, Salatiga. 2012
7. Firmanda R (2019) Penyimpanan Energi Listrik Dari Konversi Energi Panas Menjadi Energi Listrik Menggunakan Thermoelectric Generator. Skripsi. Teknik Elektro. FTE-Universitas Telkom, Bandung
8. Nandy PR, Adhitya M (2009) Potensi Pembangkit Daya Termoelektrik Untuk Kendaraan Hibrid. Universitas Indonesia, Depok
9. Shanti Candra Puspita (2017) Hasto Sunarno,: Generator Termoelektrik untuk Pengisisan Aki. Departmen FisikaFMIPA, Institut Teknologi Sepuluh Nopember (ITS), Kampus ITS, Sukolilo, Surabaya
10. Andreas S, Taryono, MR (2012) Perancangan, Pembuatan dan Pengujian Prototipe Generator Termolektrik Berbahan Bakar Gas, ISSN 1978–2365, Vol. 11 No 1 Juni 2012: 1–10, Universitas Kristen Satya Wacana, Salatiga
11. Eky I, Abrar TA (2017) Rancang Bangun dan Realisasi Alat Ukur Performasi Pendingin Termoelekrik. Universitas Telkom, Bandung
12. Working Principle of Thermocouples. https://assets.omega.com/resources/how-thermocouples-work-1.jpg. Last accessed 10 March 2020
13. Alfiyyah K (2019) Konversi Energi Panas Menjadi Energi Listrik Menggunakan Termoelektrik Generator. Skripsi. Teknik Elektro. FTE-Universitas Telkom, Bandung
14. Faris A, Ramdlan M, Porman P (2018) Pemanfaatan Thermoelectric Cooler Pada Photovoltaic Sebagai Pembangkit. ISSN: 2355–9365, e-Proceeding of Engineering: Vol .5, No. 3 December 2018|Page 3965 Telkom University, Bandung

Cross-Gender and Age Speech Conversion Using Hidden Markov Model Based on Cepstral Coefficients Conversion

Meisi Aristia H. Gultom, Raditiana Patmasari, Inung Wijayanto, and Sugondo Hadiyoso

Abstract Animation movies often use children's characters and they need children aged 5–10 to do a dubbing. For cost efficiency, a speech conversion can be done to support dubbing a children's speech. To deal with it, in this research we propose the method to converting an adult's speech to children's speech. The contribution of this study is to design a signal processing algorithm to perform the conversion. In this study we propose a conversion method using the Hidden Markov Model (HMM) based on Cepstral Coefficients Conversion. The input is the speech of source speakers and the target speakers that using similar sentences. Features extraction, which is used is by extracted pitch (f_0) and cepstral in conversion process, and the modeling method is HMM. System output is converted speech signals that has similar characteristics with target speech signal. From the testing results, the most optimal HMM parameter is using 4-state. The highest increase of cepstral Root Mean Square Error (RMSE) before conversion and after conversion is equal to 32.35% and an average 25.83% which obtained from 400 samples. Mean Opinion Score (MOS) on a scale from 1 (converted speech is very dissimilar with the target speech) to 5 (converted speech is very similar with the target speech). It resulted an average value of 2.505 in terms of similarities and has an average value of 2.805 in terms of quality which obtained from 30 respondents. The proposed method is expected to be used in the animation film industry in order to simplify and make efficient the dubbing process.

Keywords Cepstral analysis · HMM · Speech conversion

M. A. H. Gultom · R. Patmasari (✉) · I. Wijayanto
School of Electrical Engineering, Telkom University, Bandung, Indonesia
e-mail: raditiana@telkomuniversity.ac.id

S. Hadiyoso
School of Applied Science, Telkom University, Bandung, Indonesia

H. Triwiyanto et al. (eds.), *Proceedings of the 1st International Conference on Electronics, Biomedical Engineering, and Health Informatics*, Lecture Notes in Electrical Engineering 746, https://doi.org/10.1007/978-981-33-6926-9_13

1 Introduction

In the film industry, it often needed voice conversion, or commonly known as dubbing [1, 2]. It often applied a language translation and conversion to children's voices [3]. In the case of child voice-overs, several problems are often encountered, including limited resources and sometimes depending on their mood when recording. At the same time, today, many film industries play on animated films that require the character of children aged 5–10 years with a unique voice to both boys and girls. With these problems, it takes a longer time to produce the films.

Digital voice conversion is a digital signal processing application that can convert a voice into a designated output. With a voice conversion system, the source speaker sound can be converted into the target speaker sound so that it will sound similar to the listener [4–6]. Sound signals can be changed in parameters, such as pitch, frequency, and other essential parameters, so that they can produce sounds similar to the sounds of other individuals (target speakers). The most important part of the voice conversion process lies in modeling the target signal so that a new input signal can be converted similarly with the target signal.

Some studies have proposed a method or algorithm for voice conversion in the digital domain. Some of them use conventional methods, and others use digital signal processing. The male (female) to female (male) voice conversion algorithm was proposed in the study [7–9]. Basically, they focus on modifying the pitch using the proposed algorithm. Other studies are dubbing with a simple technique called voice-over [10–12]. This is performed by removing the original recorded sound. However, this technique is certainly not flexible because it requires many human resources. Another way is by applying the text to speech, as reported in the study [13–15]. However, this method has drawbacks, one of which is that the sound is flat because it cannot play intonation and pitch. Digital signal processing for implementing speech conversion from adults to children's voices has been reported in several studies [16–18]. Voice conversion using the deep neural network approach was also recently proposed in the study [19]. These studies have succeeded in simulating a system for voice conversion. However, there are still gaps in the development of methods since the intonation and pronunciation vary greatly between ethnicities.

Indonesia is known as one of the most diverse countries which have more than 600 ethnicities and more than 731 languages with around 1100 dialects. Thus, each dialect, intonation, and accent in Indonesian's language is very important and unique. Therefore, there is a need to develop a voice conversion system that matches the Indonesian language's characteristics. To deal with the problems and drawbacks in previous studies, we designed an algorithm to convert adult speakers to children speakers in Indonesian's language. Children's sound targets are designed in the age range of 5–10 years. In this study, Hidden Markov Model (HMM) and cepstral coefficients conversion are used to model and convert sound signals. The novelty of this study is the use of the cepstral coefficients approaches in adjusting the HMM model parameters to obtain the target sound. The system's output is measured using the Root Mean Square Error (RMSE) and subjective assessment in the form of Mean Opinion Score (MOS).

2 Materials and Methods

2.1 System Design

The workflow of proposed system is presented in Fig. 1a. System input is the speech of source speakers and target speakers using similar sentences. The speech of the source speaker comes from two men and two women. The speech of target speakers comes from five girls aged 5–10. In the recording, the sampling frequency that used is 22 kHz and the file is in wavelength format. Each of the speaker pronounce five sentences in Indonesian language: (a) "balonku ada lima"; (b) "selamat pagi ibu guru"; (c) "selamat ulang tahun"; (d) "libur telah tiba", and (e) "aku anak Indonesia".

There are three steps in the preprocessing stage. They are resampling, DC removal, and normalization. In the resampling process, the signal sample is reduced, and the frequency is changed into 16 kHz. The DC removal is done by using Eq. (1).

$$S_a = S_{in} - mean(S_{in}) \tag{1}$$

Here, the S_a is the output signal, and the S_{in} is the input signal. The normalization process is done to make sure that the subsequent signal processing is not affected by signal amplitude, which is too high or too low. The output of this process is a signal with amplitude range $-1 < S_n + 1$.

The feature extraction stage which shown 1b, begins with pitch f_0 detection to find speech components. After that, Speech Transformation and Representation by

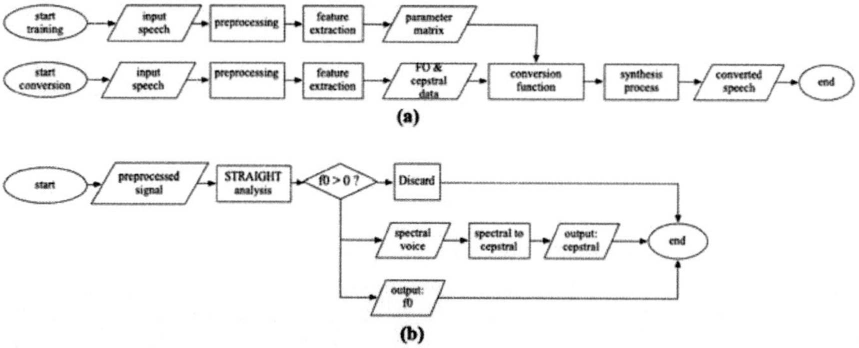

Fig. 1 (**a**) Workflow of proposed system. (**b**) Feature extraction process

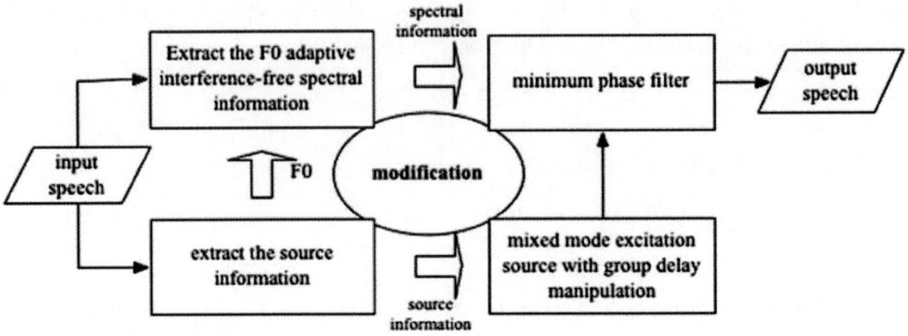

Fig. 2 Schematic diagram of STRAIGHT

Adaptive Interpolation of weighted spectrum (STRAIGHT) analysis is done to obtain signal spectrally, which shown in Fig. 2 [20]. The next process is transforming the spectral into a cepstral component. The frame with a value of $f_O > 0$ is taken for the next process, while another frame with value $f_O = 0$ discarded. There are 513 data in a frame of a spectral component. Spectral is sampling into cepstral, which consists of 25 samples. So the output of this process is 25 $\times$ N cepstral matrix and 1 X N matrix f_O where N is the number of frames.

2.2 *Modeling Using HMM*

Dynamic Time Warping (DTW) is done before the system is modeled. DTW is used to compare the similarities between two signals in the time domain, both of which have different lengths. In this study, DTW used for synchronizing source speech cepstral and target speech cepstral in the time domain. The first steps of DTW calculation is started by matching each index of the first value with one or more subsequent order indexes and vice versa (Fig. 3). The second step is to make sure that the last index of the first order have to be matched to the last index of the other order (but it does not have to be the only match). The last step is by checking he mapping of indices from the first order to the index of another order must be increased monotonically, and vice versa, that is, if j > i is the index of the first order, there cannot be two indexes l > k in the other order., so that index i is matched to index l and index j matches index k, and vice versa.

Cepstral, which resulting from DTW are combined so that we get training data $Z_r = [X_T Y_T]$. Modeling using HMM is only used in cepstral, whereas f_O using mean and variance calculation. A 25 $\times$ N cepstral matrix of source speech and 25 $\times$ M cepstral matrix of target speech are combined through the DTW process so that we get 50 $\times$ T matrix. This study use left-right HMM topology with four states because we get high modeling probability and convergence. The HMM topology used in this study is shown in Fig. 1. The measured HMM parameters include the initial state probability vector (Π), the transition state probability matrix (A = [aij]) and the

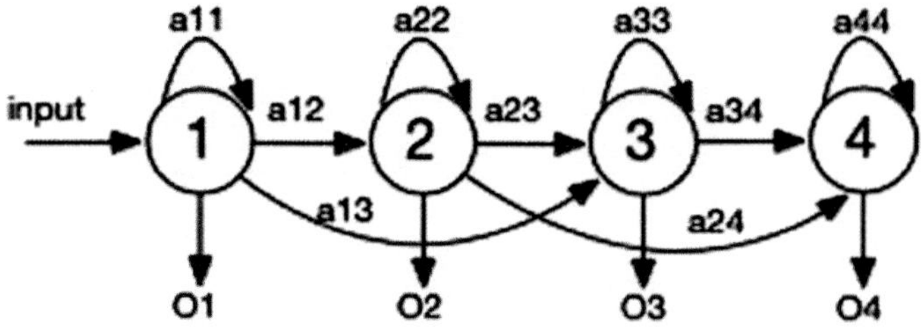

Fig. 3 Left-Right HMM models with 4-states

observable symbol probability matrix (B = [bj(m)]).The output of the modeling process is conversion parameter matrix sized 50 × 4 and a weighted parameter, which shows mixture probability.

2.3 Conversion and Synthesis

Figure 4 presents the main processes of conversion and synthesis. The main idea of this process is to convert pitch (f_0) and cepstral parameters between source speech and target speech. After conversion is done, then we synthesize signals using STRAIGHT algorithm. Conversion process is divided into f_0 conversion and cepstral conversion. The f_0 is converted by linear conversion method according to the Eq. (2).

$$f_{con}(t) = \mu_t + \frac{\sigma_t}{\sigma_s}(f_{source}(t) - \mu_s) \quad (2)$$

Here the $f_{source}(t)$ and $f_{con}(t)$ are the f_0 value before and after conversion. respectively. The μ is the f_0 mean, while the σ is the f_0 standard deviation. For cepstral conversion. we use conversion equation which based on conditional expectation of Gaussian distribution as shown in Eq. (3).

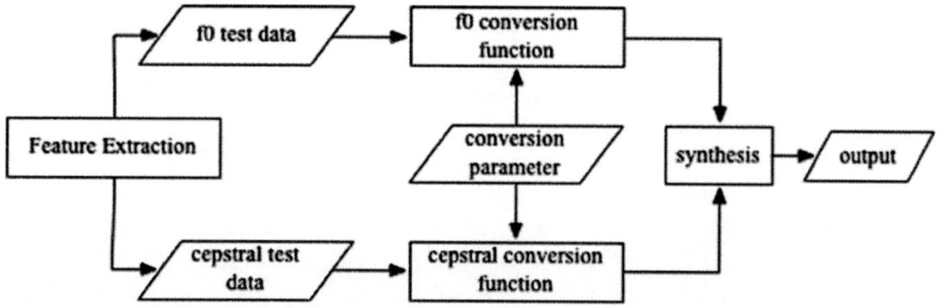

Fig. 4 Conversion and synthesis process

$$\widehat{y} = \sum_{k=1}^{M} P_k(X) * \left[\mu_t + \frac{\sigma_t}{\sigma_s}(f_{source}(t) - \mu_s)\right] \tag{3}$$

where

$$P_k(X) = \frac{\alpha_k * N(X_k \cdot \mu_k \cdot \sigma_k)}{\sum_{j=1}^{M} \alpha_j * N(X_j \cdot \mu_j \cdot \sigma_j)} \tag{4}$$

where, the X and $\widehat{y}$ are the cepstral value before and after conversion, respectively.

2.4 System Performance

The output of this system is converted speech signal with similar words used by source speaker and target speaker but has similar characteristics with target speech signal. Root Mean Square Error (RMSE) is used for system performance testing by comparing the difference between source speech cepstral and converted speech cepstral. RMSE is calculated using Eq. (5).

$$RMSE = \sqrt{\sum_{i=1}^{n} \frac{(x_i - y_i)^2}{n}} \tag{5}$$

where the y_i is the conversion value, x_i is the observed value, and n is the number of samples.

Furthermore, the system performance also presented subjectively by Mean Opinion Score (MOS). Two criteria being tested. the similarity, and the quality of the result compared with the source. The MOS is a quantitative method to score a subjective judgement by human, the value is judged on a scale from 1 (converted speech is very dissimilar with the target) to 5 (converted speech is very similar with the target).

3 Result and Discussion

The first process is done by finding the best HMM state by observing the highest modeling probability. We conduct ten experiments, where we found the highest probability lies in state 8 (2.885×10^5). The source speaker comes two males (S1 and S2) and two women (S3 and S4), while the target speaker is a girl voice (T1–T5).

Table 1 shows that the system successfully performs the conversion of the magnitude of the fundamental frequency f_0. It can be seen from the RMSE f_0 value

Table 1 Results of f_0 and cepstral testing

Source	Target	RMSE f_0			RMSE cepstral		
		Before	After	Imp. (%)	Before	After	Imp. (%)
S1	T1	96.5	35.95	62.75	0.24	0.17	27.65
S1	T2	98.84	37.73	61.83	0.26	0.18	30.61
S1	T3	71.24	38.97	45.3	0.26	0.19	27.88
S1	T4	86.18	26.62	69.11	0.23	0.17	26.90
S1	T5	71.06	49.48	30.37	0.22	0.16	30.11
S2	T1	95.58	37.32	60.95	0.23	0.19	18.05
S2	T2	97.86	37.73	61.45	0.23	0.18	23.36
S2	T3	70.51	40.47	42.61	0.26	0.21	20.66
S2	T4	83.83	26.39	68.52	0.23	0.18	21.41
S2	T5	69.13	44.49	35.64	0.21	0.16	22.75
S3	T1	44	41.24	6.26	0.23	0.16	26.91
S3	T2	45.39	37.36	17.69	0.24	0.16	32.34
S3	T3	40.59	42.79	−5.41	0.25	0.19	25.27
S3	T4	36.31	30.48	16.05	0.23	0.16	29.24
S3	T5	42.36	44.32	−4.64	0.21	0.15	28.65
S4	T1	44.51	35.71	19.77	0.23	0.18	20.59
S4	T2	47.38	38.47	18.81	0.23	0.18	22.00
S4	T3	40.73	41.62	−2.18	0.26	0.19	28.02
S4	T4	37.62	29.12	22.58	0.22	0.17	25.05
S4	T5	42.31	42.87	−1.31	0.20	0.14	29.17
		Average		31.31	Average		25.83

after conversion is smaller than RMSE f_0 before conversion. Average f_0 improvement is equal to 31.31%. Before conversion, source speech (S1 and S2) comes from male speakers and whole target speech, which comes from female speakers. RMSE f_0 values higher than the source speech (S3 and S4), a female speaker. This is because the female pitch value is higher than the male pitch so that it will produce a higher error value. There are four results of RMSE f_0 values after conversion is higher than before conversion (negative values). This occurs most likely because of an error f_0 detection, where the possibility of noise detection is considered a component of speech.

In Table 1, the system successfully performs conversion visible from after conversion is smaller than RMSE cepstral before conversion. The highest increase of cepstral RMSE before conversion and after conversion is equal to 32.34%. the lowest is 18.05%, and an average 25.83%, which obtained from 400 samples.

We also conduct a MOS testing to quantify a subjective measurement. Thirty respondents assess the converted speech compared to the target speech in terms of similarity and quality. The scoring is done following five scales from 1 (converted speech is very dissimilar with the target speech) to 5 (converted speech is very similar with the target speech. The MOS resulting an average value of 2.505 in terms of similarities and has an average value of 2.805 in terms of quality. It can be concluded that the conversion has a quite similar result with the target speech and can be heard well enough.

4 Conclusion

This study performs a speech conversion to convert a source speech into a specific target speech using a Hidden Markov Model (HMM). The input is recording from two men and two women, while the target speech is five girls aged 5–10 years old. The input speech is extracted using the STRAIGHT analysis to obtain the spectral of the signal, which then converted into a cepstral component. The modelling uses a four-state of HMM, which obtained by analyzing the log sum of probability. From the experiments, we achieve the average increase of RMSE by 25.83%, which obtained from 400 speech samples. For a subjective measurement, we calculate the similarity and quality based on the MOS. The MOS measurement of the converted speech achieves 2.505 for similarity and 2.805 for the quality value. From the result, we can conclude that the proposed method is suitable to be applied in cross gender and age voice conversion. However, the study about voice conversion in Indonesian's language still needs a large amount of speech data. Furthermore, the development of multi-target speech remains an open challenge.

References

1. Haikuo Yu (2013) English-Chinese Film Translation in China. J Transl 9(2):55–65
2. Ban R, Dıaz-Cintas J (2017) Language and translation in film. The Routledge Handbook of Translation Studies and Linguistics, (January):313–326)
3. de Reyes Lozano J, Julio de los Reyes Lozano (2017) Bringing all the Senses into Play: the Dubbing of Animated Films for Children. Palimpsestes 30:99–115
4. Ye H, Young S (2004) Voice conversion for unknown speakers. In: 8th International Conference on Spoken Language Processing, ICSLP 2004, number June, pp 1161–1164)
5. Stylianou Y, Olivier C (1998) A System for Voice Conversion Based On Probabilistic Classification and a Harmonic Plus Noise Model. In Proceedings of the 1998 In: IEEE International Conference on Acoustics, Speech and Signal Processing, ICASSP 98, pp 281–284
6. Yathigiri A, Bathula M, Kothapalli S, Vekkot S, Tripathi S (2017). Voice transformation using pitch and spectral mapping. In 2017 International Conference on Advances in Computing, Communications and Informatics, ICACCI 2017, volume 2017-Janua, pp 1540–1544
7. Lawlor B, FaganAD (1999). A Novel Efficient Algorithm for Voice Gender Conversion. In International Congress of Phonetic Sciences, pp 77–80
8. Bharti SK, Koolagudi SG, Sreenivasa Rao K, Choudhary A, Kumar B. Voice conversion using linear prediction coefficients and artificial neural network. In: ACM International Conference Proceeding Series, pp 240–245

9. Mousa Allam (2010) Voice Conversion using Pitch Shifting Algorithm by Time Stretching with PSOLA and Re-Sampling. J Electr Eng 61(1):57–61
10. Kianbakht Sajjad (2016) Dubbing and subtitling american comedy series. Eur J Engl Lang Lit Stud 4(4):65–80
11. Moh Supardi and Dea Amanda Putri (2018) Audio-Visual Translation Techniques: Subtitling and Dubbing of Movie Soundtrack in Frozen: Let it Go. Buletin Al-Turas 24(2):399–414
12. Piazza Roberta (2010) Voice-over and self-narrative in film: A multimodal analysis of Antonioni's When Love Fails (Tentato Suicidio). Lang Lit 19(2):173–195
13. Szarkowska A, Jankowska A (2012). Text-to-speech audio description of voiced-over films . A case study of audio described Volver in Polish. Emerging topics in translation: Audio description, pp 81–98
14. Fernandez-Torn′A, Matamala A (2015). Text-to-speech vs. Human voiced audio descriptions: A reception study in films dubbed into Catalan. J Speclsed Transl 24(July):61–88
15. Jacob A, Mythili P (2008) Developing a Child Friendly Text-to-Speech System. Advances in Human-Computer Interaction, 1–6)
16. Watts Oliver, Yamagishi Junichi, King Simon, Berkling Kay (2010) Synthesis of child speech with HMM adaptation and voice conversion. IEEE Trans Audio Speech Lang Process 18(5): 1005–1016
17. Watts O, Yamagishi J, King S, Berkling K. HMM Adaptation and voice conversion for the synthesis of child speech: A comparison. In: Proceedings of the Annual Conference of the International Speech Communication Association, INTERSPEECH, pp 2627–2630
18. Reima Karhila DR, Sanand, MK, Smit P. Creating synthetic voices for children by adapting adult average voice using stacked transformations and VTLN. In: ICASSP, IEEE International Conference on Acoustics, Speech and Signal Processing—Proceedings, number March, pp 4501–4504
19. Prashanth Gurunath Shivakumar and Panayiotis Georgiou (2020) Transfer learning from adult to children for speech recognition: Evaluation, analysis and recommendations. Comput Speech Lang 63:1–15
20. Banno H, Hata H, Morise M, Takahashi T, Irino T, Kawahara H (2007) Implementation of realtime STRAIGHT speech manipulation system: Report on its first implementation. Acoust Sci Technol 28:140–146

Design of Electric Wheelchair with Joystick Controller as Personal Mobility for Disabled Person

Hanifah Rahmi Fajrin, Thony Ary Zain, and Muhammad Irfan

Abstract The movement aids for people with motor system disability, especially the legs, has been currently very essential, because they also surely want to move freely from a place to another without bothering their family or closest friends. Therefore, this electric wheelchair research was made to facilitate the movement of people with disabilities within their activities, such as going to certain places or doing something. The design of the electric wheelchair was arranged in such ways to assist the body movements using joystick control connected to microcontroller Arduino. If the joystick lever was directed forward, backward, left and right, then the joystick command would be processed by the Arduino, so that it provided voltage to the motor driver, and the wheelchair could move forward, backward, turn left, and turn right. From 25 joystick command tests, it was shown the forward accuracy was 88%, the backward was 100%, the left turn was 100%, and the right turn was also 100%. Based on the test that have been conducted, the accuracy values represented that this electric wheelchair using joystick controller can be implemented as its function.

Keywords Wheelchair · Disabilities · Joystick · Ultrasonic

1 Introduction

The use of a wheelchair in general is to facilitate the patients who suffer from motor system disorders in their legs. Based on the results of a survey has been conducted in several places such as hospitals and homes for people with disabilities, it was found that the appreciation of people with disabilities for the need of more attractive

H. R. Fajrin (✉) · T. A. Zain
Department of Medical Electronics Technology, Universitas Muhammadiyah Yogyakarta, Jalan Brawijaya, Kasihan, Bantul, Yogyakarta, Indonesia55183
e-mail: hanifah.fajrin@vokasi.umy.ac.id

M. Irfan
PKU Gamping Hospital, Bantul, Yogyakarta, Indonesia

H. Triwiyanto et al. (eds.), *Proceedings of the 1st International Conference on Electronics, Biomedical Engineering, and Health Informatics*, Lecture Notes in Electrical Engineering 746, https://doi.org/10.1007/978-981-33-6926-9_14

and automatic wheelchairs is very high. This was because they were less satisfied with the present incomplete (58.3%) and uncomfortable (25%) wheelchairs, and for their difficult operation (4.1%). They also stated that manual wheelchairs currently could not make them carry out their activities like normal people (12.6%) [1]. There is high awareness of the people with disabilities towards the wheelchairs which are less able to facilitate their activities disabilities who want to move dynamically to the place they want to go without spending so much energy and do not want to continue to depend on their families and surrounding communities [2].

Based on field observations, wheelchairs on the public markets still use manual controls that require power to move/push from the users. Therefore, the persons with disabilities on hands cannot move the wheelchairs for themselves [3].

Many researchers have proposed various methods of electric wheelchair control systems, including voice recognition system, EEG (Electro-Encephalo-Gram) for brain wave detection, EOG (Electro-Oculo-Gram) for eye movements, and EMG (Electro-Myo-Gram) for detection of muscle movements [3–12]. The problems that are often faced by the electric wheelchairs that use voice recognition system is an error in speech recognition because at the time of testing, the form of words used is more than one word and has similarities. So that voice recognition commands are often recognized by other words as well as in voice recognition, the noise level and the type of microphone used greatly affect speech recognition [13]. Meanwhile, the weakness of EMG based-wheelchair is the placement of the muscle leads must be properly placed because the tapped signal through the electrodes is prone to noise and has a tiny amplitude [14, 15]. In addition, wheel chair using EOG system that uses eyes movement will result in failure because it is affected by the intensity of light captured by the eye, both indoors and outdoors [16, 17]. Furthermore, EEG's wheelchair EEG requires high accuracy for its movement to be smooth because there is a lot of noise in the brain waves that forces the brain to work in full concentration [18, 19].

Based on the problem above, an electric wheelchair is designed with a joystick controller, it is placed on the right-hand grip of the wheelchair used to control the movement of the wheelchair so that it can move forward, backward, turn left and turn right and control the rotation of the motor in a wheelchair. The use of joysticks can facilitate the activities of people with disabilities without spending a lot of time and energy and is considered more efficient [4, 5, 11, 20, 21].

2 Materials and Method

The methods used in this research are consisted of several stages, namely: software design, hardware design, and tool design.

2.1 *Software Design*

Based on the flow chart in Fig. 1, the process began with the initialization of the joystick or the installation of the joystick module in the right-hand grip of the wheelchair. Then, the module would read the patient's hand movements, if the user moved the joystick lever forward, it would cause the wheelchair to move forward; if the user's hand moved the joystick backward, it would cause the wheelchair to move backward, and if the joystick was pointed left or right, it would cause the wheelchair to turn left or right.

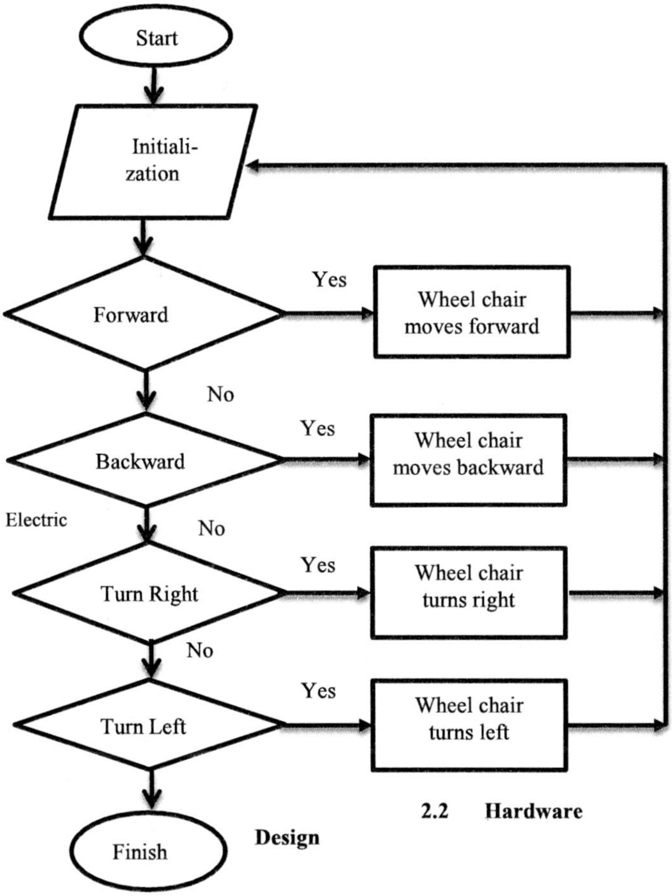

Fig. 1 Flow chart of electric wheelchair

2.2 Hardware Design

Electric

2.2 *Hardware Design*

The entire range of electric wheelchair using a joystick included the microcontroller Arduino series, motor drivers, and joystick module, as can be seen on Fig. 2. The Arduino was connected to the Accelerometer sensor and the Joystick module were connected to ports A0, A1, A2 and A3, the relay driver was connected to pins 8, 9, 10 and 11. The joystick is consisted of 5 pins; the first was connected to ground, the second was connected to VCC, the third was connected to A0, and the fourth was connected to A1 which was an analog microcontroller port. The joystick module served to regulate the direction of motion of electric wheelchairs, and the commands on the joystick were controlled by the user's hand that was still functioning [22]. Options for electric wheelchair movements were forward, backward, turn left, and turn right [23]. Meanwhile, The motor driver circuit was a DC motor drive switch that functioned to move the motor when the tool was used and connected to the joystick as a controller for motor movement [24]. When the joystick was directed forward, the driver circuit got voltage from pins 8 and 9, so that the motor would rotate clockwise, otherwise if the driver circuit got the voltage from pins 10 and 11, the driver circuit would instruct the motor to rotate counterclockwise. The driver circuit as a switching motor served to rule the motor in getting the voltage, so that the motor could spin to move the electric wheelchair. When the transistor got the power from the microcontroller, it then activated the relay, so that the NC (Normally Close) moved to NO (Normally Open). NO and NC here were connected directly to the battery. NO was connected with positive voltage, and NC was connected to negative one. When NC to NO transfer occurred, the motor would get the power and then rotated [25].

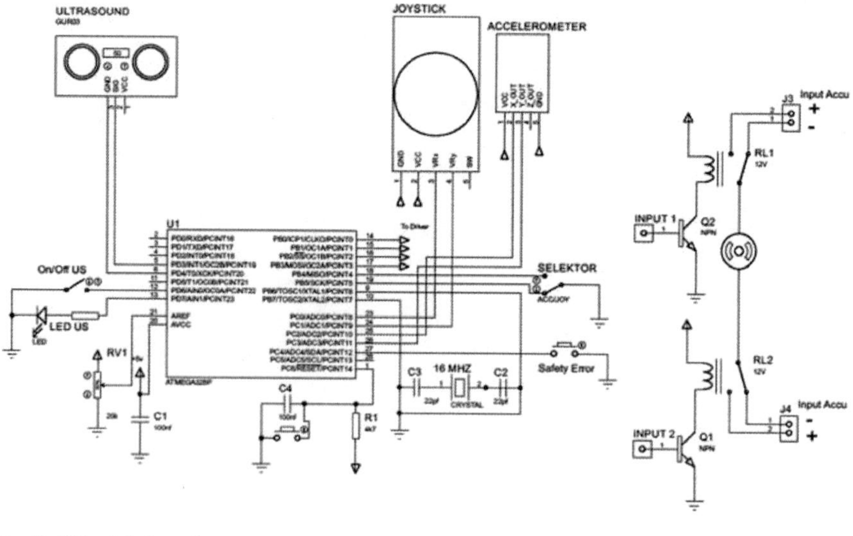

Fig. 2 Wheelchair series

2.3 Electric Wheel Chair Design

For the tool design of electric wheelchair, the authors used some following materials, namely joystick module, wheelchairs, batteries, microcontroller Arduino, motor drivers, and DC motors. The illustration of the tool design could be seen in Fig. 3.

3 Result and Discussion

The testing and measurement of electric wheelchair using Joystick comprised several tests. The first test was assessing the joystick command, the second was testing the speed of wheelchair and the last was testing automatic braking system.

3.1 Testing of Wheelchair Movement/Joystick Commands

Table 1 is the result of testing the joystick execution command on the electric wheelchair with the execution commands of moving forward, backward, turn left, and turn right. The tests were carried out five times for each command, with the patient's weight of 55 kg, and the results of the test are calculated using the accuracy and error formula. The percentage of accuracy that was achieved on each command is: moving forward 88%, backward 100%, turn left 100%, and turn right 100%. 12% error for forward direction which was the movement recognized as turn right and turn left was caused by the bad conditions of the road during the assessment, so that the joystick control trembled resulting in the program setting to be incompatible with the instructions made [5]. Besides, the use of an electric wheelchair with joystick control requires attention to the direction of the joystick lever in four directions, namely: front, back, left and right. The accuracy obtained represents a pretty good value, more than 80% for this wheelchair can be used as

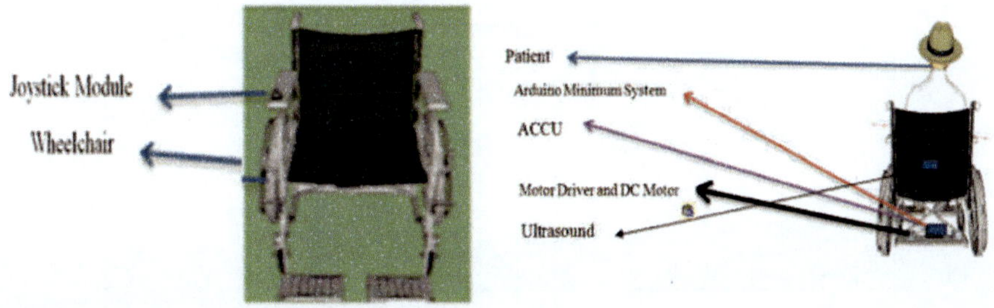

Fig. 3 Wheelchair design

intended. Furthermore, errors could be obtained because the joystick axis interpretation for the forward direction was a little imprecise [11, 23]. However, the joystick controller is more effectively implemented and the movement is smoother because it is not affected by internal noise such as using the ECG, EMG or EOG systems [13, 26, 27].

3.2 *Testing of Wheelchair Speed*

The speed testing was carried out to check the speed of the electric wheelchair. Table 2 shows the results of speed and average testing on the electric wheelchair with the distance of 10 meters. The average time taken by the electric wheelchair with the patient's weight of 50 kg and 10 meter-distance was 15.43 s, so that the average speed of the wheelchair was 0.64 meters/second. The average time taken by the electric wheelchair with the patient's weight of 50 kg and 10 meter-distance was 15.42 s, so that the average speed of the wheelchair was 0.64 meters/second. The average time taken by the electric wheelchair with the patient's weight of 60 kg and 10 meter-distance was 16.05 s, so that the average speed of the wheelchair was 0.62 meters/second.

Table 1 Testing of joystick commands

Command		Forward					Turn Right					Turn Left					Backward					Accuracy (%)
		1	2	3	4	5	1	2	3	4	5	1	2	3	4	5	1	2	3	4	5	
Forward	1	√	√	√	√	√																88
	2	√		√	√	√		√														
	3	√	√	√	√	√																
	4		√	√	√	√	√															
	5	√	√		√	√								√								
Turn Right	1						√	√	√	√	√											100
	2						√	√	√	√	√											
	3						√	√	√	√	√											
	4						√	√	√	√	√											
	5						√	√	√	√	√											
Turn Left	1											√	√	√	√	√						100
	2											√	√	√	√	√						
	3											√	√	√	√	√						
	4											√	√	√	√	√						
	5											√	√	√	√	√						
Backward	1																√	√	√	√	√	100
	2																√	√	√	√	√	
	3																√	√	√	√	√	
	4																√	√	√	√	√	
	5																√	√	√	√	√	

Table 2 Testing of wheelchair speed

Weight (kg)	Distance (meters)	Average time (s)	Speed (m/s)
50	10	15,43	0,64
55	10	15,42	0,64
60	10	16,05	0,62

Table 3 Testing of automatic braking system

Test	Stop for two seconds	Accuracy (%)
1	Successful	100
2	Successful	
3	Successful	
4	Successful	
5	Successful	

The results from testing the speed of a wheelchair with a patient's body weight of 50 kg and 55 kg were the same, namely 0.64 meters/second so that the use of power and torque in patients weighing 50 kg and 55 kg was not much different. Meanwhile, with a body weight of 60 kg the speed results obtained were 0.62 meters/second. This difference in speed was due to the power and torque when using an electric wheelchair affected the patient's body weight of 60 kg so that the use of power and torque increased resulting in a lower speed at this body weight [28]. The average speed obtained was 0.64 meters/second. The speed of an electric wheelchair might change depending on the patient's weight and power [8, 20]. The heavier the weight of the patient, the velocity of wheelchair will significantly decrease.

3.3 *Testing of Automatic Braking System*

The automatic braking test with a safety distance of one meter was carried out five times. Table 3 is the results of the test stopping for two seconds when there was an object behind wheelchair with one-meter distance. The results show that the test was successful with the accuracy of 100%. So that, wheelchair could stop automatically with high accuracy for avoiding the obstacle behind

4 Conclusion

The Electric Wheelchairs Using Joystick have functioned well after being tested and the accuracy values have been measured. The accuracy in forward movement was 88%, turn right 100%, turn left 100%, and backward 100% for each experiment carried out five times. When the electric wheelchair at the distance of 1 m, it will stop for 2 s, and this braking test was carried out five times with the accuracy of 100%. Moreover, the speed of the electric wheelchair is 0-0.64 m/s, it depends on the user's weight. For the next improvement, we will focus on the ergonomic design for user's convenience.

Acknowledgements The authors gratefully acknowledge the support of Lembaga Penelitian, Publikasi dan Pengabdian Masyarakat (LP3M), Universitas Muhammadiyah Yogyakarta, Indonesia.

References

1. Krishnan RH, Pugazhenthi S (2014) Mobility assistive devices and self-transfer robotic systems for elderly, a review. Intell Serv Robot 7(1):37–49
2. Hunt ALE, Galea ER, Lawrence PJ, Frost IR, Gwynne SMV (2020) Simulating Movement Devices Used in Hospital Evacuation. Fire Technol 56(5):2209–2240
3. Hamatani S, Murakami T (2015) A novel steering mechanism of two-wheeled wheel chair for stability improvement. *IECON 2015—41st Annu Conf IEEE Ind Electron Soc*, 2154–2159
4. Cooper RA, Spaeth DM, Jones DK, Boninger ML, Fitzgerald SG, Guo S (2002) Comparison of virtual and real electric powered wheelchair driving using a position sensing joystick and an isometric joystick. Med Eng Phys 24(10):703–708
5. Rabhi Y, Mrabet M, Fnaiech F, Gorce P, Miri I, Dziri C (2018) Intelligent Touchscreen Joystick for Controlling Electric Wheelchair. Irbm 39(3):180–193
6. Rabhi Y, Mrabet M, Fnaiech F (2018) A facial expression controlled wheelchair for people with disabilities. Comput Methods Programs Biomed 165:89–105
7. Alqudah M, Abdelfattah M, Boiko I, Alhammadi K (2017) Dynamic modeling and control design for a self-balancing two-wheel chair. Comput Methods Programs Biomed 2:1–4
8. Song JS, Baek MJ, Noh HJ, Cho SH, Mok HS, Kim CW (2015) Analysis of in-wheel motorized wheelchair cornering performance with electro-mechanical co-simulation. Int J Precis Eng Manuf 16(3):501–507
9. Purwanto D, Mardiyanto R, Arai K (2009) Electric wheelchair control with gaze direction and eye blinking. Artif Life Robot 14(3):397–400
10. Nasif S, Khan MAG (2018) Wireless head gesture controlled wheel chair for disable persons, *5th IEEE Reg. 10 Humanit. Technol. Conf. 2017, R10-HTC 2017*, 2018:156–161
11. Choi JH, Chung Y, Oh S (2019) Motion control of joystick interfaced electric wheelchair for improvement of safety and riding comfort, *Mechatronics*, 59:104–114, September 2018
12. Paulite YVP, Carandang NJC, Arboleda ER (2018) Smart wheelchair with dual control using touchpad and android mobile device. Indones J Electr Eng Informatics 6(1):86–96
13. Velázquez R, Gutiérrez CA (2014) Modeling and Control Techniques for Electric Powered Wheelchairs : An Overview. In 2014 IEEE CENTRAL AMERICA AND PANAMA CONVENTION (CONCAPAN XXXIV), no. Concapan Xxxiv, pp 6–11
14. Hardiansyah R (2020) The Electric Wheelchair Control Using Electromyography Sensor Of Arm Muscle, in *2016* International Conference on Information, Communication Technology and System (ICTS), pp 129–134
15. Nudra IW, Pradivta B (2019) Design of Myoelectric Control Command of Electric Wheelchair as Personal Mobility for Disabled Person MCU1. IBITeC 2019:112–117
16. Hirshkowitz M (2014) Polysomnography: Understanding this technology's past might guide future developments. IEEE Pulse 5(5):26–28

17. Rokonuzzaman M, Ferdous SM, Tuhin RA, Arman SI, Manzar T, Hasan MN (2011) Design of an autonomous mobile wheel chair for disabled using electrooculogram (EOG) signals. Mechatronics Recent Technol Sci Adv, 41–53
18. Wangchuk J, Machangpa W, Singh T, Chingtham S (2018) Science Direct Head Gesture Controlled Wheelchair for Quadriplegic Patients. Procedia Comput Sci 132:342–351
19. Gentiletti GG, Gebhart JG, Acevedo RC (2009) Command of a simulated wheelchair on a virtual environment using a brain-computer interface. IRBM 30:218–225
20. Clearesta E, Wardhana AA, Widyotriatmo A, Suprijanto S (2013) Adaptive control for velocity control of an electric wheelchair. *Proc 2013 3rd Int Conf Instrumentation, Control Autom ICA 2013*, 222–226
21. Pu J, Jiang Y, Xie X, Chen X, Liu M, Xu S (2018) Low cost sensor network for obstacle avoidance in share-controlled smart wheelchairs under daily scenarios. Microelectron Reliab 83(March):180–186
22. Rahman JRB, Rahman MS (2019) Joystick controlled industrial robotoc system with robotic arm. In 2019 IEEE International Conference on Robotics, Automation, Artificial-intelligence and Internet of Things (RAAICON), pp 10–13
23. Rabhi Y, Mrabet M, Fnaiech F (2016) Optimized joystick control interface for electric powered wheelchairs. 16th Int Conf Sci Tech Autom Control Comput Eng STA 2015, 201–206
24. Palya WL, Doyle AF (1978) A relay driver and contact closure sensing interface for an LSI-11 DRV11 parallel I/O board. Behav Res Methods Instrum 10(4):485–487
25. Morarka AR (2016) Demonstration model of self inductance using relay. Resonance 21 (5):457–465
26. Rathore DK (2014), A Novel Multipurpose Smart Wheelchair. In 2014 IEEE Students' Conference on Electrical, Electronics and Computer Science, pp 2–5
27. Sreejith T (2018) Trackball Controlled Novel, Cost Effective Electric Wheelchair. In 2018 International Conference on Control, Power, Communication and Computing Technologies (ICCPCCT), pp 205–209
28. Rahulanker R, Ramanarayanan V (2006) Battery assisted wheel chair. Proc India Int Conf Power Electron IICPE 2006(3):167–171

Comparison of the Effects of Feature Selection and Tree-Based Ensemble Machine Learning for Sentiment Analysis on Indonesian YouTube Comments

Siti Khomsah, Ahmad Fathan Hidayatullah, and Agus Sasmito Aribowo

Abstract The main problems in sentiment analysis models on Indonesian YouTube comments are unstructured data and low classification accuracy. Sentiment analysis for Indonesian, which is different from English, requires proper preprocessing and classification methods. Previous research usually using Linear Support Vector Machine (SVM), Naïve Bayes and Decision Tree. Although the accuracy of SVM is better than other algorithms, it still needs to be improved. This study aims to compare the performance of the tree-based ensemble method and feature selection to improve the sentiment analysis model for Indonesian YouTube comments. This research crawled Indonesian YouTube comments from different domains and produce ten datasets. The preprocessing's method in this research was removed stopword, convert slang words, and stemming. For feature selection, we tested two vectorizer method, i.e. Term Frequency (TF) or Term Frequency/Inverse Document Frequency (TF-IDF). The model build using six machine learning, consist of four tree-based ensemble machine learning to raise better accuracy, Linear SVM and Decision Tree. We use tree-based ensemble machine learning, they are Random Forest, and Extra Tree represents bagging ensemble. AdaBoost and Gradient Boosting represent boosting ensemble. SVM and Decision tree as a comparison. Based on experiments by combining feature selection and ensemble machine learning, it can be concluded that the type of vectorizer has little effect on

S. Khomsah (✉)
Department of Data Science, Institut Teknologi Telkom Purwokerto, Jawa Tengah, Indonesia
e-mail: siti@ittelkom-pwt.ac.id

A. F. Hidayatullah
Department of Informatics, Universitas Islam Indonesia, Daerah Istimewa Yogyakarta, Indonesia
e-mail: fathan@uii.ac.id

A. S. Aribowo
Department of Informatics, Universitas Pembangunan Nasional Veteran Yogyakarta, Daerah Istimewa Yogyakarta, Indonesia
e-mail: sasmito.skom@upnyk.ac.id

H. Triwiyanto et al. (eds.), *Proceedings of the 1st International Conference on Electronics, Biomedical Engineering, and Health Informatics*, Lecture Notes in Electrical Engineering 746, https://doi.org/10.1007/978-981-33-6926-9_15

classification accuracy. In all experiments, the best machine learning methods are Extra Tree with an accuracy of 93.39% and AdaBoost with an accuracy of 92.53%. Whereas, the use of TF or TF-IDF does not significantly affect accuracy.

Keywords Sentiment analysis · Indonesian YouTube comments · Tree-based ensemble machine learning · Feature selection · TF-IDF

1 Introduction

Extracting the sentiment from Indonesian YouTube comments is still a challenge. The comments on each video contain a lot of slang word, incomplete written word, expression word, emoticon, which is a challenge in text preprocessing [1]. The stages in sentiment analysis are text preprocessing, namely stopword removal, slang words conversion, tokenizing, and stemming. In previous research, we have conducted several preprocessing models [2], focusing on slang word handling solutions. That research proves that the conversion of slang words into vocabulary, according to KBBI (Indonesian dictionary) rose accuracy. We continue our previous study in this research, focus on feature selection and the machine learning phases. The feature selection phase is text vectorization, which is converting Bag Of Word (BoW) into vectors and calculating the weight of its vectors. The vector having high weight is a selected feature. Feature selection can affect the performance of the model in carrying out the classification process. The most popular Bag of Word (BoW) vectorizations is the Term- Frequency (TF) and Term-Frequency-Inverse Document Frequency (TF-IDF) [3]. The datasets of each domain have their typical features, which is a problem on the vectorization stage that must be resolved. Hence, the research to choose a vectorization method has to do to find out which is method produces the right features to gain high accuracy.

The modelling stage is an essential part of the sentiment analysis. At this stage, choosing the right machine learning for a dataset is a problem that needs to be solved. The machine learning method in sentiment analysis affects the performance of the model, especially for the Indonesian language corpus. Researcher develops many kinds of machine learning algorithms. However, the stability of machine learning also needs to be tested on the sentiment analysis model. Kanakaraj and Guidetti [4] investigated that ensemble machine learning better than standard machine learning. Ensemble increases the accuracy of the classification model on independent features.

Our research uses opinion datasets downloaded from YouTube video comments in Indonesian, which are obtained from two major domains, namely the political domain (elections) in Indonesia and the domain of Indonesian government policies related to the handling of the COVID-19 pandemic in Indonesia. We choose five different datasets from each domain. Overall, we will process ten datasets. In feature selection stage uses two methods, namely TF and TF-IDF. Several ensemble machine learning applies in each selected feature to investigate the best combination of feature selection and machine learning methods that increase accuracy.

This study will evaluate the accuracy of four decision tree-based ensemble machine learning models for five opinion datasets in Indonesian. The ensemble machine learning methods which will be assessed are Random Forest, AdaBoost, Gradient Boosting, and Extra Tree. We use SVM and Decision Tree as a comparison from previous studies. The expected result is a new model, which is a combination of the best preprocessing model of the previous research [5], the best vectorization methods, and the best machine learning of tree ensemble-based machine learning. We aim to raise accuracy by more than 85% on most of the tested datasets.

2 Literature Review

This section presents several articles related to sentiment analysis on YouTube video comments in Indonesian, in the last five years. The first research is the use of word embedding with the convolutional neural networks (CNN) for sentiment analysis in Indonesian. This research also applies to TF-IDF vectorization. The accuracy only reaches 76.2% [5]. These results require better methods for increasing accuracy.

Another study is sentiment analysis on YouTube comments using SVM. This research uses 1000 samples data and gets an accuracy of 84%, precision 91%, and recall 80% [6]. It needs to be tested on various types of datasets with more records. The next research is the use of SVM for YouTube comments for cyberbullying classification. This research shows the result of accuracy only 79,412% [7]. Other study using SVM with linear kernel function, yield accuracy only 62.76% [8].

Other studies in sentiment analysis usually apply to a single domain. This study uses lazy machine learning, such as K-Nearest Neighbor gets an accuracy of 95% [9]. These results need to be attempted on many kinds of datasets from different domains. Another study developed a combination of K-Nearest Neighbor and Levenshtein Distance. This combination only gets an accuracy of 65,625% [10]. Another study that combines several machine learning methods is the combination of the Naive Bayes and Decision Tree Classifier but does not report its accuracy [11]. Combining Naive Bayes and SVM produces an accuracy of 91%, recall of 83%, and F1-score of 87%, but has not yet been tested on datasets from several domains [12]. In similar research, using Naive Bayes for sentiment analysis in the data movie trailer achieves accuracy, precision, and recall, respectively, 81%, 74.83%, and 75.22% [13]. In categorizing sentiment-fanaticism uses tree-based machine learning, Random Forest reaches an accuracy of 91.8%. However, this research also has not yet been conducted on data from multiple domains [14].

Based on the literature review above, most of the previous studies used Naive Bayes and SVM as classifier and TF-IDF as vectorizer. Usually, SVM provides high accuracy [15], so this research use SVM methods as a comparison of tree ensemble-based methods such as Random Forest, AdaBoost, Gradient Boosting and Extra Tree Classifier. We expect these tree ensemble-based methods to achieve high accuracy in the sentiment analysis of Indonesian languages. Bootstrap Aggregating (Bagging) is one of the ensembles using a voting mechanism to increase accuracy [16] if combining with certain feature-selection. Furthermore, boosting such as AdaBoost or Gradient Boosting is the best ensemble's technic to increase accuracy [17]. The boosting theory works by finding weak learning conditions and then fix them to become robust learning. Otherhand, AdaBoost has the capability to mapping data, which is hard to classify into class [18]. Gradient boosting works well when it is using uni-gram features [19].

3 Method

This research aims to compare effect using different feature selection and classification model using tree-based ensemble machine learning in sentiment analysis model. The research steps consisted of data preparation, features word selection, and build a classifier model. The research steps begin with data-crawling followed by labelling, data cleaning, vectorization, modelling, and evaluation, as shown in Fig. 1.

3.1 Data Preparation

This study uses comment's datasets from YouTube. Data preparation consists of data crawling and labelling.

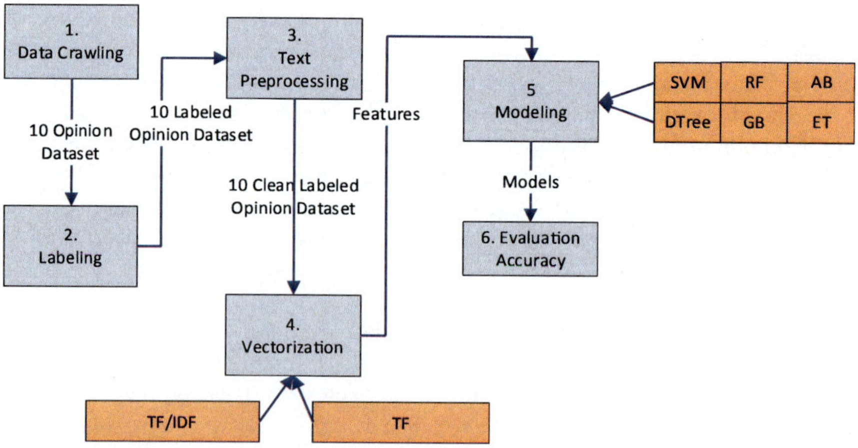

Fig. 1 Research steps

Data Crawling. We choose the YouTube channel of national news office and television station, and they are Metro TV News, TribunNews, Kompas TV, and VIVA.co.id as the data source. There are two groups of datasets used in this study. In the first group datasets, we download comments on the video about government policies related to COVID-19. First, we search from those channel based on keywords from five policies and regulations in Indonesia related to the COVID-19 pandemic. The five keywords are (1) psbb or policy about large-scale social restrictions, (2) listrik gratis or policy about free electricity programs, (3) bantuan tunai or policy about cash donations, (4) import obat or rule about import drugs, and kartu prakerja or pre-employment card. The dataset obtained with the keyword psbb is stored under the name covid 1, dataset from keyword listrik gratis stored as covid 2, the dataset from the keyword bantuan tunai named as covid 3, the dataset from the keyword import obat named as covid 4, and dataset from the keyword kartu prakerja named as covid 5. The second group dataset is crawled from the videos of the 2019 Indonesian presidential candidates debate, namely debate 1, debate 2, debate 3, debate 4, and debate 5.

Data Labeling. Data-labeling is a process of marking the type of sentiment for each comment. We use two sentiment labels, positive and negative. The annotation method refers to previous research [2]. In [2], some comments are labelled by annotators who understand Indonesian. Then, the researcher makes a program logic that is formed based on some of the labelled data, and then the program is used to determine other unlabeled comment data. A summary of the dataset after labelling is shown in Table 1.

3.2 Text-Preprocessing and Vectorization

Text Preprocessing. Text-preprocessing is a step to clean data from noise, including punctuation, converting slang words to formal word, remove stop word, and stemming as in research [2].

Vectorization. For vectorization of feature uses unigram. Unigram is a single word feature. For example, the sentence psbb policy makes you confused produces four features, namely policy, psbb, you, makes, confused. Furthermore, all features will be converted into a vector in numbers to represent them.

This study uses two vectorizations, namely the frequency of the terms (TF) and Term-Frequency-Inverse-Document-Frequency (TF-IDF). These vectorization techniques will be investigated toward their effects on classifiers. The equations of two types of vectorization are shown in Eqs. (1), (2), and (3).

$$TF(i,j) = \frac{Term\, i\, frequency\, in\, document\, j}{Total\, words\, in\, document\, j} \tag{1}$$

Table 1 Datasets

No	Dataset	Positive	Negative	Total
1	Covid 5	874	590	1464
2	Covid 4	1029	661	1690
3	Covid 3	1368	371	1739
4	Debate 2	1351	866	2217
5	Debate 4	1878	1235	3113
6	Covid 1	2462	2382	4844
7	Covid 2	3211	1651	4862
8	Debate 3	3868	2219	6087
9	Debate 1	4345	3061	7406
10	Debate 5	10,987	8852	19,839

Notes
Covid 1: local lockdown dataset
Covid 2: electricity subsidies for the people's dataset
Covid 3: cash donations for poor people's dataset
Covid 4: drugs import's dataset
Covid 5: Unemployed card's dataset
Debate 1: The first round of the Indonesian presidential candidate debate, 2019
Debate 2: The second round of the Indonesian presidential candidate debate, 2019
Debate 3: The third round of the Indonesian presidential candidate debate, 2019
Debate 4: The fourth round of the Indonesian presidential candidate debate, 2019
Debate 5: The fifth round of the Indonesian presidential candidate debate, 2019

$$IDF(i) = \mathrm{Log}_2\left(\frac{Total\,documents}{documents\,with\,term\,i}\right) \tag{2}$$

$$TF - IDF(Score\,for\,term\,i\,in\,document\,j) = TF(i,j) * IDF(i) \tag{3}$$

where:
TF = Term Frequency
IDF = Inverse Document Frequency
t = Term
j = Document

3.3 Modelling

This research will evaluate tree-based ensemble machine learning in several datasets. We compare several algorithms, such as Decision Tree, Random Forest, AdaBoost, Gradient Boosting, and ExtraTree.

Decision-Tree algorithm that will arrange the features of the training data into a tree model for classification (see Fig. 2). Decision-trees branches are a classification question. The arrows are the values of the answers, and the leaves are the classes.

The foremost step in building a tree structure is to choose the main attribute as root, create a branch for each value, then divide the data into the branches that are created. The process is repeated in all branches until all data in the branch has a homogeneous class. Decision Trees usually overfits the data it is learning from because it learns from only one pathway of decisions. Predictions from a single Decision Tree usually do not make accurate predictions on new data [20].

Bootstrap aggregating (Bagging) is an ensemble learning method that aims to enhance the predictive performance by combining classifiers trained on different training sets obtained from the original training set by sampling with replacement. Example of the bagging algorithm is Random Forest and Extra Tree. Random Forest is the enhance of a Decision Tree. Random Forest builds many trees in the same way as a Decision Tree using the dataset. Random Forest reduces overfitting by building multiple trees, bootstrapping, and splitting nodes using the best split among a random subset of features selected at every node. An example of making many trees is in Fig. 2. Each data will be tested on every tree that is formed to determine its class. The final data class decision is the majority class that results from the trees (majority class).

There are several experiment result showed that sentiment analysis system using random forest give a good performance [21] (Fig. 3). Extra Tree algorithm or known as well Extremely Randomized Trees. This algorithm is almost like a Random Forest, divide the dataset into clusters to build many trees and split nodes randomly, but not using bootstrap (sample without replacement), and nodes are divided using random splits, not by the best split. The final classification is the majority class that results from these trees [22].

Boosting algorithm is an ensemble learning which aims to enhance the predictive performance by training the algorithms recursively on different sampling distributions. Gradient boosting generates learners during the learning process, it builds the first learner to predict the values/labels of samples and calculates the loss sample, which is different between the outcome of the first learner and the real value. It then builds a second learner to predict the loss after the first step. The step

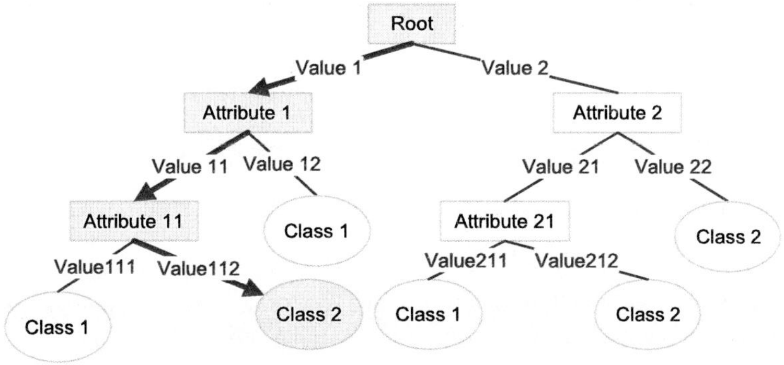

Fig. 2 Decision tree

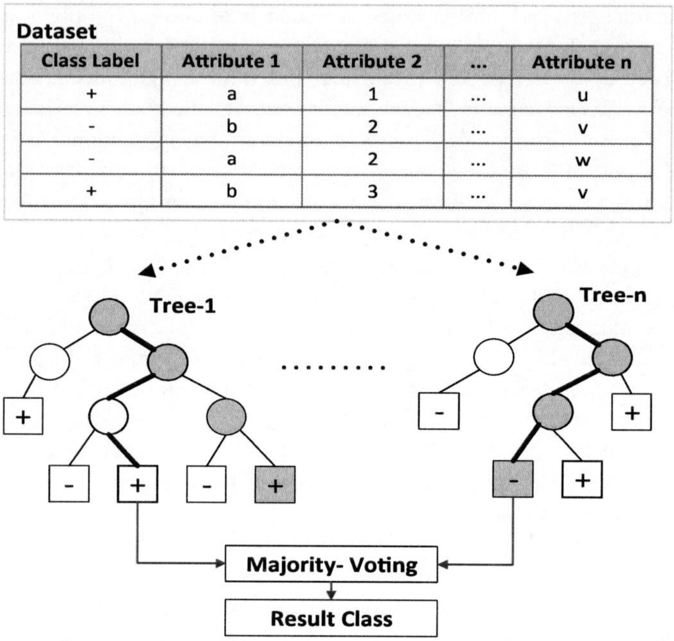

Fig. 3 Random forest

continues to learn the third, fourth, and so on, until a certain threshold. AdaBoost is an algorithm ensemble that uses loss functions to improve accuracy. Adaboost has the characteristics of speed, durability, and simplicity. AdaBoost requires users to specify a set of weak learners. Alternatively, AdaBoost will randomly generate a set of weak learners before the real learning process. It will learn the weights of how to add these learners to be a strong learner. The process is repeated until convergence [17, 18].

3.4 Evaluation Accuracy

The dataset is divided into 80% as training data and 20% as testing data. Data training is used for modelling and testing data to evaluate model performance. The confusion matrix (Table 2) used to compare the predicted results and the actual conditions of the model results.

From the confusion matrix, accuracy values will be calculated using Eq. (4). Accuracy is a measure of how many actual class values are the same as the predicted class, the number of true positive (TP), and true-negative (TN).

Table 2 Confusion matrix

		Actual Class	
		Positive	Negative
Predicted class	Positive	True Positive (TP)	False Positive (FP)
	Negative	False Negative (FN)	True Negative (TN)

$$Accuracy = \frac{(TP + TN)}{(TP + FP + TN + FN)} \quad (4)$$

4 Results and Discussion

Table 3 shows that in the experiment using TF, the best machine learning is Extra Tree with a maximum accuracy of 93.39%. Extra tree achieves the maximum accuracy on 5 of 10 datasets. Compared to SVM, only the AdaBoost and ExtraTree methods have better accuracy on all datasets. The results of the second scenario experiment for the TF-IDF feature extractor on 10 (ten) datasets with 6 (six) machine learning models are in Table 4.

Table 3 shows that in an experiment using TF, the best machine learning accuracy is Extra Tree. Maximum accuracy is 93,39%, and extra tree reaches the maximum accuracy on 5 of 10 datasets. The highlight marks in Table 3 indicate the maximum accuracy in each dataset. When compared to SVM, only the AdaBoost and ExtraTree methods have better accuracy in all datasets. The results of the

Table 3 Accuracy results of sentiment analysis models using TF feature extractor and six machine learning on ten datasets

Dataset	Non-ensemble		Ensemble			
	SVM (%)	Decision tree (%)	Random forest (%)	Gradient boosting (%)	AdaBoost (%)	Extra tree (%)
Covid 1	83.90	84.93	85.45	84.11	*89.68*	89.58
Covid 2	84.69	82.32	76.36	76.46	*86.33*	86.23
Covid 3	88.51	92.24	89.37	84.20	92.53	*93.39*
Covid 4	85.50	89.64	89.35	87.87	*90.83*	90.24
Covid 5	78.16	82.25	80.20	80.20	84.64	*86.35*
Debate 1	85.02	85.76	85.09	84.41	88.53	*88.66*
Debate 2	76.35	83.33	80.86	82.43	84.68	*85.36*
Debate 3	84.24	85.71	82.68	83.66	86.86	*87.11*
Debate 4	80.90	82.34	86.52	83.47	87.96	87.48
Debate 5	88.38	87.25	86.59	85.81	89.59	89.44

Table 4 Accuracy results of sentiment analysis models using TF-IDF feature extractor and six machine learning on ten datasets

Dataset	Non-ensemble		Ensemble			
	SVM (%)	Decision tree (%)	Random forest (%)	Gradient boosting (%)	AdaBoost (%)	Extra tree (%)
Covid 1	86.38	84.42	86.79	84.21	88.24	*88.65*
Covid 2	81.50	82.43	77.29	77.70	*86.13*	85.51
Covid 3	85.63	92.82	92.53	84.77	91.67	***92.82***
Covid 4	85.80	88.46	88.17	89.94	*90.24*	*90.24*
Covid 5	77.82	82.59	82.59	81.23	84.64	*87.71*
Debate 1	85.70	84.68	83.67	84.75	87.31	*87.92*
Debate 2	80.86	83.78	80.41	82.88	83.56	83.56
Debate 3	84.56	*83.17*	83.17	83.50	*86.45*	86.29
Debate 4	82.50	81.54	85.87	83.47	86.20	*87.00*
Debate 5	88.26	86.19	87.45	85.79	*89.31*	89.16

TF-IDF feature extractor experiment on 10 (ten) datasets with 6 (six) machine learning models are in Table 4.

Table 4 shows that in the experiment using TF-IDF the best machine learning is Extra Tree with a maximum accuracy of 92.82% and extra tree achieves the maximum accuracy on 6 of 10 datasets. The highlight marks in Table 4 indicate the maximum accuracy in each dataset. When compared to SVM, only AdaBoost and Extra Tree have better accuracy in every dataset.

When compared with the research accuracy target of 85%, the Extra Tree and AdaBoost methods have provided accuracy exceeding the target in 80% of all datasets. These two algorithms are considered to achieve the target.

The accuracy of the ensemble method is substantially higher than that of the non-ensemble. The ensemble model that we propose is expected to achieve higher accuracy.

Based on all the experiments above, the machine learning that achieves the best accuracy is Extra Tree, then AdaBoost. However, the difference between the accuracy performance of Adaboost and Extra Tree is not significant. On some datasets, Adaboost is better, while Extra Tree achieves high accuracy on others. These results do not show the consistency of the performance of the two algorithms, Adaboost and Extra Tree, and this needs to be investigated further why this happens.

Target. However, in general, the accuracy of ensemble methods better than previous studies. In previous studies, using word embedding combining with CNN achieve the accuracy of 76.2% [5], while use SVM with a classification accuracy of 84% [6], 79.412% [7] and 62.76% [8]. Model in our study also better than research that was using K-Nearest Neighbor and Levenshtein Distance (65,625%) [10], and using Naive Bayes (81%) [13].

Now, if we observed in Tables 3 and 4, using TF or TF-IDF as feature extraction does not show a significant difference in the accuracy results. So that at the feature extraction stage, both methods are equally good.

5 Conclusions

This study aims to find the best method of machine learning in both non-ensemble and tree-based ensembles, and also to compare the effect of selecting a feature sections method toward sentiment analysis models on YouTube Indonesia comments. Based on the research results, several conclusions were obtained. We found that ensemble machine learning was better than non-ensemble. The Extra Tree and Ada Boost methods yield higher accuracy than Random Forest and Gradient Boosting. Meanwhile, the feature selection method, either TF or TF-IDF, has no significant effect on machine learning accuracy. In the next study, the accuracy performance of the Extra Tree should be tested on various types of dataset domains, and the amount of data varies from small to large.

References

1. Musdholifah A, Rinaldi E (2018) FVEC feature and machine learning approach for Indonesian opinion mining on YouTube comments. In: Proceeding of EECSI, pp 724–729
2. Khomsah S, Aribowo AS (2020) Text-preprocessing model youtube comments in indonesian. RESTI 4(4):648–654
3. Kaur S, Kumar P, Kumaraguru P (2019) Automating fake news detection system using multi-level voting model. Soft Comput 24(12):9049–9069
4. Kanakaraj M, Guddeti RMR (2015) Performance Analysis of Ensemble Methods on Twitter Sentiment Analysis using NLP Techniques. In: Proceedings of the 2015 IEEE 9th International Conference on Semantic Computing, IEEE ICSC 2015, pp 169–170
5. Savigny J, Purwarianti A (2017) Emotion Classification on Youtube Comments Using Word Embedding. In: International Conference on Advanced Informatics: Concepts, Theory and Applications, pp 1–5
6. Tanesab FI, Sembiring I, Purnomo HD (2017) Sentiment Analysis Model Based on Youtube Comment Using Support Vector Machine. Int J Comput Sci Softw Eng (IJCSSE) 6(8):180–185 [Online]. Available: http://ijcsse.org/published/volume6/issue8/p2-V6I8.pdf
7. Andriansyah M et al. (2018) Cyberbullying Comment Classification on Indonesian Selebgram Using Support Vector Machine Method. In: Proceedings of the 2nd International Conference on Informatics and Computing, ICIC 2017, pp 1–5
8. Rinaldi E, Musdholifah A (2017) FVEC-SVM for Opinion Mining on Indonesian Comments of YouTube Video. In: Proceedings of 2017 International Conference on Data and Software Engineering, ICoDSE 2017, pp 1–5
9. Abraham MP, Udaya Kumar Reddy KR (2020) Feature based sentiment analysis of mobile product reviews using machine learning techniques. Int J Adv Trends Comput Sci Eng 9 (2):2289–2296

10. Anggraini N, Tursina MJ (2019) Sentiment Analysis of School Zoning System on Youtube Social Media Using the K-Nearest Neighbor with Levenshtein Distance Algorithm. In: 2019 7th International Conference on Cyber and IT Service Management, CITSM 2019, May, pp 1–4
11. Maisal RA, Hidayanto AN, Ayuning Budi NF, Abidin Z, Purbasari A (2019) Analysis of Sentiments on Indonesian YouTube Video Comments: Case Study of the Indonesian Government's Plan to Move the Capital City. In Proceedings—1st International Conference on Informatics, Multimedia, Cyber and Information System, ICIMCIS 2019, pp 121–124
12. Muhammad AN, Bukhori S, Pandunata P (2019) Sentiment Analysis of Positive and Negative of YouTube Comments Using Naïve Bayes-Support Vector Machine (NBSVM) Classifier. In: Proceedings International Conference on Computer Science, Information Technology, and Electrical Engineering, ICOMITEE 2019, vol 1, pp 199–205
13. Risky Novendri CEP, Syafarani Callista A, Naufal Pratama D (2020) Sentiment Analysis of YouTube Movie Trailer Comments Using Naïve Bayes. Bull Comput Sci Electr Eng 1(1):1–5
14. Aribowo AS, Basiron H, Herman NS, Khomsah S (2020) Fanaticism Category Generation Using Tree-Based Machine Learning Method. J Phys: Conf Ser 1501(1)
15. Sultana N, Islam MM (2020) Meta Classifier-Based Ensemble Learning For Sentiment Classification. In: Proceedings of International Joint Conference on Computational Intelligence, Algorithms for Intelligent Systems, pp 73–84
16. Pong-Inwong C, Kaewmak K (2016) Improved Sentiment Analysis for Teaching Evaluation Using Feature Selection and Voting Ensemble Learning Integration Chakrit. In Proceedings 2016 of 2nd IEEE International Conference on Computer and Communications, pp 1222–1225
17. Onan A, Korukoğlu S, Bulut H (2016) LDA-based Topic Modelling in Text Sentiment Classification: An Empirical Analysis. Int J Comput Linguist Appl 7(1):101–119
18. Cao Y, Miao Q-G, Liu J-C, Gao L (2013) Advance and Prospects of AdaBoost Algorithm. Acta Autom Sin 39(6):745–758
19. Alzamzami F, Hoda M, El Saddik A (2020) Light Gradient Boosting Machine for General Sentiment Classification on Short Texts: A Comparative Evaluation. IEEE Access 8:101840–101858
20. Sharma H, Kumar S (2016) A Survey on Decision Tree Algorithms of Classification in Data Mining. Int J Sci Res (IJSR) 5(4):2094–2097
21. Fauzi MA (2018) Random Forest Approach for Sentiment Analysis in Indonesian Language. Indones J Electr Eng Comput Sci 12(1):46–50
22. Vanegas MI, Ghilardi MF, Kelly SP, Blangero A (2018) Machine learning for EEG-based biomarkers in Parkinson's disease. In: 2018 IEEE International Conference on Bioinformatics and Biomedicine (BIBM), pp 2661–2665

Assessing Beads Generation in Fabricating Nanofiber Bioactive Material-Based Associated with Its Fluid Factors

Muhammad Yusro

Abstract Nanofiber materials for biomedical applications inevitably need to control their morphology to reach their best performance. However, it has a challenge regarding occurring beads formation during the fabrication process. Even though beads shape has already observed in numerous nanofiber experiments, a deeper study regarding a bead formation particularly related to fluid factors in bioactive materials have not reported yet. The main objective of this report is to elaborate the beads development particularly in fabrication nanofiber bioactive material-based and to investigate the result associated with the fluid factors (viscosity, conductivity, and surface tension). In this research, bioactive material chitosan (positive charge) and pectin (negative charge) are mixed with PVA (an electrospinnable polymer) in assorted composition PVA/Chitosan-Pectin (v:v) specifically 90/10, 80/20, 70/30, and 60/40. Based on quantification, 90/10 had 15 beads and got 92.7±19.59 μm^2 of average area. In 80/20 composition, it had 57 beads with 121.83±19.78 μm^2 average area. For 70/30, it had 86 beads with 111.6±24.46 μm^2. And 60/40 had 117 beads with 129.8±19.13 μm^2 average area. The result showed that the bigger bioactive material added to system, the more beads are formed. Regarding fluid factors, viscosity found that it had an opposite correlation with beads formation. Meanwhile, the relationship between conductivity and surface tension were observed complemented associated with beads formation. In the bead precision perspective, interestingly, the non-uniformity of the bead shape had no relation with fluids factors proofed by its average area and standard deviation in respective composition.

Keywords Bead · Electrospinning · Nanofiber

M. Yusro (✉)
Department of Biomedical Engineering, Institut Teknologi Telkom Purwokerto, Kawasan Pendidikan Telkom, Jl. D.I. Panjaitan No 128, Jawa Tengah, Indonesia
e-mail: yusro@ittelkom-pwt.ac.id

H. Triwiyanto et al. (eds.), *Proceedings of the 1st International Conference on Electronics, Biomedical Engineering, and Health Informatics*, Lecture Notes in Electrical Engineering 746, https://doi.org/10.1007/978-981-33-6926-9_16

1 Introduction

In biomedical application, it is common to use bioactive material as a substance to create medical product. The reason behind that, it is because by using bioactive material the functionality of medical product become higher comparing to the conventional material. For instance, it has been known that by using material which has positive charge such as Chitosan attracts more osteoblast cell [1] and could promote wound healing faster [2].

It also has been reported that bioactive material is used in fabricating nanofiber material using electrospinning method for various application. The fabrication nanofiber based on biomaterial needs to manage influenced factor particularly fluids factor [3]. Fluid factor is the parameter that come out based of material characteristic that are dissolved by a specific solvent to make a solution. Viscosity, conductivity, and surface tension has been reported as the big three factors that affect the fiber result [3]. Even tough electrospinning is mentioned as the most effective way to fabricate nanofiber, the product of this method confronts the challenging problems such as bead formation. Fabricating nanofiber by electrospinning is tricky caused by variables that have to be controlled to achieved proper result.

This report studies the relationship between beads formation and three fluid parameters to see the association between them in bioactive material solution. Bead is the morphological shape that commonly occur in the process of fabrication nanofiber that generate by certain influenced factor. It has been reported that surface tension is the factor that contribute to this event and the answer to tackle this problem is by engineered the solvent [4–6]. In biomedical implementation, increasing chemical liquid similar to the solvents into the living system is creating a new problem because it makes a toxic environment to surrounding life cells. In this research the solvent had minimum concentration that was 1.5% acetic acid. This research design imposes finding alternative solution through fluid factor assessment to reduce bead development. Hopefully, this study could help the community to decrease the result instability and gain the better product in morphological perspective especially in implementing bioactive material for biomedical application.

2 Material and Method

2.1 Electrospinning Set up

In this research, the electrospinning is assembled by three components, namely: (1) High power supply, (2) Syringe Pump, and (3) Flat Collector. This machine is built by Hakaku Instrument and it is placed in Laboratorium Penelitian Terpadu Universitas Gadjah Mada (LPPT UGM), Indonesia.

In this study, the setting variable is suited based on recommended value which is usually make stable result in that laboratory. The distance between needle and collector is set in 12 cm. The power supply is fixed in stable value which is 15 kV. The flow rate of solution is situated around 1.5 ml/hour. Regarding the dimension of needle, the 0.55 mm diameter is chosen as recommended size.

2.2 *Making the Liquid Solutions*

Assorted mixed solution is created to see the limitation of nanofiber production. Chitosan-Pectin is mixed in 1:1 (v:v) composition based on reported value in particular biomedical application [1]. To enhance the liquid ability to transform into the fibers, PVA, the well- known electrospinnable and biocompatible material, has been added to the liquid composition. It can be seen in Fig. 2 that the various composition has designed to understand the boundary of this experiment.

The material of solution consists of (1) Local Chitosan with Degree of deacetylation $\geq 90\%$ made by Medical Grade PT. Biotech Surindo, Cirebon, Indonesia. (2) High Metoxyil Pectin with Degree of Esterification > 50 made by Cargill, Germany. (3) PVA Gohsenol with production code C1210A57 from P.T. Brataco. (4) 1.5% Acetic Acid that is used as a solvent diluted from Acetic Acid (Glacial) 100% Merck KgaA, Germany, and last component (5) Aquabidest Sterile Water for Irrigation U.S.P. from PT. Otsuka Indonesia.

In Fig. 1, it can be seen that the research design is starting with making a solution composition from 100% PVA as a control then it is reduced by following composition 90/10 until pure chitosan-pectin 100%. Then, the liquid is loaded into electrospinning to create the nanofiber. The liquid compositions also have been investigated by their fluid parameters namely viscosity, conductivity, and surface tension. In this research the mixed composition only assessed until 50/50 because in

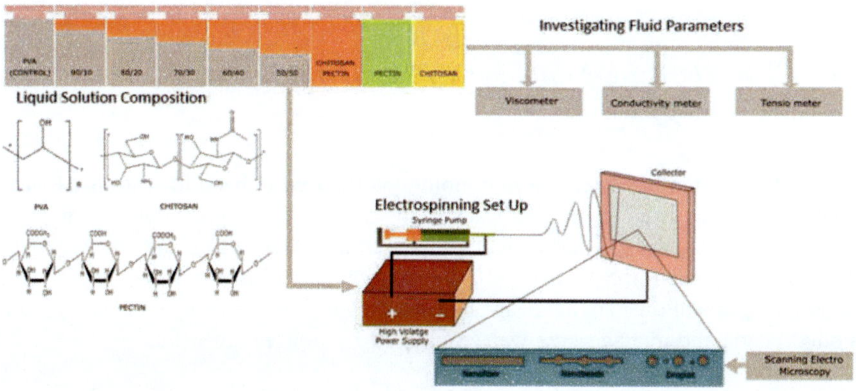

Fig. 1 Schematic research design

that property, the liquid cannot transform to the fiber. The reason behind that it is because the conductivity is too high so the process elongation and stretch make the fiber discontinued [3]. Finally, the result of the electrospinning process is observed in SEM to see their morphology that can be as a nanofiber, beads, or the droplet.

2.3 Investigating Solution Parameters

One of the objectives of this report is to understand the relationship between beads formation and parameters which are viscosity, conductivity, and surface tension. Viscosity parameter is counted by Ostwald viscometer. The density of certain liquid counted by deducting mass of pycnometer filled by certain liquid with empty pycnometer. The prepared liquid is filled in capillary pipe and then the duration of moving liquid from up line to bottom line is counted as flow of water. This measurement is conducted in three repetitions. The viscosity value can be counted with formula if liquid density and duration is counted. Conductivity is related to magnitude of charge density in liquid. Initial procedure to measure conductivity are doing calibration and then the sample solutions are poured to the beaker glass. The top of rod of conductivity meter is dipped to prepared solutions. The value of conductivity will be show in the screen. This counting method conducted in three repetitions and for each repetition, the top of the rod is cleaned by aquabidest until it is shown 0 μS. This step is necessary to prevent error in counting. Surface tension is measured by Du-Nouy ring method. This method employing force which is pulled from the ring. This force is equivalent with surface tension of the solution [7]. The initial procedure in this step is calibrating the surface potentiometer and preparing solution in beaker glass then loaded to surface tensiometer. The ring of surface tensiometer dipped until the increasing of the surface tensiometer becoming stable. This procedure conducted in three repetitions. For sterilization, the ring need to be burned by 70% alcohol.

2.4 Characterizing Nanofiber by Scanning Electron Microscopy (SEM)

In this research the investigating morphology is focused in bead formation. SEM is a tool that can be used to see the beads shape and size. The procedure of this step can be conducted by preparing the sample around 4 × 6 mm and coated with platinum and loaded in 5 V. SEM characterization is worked on 5000, 10,000, and 20,000 magnification. To have an analysist regarding the bead generation, the spotted beads and average area were examined by imageJ software.

3 Results

3.1 Bead Formation Increase Assorted Composition

It can be seen in Fig. 2 that the number of beads is increasing following assorted composition. For the first study, the number of beads is plotted by white spot to make investigation regarding beads distribution to be more clearly. ImageJ software is used to assessed number and size in bead generation.

To get deeper understanding regrading beads distribution, the quantification regarding bead formation is elaborated by seeing the relationship between number of beads for each composition and the area (μm²). Furthermore, each composition is separated to see the precision of shape. In this investigation, three lines is made by using standard deviation (σ). Acceptance limit line is group that has shape in region of average bead shape ±1 σ value. In this graphic, it is noted as green dots. Another group, which is warning limit line, is the region which has average ±2 value. This classes spotted as yellow dots. Meanwhile if the bead shape has a dimension more than ±2 value, it can be noticed in red dots (Fig. 3).

According to this figure, the number of beads rose following assorted composition. Based on quantification, 60/40 had the highest number of beads with 117 beads. This composition had 129, 8±19.13 μm². Meanwhile 70/30 composition reported had 86 beads and got 111, 6±24.46 μm² regarding its average area. In 80/20 composition, the number of beads was founded 57 number of beads with 121, 83 ±19.78 μm² average area. And the last one that was 90/10 composition reported that it had 15 beads and 92.7±19.59 μm² of average area. Another analysis that also can be concluded from the result was that it also could be seen that in 60/40, 70/30, and 80/20 that there were four red dots that was over warning limit line. Meanwhile in 90/10 composition there was no data that over that value. It meant that 90/10 had the most stable result regarding bead shape. To study more deeply regarding the

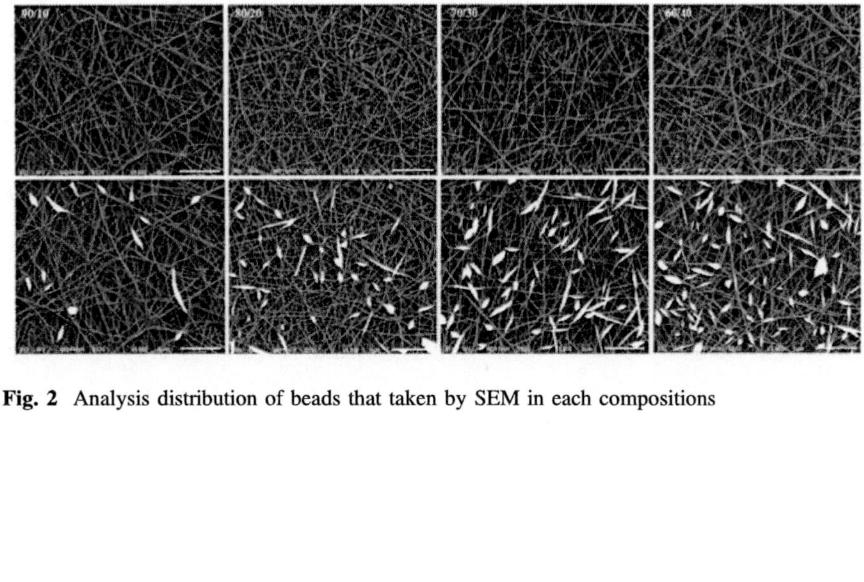

Fig. 2 Analysis distribution of beads that taken by SEM in each compositions

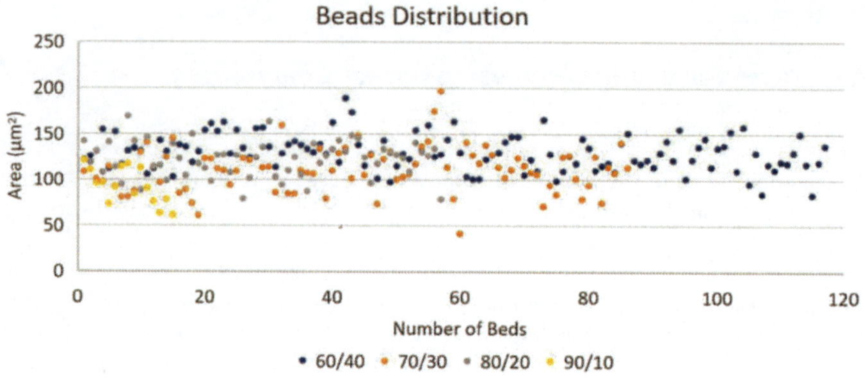

Fig. 3 Beads distribution in bioactive material system

factor that influences the result. Three parameters were investigated to see the relationship between result and the parameters and will be discuss in the following section of this report (Fig. 4).

3.2 *Investigating the Relationship Between Beads and the Parameters*

It has been informed in the previous author report that fluid parameters are the most influenced factor in bioactive material system [2]. In PVA/Chitosan-Pectin composition, fabrication nanofiber was strongly affected by conductivity. The reported analysis regarding beads formation versus three fluids factor that are viscosity, conductivity, and surface tension can be seen exclusively in Fig. 5.

Viscosity is parameter that strongly related to nanofiber formation, in the Fig. 4 blue line and orange line is opposite each other meaning that it had contrary effect to number beads generation. Another parameter conductivity is reported in the previous worked that had strongly effect related to the stretching and elongating the fibers, in material properties perspective the increasing positive charges in solution can be promoting shear flow that caused beads generation. In Fig. 4 conductivity has the same trend with beads generations. Surface tension, the most suspected parameters in this research design, based on literature regarding beads formation is made by shear flow between fluid (air) and liquid [8]. According to the figure it can be clearly seen that surface tension trend was complemented to bead generation.

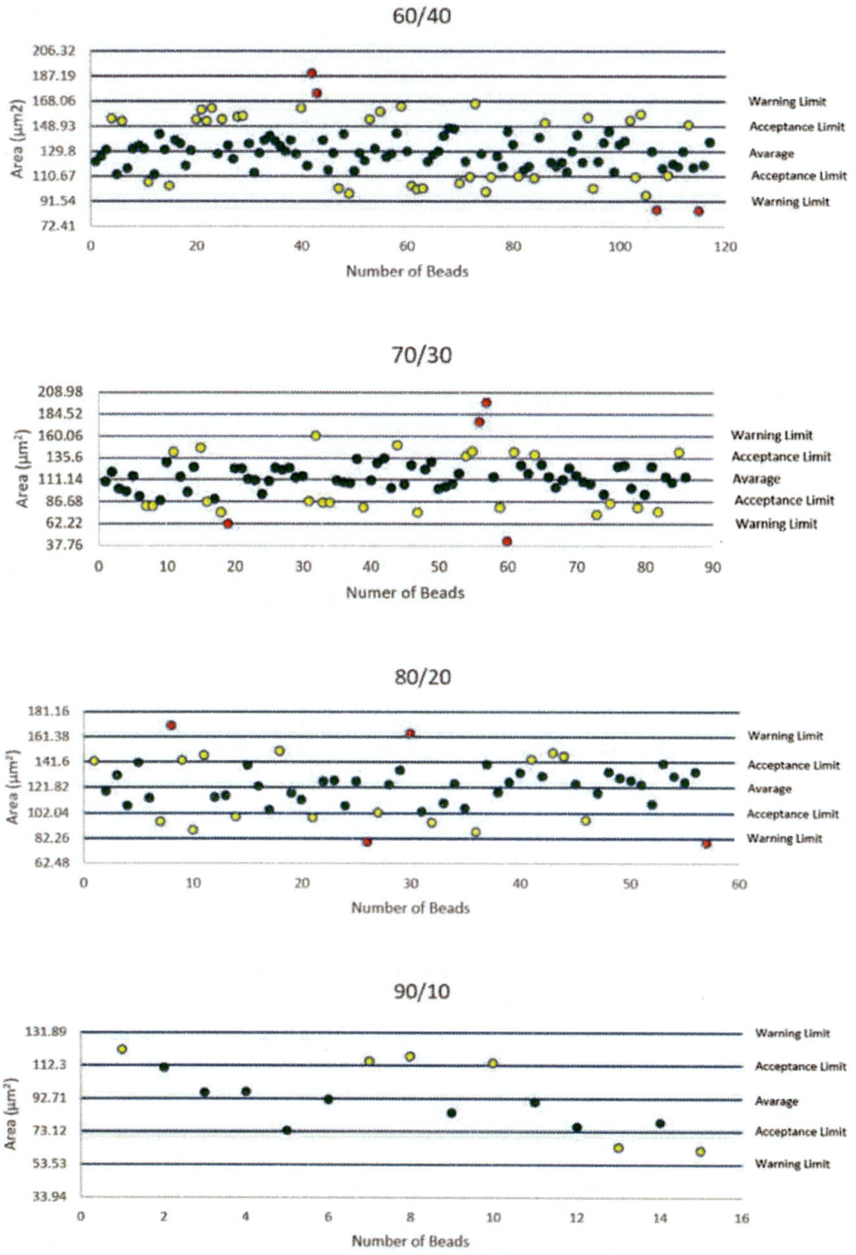

Fig. 4 Beads distribution in each composition and their classification

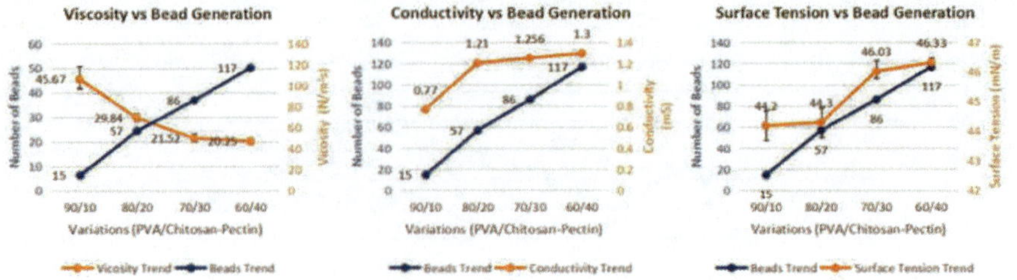

Fig. 5 The relationship between number of beads and fluid parameters

3.3 Various Bead Shape in Fabrication Process: Analytical Perspective

In electrospinning fabrication, beads dimension had been observed by SEM having various size and shape. The type of bead shape can be a ball or in a spherical form. It has been measured for consecutive sample (from 60/40 to 90/10) that the value for average area is 129.8±19.13 μm^2, 111.6±24.46 μm^2, 121.83±19.78 μm^2, and 92.7±19.59μm^2. Based on this observation, interestingly the area of fiber and standard deviation did not correlate to three parameters.

The illustration regarding interaction between three parameters and bead generation can be seen in Fig. 6. Viscosity is the parameters that related to fluid which has role to stabilize the form of fiber. When viscosity is decreasing and it became less consist, the effect of shear flow is stronger compared to condition when the viscosity restrains the fluid flow. Conductivity, the most influenced factor in bioactive material system, plays a role in rising electrostatic forces caused by its electric charge. When the electrostatic force is increasing the stretching events raising affected the shear flow. Based on Fig. 5 conductivity has the same trends with beads generation. In this bioactive composite system, the trend of surface tension is complemented with beads generation. Surface tension is the reason why fiber become spherical shape caused it is held by force that come from surface tension when it is contacted to shear flow.

4 Discussion

Bead formation is created from interaction between shear flow from the air and elongated liquid as fluid. Even though viscosity has role to hold the structure of liquid become a fiber and conductivity also plays in how strong force that is pulled to the collector, interaction between these two surfaces of fluids mainly because of their surface tension (Fig. 6). Regarding the bead distribution in this experiment, it can be seen that the higher composition of bioactive material the bigger number of beads developed. It can be correlated from Fig. 5 that conductivity and surface

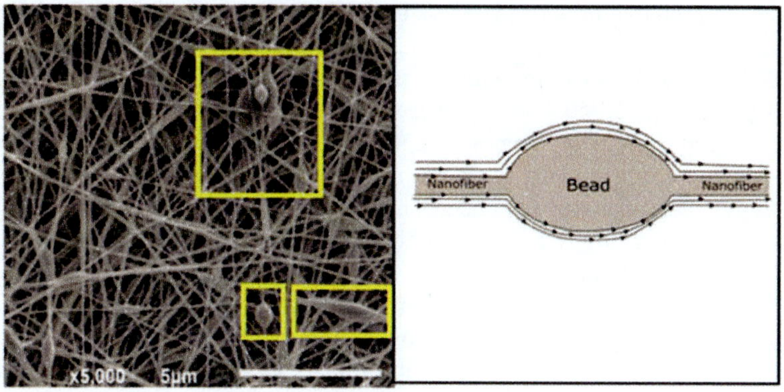

Fig. 6 Various bead size and shape and its illustration

tension are in line with bead generation. It means that in this bioactive material liquid system adding forces that caused by conductivity gain the shear flow between two fluids. Meanwhile associated with surface tension, in this system, that variable also play the biggest role. On the other hand, viscosity has opposite relation with bead generation. It is caused more viscous the liquid, the more holding power that can stabilize the fiber.

Interesting result also come up in this work related to precision beads shape. Based on this result the average area of fiber for respective compositions had no clear pattern, When the bead distribution is elaborated using the quality standard of precision, by adding $\pm 1\sigma$, $\pm 2\sigma$, and $\pm 3\sigma$, there is no significant profile that can be concluded regarding their relationship.

Understanding the event of the fabrication process, it can be seen by the forces point of view. Basically, nanofiber fabrication process is balancing three forces between electrostatic (Coulomb), hydrodynamic forces, and surface tension [9]. Furthermore, the forces also can be derived to another parameter. Electrostatic force for instance is influenced by potential differences, distance, and conductivity. Moreover, all those variables can be acquired from material characteristic, fluid properties, and instrumentation setting. It can be suggested for the theoretical force that another parameter plays in this precision and bead shape. The stability of power supply that create 15 kV potential difference can be suggested to be explore as the manipulated variable to see its effect in future research design.

5 Conclusion

It can be concluded from the experiment that investigating beads formation in bioactive material system appears with three conclusions. Firstly, bead development is increasing following the assorted composition. The higher composition of bioactive material the more bead generation is produced. For detailed, 90/10 had 15 beads and got 92.7±19.59 μm^2 of average area. In 80/20 composition, it had 57 beads with 121.83±19.78 μm^2 average area. For 70/30, it had 86 beads with 111.6 ±24.46 μm^2. And 60/40 had 117 beads with 129.8±19.13 μm^2 average area. Secondly, even though fabrication nanofiber bioactive material was reported has highly influences to conductivity. In this research, conductivity parameters reported that it is not the strongest parameters correlated to bead formation. It could be concluded, by observing relationship between surface tension and beads generation trends, that beads formation in bioactive material system was mostly influenced by surface tension. To reduce bead formation in this system, increasing viscosity could be suggested to gain more stable fiber by adding more concentration. It is can be clearly seen that the highest viscosity in the system the lowest bead formation in the result fabrication. And thirdly, regarding beads shape investigation, interestingly, those three parameters did not correlate with precision of their geometry. In the future, the following research can be conducted to see more deeply to uncover the influenced factor that affect the non-uniformity of beads dimension.

References

1. Januariyasa IK, Ana ID, Yusuf Y (2020) Nanofibrous poly(vinyl alcohol)/chitosan contained carbonated hydroxyapatite nanoparticles scaffold for bone tissue engineering. Mater Sci Eng C 107:110347. https://doi.org/10.1016/j.msec.2019.110347
2. Archana D, Dutta J, Dutta PK (2013) Evaluation of chitosan nano dressing for wound healing: Characterization, in vitro and in vivo studies. Int J Biol Macromol 57:193–203. https://doi.org/10.1016/j.ijbiomac.2013.03.002
3. Yusro M, Martien R (2020) Investigating Fluid Parameters in Nanofiber Biomaterial Fabrication using Electrospinning. J Energy Mech Mater Manuf Eng 5(1):11. https://doi.org/10.22219/jemmme.v5i1.11226
4. Mansouri F (2007) Deakin Research Online. Ethos 15(3):15–18
5. Uyar T, Besenbacher F (2008) Electrospinning of uniform polystyrene fibers: The effect of solvent conductivity. Polym (Guildf) 49(24):5336–5343. https://doi.org/10.1016/j.polymer.2008.09.025
6. Zuo W, Zhu M, Yang W, Yu H, Chen Y, Zhang Y (2005) Experimental study on relationship between jet instability and formation of beaded fibers during electrospinning. Polym Eng Sci 45(5):704–709. https://doi.org/10.1002/pen.20304
7. Indarniati I, Ermawati FU (2008) Perancangan Alat Ukur Tegangan Permukaan dengan Induksi Elektromagnetik. J Fis dan Apl 4(1):080105. https://doi.org/10.12962/j24604682.v4i1.948
8. Fong H, Chun I, Reneker DH (1999) Beaded nanofibers formed during electrospinning. Polym 40(16):4585–4592
9. Harsojo K, Triyana (2013) Harini. Studi Pembuatan PVA Nano Fiber dengan Electrospinning. Pros. Pertem. Ilm. XXVII HFI Jateng DIY, pp 16–19

Intelligent System of Handling In Vitro Fertilization (IVF) Patients Post Embryo Transfer to Reduce the Level of Patient Anxiety and Help Fertility Doctors Quickly Answer Patient Questions

Paminto Agung Christianto, Eko Sediyono, Irwan Sembiring, and Sutarto Wijono

Abstract 77.7% of IVF patients have high anxiety and 83.3% of patients have failed IVF programs. The strong desire to have a biological child and the process of IVF that is not easy, makes patients protective of the IVF process that is being undertaken. If patients experience health complaints, then patients immediately communicate with fertility doctors through the existing communication media. However, the slow time doctors give answers to patients, is a cause of increased anxiety of patients. Doctors have a strong desire to be able to quickly answer questions from patients, but are constrained by other medical activities that are the responsibility of doctors. Research aims to find a smart system method that can help IVF patients control anxiety and help fertility doctors answer questions from IVF patients. Primary data triangulation to obtain valid data, strengthened by validity testing and reliability testing. Secondary data to obtain evidence of the accuracy of a case-based reasoning (CBR) smart system and the challenges of producing quality system outputs. Based on the results of primary and secondary data analysis, a CBR modification was carried out by adding the role of patient feedback as a quality controller for system output. Anova test resulted in the value of F = 9902 and the coefficient test resulted in a value of t = 3147. The result of the research is a modified CBR for a smart system that helps IVF patients control anxiety and helps fertility doctors answer IVF patient anxiety questions quickly and accurately.

Keywords CBR modification · Intelligent system · IVF patients

P. A. Christianto (✉)
Department Computer Science, STMIK Widya Pratama, Pekalongan, Indonesia
e-mail: p_a_chr@stmik-wp.ac.id

E. Sediyono · I. Sembiring
Department Computer Science, Satya Wacana Christian University, Salatiga, Indonesia

S. Wijono
Department Psycology, Satya Wacana Christian University, Salatiga, Indonesia

H. Triwiyanto et al. (eds.), *Proceedings of the 1st International Conference on Electronics, Biomedical Engineering, and Health Informatics*, Lecture Notes in Electrical Engineering 746, https://doi.org/10.1007/978-981-33-6926-9_17

1 Introduction

Every married couple certainly crave the presence of biological children, but not all married couples get biological children. Married couples who have regular sexual relations without using contraception, as much as 2–3 times every week for 1 year, but the wife has not been declared pregnant, so the husband and wife have infertile problems. Infertile problems can occur wife or husband or both. The solution for infertile couples to have biological children is the IVF program [1]. IVF program is the process of fertilization of an egg cell by sperm which is carried out outside the wife's body, after forming an embryo then the embryo transfer process is continued to the wife [2]. In 1988, IVF program services began in Indonesia and the number of IVF patients continued to increase every year. The IVF program has several challenges: the success rate of IVF programs is still low, namely 29% [3], 83.3% of IVF patients have failed IVF programs [4] and 17% of IVF patients have miscarriages [5].

77.7% of IVF patients have a high level of anxiety [4] and high anxiety has a negative impact on the health of IVF patients. Traumatic experiences of patients such as a history of recurrent miscarriage and the pressure of having a biological child because the age of marriage past 4 years or the age of women has exceeded 34 years are triggers for the high anxiety of IVF patients [6]. When IVF patients are declared pregnant, IVF patients become protective of their pregnancy.

The protective attitude of IVF patients towards pregnancy, encourages IVF patients to actively ask fertility doctors about all health complaints through existing communication media (SMS, telephone, WhatsApp). Good communication between fertility doctors and IVF patients can reduce misunderstanding of information [7], thereby helping to reduce the level of anxiety of IVF patients. Fertility doctors have the desire to quickly answer all anxiety questions of IVF patients, because fertility doctors fully understand the protective attitude of IVF patients. However, fertility doctors have several obstacles, such as: fertility doctors have to do other medical activities, fertility doctors are sick and fertility doctors are carrying out religious obligations. The obstetrician's obstacle causes IVF patients to have to wait for an answer for relative time. The relatively long waiting time causes the increased anxiety of IVF patients.

Telemedicine services have developed rapidly, telemedicine services can provide medical services that are fast, easy and inexpensive [8]. Telemedicine services can operate properly, if there is a doctor in charge of providing telemedicine services to patients. Existing research recommendations, telemedicine services developed into an online service system that can work automatically to deal with patient diseases [9]. Research on mobile-based case-based reasoning (CBR) intelligent systems provides evidence that the CBR intelligent system can handle health checks for pregnant women, because CBR intelligent systems have the same capabilities as obstetricians. CBR intelligent system produces good system output with an accuracy rate of 87.5%. CBR intelligent systems do not replace medical procedures, but CBR intelligent systems play an important role in providing early recommendations to pregnant women and assisting doctors' duties [10]. Other research on CBR intelligent systems, provides evidence that CBR intelligent systems are capable of carrying out fetal health checks and provide accurate information on fetal health conditions [11].

The main challenge of intelligent systems is to produce good quality system outcomes to patients without the constraints of time and place [12]. To get a good quality system output, an intelligent system must involve patients [13] through feedback to the system [7]. CBR for the intelligent system of handling the health of pregnant women and the intelligent system of diagnosis of fetal health have been proven to produce accurate system outputs. But intelligent systems do not yet involve the role of patient feedback to control the quality of the system's output.

Based on the problems of fertility doctors, the problems of IVF patients, the potential of telemedicine, the potential of the CBR intelligent system and the challenges of the intelligent system, this study will modify the CBR smart system by adding the role of patient feedback to the CBR intelligent system. The logic flow of the CBR intelligent system modification is different from the existing CBR intelligent system the logic flow. The results of the modification of the CBR intelligent system are an answer to the challenges of developing intelligent systems [7, 12, 13], while adopting the potential of telemedicine services, so that the CBR intelligent modification system has the ability to help IVF patients control anxiety and assist the task of fertility doctors, through system outcomes intelligent who gives answers to IVF patients who are not only fast, but also accurate.

This paper is structured as follows, Sect. 2 presents research materials and methods to find a smart system method that can help IVF patients control anxiety and help fertility doctors answer questions for IVF patients. Section 3 describes the research data used to modify the smart system CBR and validate the results. Section 4 provides conclusions and further research opportunities.

2 Methodology

The first stage of research is used to determine the scope of research, determine the topic of literature, compile a list of questions, compile an implementation plan, determine resource persons, determine data collection methods and determine methods of statistical processing. Literature study was conducted to obtain case-based reasoning (CBR) data applied to health intelligent systems and obtain information about the challenges of developing smart systems. CBR works to imitate the way humans solve problems, namely by remembering similar experiences of the past and adjusting to overcome current problems [12]. Desired data is proof of the accuracy of CBR-based intelligent system output and understanding of CBR stages (retrieve stage, reuse stage, revision stage and retain stage) [13]. Based on an understanding of the stages of the CBR and the challenges of developing smart systems [10], a hypothesis is developed:

Hypothesis 1. Test the influence of IVF patients through user feedback on intelligent systems
The challenge of developing intelligent systems now is to involve IVF patients [11], through IVF patient feedback [7] to the smart system. IVF patient feedback is used as a quality control system output [10]. If there is a lot of negative feedback from IVF patients, it will certainly reduce the quality of the existing system output, so the related system's output must be reviewed by fertility doctors who are expert users on the smart system. Testing this hypothesis will prove whether there is a significant influence on IVF patient variables through IVF patient feedback with intelligent system variables.

There are two groups of respondents: fertility doctor respondents and IVF patients. The fertility doctor respondents consisted of two fertility doctors from two different hospitals in different provinces (Fig. 1). With two fertility doctors, a cross check can be made of the data obtained. Interviews with two fertility doctors were carried out at different times (30 September 2019 and 9 October 2019).

Interviews with two IVF patients from different cities and different implementation times (August 19, 2019 and August 23, 2019). The questionnaire was prepared using a Likert scale of 5, namely: strongly agree, agree, neutral, disagree and strongly disagree. Distribution of questionnaires using Google Forms with a duration of 1 week (October 21, 2019–October 28, 2019). The questionnaire was distributed to members of the Permata Hati Tough Fighting Community, which is a community of IVF patients.

Research uses quantitative and qualitative approaches [14]. Triangulation is used to compare qualitative research results with quantitative research results, so that valid and unbiased results are obtained [15]. Triangulation uses the same object, but researched with different methods [16]. Triangulation will compare 4 data, namely: the results of interviews with 2 IVF patients, the results of interviews with 2 fertility doctors, the results of questionnaire processing for IVF patients and the results of literature studies. Based on the results of data analysis, case based reasoning was modified which was then continued with hypothesis testing. The final stage of the research is compiling a research report Fig. 2 is a summary of the stages of the study:

1. There are several tests using SPSS software version 23.
2. Testing the validation of research data to get the Pearson coefficient with a target value of > 0.3 and a sign value with a target value of ≤ 0.05.

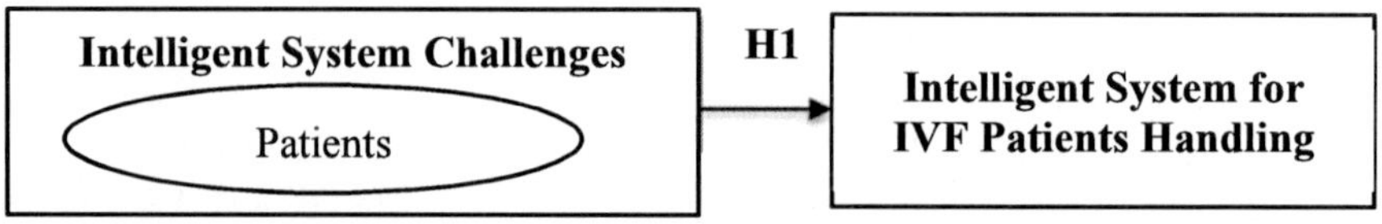

Fig. 1 Research hypothesis

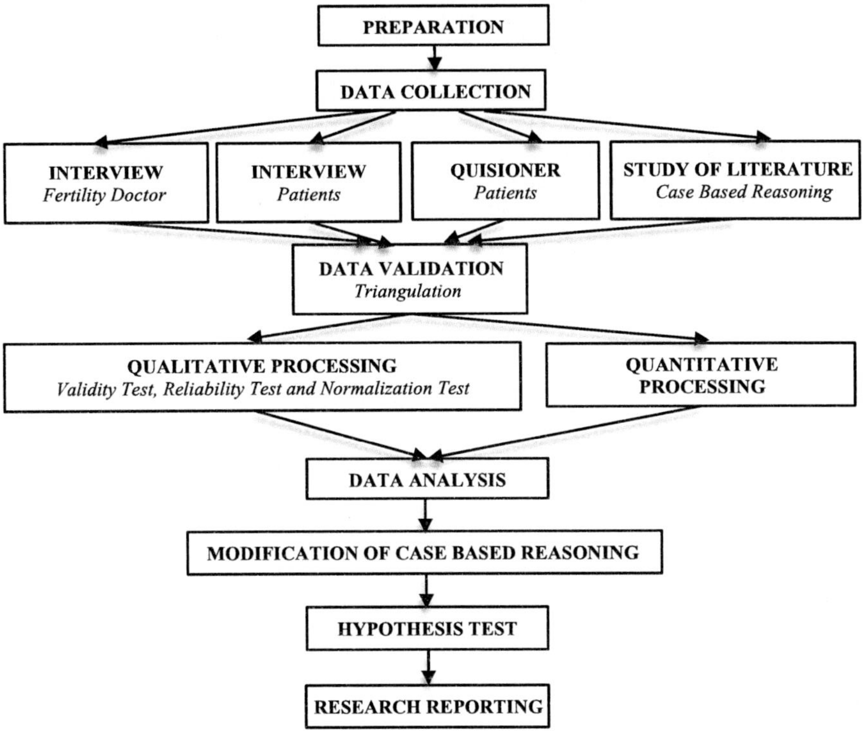

Fig. 2 Research stages

3. Testing the reliability of research data to get Cronbach's Alpha value with a target value of $\geq$ 0.6.
4. Testing the normalization of research data to get the significance value of the Kolmogorov-Smirnov test with a target value > 0.005.
5. Hypothesis testing using ANOVA testing to get the F value with a target significance value < 0.005 and coefficient testing.

The results of hypothesis testing which prove that IVF patients have a significant effect on the smart system is a factor that strengthens the CBR modification results on the smart system that will be used to help IVF patients and help fertility doctors. The final step of the research is to compile a research report and provide suggestions for further research to strengthen the results of this study.

3 Result and Discussion

The results of data processing with SPSS software, states that the questionnaire data are worthy of being research data, such as Table 1.

The Pearson coefficient and the sign value provide evidence that the research data obtained is valid. In addition to being valid, Croncbach's alpha value proves the research data has high reliability and normal data distribution is based on the significance value of the Kolmogorov-Smirnov test.

Data analysis found several facts:

1. Table 2 shows the fact of the ability of the CBR-based health intelligent system and the use of user feedback as a quality controller for the output of smart systems.

Table 2 shows scientific evidence that a smart CBR system produces good system outcomes and can be applied to the health sector. However, from 4 research

Table 1 Feasibility of research data

Test result	Standard value	Conclusion
Pearson correlation coefficient value lowest = 0.458	>0.3	Valid data
The highest sign value = 0.025	≤ 0.05	Valid data
Cronbach's alpha value = 0.794	≥ 0.6	Reliable data
The significance value of the Kolmogorov-Smirnov test = 0.201	>0.05	Normal data

Table 2 Facts of intelligent system capabilities and use of feedback to intelligent systems

Research	Accuracy of results	System output quality
Malathi D. et al.	Having good system output accuracy in predicting complex disease problems due to the automatic learning feature of the available rules [17]	Does not involve user feedback as a quality controller for system output
Juan Ramos Gonzales et al.	Able to solve various diagnostic problems in the medical domain [18]	Does not involve user feedback as a quality controller for system output
Lucky Gagah et al.	In testing using 60 medical record data from RSUD dr. Soetrasno Rembang consisting of 40 old cases and 20 new cases, obtained an accuracy rate of intelligent system diagnosis of 95% [19]	Does not involve user feedback as a quality controller for system output
Kehui Song et al.	Able to carry out a diagnosis of fetal health, so that it can decide the condition of a healthy fetus and the condition of the fetus that requires medical treatment [11]	Does not involve user feedback as a quality controller for system output

Table 3 Facts on the level of confidence of IVF patients in fertility doctors

Fertility Doctor 1	Fertility Doctor 2	IVF Patient 1	IVF Patient 2	Questionnaire results
Yes	Yes	Yes	Yes	59% of respondents expressed strongly agree and 35% of respondents agreed

results [11, 19], there has been no research result involving feedback from smart system users to control the quality of intelligent system output, whereas previous research results [7, 13] prove that patients play a role in maintaining the quality of the system output.

2. Table 3 shows the fact of the level of confidence of IVF patients to fertility doctors.

The results of interviews with two fertility doctors and two IVF patients, and the results of a questionnaire survey to the IVF patient community, for the same question: "Do IVF patients trust the fertility doctor more than other obstetricians?":

The statement of 2 IVF patients who agreed that IVF patients had more trust in fertility doctors than other obstetricians was confirmed by 2 fertility doctors' statements and strengthened by the results of questionnaire processing with IVF patient respondents. IVF patients have more confidence in fertility doctors, because the process of IVF is not easy, IVF patients are handled by a fertility doctor from the beginning of the IVF program, so that fertility doctors will best understand the medical conditions of IVF patients. The fertility doctor has an important position for IVF patients, all health complaints of IVF patients must immediately be asked to the fertility doctor, the fertility doctor's answer will give IVF patient peace of mind.

3. Tables 4, 5, and 6 show the fact the importance of IVF patient communication with fertility doctors.

Table 4 Facts of IVF patients protective with pregnancy

Fertility Doctor 1	Fertility Doctor 2	IVF Patient 1	IVF Patient 2	Questionnaire results
Yes	Yes	Yes	Yes	82% of respondents expressed strongly agree and 18% of respondents agreed

Table 5 Facts on the length of time receiving an answer increases the anxiety of IVF patients

Fertility Doctor 1	Fertility Doctor 2	IVF Patient 1	IVF Patient 2	Questionnaire results
Yes	Yes	Yes	Yes	41% of respondents stated strongly agree and 53% of respondents agreed

Table 6 Facts on easing of anxiety of IVF patients after receiving answers

Fertility Doctor 1	Fertility Doctor 2	IVF Patient 1	IVF Patient 2	Questionnaire results
Yes	Yes	Yes	Yes	65% of respondents stated strongly agree and 35% of respondents agreed

Facts were obtained from the results of interviews of two fertility doctors and two IVF patients, as well as the results of a questionnaire survey to the IVF patient community for the same 3 questions. Table 4 shows the answer to the first question: "Are IVF patients more protective of their pregnancy and actively ask fertility doctors?".

The statements of 2 IVF patients, the statements of 2 fertility doctors and the results of questionnaire processing with IVF patient respondents, confirmed that IVF patients were more protective of their pregnancies and actively asked fertility doctors. This condition makes IVF patients anxious easily and the long wait for an answer from the fertility doctor increases the anxiety of IVF patients. Table 5 shows the answer to the second question: "Does the length of time given by the fertility doctor increase the anxiety of IVF patients?".

The statements of 2 IVF patients, the statements of 2 fertility doctors and the results of questionnaire processing with IVF patient respondents, confirm that the length of time the fertility doctor answers will increase the anxiety of IVF patients. Fertility doctors have a strong commitment to immediately answer questions from IVF patients, but there are several conditions that become obstacles for fertility doctors, such as: the fertility doctor has to do other medical activities, the fertility doctor is sick and the fertility doctor is carrying out religious obligations. Table 6 shows the answer to the third question: "Can the answers received from fertility doctors ease the anxiety of IVF patients?".

The statement of 2 IVF patients, the statement of 2 fertility doctors and the results of questionnaire processing with IVF patient respondents, confirmed that the fertility doctor's answer relieved the anxiety of IVF patients. So that to help IVF patients control anxiety and help fertility doctors overcome obstacles to be able to immediately answer IVF patient questions, a smart system is needed to help, as in the results in Fig. 3.

4. Facts on IVF patients' needs for intelligent systems handling IVF patients after embryo transfer.

Figure 3 is the result of a questionnaire survey to the IVF patient community for the question: "Is there a need for an intelligent system capable of duplicating the ability of fertility doctors, so that they can quickly answer all IVF patient questions?" The result: 53% of respondents strongly agreed, 35% of respondents agreed, 6% of respondents stated neutral and 6% of respondents stated disagree. So based

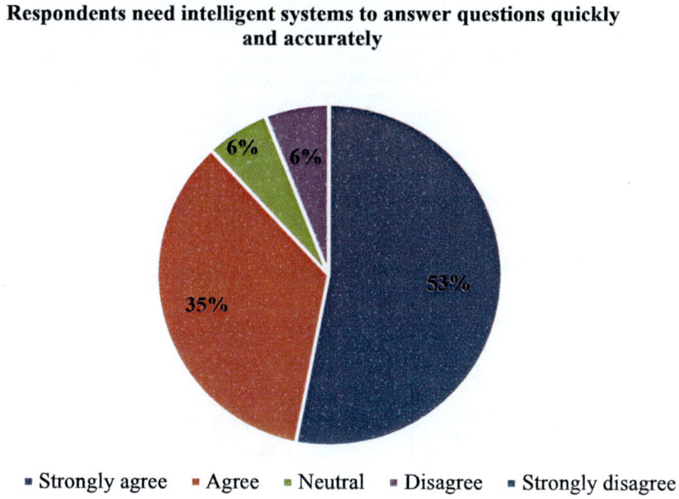

Fig. 3 Patients in IVF need an intelligent system

on these results, it can be seen that IVF patients need an intelligent system, which not only quickly provides answers to IVF patients, but also provides accurate answers.

The facts found produce one important point that must be resolved: CBR applied to intelligent systems produces reliable system outputs, but it needs to be improved by involving patient feedback as a quality controller for system outputs. The improvement of the CBR is an answer to the results of previous research on the requirements to get quality system output [7, 11]. High-quality system output is very necessary for IVF patients to help control anxiety and fertility doctors to answer all anxiety questions of IVF patients.

To resolve this important point, a CBR modification was carried out by involving patient feedback as an intelligent quality control system. IVF patient feedback will be the determinant of the feasibility of the solution before it is given to IVF patients. CBR modification can be applied to an intelligent system handling IVF patient after embryo transfer, so that the intelligent system has the ability to answer IVF patients' questions quickly and accurately. Figure 4 shows the difference between the original CBR and CBR modification.

The main differences between the original CBR and CBR modifications:

1. Original CBR [11, 17–19]: the patient only inputs the problem to the system and then receives the system output. The system has only one determinant of the feasibility of a system outcome before it is given to the patient: the feasibility of similarity between the old case and the patient's problem.
2. Modification of CBR: patients not only provide input problems to the system, but also provide feedback to the system after receiving system outputs. Patient feedback acts as a determinant of the feasibility of the system output before it is

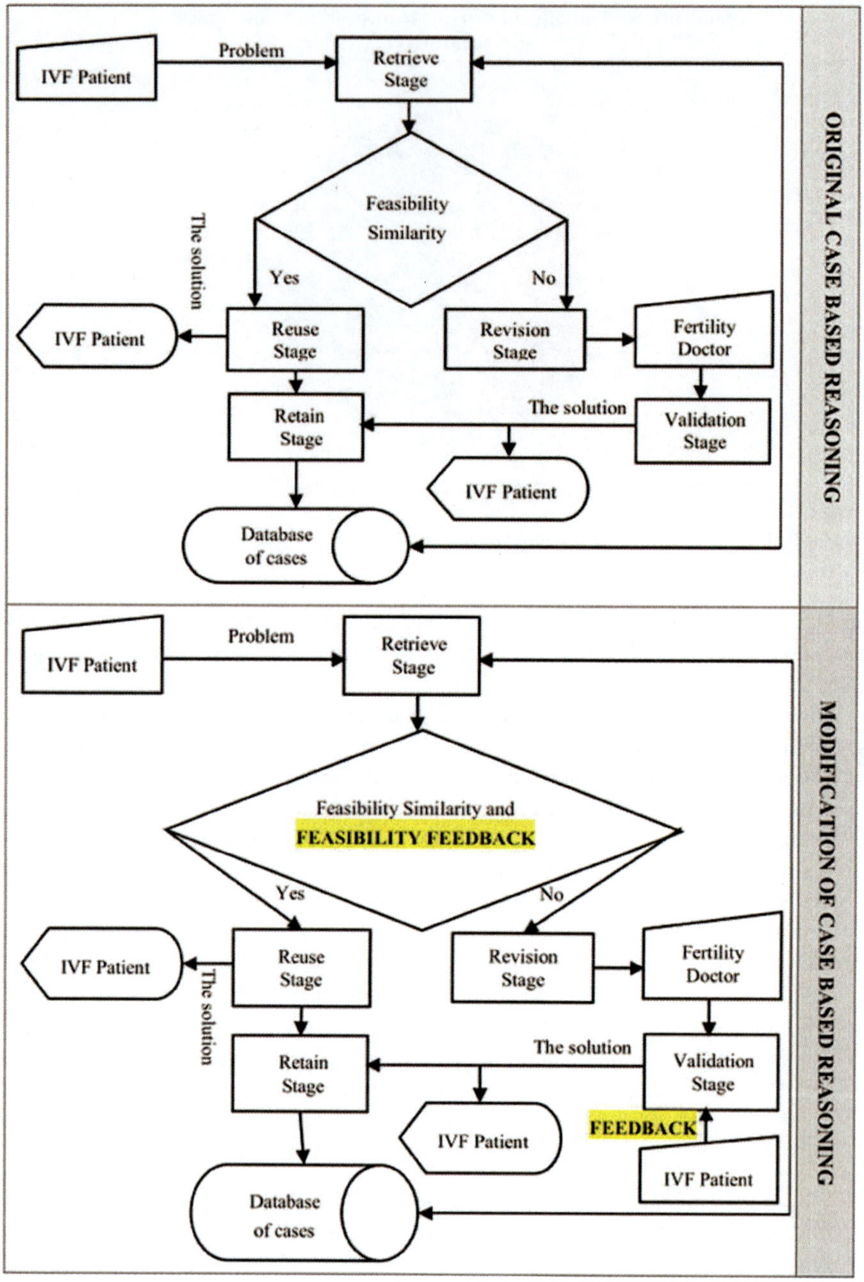

Fig. 4 Difference between the original CBR and CBR modification

given to the patient. So that the CBR modification has two determinants of eligibility: the appropriateness of the similarity between old cases with patient problems and the feasibility of patient feedback.

Explanation of the phases in CBR modification:

1. IVF patients enter anxiety questions into the smart system.
2. The intelligent system responds to IVF patient anxiety questions by looking for similarities between IVF patient anxiety questions and the old case database (stage retrieve).
3. After finding the old cases that are most similar to the anxiety questions of IVF patients, the similarity and feedback feasibility were tested (there were no negative complaints of IVF patients to the solution that would be given to answer the anxiety questions of IVF patients).

    3a. If both eligibilities are met, then the intelligent system can directly provide solutions to IVF patients (reuse stage).
    3b. If there is one eligibility not met or each eligibility is not met, then the solution must be checked and validated by the fertility doctor (revision stage) before being given to IVF patients.

4. All solutions given to IVF patients are saved to the case database (retain stage), so they can be used again to answer the next anxiety questions.
5. After getting answers, IVF patients provide feedback to the system.

Modified CBR has similarities and differences with CBR in previous studies, as seen in Table 7.

Table 7, shows the intelligent CBR system output given to patients based solely on the similarities between the problem and the old cases stored on the system. Meanwhile, CBR modification provides the role of user feedback to the system, by providing a user feedback path to the system and as one of the feasibility values for the system output before being given to IVF patients. The results of hypothesis testing provide evidence that IVF patients have a significant influence on intelligent systems, Table 8 shows the results of anova testing.

Table 7 Similarities and differences

Intelligent system model	Feasibility similarity	Feasibility feedback	The flow of user feedback into intelligent systems
Malathi D. et al.	Yes	No	No
Juan Ramos Gonzales et al.	Yes	No	No
Angelo Costa et al.	Yes	No	No
Lucky Gagah et al.	Yes	No	No
Kehui Song et al.	Yes	No	No
Modified CBR	Yes	Yes	Yes

Table 8 Anova test results

Model		Sum of squares	df	Mean square	F	Sig.
1	Regression	4725	1	4725	9902	0.007[b]
	Residual	7157	15	0.477		
	Total	11,882	16			

[b]Predictors: (Constant), IVF patient

Table 9 Coefficient test results

Model		Unstandardized coefficients		Standardized coefficients	t	Sig.
		B	Std. error	Beta		
1	(Constant)	−2945	2325		−1266	0.225
	Pasien IVF	0.398	0.126	0.631	3147	0.007

Anova test results are the value of F = 9902 with a significance level of 0.007 < 0.005. So the ANOVA test results state that there is a significant influence of IVF patients on the intelligent system of handling IVF patients post embryo transfer. These results corroborate the results of the CBR recommendations which provide the role of feedback for IVF patients to the smart system. Table 9 shows the results of testing the coefficients.

The coefficient test produces a constant (a) of −2945 and an IVF (b) value of 0.398, so a regression equation is produced: Y = a + bX or −2945 + 0.398X. Coefficient b is a regression direction coefficient which states the average change of the intelligent system for each change in IVF patients by one unit.

1. A constant of −2945 states that if there are no IVF patients, an intelligent system is worth −2945 or not needed.
2. The regression coefficient X of 0.398 states that for each addition of 1 IVF patient value, the value of the intelligent system increases by 0.398.

The test results prove that the more IVF patients the more intelligent systems are needed to handle IVF patients after embryo transfer. In column t, known t value of 3.147 with a significance value of 0.007 < 0.05, which indicates the real influence of IVF patients on the intelligent system of handling IVF patients after embryo transfer. Anova test results and coefficient testing become proof of case-based reasoning modification that involves IVF patient feedback to the intelligent system of handling IVF patients post embryo transfer.

4 Conclusion

The results of the research are in accordance with the research objectives to find a smart system method that can help IVF patients control anxiety and help fertility doctors answer questions from IVF patients. Research results in the form of CBR modification in a smart system can help IVF patients control anxiety and help fertility doctors answer all the anxiety questions of IVF patients quickly and accurately. Modification of the CBR gives the influence of IVF patient feedback on the assessment of the feasibility of the solution before it is given to IVF patients. ANOVA test results and coefficient testing reinforce the truth of case-based reasoning modification, because it becomes evidence that IVF patients have a significant influence on intelligent systems.

Further research needs to be done to examine the exact formula to calculate the value of IVF patient feedback, so that it can appropriately assess the feasibility of the solution before it is given to IVF patients and as a complement to the results of CBR modification.

References

1. Indarwati I, Budihastuti UR, Dewi YLR (2017) Analysis of factors influencing female infertility. J Matern Child Heal 2(2):150–161
2. Adnyana P (2018) In Vitro Fertilization Indicatin—Procedure—Monitoring. In 14th HKKI CONFERENCE Driving Impacts in Laboratory Medicine, pp 1–68
3. Merck (2018) Merk dan PERFITRI Sosialisasikan Byi Tabung/In Vitro Fertilization (IVF) sebagai Solusi Masalah Kesuburan di Indonesia, pp1–4
4. Nuryati S (2014) Hubungan Tingkat Kecemasan dengan Tingkat Keberhasilan Bayi Tabung pada Perempuan Usia 25–38 Tahun yang Mengikuti Program Bayi Tabung di Klinik Permata Hati RSUP Dr. Sardjito Yogyakarta, Yogyakarta
5. Hanoum IF, Boediono A, Pangestu M, Haryadi D, Widad S, Dasuki D (2015) Microvolume of 0.1Ml Gama Sleeved Cryoloops for Blastocyst Vitrification of Assisted Reproductive Technology Patients. J Kesehat Reproduksi 2(1):47–52
6. Gao L, Qu J, Wang AY (2019) Anxiety, depression and social support in pregnant women with a history of recurrent miscarriage: a cross-sectional study. J Reprod Infant Psychol, pp 1–12
7. Lu X, Zhang R (2019) Impact of physician-patient communication in online health communities on patient compliance: Cross-sectional questionnaire study. J Med Internet Res, 21(5)
8. Prawiroharjo P, Pratama P, Librianty N (2019) Layanan Telemedis di Indonesia: Keniscayaan, Risiko, dan Batasan Etika. J Etika Kedokt. Indones 3(1):1
9. Hamrioui SGA, López-Coronado M, Berbey A (2018) Isabel de la Torre Díez What Is the Evolution of Telemedicine And e-Health in North Africa? A Systematic Review Wings to the Research, Trends Telemed. E-health, pp 1–6
10. Akbulut A, Ertugrul E, Topcu V (2018) Fetal health status prediction based on maternal clinical history using machine learning techniques. Comput Methods Programs Biomed 163:87–100
11. Song K, De Jonckheere J, Zeng X, Koehl L, Yuan X, Zhao X (2019) Development of a data-based interactive medical expert system for supporting pregnancy consultations: General architecture and methodology. IFAC-Papers Online 52(19):67–72

12. Hopfe M, Prodinger B, Bickenbach JE, Stucki G (2018) Optimizing health system response to patient's needs: an argument for the importance of functioning information. Disabil. Rehabil. 40(19):2325–2330
13. Graffigna G, Barello S, Bonanomi A, Riva G (2017) Factors affecting patients' online health information-seeking behaviours: The role of the Patient Health Engagement (PHE) Model. Patient Educ Couns 100(10):1918–1927
14. Brown D, Aldea A, Harrison R, Martin C, Bayley I (2018) Temporal case-based reasoning for type 1 diabetes mellitus bolus insulin decision support. Artif Intell Med 85:28–42
15. Zhang H, Dai GL (2018) Research on traffic decision making method based on image analysis case based reasoning. Optik (Stuttg) 158:908–914
16. Zainuddin Z, Perera CJ (2019) Exploring students' competence, autonomy and relatedness in the flipped classroom pedagogical model. J Furth High Educ 43(1):115–126
17. Morgan DL (2019) Commentary—After Triangulation, What Next? J Mix Methods Res 13(1):6–11
18. Ramos-González J, López-Sánchez D, Castellanos-Garzón JA, de Paz JF, Corchado JM (2017) A CBR framework with gradient boosting based feature selection for lung cancer subtype classification. Comput Biol Med 86:98–106
19. Vedayoko LG, Sugiharti E, Muslim A (2017) Expert system diagnosis of bowel disease using case based reasoning with nearest neighbor algorithm. Sci J Informatics 4(2):2407–7658

Object Detection for Using Mask in COVID-19 Pandemic with Faster R_CNN Inception V2 Algorithm

Apri Junaidi and Jerry Lasama

Abstract When this research was done, based on data from https://covid19.go.id/, the number of positive patients reached 127,083, the increasing number of COVID-19 patients in Indonesia, and the new normal period had been imposed, making people more concerned about the health and the danger of spreading COVID-19 virus. New normal means were starting a new habit that is the habit of washing your hands and use a mask. Everyday activities in normal times require us to work as usual, in an atmosphere with other people. Everyone is required to use a mask to support the policy of using a mask, a system that can detect whether someone is wearing a mask or not. This research aims to be able to identify the use of masks in public areas. The dataset used is 5000 images of people wearing masks. This research uses the Faster R_CNN Inception V2 Algorithm. And then the results were evaluated using COCO mAP Score yielding in 0.58 mAP, with 0.78 mAP for large objects, 0.65 mAP for medium objects, and 0.48 mAP shows this research can contribute to the community to care in the use of masks. The model that has created in this study is used to detect the use of masks in public areas by using an image captured by a camera mounted in a particular place.

Keywords COVID-19 · Wearing mask · R_CNN inception V2 Algorithm

1 Introduction

In December, 2019, a series of pneumonia cases of unknown cause emerged in Wuhan, Hubei, China, with clinical presentations greatly resembling viral pneumonia [1]. According to reports, the virus is spreading rapidly to various countries,

A. Junaidi (✉) · J. Lasama
Institut Teknologi Telkom Purwokerto, Jl. DI Panjaitan no. 128 Purwokerto, Purwokerto, Indonesia 53147
e-mail: apri@ittelkom-pwt.ac.id

J. Lasama
e-mail: 18102018@ittelkom-pwt.ac.id

H. Triwiyanto et al. (eds.), *Proceedings of the 1st International Conference on Electronics, Biomedical Engineering, and Health Informatics*, Lecture Notes in Electrical Engineering 746, https://doi.org/10.1007/978-981-33-6926-9_18

so it is necessary to take strict control measures to prevent transmission by locking their borders and closing airports and internal transportation networks [2]. In Indonesia, to prevent the spread of a lockdown known as large-scale social restrictions. During this pandemic, the order recommends complying with health protocols for all Indonesian citizens. The COVID-19 pandemic has affected human life, stressed health care capacity, and delayed the usual delivery of care. As we enter a deceleration or indolent phase of the disease and a return to a "new normal" for the foreseeable future [3]. New normal means were starting a new habit that is the habit of washing your hands and use a mask. Everyday activities in normal times require us to work as usual, in an atmosphere with other people. Everyone is required to use a mask to support the policy of using a mask, a system that can detect whether someone is wearing a mask or not.

When this research was done, based on data from https://covid19.go.id/, the number of positive patients reached 127,083, 39,082 patient in medical care, 82,236 get well and 5765 pass away. The increasing number of COVID-19 patients in Indonesia, and the new normal period had been imposed, making people more concerned about the health and the danger of spreading COVID-19 virus.

Figure 1, an overview of the spread of COVID-19 in Indonesia, this data is updated every day at URL https://covid19.go.id/ that is the official website of the Government of Indonesia for handling COVID-19 information.

Figure 2, describes information on the global spread of COVID-19 on the WHO Coronavirus Disease (COVID-19) Dashboard, on this website, we get information about the development of the spread of COVID-19 by country.

Recommendation of World Health Organization (WHO), the use of masks is part of prevention and control that can limit the spread of viral diseases, including COVID-19, masks can be used for the protection of healthy people or handling infected people [6]. Face mask usage by the healthy population in the community to reduce the risk of transmission of respiratory viruses [7]. In another study, the recommendation to use masks in public areas such as high-risk public transportation areas against COVID-19, for passengers to use masks in open vehicles [8]. In another research recommends that the public should wear masks during the COVID-19 pandemic according to the local context. Also, give recommendations

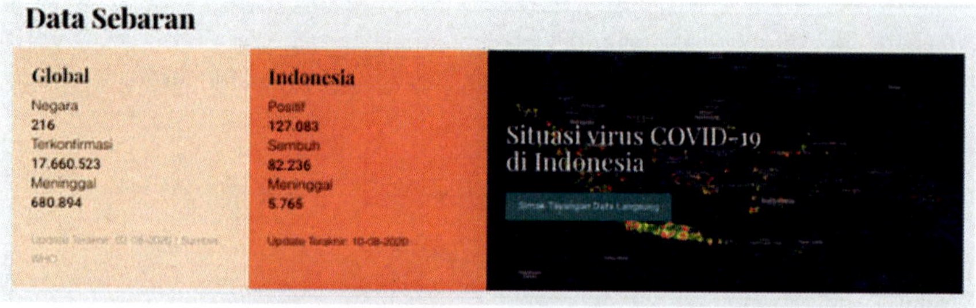

Fig. 1 Spread of COVID-19 in Indonesia [4]

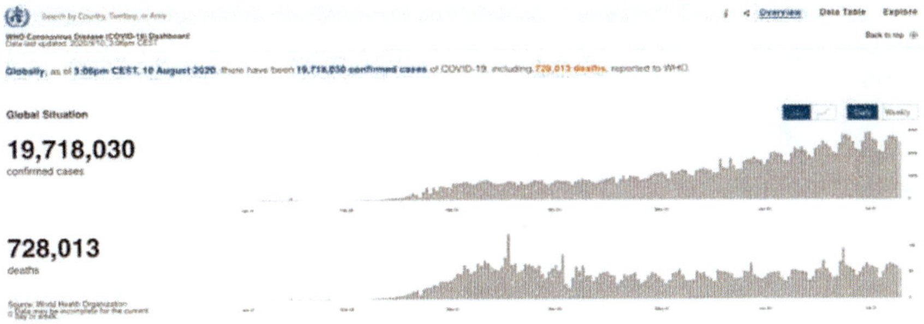

Fig. 2 Global situation of COVID-19 by WHO [5]

to the government must establish a risk-adapted strategy for using masks to scientifically publicize the use of masks, ensure an adequate supply of masks, and work together to reduce inequality of health resources [8].

Based on the recommendations of several studies on the importance of using masks during the COVID-19 pandemic, this research focused on the role of machine learning in object detection to identify people who are wearing masks or are not wearing masks.

2 Method

2.1 Materials

The development of science, especially in the fields of machine learning and computer vision, can solve several problems [9] such as computers that can improve sensory abilities aided by several tools such as cameras. Machine learning capabilities continue to improve with several studies such as face detection, which is detecting a human face in an image [10], vehicle detection [11], seagrass detection from underwater digital Images [12], detecting advertising on building [13], fruit detection [14] and many other studies are still developing.

The development of object detection methods currently shown by the trend in the use of deep learning techniques, one of which is the Convolutional Neural Network (CNN). The method itself has evolved from an architectural perspective, which aims to reduce the complexity of the search for features [15]. Faster R-CNN is a region-based object detection network that proposed by Shaoqing Ren et al. (Figure 3). Object detection networks depend on region proposal methods to hypothesize object locations. At the same time, the original techniques typically rely on inexpensive features and implemented on the CPU, which makes the running time of the proposal step intolerable. Faster R-CNN proposed to lead to an elegant and effective solution to this problem [16].

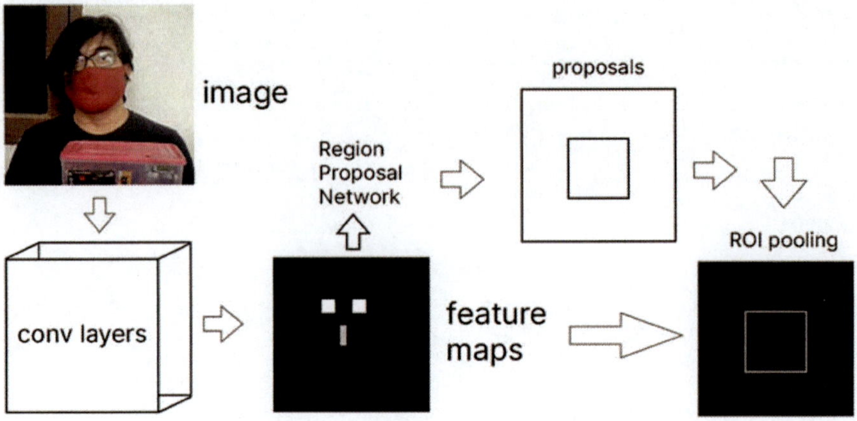

Fig. 3 Faster R-CNN architecture

2.2 *Procedure*

Some of the procedures carried out in this study started from gathering images via google image using a browser extension called Fatkun Batch to modeling, and the results of each method obtained as shown in the Fig. 4.

Based on Fig. 3, each step can describe as follows: Gather masks images and people images are the first steps to get the data set. To collect dataset, this research using google image and install an extension in browser to college images. Several keywords were used, such as using a mask, wearing masks, and others until you get 5000 images.

After the image collection stage continues with labeling each image using labeling software, this process is quite time-consuming. Next step, research will continue to converting images file into CSV file using pandas and tensor flow, the next step is to create a label map and training configuration, then proceed to load the trained algorithm and train model. The next step is to freeze the model graph after training for inference using tensor flow and finally predict images from the camera using OpenCV and tensor flow.

3 Result and Discussion

This study produces a model that can predict whether someone is wearing a mask, as seen in Fig. 3 about the results of recall, precision, and loss. The accuracy metric was computed using COCO mAP Score. As shown in Fig. 5 that the mAP for large objects has high difference with the mAP for small objects, this is likely caused by a

Fig. 4 Research method

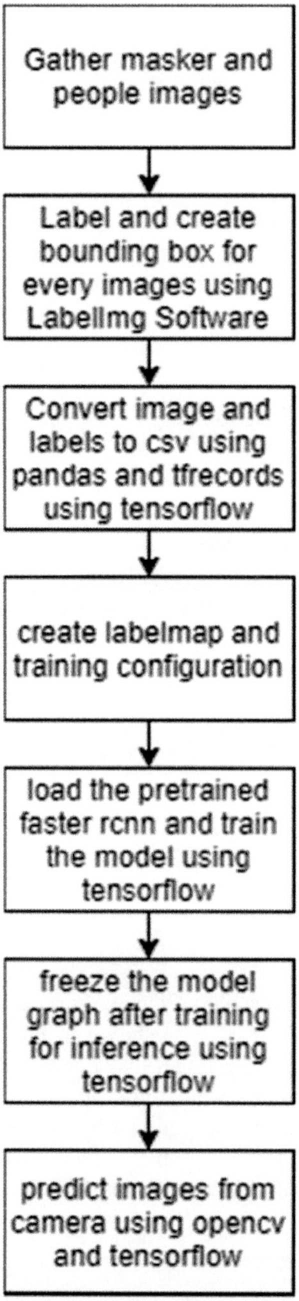

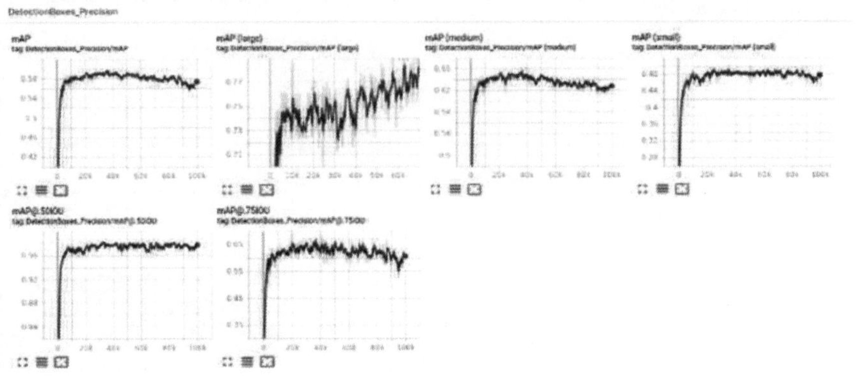

Fig. 5 Precision

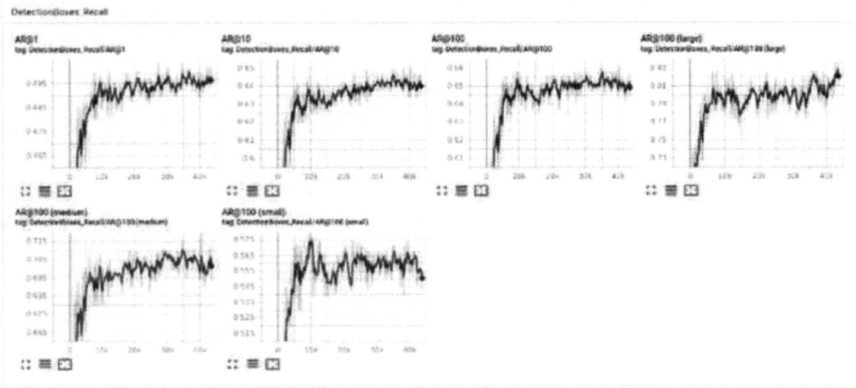

Fig. 6 Recall

minscule variance of objects sizes in the training set. Similar case was also found in the Recall as shown in Fig. 6.

The model takes an image input from camera, and then predict the image, after masks were found in the image, the program would draw a bounding box around the mask along with the confidence rate of the prediction. Figures 7 and 8 shown an example of the model predicting mask in an image taken from camera with the confidence rate of 100%.

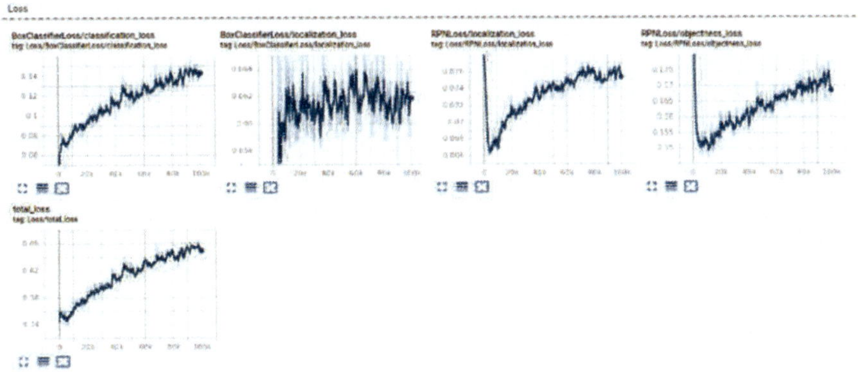

Fig. 7 Loss

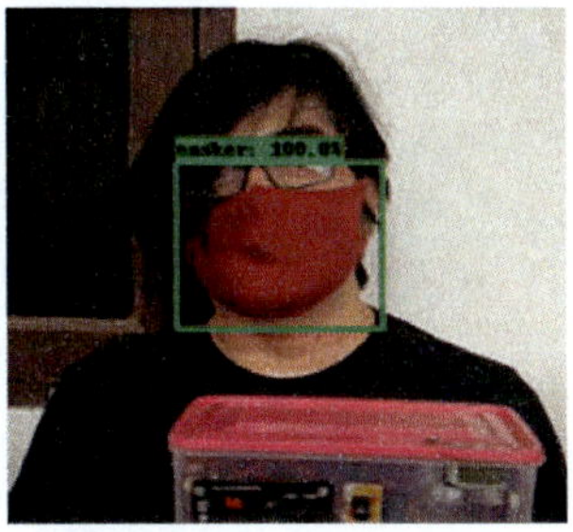

Fig. 8 Prediction result from model

4 Conclusion

An object detection model was trained using Faster R-CNN Inception V2 Algorithm. The model yields an average of 0.58 mAP, with 0.78 mAP for large objects, 0.65 mAP for medium objects, and 0.48 mAP for small objects. The high difference in the mAP score is caused by the lack of variance in object sizes in the dataset. It is advised for the next research to ensure the quality of source dataset so the model can be trained to be more accurate

References

1. Huang C et al. (2020) Clinical features of patients infected with 2019 novel coronavirus in Wuhan. Lancet 395(10223):497–506, China
2. Manoj MG, Satheesh Kumar MK, Valsaraj KT, Sivan C, Vijayan SK (2020) Potential link between compromised air quality and transmission of the novel corona virus (SARS-CoV-2) in affected areas. Environ Res, 110001

3. Zoghbi WA et al (2020) Multimodality Cardiovascular Imaging in the Midst of the COVID-19 Pandemic: Ramping Up Safely to a New Normal. JACC Cardiovasc. Imaging 13(7):1615–1626
4. Gugus Tugas Percepatan Penanganan COVID-19. [Online]. Available: https://covid19.go.id/. Accessed 10 August 2020
5. WHO Coronavirus Disease (COVID-19) Dashboard. [Online]. Available: https://covid19.who.int/. Accessed 10 August 2020
6. Organización Mundial de la Salud (2020) Advice on the use of masks in the context of COVID-19: interim guidance-2. Guía Interna la OMS, April, pp 1–5
7. Cheng VCC et al (2020) The role of community-wide wearing of face mask for control of coronavirus disease 2019 (COVID-19) epidemic due to SARS-CoV-2. J Infect 81:107–114
8. Filipczak NPJSKYSTV (2020) Adherence to social distancing and wearing of masks within public transportation during the COVID 19 pandemic. Adv Drug Deliv Rev, 40
9. Esposito F, Malerba D (2010) Applied Artificial Intelligence: an machine learning in computer vision, April 2013, pp 37–41
10. Jiang H, Learned-Miller E (2017) Face Detection with the Faster R-CNN. In: Proc—12th IEEE Int Conf Autom Face Gesture Recognition, FG 2017—1st Int. Work. Adapt. Shot Learn. Gesture Underst. Prod. ASL4GUP 2017, Biometrics Wild, Bwild 2017, Heteroge, pp 650–657
11. Yang W, Li Z, Wang C, Li J (2020) A multi-task Faster R-CNN method for 3D vehicle detection based on a single image. Appl Soft Comput J 95:106533
12. Moniruzzaman M, Islam SMS, Lavery P, Bennamoun M (2019) Faster R-CNN Based Deep Learning for Seagrass Detection from Underwater Digital Images. Digit Image Comput Tech Appl DICTA, 1–7
13. Bochkarev K, Smirnov E (2019) Detecting advertising on building façades with computer vision. Procedia Comput Sci 156:338–346
14. Wan S, Goudos S (2020) Faster R-CNN for multi-class fruit detection using a robotic vision system. Comput Networks 168:107036
15. Ren S, He K, Girshick R, Sun J (2017) Faster R-CNN: Towards Real-Time Object Detection with Region Proposal Networks, IEEE Trans Pattern Anal Mach Intell 39(6):1137–1149
16. Zhu B, Wu X, Yang L, Shen Y, Wu L (2016) Automatic detection of books based on Faster R-CNN, 2016. In: 3rd Int Conf Digit Inf Process Data Mining, Wirel Commun DIPDMWC, pp 8–12

Long Range Ultrasonic Testing System Based on Lamb Wave Method for Validation an Optimized Piezoelectric Sensor Gap Array

Kharudin Ali, Johnny Koh Siaw Paw, Damhuji Rifai, Nur Amalina Awang, Ahmed N. AbdAlla, Abdul Rahim Pazakadin, and Chong Kok Hen

Abstract Non-Destructing Testing (NDT) is crucial in the oil and gas industry to avoid fatal pipeline accidents and alarming property damage. Its general applications include the detection of pipeline defects in nuclear power plants, steam generator tubing, aircraft etc. Meanwhile, the Piezoelectric with Lamb Wave method testing system (PZ-LW), also known as Long Range Ultrasonic Testing (LRUT) is one of the methods in NDT used for crack detection on long-distance surface area. The current research proposed the ultrasonic testing probe design for the ideal gap between Piezo sensor resulting in reflection signal optimization for Piezoelectric sensor array in carbon steel pipe inspection. Response Surface Methodology (RSM) used the signal wave frequency excitation and the distance between the sensors array were optimized for appropriate multiple defect detection on 60 mm diameter carbon steel pipe sample. An Artificial Axial and Hole defect was utilized to test its efficiency. The analysis of the experimental results suggests the accuracy of PZ-LW system to amount to 98.55% when determining the defect location (hole defect), above 96.05% (axial defect measurement), while 98% and beyond (identification of defect shape). The inspection position is achievable until 311,399 m on free damaged pipe, 64,377 m (axial damage) and 61,267 m (hole crack defect damage). The reflection signal on PZ-LW inspection indicated good

K. Ali (✉) · D. Rifai · A. R. Pazakadin
Faculty of Electrical and Automation Engineering Technology, UCTATI, 24000 Terengganu, Malaysia
e-mail: kharudin@uctati.edu.my

J. K. S. Paw · C. K. Hen
UNITEN, Institute of Sustainable Energy (ISE), 43000 Selangor, Malaysia

N. A. Awang
Akademi Pengajian Bahasa, UiTM, Cawangan Kelantan, Bukit Ilmu, 18500 Machang, Kelantan, Malaysia

A. N. AbdAlla
Faculty of Electronic Information Engineering, Huaiyin Institute of Technology, Huai'an Jiangsu, China

H. Triwiyanto et al. (eds.), *Proceedings of the 1st International Conference on Electronics, Biomedical Engineering, and Health Informatics*, Lecture Notes in Electrical Engineering 746, https://doi.org/10.1007/978-981-33-6926-9_19

feedback signal amplitude with high distance detection in axial crack defect. The comparison of experimental and simulation results in Simulation of Non-Destructed Testing (SIMNDT) has successfully proven the consistency and accuracy of the proposed PZ-LW system for carbon steel pipe inspection.

Keywords Piezoelectric sensor · NDT · Ultrasonic testing · Amplitude · Artificial crack defect · Sensor gap

1 Introduction

Ultrasonic testing technique is one of the most widely used method of NDT for structure integrity assessment. Since ultrasonic wave can pass through most materials, this technique can be applied to defect detection, material characterization and imaging. The common technique of ultrasonic testing is categorized under three properties of the wave. The through transmission wave technique was the first practical applications of ultrasonic NDT technique for material assessment [1–3]. For this method, good and consistent acoustic coupling must be ensured in order to confirmed the receive signal is generating by the presence of the defect.

The second method is pulse echo technique which offers greater versatility considering that its result is easier to interpret [4–7] whereby it involves typical defects including welds, cracks, porosity, and others. The whole idea of this technique is to send a short burst of ultrasonic wave into structure or sample material in order to measure the echoes signal which returns from the defect. More importantly, it should be noted that one of the advantages of pulse echoes technique is the fact that access is only required from one side surface which is important for inspection, particularly for complex structure that has limited access. Next, the third technique is resonance technique which is mostly similar to the pulse-echo technique because it is dependent on the reflections of ultrasonic wave from the defect [8–11]. However, the difference is that the transmitted and reflected waves for this technique are superimposed and only able to form stationary wave.

Ultrasonic Testing (UT) is considered to be more advantageous for long surface area structure such as pipeline compared to other techniques due to the ability of the UT to examine the long-distance surface area over up to 20 m for the steel material. Meanwhile, it should be noted that this technique is also known as Long Range Ultrasonic Testing (LRUT). Existing research in the literature recognizes the critical role played by the application of LRUT for structural integrity assessment. Accordingly, an array of transducer was proposed which is able to generate selected guided wave for long-range inspection on railway track [12]. The experimental results showed that the LRUT is able to detect defect in rails. In another study, an intelligent signal processor was utilized to improve defect detection in railway track by reducing the influence of high-level dispersive wave modes of LRUT during rail inspection [13]. Regarding this matter, the defect signal wave analysis showed that the proposed method is able to reduce the effect of dispersion to a greater extent, even in the case of extremely high Signal to Noise Ratio (SNR) level. Meanwhile, past research also investigated the effect of shift ultrasonic wave distance on defect detection of brass plate [14, 15]. The experimental result revealed that the increase of ultrasonic beam shift can improve the ultrasound transmission.

On a similar note, another study proposed a semi-analytical algorithm based on finite element methods for dispersion curves using higher-order elements for long-range ultrasonic testing. The simulation analysis proved that the proposed method can improve the efficiency of LRUT technique [16]. In summary, a great amount of interesting results clearly indicates the potential of LRUT technique for long-distance surface area. However, most of the studies in the open literature has not been able to simultaneously examine the optimization of LRUT probe design.

Therefore, the present study aims to optimize and correct the amplitude reflection signal of PZS using Fuzzy Logic for long-range ultrasonic testing probe design based on Piezoelectric Sensor (PZS) array. In addition, the current work will identify the optimum distance between the sensor array and the probe distance to the defect location. Next, the effect of attenuation based on the defect distance positioning will be analyzed for error compensation in Fuzzy Logic System. Finally, the response surface method will be utilised in order to optimise sensor array distance as well as the most effective distance of probe and defect location for 60 mm carbon steel pipe inspection.

2 Material and Method

Sensor array was one of mostly used methods in inspection. This method has always been applied in automotive industrial either for aircraft or also in train (railway rail inspection). The effect of this method provided the actual positioning of defect based on time response and according to the time responses for all sensors, it was tabled and from here the shape of defect was identified. From here, the shape of defect and long of defect was drawn after signal has plotted by base on time respond. Figure 1 shows array of the sensor on the PZ-LW system. Specifically, this array used 10 pairs of Piezoelectric Sensors with a diameter of 10 mm each. The selection of 10 pairs of Piezoelectrics were based on the size of gas pipe used in industrial (diameter 60 mm and 5 mm thickness). According to the RSM for optimisation, the gaps of between sensors contributed to the total pairs of Piezoelectric Sensor within the max gaps was 2.5 mm. The operating frequency of the sensor supported up to 4 MHz with a thickness of 1 mm. Meanwhile, it should be noted that the switching technique was used as the activation technique of the sensor whereby only one pair of Piezoelectric Sensors was activated at a time. Moreover, the activation method was controlled based on the programming for the multiplexer. The reflected signal was received through the DAQ module and then displayed on the PC through QuickDAQ software. The received signal was analysed using the Simulink feature of the MATLAB software for error compensation using Fuzzy Logic method.

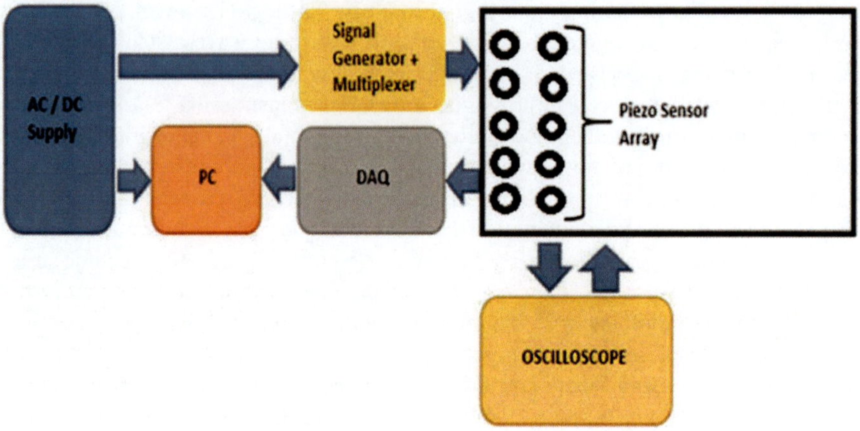

Fig. 1 Piezoelectric lamb wave inspection system

2.1 Experiment Setup

As a whole, it is crucial to note that the PZ-LW full system devices development has five major parts. The first part is the Atmega328 controller and National Instrument DAQ (DT9816) which is used as the controller device in data input processing and output display. Next, the second part concerns the input device whereby the piezoelectric is used as a sensor and actuator for defect measurement. The third part refers to the output display for PZ-LW which appears on the LCD display. Specifically, the width of the defect displayed will be based on the amplitude as well as time response from sensor. In the fourth part, the Gausses sine pulse excitation signal for piezoelectric actuator is used as the signal from the signal generator. The final part of the testing is done using the calibration block for the purpose of ensuring that the depth of defect being displayed is correct. Figure 2 shows the PZ-LW system device setup for inspection testing. The experimental setup consists of six items, namely Oscilloscope, Signal Generator, DC Power supply, Piezoelectric actuator, receiver Controller, and PC for data analysis including Simulink Interfacing software.

The four sets sample of carbon steel pipe which are in axial, gradient axial, and hole defects are made using electrical discharge machining (EDM) as well as the turning machine. In the case of the present study, it can be observed that both samples have a 5 mm depth intrusion inside of the pipeline wall for the defect detection testing with the proposed PZ-LW probe. Figure 3 presents the carbon

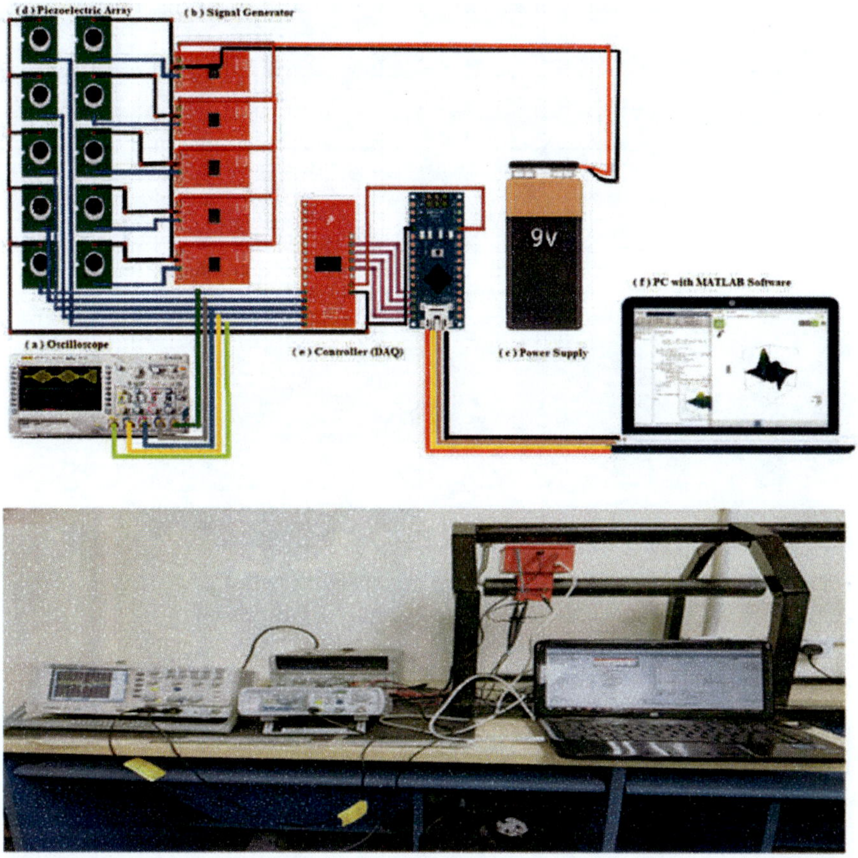

Fig. 2 Piezo Lamb Wave testing inspection system (PZ-LW)

steel pipe sample and the layout of the axial and hole defect positions. The dimension of the axial defect of 2.0 mm (width) and 40 mm (height) and the hole size 4 mm is clearly illustrated in Fig. 3a, while the size of the hole defect shown in Fig. 3b is 4 mm and 6 mm in diameter.

Figure 4 shows the artificial cracks with the size of 40 mm for the axial defect and the width defect of 2 mm. Figure 4b represents the crack for the hole and angle defect. As can be clearly seen, the hole defect diameter is 4 mm, while the angle defect of 45° within the high is 50 mm and 2 mm width. The influence of time response and defect amplitude on defect measurement in piezoelectric was tested using the proposed PZ-LW probe.

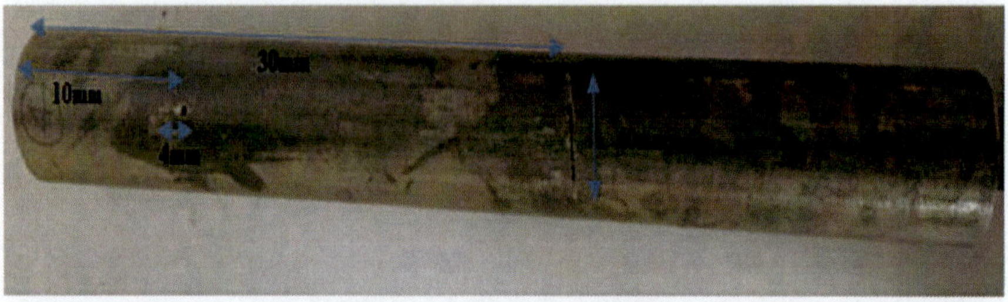

(a)

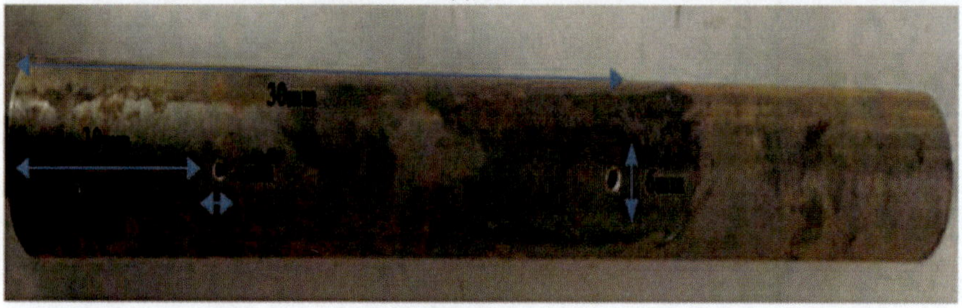

(b)

Fig. 3 The geometrical dimension of (**a**) Combining Hole and Axial defect on carbon steel pipe (**b**) Hole defect on carbon steel pipe

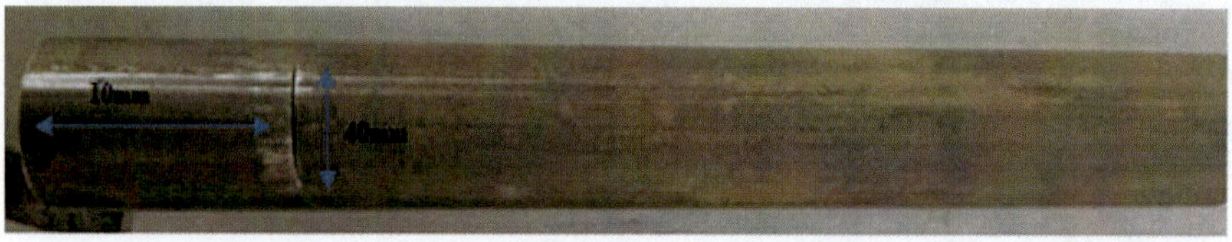

(a)

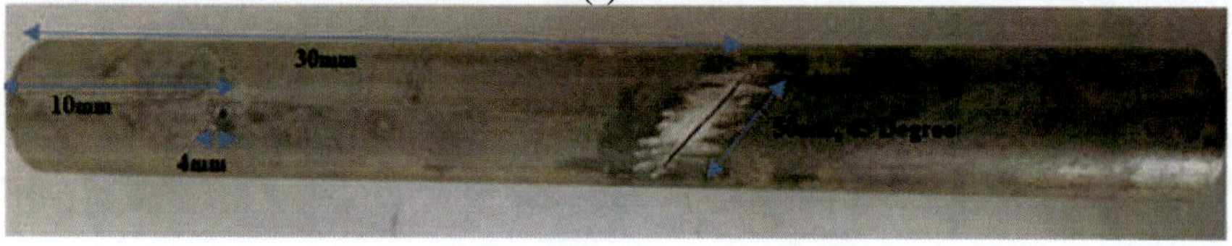

(b)

Fig. 4 Carbon steel calibration pipe (**a**) The single axial defect (**b**) The hole defect and axial defect with a gradient (angle defect)

3 Result

3.1 Sensor Array Detection Result

The experiment for sensor array result was carried out based on the arrangement of six pairs of sensors in the circumference of pipeline with different types of artificial defect which included hole, axial, gradient axial, and multi defect. The size of pipe was 500 mm in length, followed by the pipe thickness of 5 mm, and the inner and outer diameter of 55 mm and 60 mm respectively. Meanwhile, the excitation amplitude for Piezo Actuator was set at 10Vpp.

In the hole defect, the higher signal could be obtained if the positioning of PZ-LW sensor was against the defect. In this case, the amplitude of defect was reduced because the PZ-LW sensor was not in line with the defect position. As could be observed in Fig. 5a, the amplitude received was 2.0Vpp when the positioning of PZ-LW sensor was against the defect, whereas the signal reflecting was reduced to 0.05Vpp if the PZ-LW was not in line with the gap of 22 mm. As shown in the Fig. 5a, the amplitude obtained was 0.1Vpp when the gap of PZ-LW sensor was 12 mm.

Finally, the test was made for multiple defects with three types of defect namely hole defect, axial defect, and gradient axial defect on the pipeline inspection. The results presented in Fig. 5b showed two signals where the highest was 0.5Vpp and the lowest was 0.08Vpp, particularly when the positioning of PZ-LW sensor on the gap of 22 mm with the right side. Moreover, this signal came from the hole and axial defect with different position based on the time response. Furthermore, two high signal amplitudes could be observed when the positioning of PZ-LW sensor of 12 mm was at the right side, in which the first signal was 0.32Vpp and the second signal was 0.64Vpp. Specifically, this signal came from the hole and axial defect at different positions, whereas the PZ-LW sensor was more against the axial defect position. The higher signal in this experiment was 1.73Vpp while the signal came from axial defect whereby the PZ-LW sensor was completely against it.

3.2 Relation Piezoelectric Sensor Array Gap and Reflection Amplitude Signal Result

Table 1 shows that all of the independent variables, the number of distances, and the sensor gap are significant ($p < 0.05$). The model for F-value is equal to 170.48 which implies the significance of the model. In this case, there is only a 0.01% chance that the "Model F-Value" is obtained as a result of noise. The values of "Prob > F" which is less than 0.0500 produces a significant term of the model. Meanwhile, the values of A, B, AB, and A2 indicate significant model terms, whereas insignificant model terms are indicated if the values are greater than 0.1000. Therefore, model reduction may be able to improve the model if there are many insignificant model terms (not counting those required to support hierarchy).

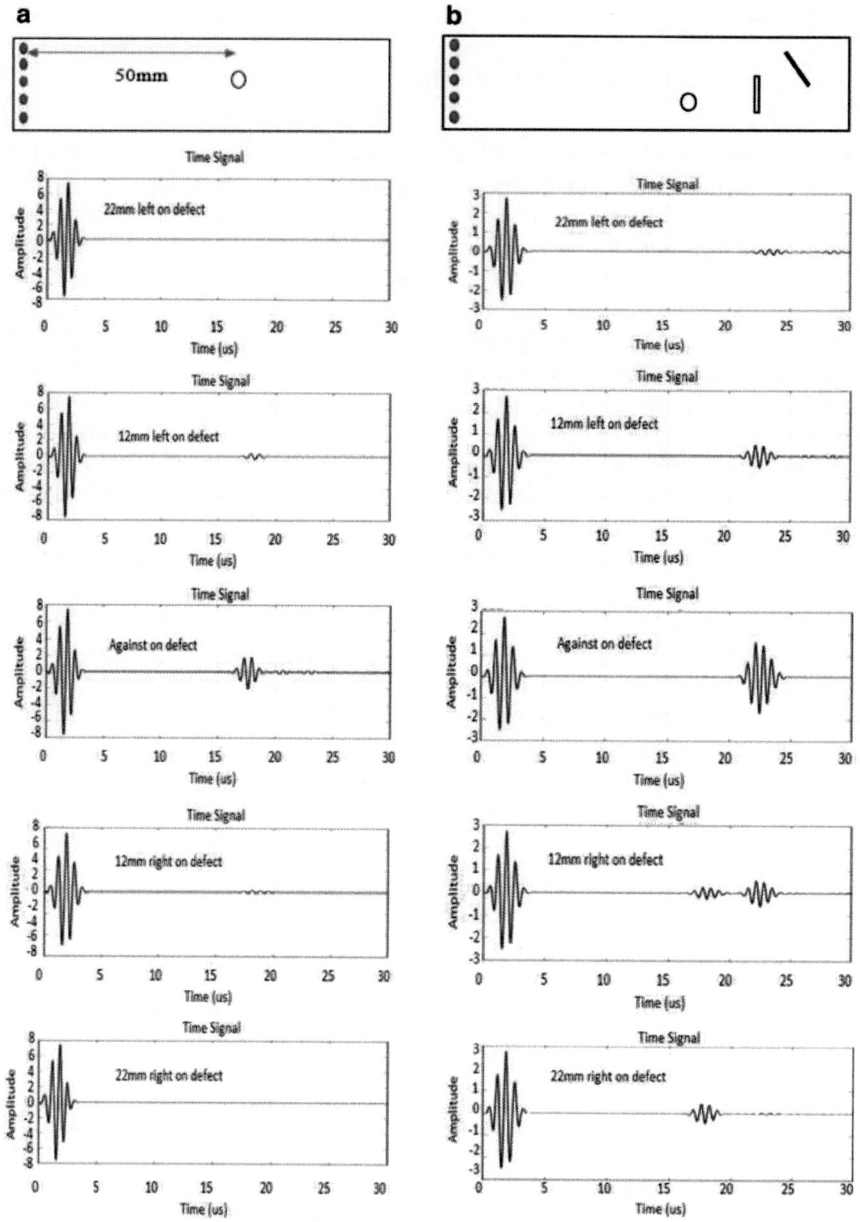

Fig. 5 Result of crack defect using PZ-LW sensor array system (**a**) Hole Crack Defect (**b**) Multiple Crack Defect

Table 1 ANOVA table for amplitude defect detection response in surface quadratic model

Analysis of variance table [partial sum of squares—Type III]						
Source	Sum of squares	df	Mean square	F value	p-value prob > F	
Model	118.442396	4	29.61059899	170.484984	<0.0001	Significant
A-Distance	90.75	1	90.75	522.4991329	<0.0001	
B-Gap	16.62651793	1	16.62651793	95.72827772	<0.0001	
AB	8.798132945	1	8.798132945	50.65583289	<0.0001	
A^2	2.11316886	1	2.11316886	12.16670961	<0.0040	
Residual	2.257898484	13	0.173684499			
Cor Total	120.7002944	17				

Table 1 presents the ANOVA analysis which shows that R-Squared is 0.9813. Other than that, the Pred. R- Squared" of 0.9600 is in a good relationship with the "Adj. R-Squared" of 0.9755 with a difference of < 0.01. In this case, it can also be observed that the Std. Dev. is 0.42 which indicates that the analysis data is significant. The implementation of RSM led to the following regression equation which is considered as an empirical relationship between the amplitude of defect as well as the independent parameters as described in Eqs. 1 and 2 as their actual values. The following equations describe the mathematical modelling for probe optimising based on the probe parameters design as well as to predict the amplitude of defect detection.

$$\text{Amplitude} = +7.50 - 2.75 * A - 1.41 * B + 1.25 * A * B + 0.76 * A^2 \tag{1}$$

$$\begin{aligned}\text{Amplitude} = &+21.38753 - 0.29395 * \text{Distance} - 1.66035 * \text{Gap} \\ &+ 0.019923 * \text{Distance} * \text{Gap} + 1.21944E - 003 * \text{Distance}^2\end{aligned} \tag{2}$$

Figure 6 clearly illustrates the interaction graph between the distance and gap of the sensor for amplitude measurement. As can be observed in the graph, the value of sensor gap B decreases when the distance of defect position increases. Accordingly, this will pose an effect that may reduce the amplitude. In addition, it can be clearly seen that the minimum and maximum distance defects are tested only from 30 mm until 80 mm.

Finally, Fig. 7 presents the 3-D surface that explains the effect of the defect distance and sensor gap in the array sensor which are related to the detection effectiveness for the amplitude defect in the inspection of the carbon steel pipe. In this case, the sensor gap starts from 2.50 mm with a defect distance of 42.50 mm, which leads to high amplitude of defect. Moreover, the amplitude of the signal becomes low when the sensor gap increases. Therefore, it should be understood that the sensor gap is inversely proportional to the amplitude of signal defect.

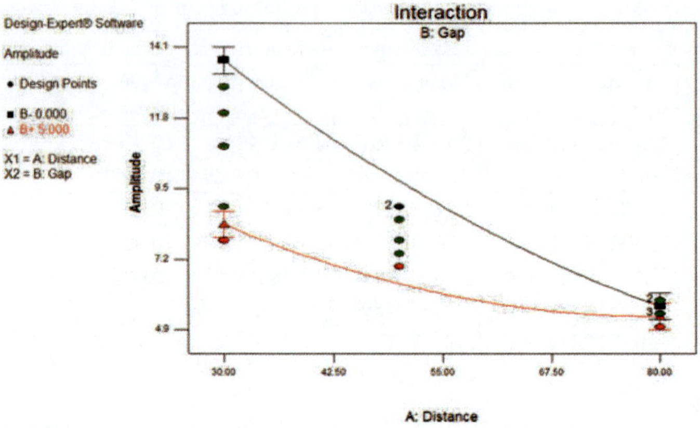

Fig. 6 Interaction of probe design factors between distance and the sensor gap

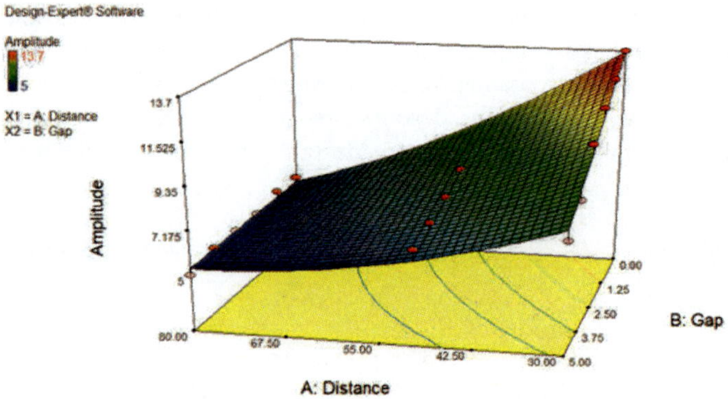

Fig. 7 The 3-D surface plot for the influence of excitation frequency and defect distance in amplitude defect detection

For instance, the ToF obtained in circumference cracked pipe is 0.000077 s. Accordingly, this value is multiplied in the group of speed (5400 m/sec) which makes it possible to obtain the location of the crack after dividing the result by two. Therefore, the location of the crack in the mentioned case is $(0.000077 \times 5400)/2 = 0.2079$ m. Table 2 illustrates the obtained results of ToF, distance calculated, actual distance, and relative error after the four cases are tested. This Table 2 also showed the maximum distance pipe that could be inspected for crack identification based on 5Vpp excitation signal with Gausses sine wave signal. From here, the LRUT maximum distance pipe for inspection could be reached until 311399 mm based on free damaged pipe. The 0-signal amplitude is occurring when there is no crack on pipeline. In the experiment, the amplitude 1.66667E-06 was assumed as 0 signal. Based on the calculation of the free damage pipe, the experimental result

Table 2 Comparison of experimental and simulation distance with the actual distance

Free damaged pipe		
Description	Experimental	Simulation
Time of flight (ToF) (sec)	0.000368	0.000369
Distance calculation (mm)	993.6	996.3
Actual distance (mm)	1000	1000
Relative error (%)	0.64	0.37
Axial damaged pipe		
Description	Experimental	Simulation
Time of flight (ToF) (sec)	0.000077	0.000075
Distance calculation (mm)	207.9	202.5
Actual distance (mm)	200	200
Relative error (%)	3.95	1.25
Hole damaged Pipe		
Description	Experimental	Simulation
Time of flight (ToF) (sec)	0.000073	0.000074
Distance calculation (mm)	197.1	199.8
Actual distance (mm)	200	200
Relative error (%)	1.45	0.1

showed the maximum signal amplitude was 5.19E-05 and the zero signal was assumed as 1.66667E-07. Thus, the gain of amplitude was achieved by dividing the experimental result of amplitude with 1.66667E-07 and the result indicated the gain of 311. From here, the distance was measured with 5.19E-05 of 1000 mm. After it was multiplied to 311 gain, the maximum distance of pipe for inspection could be reached until 311399 mm or equal to 311 m. For axial damage pipe defect, the maximum pipe that could be achieved for inspection was 64.377 m and lastly for hole defect, the maximum distance could be reached was 61.267 m. From here, it showed that the distance of defect depended on the types and width of crack.

4 Conclusion

The current work has provided a clear presentation and discussion on the effectiveness and the generality of the data-driven Piezoelectric-LRUT framework in detecting and localising different damages which include circumference, hole, and sloping in pipes. In the case of the present study, a data-driven framework based on pattern recognition and machine learning was developed in order to differentiate various types of damages. The current research also investigated the spread of missile Lamb wave to pipelines as well as their interaction with defects. Accordingly, a piezoelectric sensor network (array) was organized and surface-mounted on the pipeline for the purpose of exciting and acquiring PZ-LWs. Apart from that, several simulation trials were also performed using SIMNDT software to validate the feasibility and applicability of the modified model. Accordingly, the optimized for piezo sensor gap with optimum distance can be set on 2.50 mm with the high accuracy amplitude signal are receive from PZ-LW system. Specifically, the pattern of defect can identify base on reflection signal from Piezo sensor array on PZ-LW system. It shows that until 98% precise match of shape defect can identified. Regarding this matter, the efficiency of defect positioning can be proving by comparing between simulation and experiment where the hole defect positioning giving high accuracy comparing axial defect within 98.55 and 96.05%.

Overall, it can be concluded that the results of sensor gap and displacement-time curves in both numerical and experimental work were almost similar. In addition, the ToF, distance calculated, actual distance, and relative error summarized in Table 2 proved that the numerical simulation and experimental work led to almost very close and similar results.

Furthermore, it can be understood that the numerical simulation method is feasible and accurate which makes the relative error acceptable. Consequently, other experiments were also performed using numerical simulation.

Acknowledgements We would like to express our gratitude to TATIUC for the facilities and equipment provided in this experiment with including the grant STG: 9001-1806.We would also like to thank UNITEN for their unwavering support and assistance in the success of this research under the BOLD scholarship scheme as well as the BOLD funding scheme for UNITEN Postdoctoral Engineering. The authors also hope that more collaborative research between UNITEN and TATIUC can be conducted in the future for academic development while also contributing to the development of the country's technology.

References

1. Yu L, Giurgiutiu V (2008) In situ 2-D piezoelectric wafer active sensors arrays for guided wave damage detection. Ultrasonics 48(2):117–134
2. Kamas T, Giurgiutiu V, Lin B (2015) E/M impedance modeling and experimentation for the piezoelectric wafer active sensor. Smart Mater Struct 24(11):115040
3. Ali K et al (2018) S55c carbon steel for heat treatment process with different medium in attenuation measurement using ultrasonic testing. Int J Eng Technol 5(4):527–533
4. Zhang W, Akber MA, Hou S, Bian J, Zhang D (2019) Detection of Dynamic Modulus and Crack Properties of Asphalt Pavement Using a Non-Destructive Ultrasonic Wave Method. Appl Sci 9(1):1–12
5. Carino N (2001) The impact-echo method: an overview. Structures Congress & Exposition, p 18
6. Ali K et al. (2020) Effect of Crack on Bending Process for S55c Carbon Steel with Ultrasonic Testing on Zero Degree Probes. J Phys Conf Ser 1532(1)
7. Abdalla AN, Faraj MA, Samsuri F, Rifai D, Ali K (2018) Challenges in improving the performance of eddy current testing. Review Meas Control
8. Álvarez-Arenas TG, Camacho J (2019) Air-coupled and resonant pulse-echo ultrasonic technique. Sensors (Switzerland) 19(10)

9. Guarneri GA, Pipa DR, Neves FJ, de Arruda LVR, Zibetti MVW (2015) A sparse reconstruction algorithm for ultrasonic images in nondestructive testing. Sensors (Switzerland) 15(4):9324–9343
10. Zhang JK, Yan W, Cui DM (2016) Concrete condition assessment using impact-echo method and extreme learning machines. Sensors (Switzerland) 16(4):1–17
11. Ali K, Paw JK, Rifai D, Alla ANA, Faraj MA, Hen CK (2020) Optimization of Ultrasonic Testing for Defect Localization Signal on S55C Carbon Steel Pipe, 10(3)
12. Gharaibeh Y, Mudge P (2011) The Application of Long Range Ultrasonic Testing (LRUT) for Examination of Hard to Access Areas on Railway Tracks. in IET, pp 1–7
13. Kappatos V, Selcuk C, Gharaibeh Y (2011) Decreasing the Influence of Dispersive Wave Modes in Long-Range Ultrasonic Rail Testing Using Wavelets. In: 5th IET Conference on Railway Condition Monitoring and Non-destructive Testing (RCM 2011) 44
14. Li D, Yan X, Xu Z, Ta D (2019) Long-distance shift of ultrasonic beam using a thin plate with periodic gratings. Ultrasonics 95(March):32–36
15. Abdalla AN, Ali K, Paw JKS, Rifai D, Faraj MA (2018) A novel eddy current testing error compensation technique based on mamdani-type fuzzy coupled differential and absolute probes. Sensors (Switzerland) 18(7)
16. Otero J, Galarza N, Rubio B, Moreno E (1969) Semi-analytical finite elements methods for dispersion curves using higher order elements for long range ultrasonic testing. In: IEEE International Ultrasonics Symposium Proceedings, 2009, pp 1966–1969

Fuzzy Logic Error Compensation Scheme for Eddy Current Testing Measurement on Mild Steel Superficial Crack

Damhuji Rifai, Abdul Rahim Pazikadin, Kharudin Ali, Moneer A. Faraj, Noraznafulsima Khamsah, and Ahmed N. Abdalla

Abstract Accurate measurement the depth of defect is essential to ensure the reliability and integrity of the pipe line structure and safety of the personnel workers in the oil and gas industry. This study proposes intelligent algorithm base on Fuzzy logic scheme to compensate the depth error measurement of GMR sensor on mild steel superficial crack. Intelligent rules in Fuzzy logic scheme allows the propose method to be effective on compensate lift off effect in between 1 and 4 mm. The Eddy current testing probe is design by utilize the sensitive of GMR sensor on magnetic field in order to improve the accuracy depth crack measurement on mild steel. The Arduino Mega 2650 was used as a data processing device for receiving and transmitting of signal through the available fifty-four digital pins (as input and output) and sixteen analogue pins. MATLAB is use as a platform to design and implementation the Fuzzy error compensation. The experiment results show the proposed sensor error compensation scheme able to reduce the error measurement up to 23%.

Keywords Eddy current testing · Giant magneto resistance · Mild steel · Fuzzy logic

D. Rifai (✉) · A. R. Pazikadin · K. Ali · N. Khamsah
Faculty of Electrical and Automation Engineering Technology, UCTATI, 24000 Terengganu, Malaysia
e-mail: damhuji@uctati.edu.my

M. A. Faraj
Electrical and Electronics Engineering Department, Omar al Mukhtar University, Al Baida, Libya

A. N. Abdalla
Faculty of Electronic Information Engineering, Huaiyin Institute of Technology, Huai'an Jiangsu, China

H. Triwiyanto et al. (eds.), *Proceedings of the 1st International Conference on Electronics, Biomedical Engineering, and Health Informatics*, Lecture Notes in Electrical Engineering 746, https://doi.org/10.1007/978-981-33-6926-9_20

1 Introduction

Mild steel is a material that has high strength and cheap in terms of economic costs and it is widely used as structural building materials on less critical parts in oil and gas industry structure. Eddy current testing (ECT) is a main technique for oil and gas structure inspection, when appropriately used, can detect superficial and sub-superficial defects. For specific materials and defect types, the probe design and sensitive receiver sensor is the main factor that can improve the accurate depth measurement of the defect.

For structural integrity assessment purposes in the oil and gas industry, non-destructive testing ECT has several advantages over other non-destructive methods. Main advantages, this method has a fast and highly scalable scanning rate for inspection involving large structures such as in the oil and gas industry [1, 2]. In addition, the depth of defect scanning can be adjusted by controlling the frequency of excitation applied. The conventional ECT probe design is used a coil as a magnetic field excitation and receiver sensor generated by the structure of the tested material. This method is the main factor that cause conventional ECT coil probe less sensitive and reduces the accuracy of the measurement due to the high of Signal to Noise Ratio (SNR) [3, 4]. This limitation causes the development of the ECT method to be lagged behind compare with the ultrasonic testing (UT) method for non-destructive testing. However with the advance development of MOSFET technology and the development of Giant magneto resistance (GMR) that very sensitive to the magnetic field have been open new dimension for improvement of ECT [5]. The previous study shows the implementation of GMR sensors as a magnetic detection sensor in ECT probe design has increased the sensitivity probe to the changes of magnetic field that caused by structural defects. Enhancement of ECT probe sensitivities consequently improve the information and defect profile that can be obtained through tests conducted. There have been several studies in the literature reporting the implementation of GMR on ECT probe design. Study by [6] show the combination of GMR sensor and excitation coil in ECT probe design improve the accuracy of defect measurement. The experimental and simulation result validate the accuracy of the probe measurement. In a different study [7], examined the detection of defect on aluminum plate at low frequency. The finding of the investigation suggested that eddy current probe consisting of the GMR sensor able to detect the bipolar magnetic field up to 716 gausses with a constant field to voltage transfer function at frequencies up to 10 kHz. With the same objective [8], conducted experiments on enhance detection of deep seated flaws in 316 stainless steel plates. The result shows the EC-GMR sensor probe able to measure subsurface defect deep down to 8 mm. The above finding is consistent with the study by [9]. Karpenko et al. [9] examined the EC-GMR probe improve the inspection accuracy on riveted multilayer structures.

The previous literature above reveals that the level of sensitivity of the ECT probe can be improved through implementation of GMR sensor as a receiving sensor in ECT probe design [10, 1]. Although there were many researches on improved the accuracy of ECT inspection, many of them focus probe design. So it is necessary to do deep research on improve the accuracy of ECT inspection by improving the sensor accuracy and reduce the error of sensor measurement [3]. This paper aims to illustrate the development of intelligent GMR sensor error compensation by using Fuzzy Logic algorithm. Mild steel used as testing material in order to validate the propose method. GMR sensor are used as a magnetic field receiver sensor to improve the sensitivity limitation of coil receiving sensor in ECT probe design.

2 Types of Eddy Current Testing Probe for Surface Scanning

The magnetic field will be formed around the conductor material when the alternating current flows on the material. When this magnetic field is approached on one other conductor material, the current will be induced to the material and produces the eddy current flowing in the sphere. By analyzing changes in the shape of the magnetic field that occurs when there is a defect on the surface of the conductor, the defect profile can be identified.

In addition to the analysis of the magnetic field, analysis of impedance changes can also provide the defective information available on specimens [11, 12]. When the test is carried out, the alternating current generates a magnetic field around the conductor of the material, when the magnetic field is moved near a defective or cracked area, the magnetic field will be disturbed and also cause a change in the impedance of the coil transmitting and the coil receiver.

The main advantage of eddy current non-destructive testing techniques is the variety of checks that can be used with this technique. In addition to measuring the cracks profile on the material structure, this method can also be used to measure coating thickness, material conductivity and material permeability.

Probe for eddy current checks is available in various forms to meet different requirements of different industries and applications. Each designed probe will give optimal results if the probe is used in accordance with the application and the specimen material structure. The main difference of the design for this probe is to refer to the wired coil design and how the magnetic field change method is detected [13]. Existing probe used in industry is like absolute probe, differentiation, reflection and hybrid. Using the exact probe for each specimen can make measurements and more accurate checks.

The probe is absolutely using a reactant change to produce a defective profile on the tested specimen. The probe design has only one coil. When the alternating current through the coil, the magnetic field will be generated around the coil and when it is approached on the specimen to be tested, an induced current will be generated on the specimen [14]. This induction current will produce its own magnetic field which will reject the premier magnetic field from the coil. This rejection reaction will change the reactant and the profile of the specimen structure can be generated by measuring the reactance changes. This type of probe is widely used to measure the conductivity and thickness of coating on pipes in the oil and gas industry. This type of probe is sensitive to the impact of lift-off and permeability of the specimen material. Therefore, it can also be used to identify the material to be tested.

Probe differential has two soft iron cores wrapped in coil coils in series. When this differential probe scans an area with no defects, there is no signal difference between the two core coils. But when there is a defect on the surface of the specimen, the signal difference will be generated between these two coils, the difference in the signal is the effect of the presence of the surface defect. The defective profile can be obtained by analyzing such conditions. This type of probe is very sensitive to defect such as cracking but less sensitive to measuring defect changes. In addition, this type of probe is not suitable for detecting long defects and exceeds the distance between two coils. This is because long defects exceeding the distance of two coil will make it difficult to analyze the defective profile. The probe will only be able to scan some of the defects and this will cause trailing when the signal cancellation occurs.

Reflection probes have two coils similar to a differential probe, but one coil is used to transmit and the other is used as a receiver. These types of probes are called as transmit-receive probes [5]. The receiver coil in reflection probe is made very small so that it will be very sensitive to small defects. The use of this types probe design enhanced the SNR that improve the detection and advantageous when deeper penetration is required, such as detection of subsurface defects. The advantage is that transmit and receive coils can be optimized independently. Such probes also have a wider frequency range than other probes and larger excitation coil provide a more uniform electromagnetic field for better depth penetration. Figure 1 shows the basic configuration of ECT probe.

Figure 1b shows differential probes that have two active coils wound in opposition. When the two coils are over a flawless test sample field, there is no differential signal produced between the coils. The disadvantages of this probe is the signals may be hard to perceive. For example, if a flaw exceeds the distance between the two coils, only the leading and trailing edges signal can be identified due to the cancelation of the signal as both coils detect the defect equally. A coil pair Fig. 1c which has separate transmitting and receiving coil windings can be used for enhanced the sensitivity of the probe sensor detection if deep penetration of eddy current testing required for subsurface defect inspection.

Hybrid probes operate in the reflection mode but its sensing coils is replaced with semiconductor base magnetic sensing device such as GMR sensor. The utilization of GMR sensor improve the ECT probe sensitivity to the changes of magnetic field and improve accuracy inspection on subsurface and surface cracks detection. Hybrid probes are specially designed for a specific inspection with high sensitivity need for deep subsurface inspection.

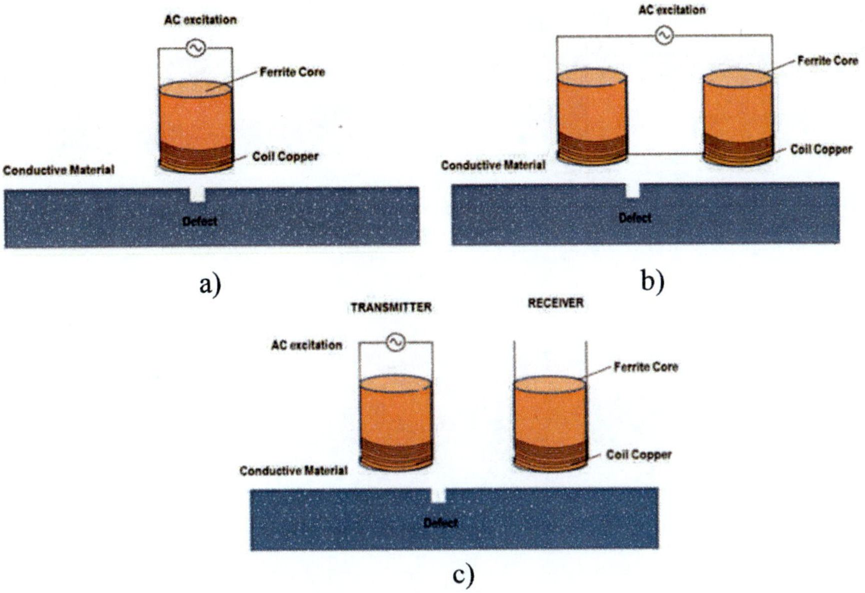

Fig. 1 ECT probe design configuration: (**a**) Single coil absolute probe (**b**) Differential probe (**c**) A Transmitter and receiver coil probe

3 Eddy Current Testing Probe Design

The design of probes is very important for proper detection of eddy currents testing. The probe coils consist of a length of wire wound around a probe core. The winding has more than one layer to increase the value of coil inductance. The core can consist of either a solid material or just air as shown in Fig. 2. The probe structure can classify coils by its core, coils with ferrous core are called ferrous coils and coils with air core are called air coils.

The propose probe design configurations parameters is shown in Table 1. All coils are wounded on carbon steel pipe and have an air core. Figure 2 shown the design of propose ECT probe design while Fig. 3 shown the realization of the ECT probe.

4 Eddy Current Testing Measurements System

The block diagram and experimental setup for the system with the A/D card is illustrated in Fig. 4. The two coils probes were excited by Keysight Function generator. The differential amplifier is a wide band amplifier that was designed to amplifies the excitation signal. The gain of the amplifier is set to 3 dB. An ideal

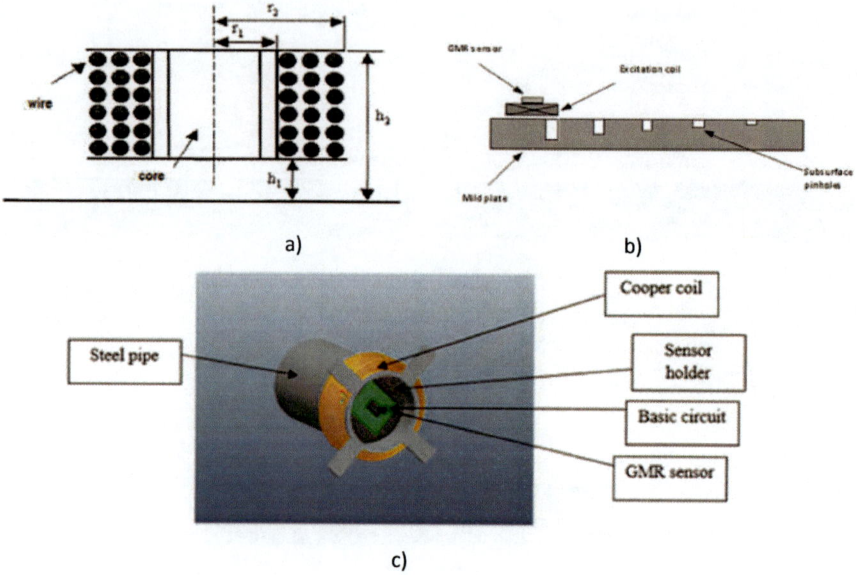

Fig. 2 The propose ECT probe design: (**a**) Diagram of a coil (**b**) Scanning diagram for surface ECT inspection (**c**) 3-D designed of GMR-Coil probe

Table 1 Parameters of the costumed coils used in the experiments

Number of coil turns, n	Inner radius, r1	Outer radius, r2	Height, h2 −h1 (mm)	Resistance, Rc (ohm)	Inductance, L (mH)
110	1.19	2.00	2.85	1.96	0.02289

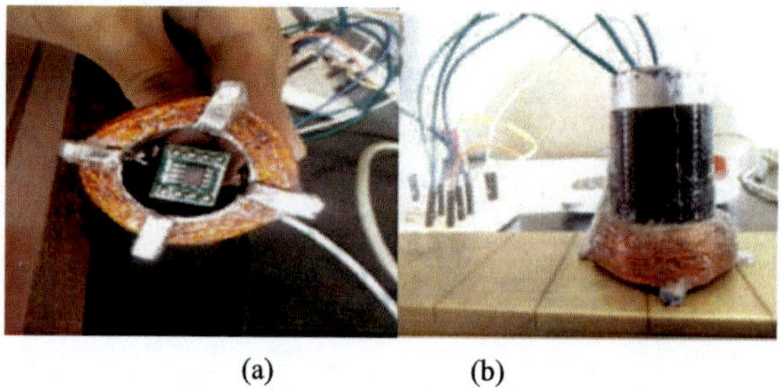

Fig. 3 Realization of ECT GMR-coil probe design; (**a**) bottom; (**b**) front

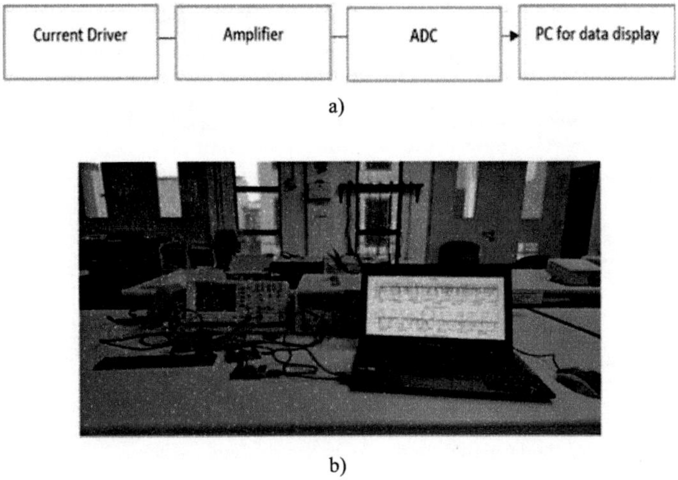

Fig. 4 (**a**) Block diagram and (**b**) Experimental setup for ECT system

voltage or current source is a very important for eddy current testing system because it will determine efficiency of the ECT probe for detection any presence defect on sample testing. The output of the amplifier was connected to a 14-bit A/D card model Compu Scope 14100 from Gage applied.

The Arduino base A/D card was used in the data acquisition system. This card can collect data in several ways. In this acquisition data, the pulse data were collected and then transferred to the host computer where they were processed. This method does not guarantee a constant interval between two sampling because it depends on the computer speed and CPU availability. This method provides a fixed time interval between two acquired pulses. The rate of data acquisition is determined by the signal from the current driver. This method gives more exact and acceptable experimental results.

In order to test the accuracy of the ECT testing system, inspection of mild steel with depth of defect 1, 2 and 3 and 4 mm are conducted. The measurements are compared to the calculations based on the analytical solutions of the coil's impedance for a given frequency of excitation. The results show very good agreement between the measurements and calculations.

5 Fuzzy Logic Error Compensation

The overall block diagram of proposed error compensation technique for the ECT measurement of depth mild steel crack is shown in Fig. 5. This technique utilized a single GMR probe operated in two different ways: one was to create a set of

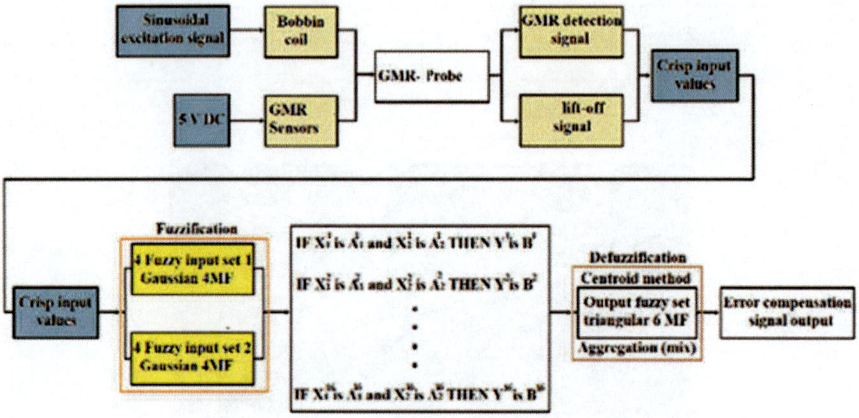

Fig. 5 The diagram of the proposed Fuzzy Logic compensation scheme

detection channels, and the other was to measure of lift-off measurement by using the impedance relationship value when there is a variation of distance between GM sensor and the surface of mild steel during the measurement. A simple relationship can be created between the two-variable using the Mamdani type fuzzy. The depth defect parameter can be quantitatively evaluated by measuring how high the peak amplitude of the GMR signal in the eddy current detection. The GMR signal can be affected by the changing in the lift-off which lead to inaccurate ECT measurement. This study proposed GMR sensor error compensation based on the Mamdani fuzzy type approach, the effect of the lift-off can be reduced. The rule for Fuzzy sensor error compensation is tabulate on Table 2.

MATLAB was utilized to process the ECT GMR sensor probe input signals with the fuzzy inference system together with the output signal. Figure 6 shows the simulation block that was used to integrate the hardware probe with MATLAB software. The ouput of GMR sensor then were then treated as input for the error compensation technique which was done using Mamdani FIS. The simulation model consisted of three parts, which were utilized for error compensation technique. The first part was the output of GMR sensor probe contain the voltage magnitude that reflect to the depth of crack on mild steel and the capacitance which were set to reflect the variation of lift of as s inputs to the Fuzzy error compensation rule. The second part was the fuzzy inference system (FIS) model, being used to compensate the errors which were introduced by the lift-offs. The output signal from fuzzy block will be brought through the error compensation equation in the signal block, and it would be fed back into the error block, and lastly forwarded into the output display.

Table 2 Rule base of Mamdani-type FIS

Rules	IF	GMR(V)	THEN	Depth of defect (mm)
1		0.88		1.5
2		0.88		1.5
3		0.88		1.5
4		0.88		2.0
5		1.75		2.5
6		1.75		2.5
7		1.75		2.5
8		1.75		3.0
9		2.63		3.5
10		2.63		3.5
11		2.63		4.0
12		2.63		4.0
13		3.5		4.0
14		3.5		4.0
15		3.5		4.0
16		3.5		4.0

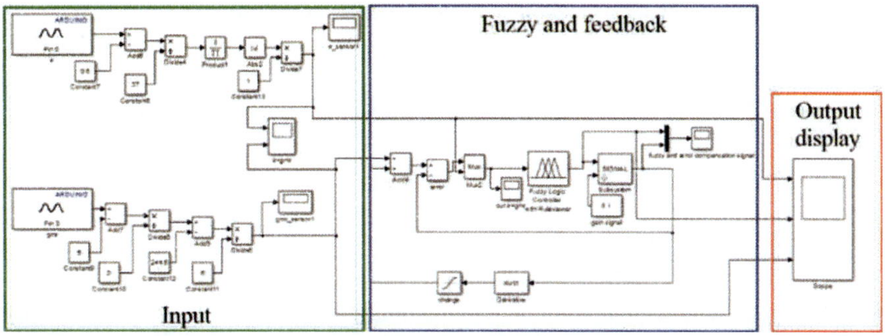

Fig. 6 MATLAB Simulink Fuzzy Logic compensation scheme schematic

6 Sample Preparation for Mild Steel Material Sensor Array Detection Result

Mild steel samples with different depth of artificial defect are used as a sample test for validation of the propose method. The process of sample preparation is shown in Fig. 7. This process is to fabricate mild steel sample testing material with 1, 2, 3 and 4 mm axial defect using EDM wire cut machine.

Wire Electrical Discharge Machine (EDM) is used to fabricate defect with different depth. The ECT sample testing block is fabricated with high accuracy dimension in order to validate the precision of the propose ECT probe.

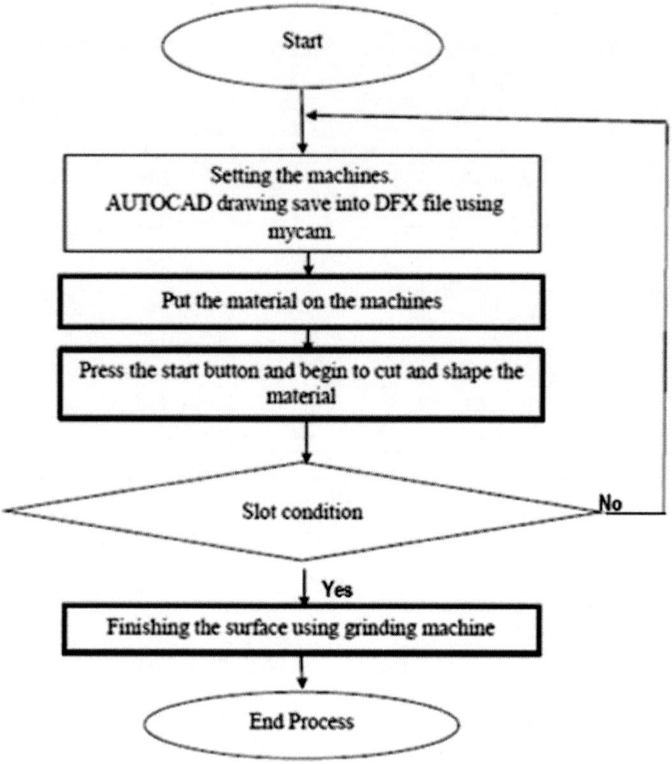

Fig. 7 EDM wire cut machine process for mild steel ECT testing sample preparation

Wire cutting by EDM uses a metal wire to cut a contour in a piece of work. The process of machining start with drilling a hole in the work piece or starting point from the edge. The wire can be rotated so that sections can cut different profiles design. Electrode and work piece do not have any mechanical contact. The wire is usually made from brass or stratified copper material and has a diameter between 0.1 and 0.3 mm. A part will either be one cut or it will be roughed and skimmed, depending on the precision and surface finish required. Ideally the wire passes through a solid part on one cut and drops a bit of slug or scrap when it is finished. The dimension for a mild steel sample defect are that used to verify the proposed ECT probe and Fuzzy Logic compensation scheme is shown in Fig. 8.

Figure 9 show a mild steel sample block during and after wire cut process using EDM wire cut machine. 5 slots of artificial defects have been created during this process.

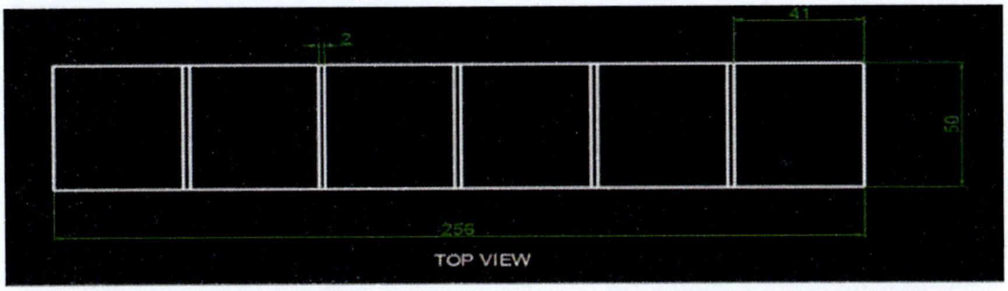

a)

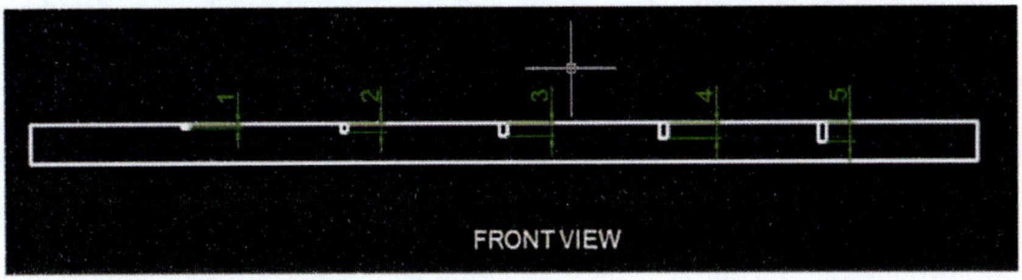

b)

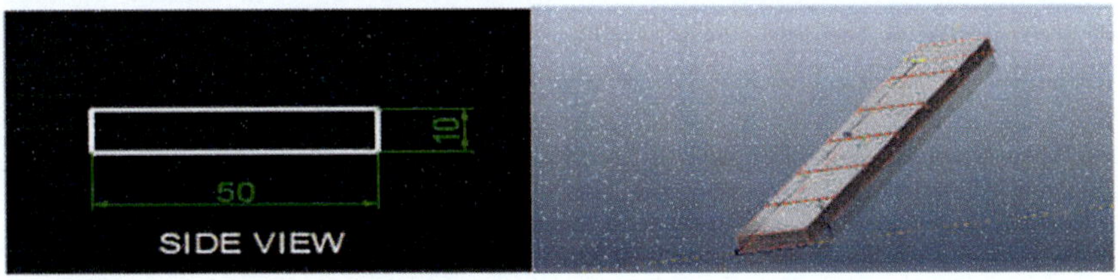

c) d)

Fig. 8 Mild steel sample for ECT inspection (**a**) Top view (**b**) Front view (**c**) Side view (**d**) 2-D design

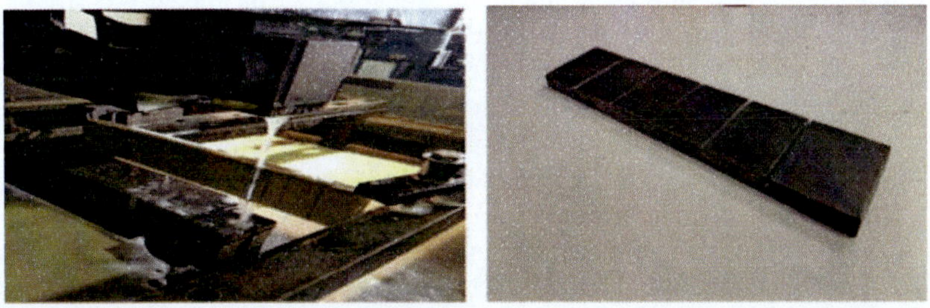

Fig. 9 Calibration block during and after wire cut process

7 Results

7.1 Mild Steel Superficial Crack Measurement

A simplified describing eddy current flow at the surface of a specimen in the vicinity of a depth crack measurement is presented. This is then used to explain the experimental results obtained. The results can be applied as a reference for cracks depth measurement on mild steel.

In this propose probe GMR-coil model, the induced eddy currents are considered in terms of a series of current loops in a thin surface layer. It may be considered that these currents are concentrated in paths that reflect the periphery of the coil and follow along boundary of the defect. The experiment results show the current distribution along length of defect is circularly symmetric around the coil axis and decays exponentially with depth. The finding is consistent with basic principle of skin depth effect on metal material, which is stated the skin effect of eddy current phenomena is decrease exponentially when the magnetic field penetrate into the mild steel material. Figure 10 shows the result of ECT depth defect measurement using propose GMR-Coil probe on mild steel.

The signal amplitude measurement of depth defect on mild steel was inversely proportional to the lift-off and was directly proportional to the depth of defects. Based on this experimental analysis, the actual measurement is obtain by calibrate signal amplitude measurement of the plate without lift-off as an actual depth of defect signal amplitude or reference value. The signal produced decreased according to the distance between the plate and the probe, as can be seen in Fig. 10.

7.2 Eddy Current Testing Crack Measurement Error Compensation Using Fuzzy

As described in the previous section, the Fuzzy Compensation scheme for ECT GMR error measurement compensation technique was developed to make corrections to the measure peak amplitude signal output of the ECT GMR probe that specifically fabricated for depth defect measurement on mild steel material. The variation changes in the lift-off measurement caused non-uniformity of distance between the ECT probe and the surface of the mild steel sample that will cause an error in the depth defect assessment. Experiments were performed with the use of ECT GMR sensor probes with proposed error compensation techniques in order to reduce the influence of lift-off in depth defect measurement using eddy current testing. The experiment was performed using the current amplitude supplied by the 8 VAC function generator, which is achieved by lowering the voltage from the main source to produce a frequency field of 30 kHz. This current amplitude and low frequency is necessary for increase the magnetic penetration in subsurface defect measurement accordance to the skin effect principle [15, 16]. Lift-offs vary in the

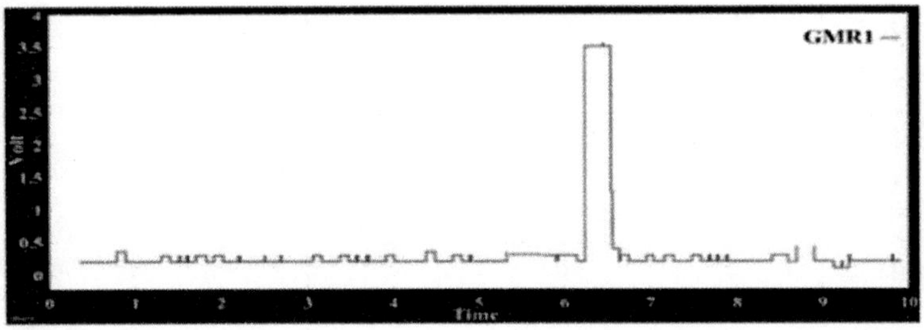

a)

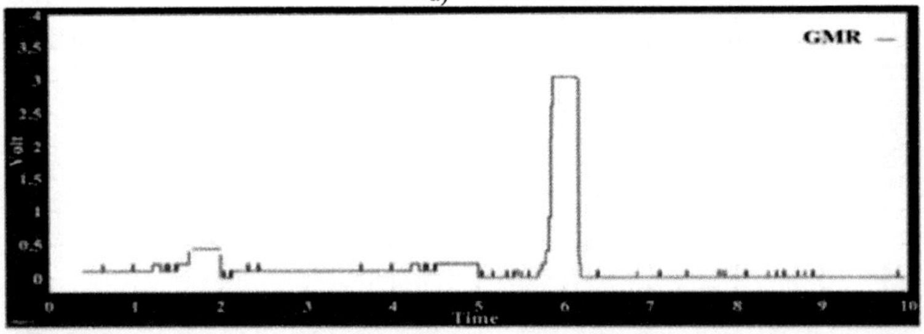

b)

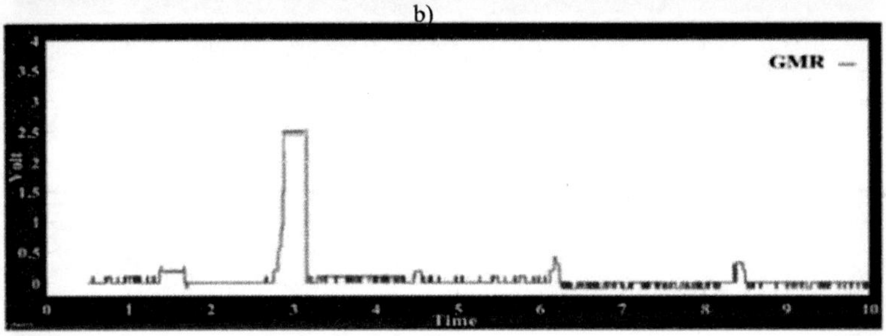

c)

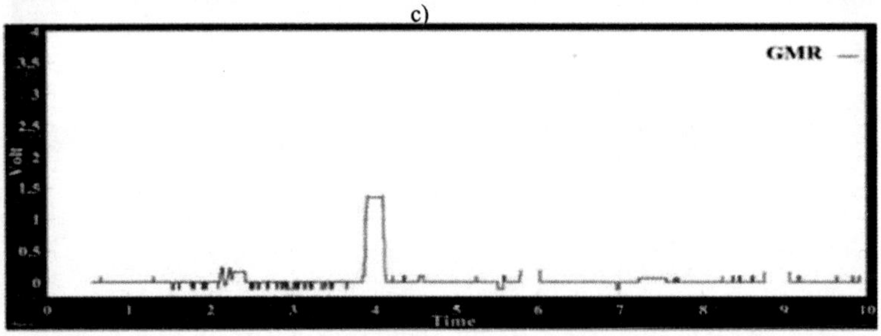

d)

Fig. 10 Mild steel superficial crack depth measurement: (**a**) 5 mm (**b**) 4 mm (**c**) 3 mm (**d**) 2 mm (**e**) 1 mm (**f**) 0.5 mm

range of 1–3 mm during experiments. Lift-offs often occur during measurements; compensation for reduction determines the actual value of the crack. Figure 11 shows the output signal for measuring 4 mm mild steel depth defect. Fuzzy Logic

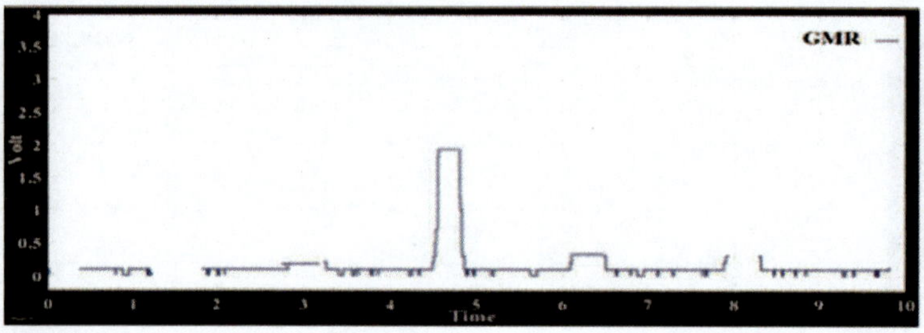

e)

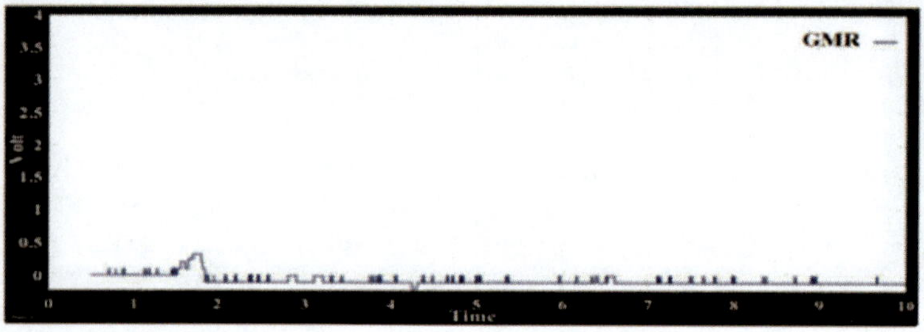

f)

Fig. 10 (continued)

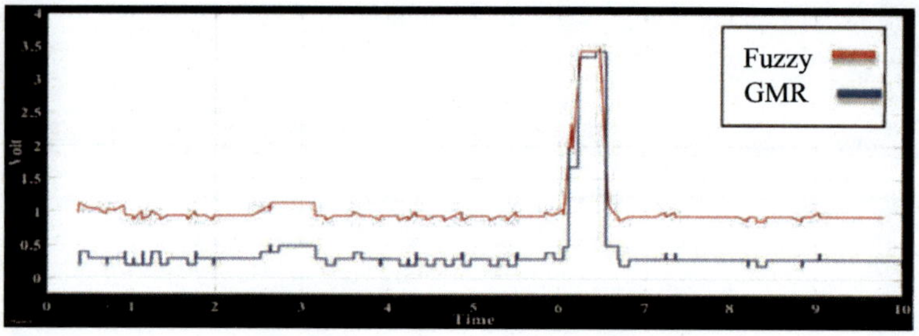

Fig. 11 Fuzzy logic for error compensation signal output without lift-off

Compensation scheme is used to correct the measurement error that caused by lift-off effect. The blue line graph is the output signal for the ECT probe and is considered as a reference value for the peak amplitude of the GMR sensor output signal. While the red signal is the signal produced by the Fuzzy Logic Compensation scheme represents the signal that has been compensated using the proposed FLC. The peak amplitude value of the GMR output signal is 3.45 V, while the FLC output value is 3.5 V.

The Fuzzy Logic compensation scheme output for the GMR sensor signal that has been compensate under different lift-offs for mild steel samples with a defect

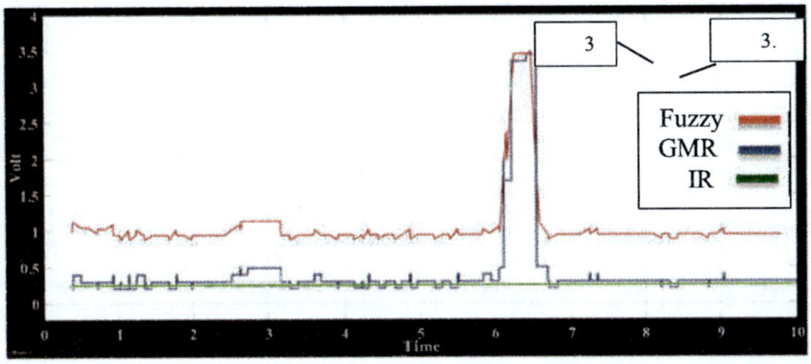

a)

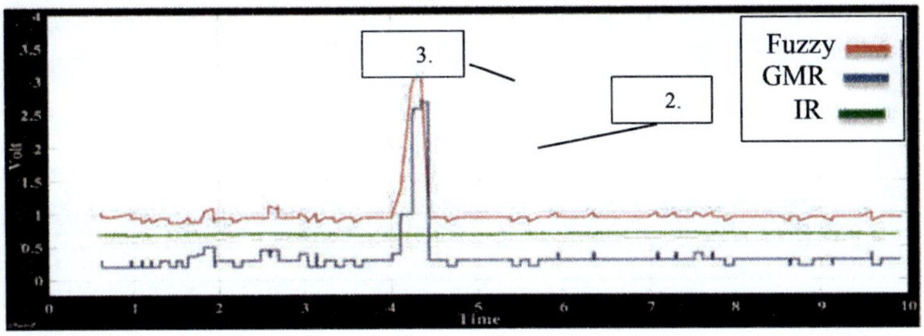

b)

Fig. 12 Fuzzy logic compensation scheme output with 4 mm axial depth defect: (**a**) 0 mm (**b**) 1 mm (**c**) 2 mm and (**d**) 3 mm lift-off

depth of 4 mm is shown in Fig. 12. The lift-off causes the GMR sensor output signal to decrease from its actual defect value. The deviation in measuring the depth of this defect will cause the structural integrity assessment to be incorrect. This is particularly critical when involving hazardous structures especially for oil and gas infrastructure. Based on Fig. 12b, the peak amplitude of the GMR sensor output signal representing a 3 mm depth defect in a light steel sample is 2.7 V. After this signal is compensated by the Fuzzy Compensation scheme, the amplitude value of this signal increases to 3.35 V. Figure 12a–c show that the amplitude of the signal that has been corrected using Fuzzy Logic error compensation can provide a more accurate measurement value of the depth defect on mild steel defect. The output values is range from 3 V to 3.5 V for defects with a depth of 4 mm. For the 3 mm lift-off as shown in Fig. 12d, the Fuzzy Logic compensation scheme increases the accuracy measurement value from 1 mm to 3 mm. Figure 12 shows the signal output of the Fuzzy Logic compensation scheme for the ECT probe signal from 1 mm to 3 mm in the 3 mm lifting case as shown in Fig. 12d.

With the initial lift-off increasing trend, the compensated peak amplitude increased marginally as can be seen in Fig. 13a–c. The value of the fuzzy outputs was 2.63 V, 2.4 V and 2.25 V which indicated a defect in depth of approximately

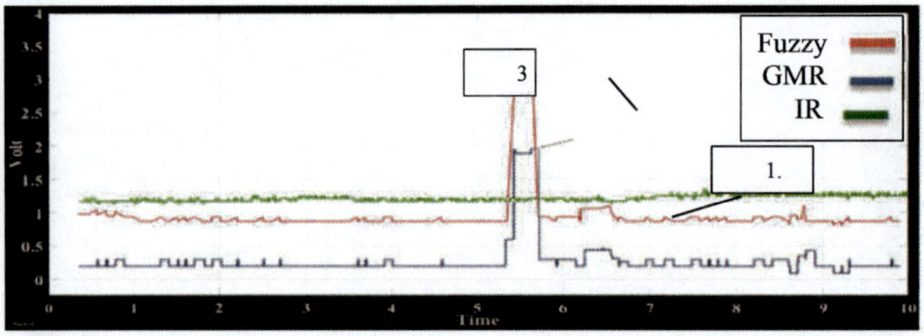

c)

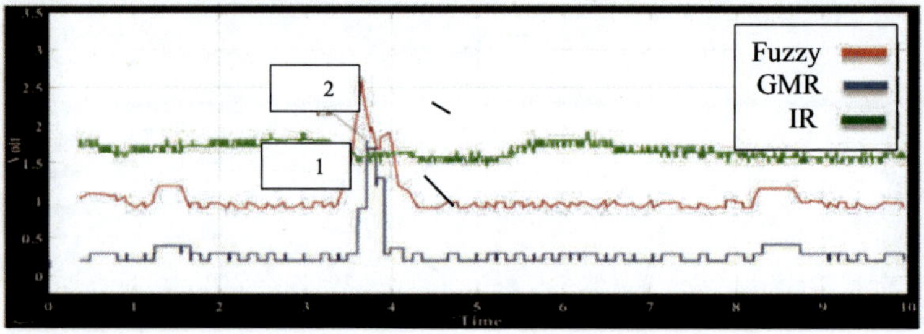

d)

Fig. 13 Continued Fuzzy logic compensation scheme output: (**a**) 0 mm (**b**) 1 mm (**c**) 2 mm and (**d**) 3 mm lift-off

3 mm. Nevertheless, the value of the fuzzy output has increased the measurement of the reference signals from 1 mm to 2 mm in the case of 3 mm lift-off as seen in Fig. 13d. Analysis of the defect signal for an axial defect with a defect in depth of 4 mm and showed that the proposed error compensation technique was accurate when the lift-off was equal to or less than 3 mm in measure.

The relationship between the compensated signal and the lift-off distance is shown in Fig. 14. The results summarize of GMR sensor and the Fuzzy Logic compensation scheme output signal are shown the signal is reduced with the increase of lift-off distance as listed in Table 3. This can explain because the magnetic density induced by the mild steel defect decreases as the distance of ECT probe and the mild steel surface increases. This condition is explained by the principle of electromagnetic skin effect. The skin effect is a phenomenon where an electric current (AC) that flows in the conductor material produces eddy current when brought close to the conductor surface. The penetration of this electromagnetic field is decreased exponentially with the depth on material conductor. The depth of the skin depends on the frequency of the electric current (AC). This is when the frequency of the alternating current increases, the current flows to the surface causing the skin depth to decrease. At the distance of the ECT probe with the sample surface of 3 mm, the percentage of error measuring this depth of defect is 26%.

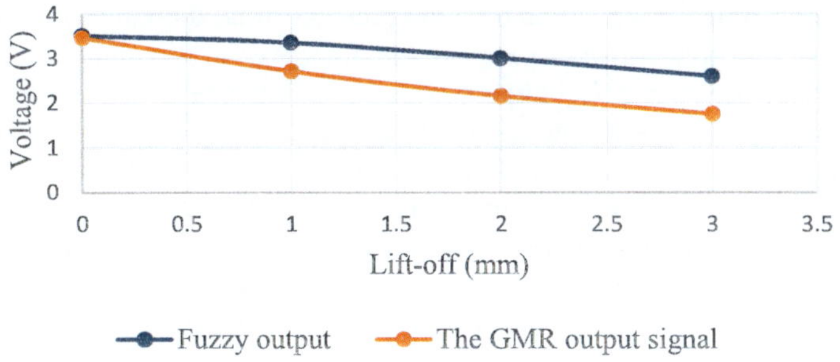

Fig. 14 Comparisons of GMR output signal (uncompensated) and fuzzy output (compensated) for depth defect of 4 mm at a range of lift-off values

Table 3 The result based on GMR-BC probe

Lift-off	Depth of defect	Signal measured	Signal measured (%)	% of error
0	1	0.88	25.14	0
0	2	1.75	50.00	0
0	3	2.63	75.00	0
0	4	3.50	100.00	0
1	1	0.75	21.40	3.74
1	2	1.50	42.80	7.20
1	3	2.40	68.50	6.50
1	4	3.35	95.70	4.30
2	1	0.60	17.10	8.04
2	2	1.35	38.50	11.50
2	3	2.25	64.20	10.80
2	4	3.00	85.70	14.30
3	1	0.55	15.70	9.44
3	2	1.10	31.40	18.60
3	3	1.80	51.40	23.60
3	4	2.60	74.20	26.00

8 Conclusion

This study proposes a sensor error compensation scheme for ECT testing. The conventional ECT coil receiver is not reliable for some mild steel's inspection as its less sensitivity to the magnetic field changes. Moreover, magnetic field has equally been obstructed by some known issues lift-off noise is one of the main factors affecting eddy current testing. In this study, an ECT probe based on bobbin coil and GMR sensor was introduced and the series of experimental on the artificial mild steel defect were performed in order to study the effectiveness the propose eddy current testing probe design. For the experimental tests, the eddy current testing inspection system was utilized to achieve the objectives of this study. Fuzzy Logic error sensor compensation technique was used to improve the accuracy of depth measurement. The proposed error compensation technique was verified experimentally and the result showed that the percentage error at 1, 2 and 3 mm lift-off were 3.74%, 8.04% and 9.44%, respectively at depth defect of 1 mm. The percentage of error for the proposed technique at 2 mm lift-off and was 11.5%. The experimental results prove the error compensation technique using the Mamdani fuzzy method generally reduces the effect of lift-off and improves the accuracy of depth defect measurement.

The outcomes of this study can be considered as reliable and supported by the previous literatures that illustrated the level of defect detection of the ECT probe can be improved through reduce the error of sensor measurement and the use of magnetic sensors in place of the conventional pickup coils

Acknowledgements We would like to express our gratitude to UC TATI for the facilities and equipment provided in this study.

References

1. Faraj MA, Samsuri F, Abdalla AN, Rifai D, Ali K (2018) Investigate the effect of lift-off on eddy current signal for carbon steel plate 06005:3–8
2. Faraj MA, Abdalla AN, Bin Samsuri F, Rifai D (2018) Construct Coil Probe Using GMR Sensor for Eddy Current Testing 02021:1–8
3. Abdalla AN, Ali K, Paw JKS, Rifai D, Faraj MA (2018) A novel eddy current testing error compensation technique based on mamdani-type fuzzy coupled differential and absolute probes. Sensors (Switzerland) 18(7)
4. Rifai D, Abdalla A, Razali R, Ali K, Faraj M (2017) An Eddy Current Testing Platform System for Pipe Defect Inspection Based on an Optimized Eddy Current Technique Probe Design. Sensors 17(3):579
5. Rifai D, Abdalla A, Ali K, Razali R (2016) Giant Magnetoresistance Sensors: A Review on Structures and Non-Destructive Eddy Current Testing Applications. Sensors 16(3):298
6. Yang G et al (2012) 3D EC-GMR sensor system for detection of subsurface defects at steel fastener sites. NDT E Int. 50:20–28
7. Jeng J-T, Lee G-S, Liao W-C, Shu C-L (2006) Depth-resolved eddy-current detection with GMR magnetometer. J Magn Magn Mater 304(1):e470–e473, September
8. Sasi B, Mukhopadhyay AVCK, RBPC (2018) Enhanced detection of deep seated flaws in 316 stainless steel plates using integrated EC-GMR sensor. Sensors Actuators, A Phys 275:44–50
9. Karpenko O, Ye C, Udpa L (2017) Dual frequency fusion for defect signal enhancement in EC-GMR inspecton of riveted multilayer structures. NDT E Int 92(July):97–103
10. Tian GY, Sophian A (2005) Reduction of Lift-Off Effects for Pulsed Eddy Current NDT. NDT E Int 38(4):319–324
11. Ali KB, Abdalla AN, Rifai D, Faraj MA (2017) Review on system development in eddy current testing and technique for defect classification and characterization. IET Circuits, Devices Syst 11(4)
12. Rifai D, Abdalla AN, Noraznafulsima, Kharudin, Ruzlaini (2016) Defect signal analysis for nondestructive testing assessment. ARPN J. Eng Appl Sci 11(4)

13. Rifai D, Abdalla AN, Khamsah N, Aizat M (2016) Subsurface Defects Evaluation using Eddy Current Testing. Indian J Sci Technol 9(March)
14. Abdalla AN, Faraj MA, Samsuri F, Rifai D, Ali K (2019) Challenges in improving the performance of eddy current testing: Measurement and Contrl 52:46–64
15. Faraj MA, Samsuri F, Abdalla AN, Rifai D, Ali K (2017) Adaptive neuro-fuzzy inference system model based on the width and depth of the defect in an eddy current signal. Appl Sci 7(7)
16. Rifai D, Abdalla AN (2015) Defect Signal Analysis for Nondestructive Testing. ARPN J. Eng Appl Sci 11(4):1–14

Development of Cutting Force Measurement Instrument for Turning Tool Post Using Arduino UNO

Wan Zulkarnain Othman, Mohamad Redhwan Abd Aziz, Nor Hana Mamat, and Ahmad Fikri Ramli

Abstract Cutting force is one of the forces occur during turning process. A measurement instrument is necessary to monitor the cutting tools performance during a turning process operation. Nowadays, dynamometers employing piezo-electric sensors embedded into the machining system, but it very expensive. The strain gauge is a cheaper approach to develop the dynamometer. The purpose of this project is to develop a measurement instrument of cutting force for turning tool post using strain gauge. Cutting force signals were captured, amplified, conditioned, converted to digital signals and read by Arduino. The measurement instrument is calibrated via increment load from 5 to 40 kg. Then, the effects of forces with two difference conditions namely dry and flood fluid condition is performed during turning process. The corresponding force readings are obtained and displayed for real time monitoring. From the observation, it is found that there is a linear relation between force and strain gauge voltage. The mathematical modelling between these force and voltage is then developed. The recent study proved that the Arduino Uno can be used in developing cheaper force instrument measurement (dynamometer) for turning process.

Keywords Cutting force · Arduino uno · Turning

1 Introduction

CNC machining is a manufacturing process in which pre-programmed computer software dictates the movement of factory tools and machinery [1]. The process can be used to control a range of complex machinery, from grinders and lathes to mills

W. Z. Othman (✉) · M. R. A. Aziz · N. H. Mamat · A. F. Ramli
Faculty of Engineering Technology, University College TATI (UC TATI), Jalan Panchor, 24000 Teluk Kalong, Kemaman, Terengganu, Malaysia
e-mail: wan_zul@uctati.edu.my

M. R. A. Aziz
e-mail: Redhwan@tatiuc.edu.my

H. Triwiyanto et al. (eds.), *Proceedings of the 1st International Conference on Electronics, Biomedical Engineering, and Health Informatics*, Lecture Notes in Electrical Engineering 746, https://doi.org/10.1007/978-981-33-6926-9_21

and routers. With CNC machining, three-dimensional cutting tasks can be accomplish in a single set of prompts. Nowadays, every manufacturer in the global market is pitted against worldwide competitors with consistently improving product quality, enhanced manufacturing productivity, elimination of inspections, and shrinking total machining costs [2]. The condition of cutting tools and the cutting process should be identified without human assistance and/or interrupting the manufacturing process operation, which is one of the most important operating criteria that influences the manufacturing quality and productivity. An automated machining process with a successful machining condition monitoring system could allow increased principal equipment utilization, hence achieving considerable cost savings for the manufacturing industry [3]. Most of manufacturers rely on machine without instruments which could detect the force applied and the condition of the tool post. The machine operator usually uses their experience to predict when the cutting should insert needs to be changed.

Cutting forces plays a vital in machining process as they provide useful information not only for the work done but also for understanding the mechanics of machining process [4]. On the other hand, the heat generated during machining process has a direct influence on cutting forces therefore accurate measurement of cutting forces in turning is essential for tool material and geometry and selection of proper cutting parameters. Available commercial dynamometers cover a wide range of machining applications but there is a lack of force measuring devices capable for cutting forces in turning process with comparatively high spindle speeds under dry cutting conditions, in this work, the development and testing of an innovative tool shank type strain gauge-based force dynamometer designed for high speed turning is discussed. The orientation of strain gauges was set to have maximum sensitivity and minimum cross sensitivity [5]. In recent, a lot of researchers focus to the miniaturization of dynamometers which coupled sensing elements, tool holders, and turning tools to measure cutting forces [6–8]. The working principle of dynamometer is the sensing of pressure by the piezoelectric material employed as the main part in the construction of the dynamometer, which is then converted to a proportional electric charge. High cost made commercial dynamometers are not fit for industrial purposes.

Hence, the purpose of this paper is to develop a measurement instrument of cutting force for turning tool post using strain gauge coupled with Arduino UNO. The developed measurement instrument will then be tested via two condition of machining of turning: dry condition and flood condition. The surface roughness will be analyzed as the response to the in which condition higher force is been applied.

2 Methodology

The methodology of this paper is divided into material used (hardware, software) and calibration of the strain gauge.

2.1 Hardware and Software

Figure 1 shows the schematic work of the project. The project consists of strain gauge, amplifier, Arduino Uno and PC. The strain gauge detects the resistance change on the cutting tool. The data collected first is to be amplified using Wheatstone bridge circuit because without amplifier, the data is too small for Arduino circuit board to be detected. Then, Arduino process the data for calibration and compile the data into the table. Finally, the result is display on PC for real time monitoring.

Strain gauge used in this project is metallic foil-type consists of a grid of wire filament of approximately 0.025 mm thickness, bonded directly to the strained surface by a thin layer of epoxy resin [9]. When a load is applied to the surface, the resulting change in surface length is communicated to the resistor and the corresponding strain is measured in terms of the electrical resistance of the foil wire, which varies linearly with strain. The foil diaphragm and the adhesive bonding agent must work together in transmitting the strain, while the adhesive must also serve as an electrical insulator between the foil grid and the surface. This module uses 24 high-precision A/D converter come with high-precision electronic scale and has two analog input channels, programmable gain of 128 integrated amplifier. The input circuit can be configured to provide a bridge voltage electrical bridge sensor model is an ideal high-precision, low-cost sampling front-end module. While the Arduino Uno R3 is a microcontroller board based on the ATmega328. It has 14 digital input/output pins, 6 analog inputs, a 16 MHz crystal oscillator, a USB connection, a power jack, an ICSP reader, and a reset button. The micro-SD Card Module is a simple solution for transferring data to and from a standard SD card. This module has SPI interface which is compatible with any SD card and it use 5 or 3.3 V power supply which is compatible with Arduino UNO/Mega. This module will greatly expand the capability an Arduino can do with its poor limited memory.

The Arduino integrated development environment is a cross-platform application that is written in the programming language Java. Arduino consists of both a physical programmable circuit board and a piece of software used to write and upload computer code to the physical board. Proteus software is used to simulate the system and as project functional testing. The strain gauge used to measure the force and the strain gauge work by varying the resistance value and send the signal

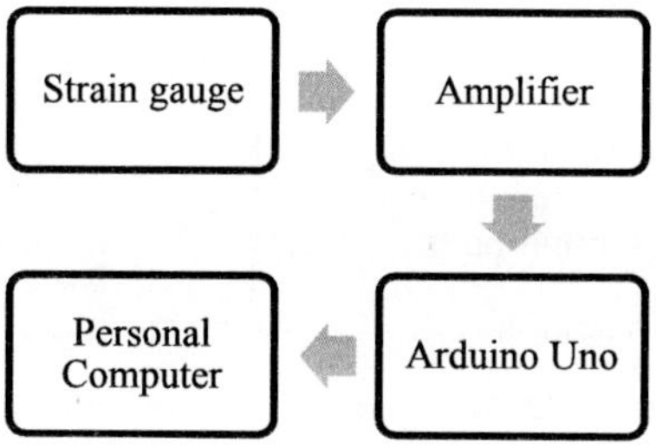

Fig. 1 Schematic diagram of the project

in voltage value to the analog input of the Arduino. As it does not exist in the simulation software, a potentiometer has been used to replace the strain gauge. The potentiometer function is almost the same as the strain gauge by the function of adjustable value of resistance which will control the output voltage that varying from 0 to 5 V. Then, a virtual terminal is added to the simulation and connected to the Arduino. The virtual terminal is used to display the output of the Arduino and collect the simulation data. For starter, the program is set to display the current date, time, value of binary data from the strain gauge and the value of voltage that generate at the analog input. The data is set to be updated every one second.

2.2 *Hardware and Software*

For a strain gauge to deliver an accurate measurement, it must be properly installed onto the measuring object. Hence the steps follow need to be done as shown in Fig. 2:

The first step of strain gauge installation is *Surface Preparation*. The tool post surface must be prepared before the strain gages and bondable terminal pads can be installed. Cleanliness is important for successful strain gage bonding. The aim of preparation is to create a smooth surface which can be wetted so it can receive the adhesive. Next is *Coarse Cleaning*. In this step, rust, scale, paint and other contaminants must be removed from the location where strain gages will be installed.

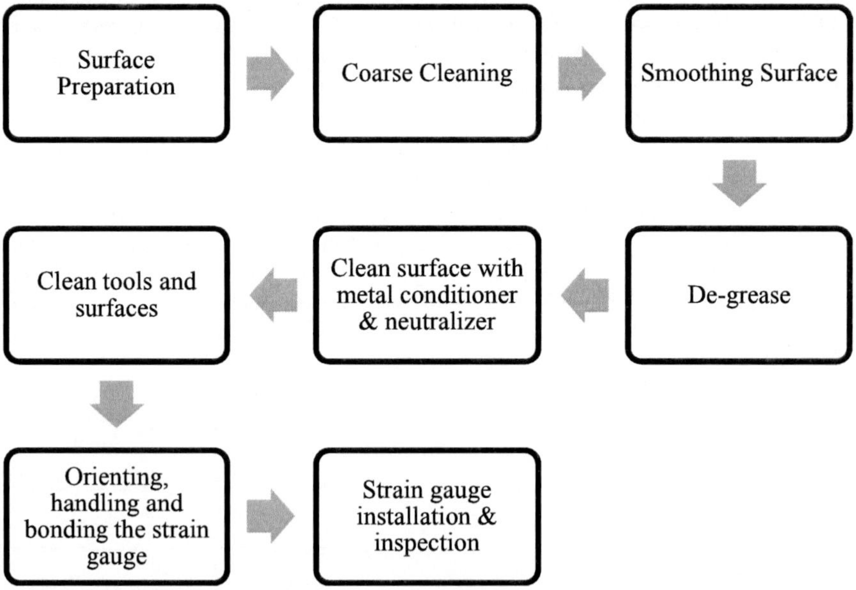

Fig. 2 Flow process of strain gauge installation [10]

Any surface coating is removed by sand blasting or by abrading with coarse grade emery paper. Smoothing Surface: Surface imperfections must be removed. Pitting, scratches, protrusions, etc. can be removed by grinding, filing or other suitable methods to smooth the surface where strain gages will be installed. Follow with a light sanding with a fine grit (240 grit) silicon carbide or emery paper. De-Grease the Surface: Use a solvent, and a soft tissue to remove all excess oil and grease. Select a solvent. Check the chemical resistance of the material, making sure that the solvent will not damage the test piece. Clean Surface with Metal Conditioner and Neutralizer: Clean the surface with a mild acid or metal conditioner. Sand lightly with the metal conditioner and wipe clean with a clean tissue or gauze pad. Clean the surface with a mild base, or metal neutralizer, wipe with a clean tissue or gauze pad. Brush with lint-free brush to remove any dust particles that may have settled. Clean Tools and Surfaces: Clean and degrease the tools that will be used to handle the strain gages. Prepare a clean and degreased work surface. A piece of glass can be used as a work surface. Do not handle the strain gages or bondable terminal pads with your hands, as introduce oils and contaminants that will cause bonding problems.

2.3 Strain Gauge Calibration

For this project, the strain gauge is been installed to the turning cutting tools. Strain gauge installation to the tool post is shown in Fig. 3a, b. First, the tool post surface is clean and, center of the tool post is identified and measured. Then, the strain gauge is to be soldered with single copper wire. The strain gauge to be glued firmly as to avoid detached later. While Fig. 4a, b show the calibration process as suggested [11]. Correct wiring is connected and it ready to test and calibrate. After full bridge, the signal is amplified by HX711 module, the data output is in form of voltage. In order to have force signal output, strain gauge first needs to be calibrated. Handheld weight scale is used to calibrate the strain gauge. Handheld weight scale is used to pull in x and y direction and the voltage output is recorded. The weight reading is taken from 5 to 40 kg with interval 5 kg each. Figure 3 depicted the steps in installation and calibration of the strain gauge.

3 Result and Discussion

The strain gauge calibration and test run using dry and wet cutting technique of turning result is reported and discussed in this section.

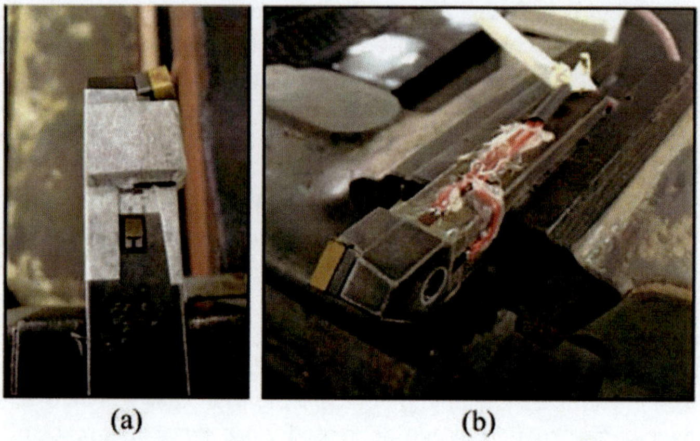

Fig. 3 Strain gauge attachment process **a** tool post cleaning and strain gauge attachment, **b** wiring of the strain gauge to the tool post

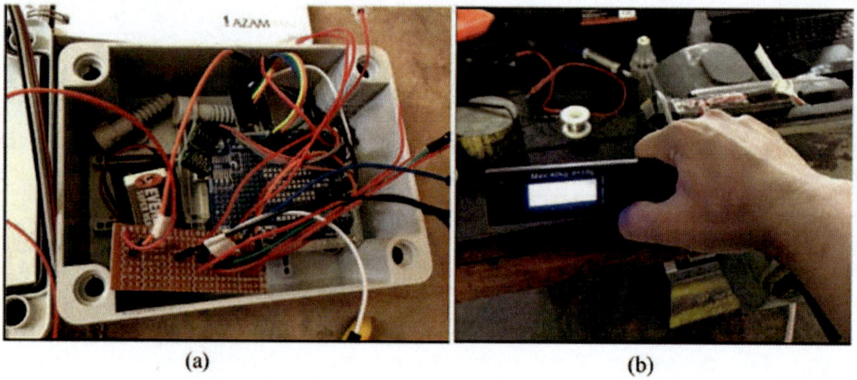

Fig. 4 Strain gauge calibration **a** setting up the Arduino Uno, **b** calibration process by using digital handheld weight scale

3.1 Strain Gauge Calibration

Strain gauge calibration work is done by collecting data between load (kg) from 5 to 40 kg versus force in x (F_x) and y (F_y) direction. Based on data collected, the resultant force (F_R) is then calculated by using formula 1.

$$F_R = \sqrt{F_x^2 + F_y^2} \tag{1}$$

Table 1 Load (kg) versus forces

Load (kg)	F_x (N)	F_y (N)	F_R (N)
5	0.00190	0.00239	0.00305
10	0.00358	0.00377	0.00520
15	0.00545	0.00571	0.00789
20	0.00735	0.00764	0.01071
25	0.00980	0.00945	0.01361
30	0.01200	0.01128	0.01647
35	0.01500	0.01316	0.01995
40	0.01590	0.01510	0.02193

Table 2 Voltage (V) versus force (N)

Voltage (V)	F (N)
0.00305	49.05
0.00520	98.10
0.00789	147.15
0.01071	196.20
0.01361	245.25
0.01647	294.30
0.01995	343.35
0.02193	392.40

Total calibration data which shows load versus force F_x, force F_y and resultant force (F_R) is tabulated in Table 1.

Based on the data collected in Table 1, the resultant force is then converted into new voltage value while the load in kg is converted into force (N) by multiplying the load with gravity (9.81 N). The voltage (V) versus load is then tabulated in Table 2. Then, graph forces against voltage is plotted which include the trend line to show the linear equation that later can be used to find force.

The graph in Fig. 5 shows the relationship between force and voltage. The graph shows the voltage is directly proportional to the force. When the voltage increase, the force is also increase. When the strain gauge is bend or deflation, it changes the resistance of the strain gauge on the Wheatstone full bridge. It creates the voltage output that getting higher when more deflation. The trend line is created and shows the linear equation ($y = 17522x + 4.3062$) that can be used to convert data voltage collected into force equivalent. Based on the result, the increment of the force is steadily increased.

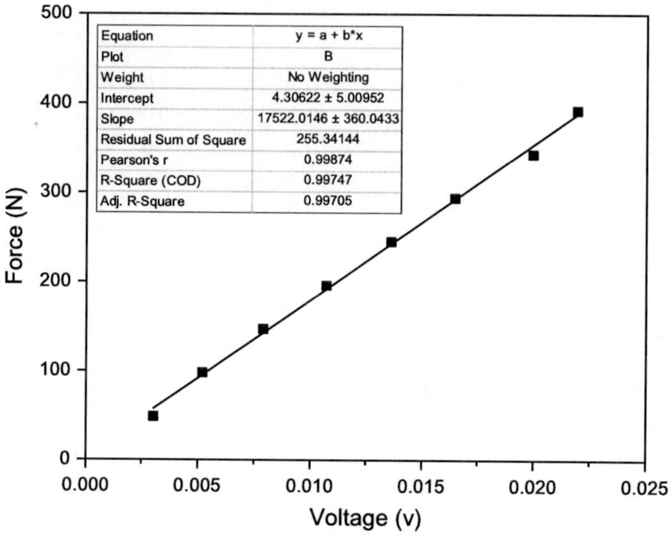

Fig. 5 Calibration chart force (N) versus voltage (V)

3.2 *Force Analysis*

In order to analyse the force, the test run is observed and collected through implementation of field test. Turning process employing an aluminium workpiece is machined in dry and wet condition. The spindle speeds (RPM), feed rate and depth of cut for a turning operation are kept constant at 1000 rpm, 50 mm/min and 0.5 mm, respectively.

The graph in Figs. 6 and 7 show the relationship between force (N) versus time for dry and wet condition, respectively. Figure 6 represent turning process via dry cutting technique shows fluctuated reading and force peak at 131 N is observed. On the other hand, Fig. 7 shows stable reading of force during cutting time. The force peak of 115 N is observed. It is also observed that the data reading starts above 25 s after the turning process. There is some lagging in output that need to be rectified. While Fig. 8 shows the comparison data between wet cutting technique versus dry cutting technique. The cutting force employing in wet condition is lower and more stable compared to the cutting force in dry condition. This is because by using the cutting liquid, the surface roughness of the workpiece is being reduced causing the cutting force decrease compared to the dry condition.

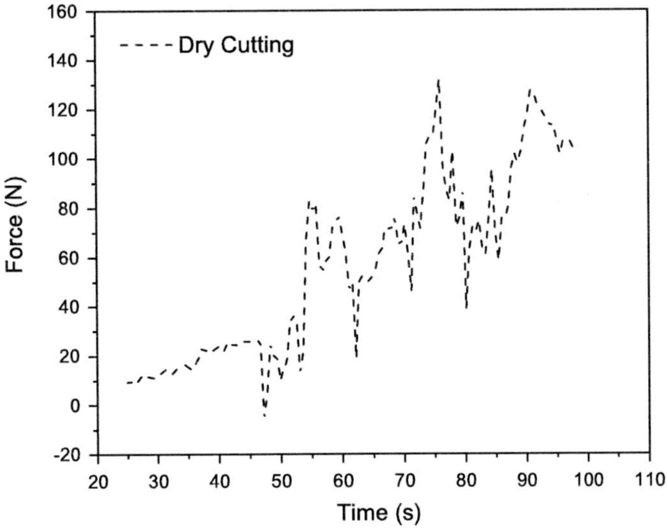

Fig. 6 Graph Force (N) versus time (s) for dry condition

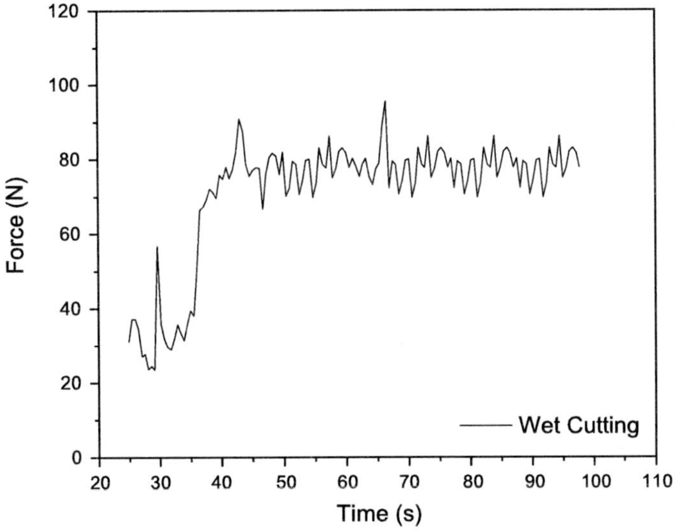

Fig. 7 Graph Force (N) versus time (s) for wet condition

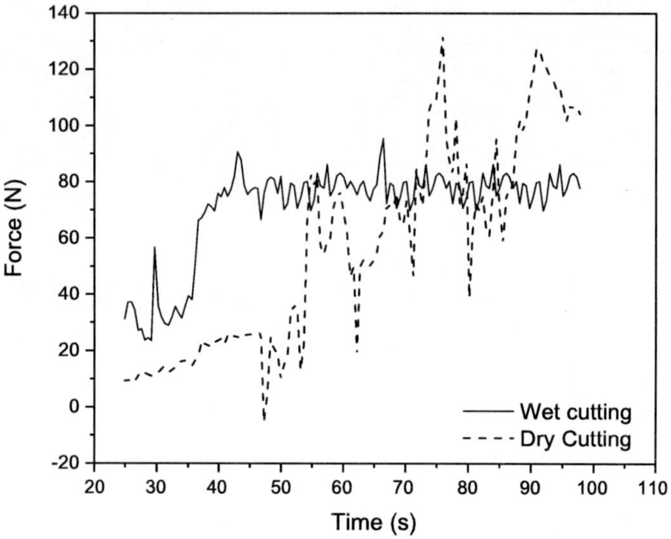

Fig. 8 Comparison graph force (N) versus time (s) for wet condition and dry cutting

4 Conclusions

The relation between the predicted and the experimental results is made by graphical representation of the radial force values. This representation clearly shows that, after getting the cutting coefficient through the calibration tests, an approximate prediction of the radial force is made by the programme created. The prediction draws a curve with the same tendency but not the exact behavior.

From the graph of dry condition and cutting fluid condition, it can be concluded that cutting force can be influenced by surface roughness. Cutting force value during turning operation using cutting fluid is lower than in dry condition. When using cutting fluid during turning operation, the surface roughness is lower than in dry condition. The recent study proved that the Arduino Uno can be used in developing cheaper force instrument measurement (dynamometer) for turning process. While there is achievement in developing low cost force measurement instrument, the respond time of the force instrument measurement need to be improved.

Acknowledgements This research is fully supported by UCTATI and UC TATI Short Term Grant (STG/9001-1902). The authors fully acknowledged University College TATI (UCTATI) for the facilities and instrumentations that make this important research viable effective.

References

1. Wright MR, Platts DE, French DB, Traicoff G, Dupont MA, Head GA (1995) CNC control system. Google Patents
2. Black JT, Hunter SL (2003) Lean manufacturing systems and cell design. Soc Manuf Eng
3. Liang Q et al (2016) Design and analysis of a sensor system for cutting force measurement in machining processes. Sensors 16(1):70
4. Thangarasu S, Shankar S, Thomas AT, Sridhar G (2018) Prediction of cutting force in turning process-an experimental approach. IOP Conf Ser: Mater Sci Eng 310(1)
5. Hanif MI, Aamir M, Muhammad R, Ahmed N, Maqsood S (2015) Design and development of low cost compact force dynamometer for cutting forces measurements and process parameters optimization in turning applications. Int J Innov Sci 3(9):306–3016
6. Öztürk E, Yıldızlı K (2017) A new static calibration methodology for strain gage integrated dynamometers. Int J Adv Manuf Technol 91(5–8):1823–1838
7. Liu M, Bing J, Xiao L, Yun K, Wan L (2018) Development and testing of an integrated rotating dynamometer based on fiber Bragg grating for four-component cutting force measurement. Sensors 18(4):1254
8. Uquillas DAR, Yeh S-S (2015) Tool holder sensor design for measuring the cutting force in CNC turning machines. In: 2015 IEEE international conference on advanced intelligent mechatronics (AIM). IEEE, pp 1218–1223
9. Kumar S (2018) Microprocessor based pressure acquisition system
10. Miles AW, Tanner KE (1992) Strain measurement in biomechanics. Springer
11. Post D, Han B, Ifju P (1994) Strain standard for calibration of electrical strain gages. In: High sensitivity moiré. Springer, pp 391–417

Spatial Mapping and Prediction of Diphtheria Risk in Surabaya, Indonesia, Using the Hierarchical Clustering Algorithm

Arna Fariza, Habibatul Jalilah, Muarifin, and Arif Basofi

Abstract Diphtheria cases in the city of Surabaya from 2015 to 2018 have increased every year. This disease can be prevented by immunizing DPT 1, DPT 2, and DPT 3 (Diphtheria, Tetanus Pertussis) given to school-age children. Immunization is the most dominant factor, where children who do not receive DPT immunization are five times more likely to be infected with diphtheria compared to children who are immunized. This paper proposes a new approach to diphtheria risk analysis in Surabaya based on multiple criteria, including DPT immunization, number of diphtheria sufferers, and population density using the hierarchical clustering algorithm. Information is presented in the form of spatial mapping of each urban village in Surabaya, Indonesia, thus, it can present information in a smaller scope. The hierarchy clustering average linkage algorithm achieves the smallest average variance value 3.3×10^{-5} and better than single linkage and complete linkage for 2016, 2017, and 2018. This developed application also provides a prediction of the next year's diphtheria risk level. The results of the 2019 predictions show a better diphtheria risk level of vulnerability using a single linkage rather than average linkage and complete linkage with the smallest variance 4.43×10^{-5}. which shows very good clustering results. The results of the knowledge shown in this application can be used as a decision support analysis for early vigilance in diphtheria in efforts to prevent and monitor diphtheria in Surabaya.

Keywords Spatial mapping · Diphtheria risk · Hierarchical clustering algorithm

---

A. Fariza (✉) · H. Jalilah · Muarifin · A. Basofi
Informatics and Computer Engineering Department, Politeknik Elektronika Negeri Surabaya, Jl. Raya ITS, Kampus PENS Sukolilo, Surabaya 60111, Indonesia
e-mail: arna@pens.ac.id

H. Triwiyanto et al. (eds.), *Proceedings of the 1st International Conference on Electronics, Biomedical Engineering, and Health Informatics*, Lecture Notes in Electrical Engineering 746, https://doi.org/10.1007/978-981-33-6926-9_22

1 Introduction

Diphtheria is an acute inflammatory disease caused by the bacterium *Corynebacterium diphtheriae* that, when coughing or sneezing, or by touching open wounds or ulcers, is transmitted from person to person through droplets [1]. Diphtheria typically occurs children 1–10 years of age, but may attack older ages. According to the World Health Organization (WHO), Diphtheria cases have increased from year to year and recorded 16,648 diphtheria cases reported worldwide in 2018 [2]. Among these figures, Indonesia contributed 1026 cases in 2018 and ranked 4th in the world after India, Yemen, and Nigeria [2]. There was an increase in cases from year to year and there were 6209 cases of diphtheria reported from 2010 to 2018. Diphtheria is a very serious fatal disease with a Case Fatality Rate (CFR) of 5–10%.

Diphtheria is a case of "re-emerging disease" in East Java Province, which ranks highest in Indonesia [3, 4]. From year to year in East Java Province, the number of Diphtheria sufferers is reported to continue to increase. In 2018, 695 cases of diphtheria were found, the most in Surabaya city with 79 cases [5]. Diphtheria cases in the city of Surabaya from 2015 to 2018 have increased every year. In 2019, diphtheria cases in Surabaya were recorded quite high at 26 cases until October 2019. Diphtheria is a disease that can be prevented by immunization and immunization against diphtheria is included in the mandatory immunization program of the Indonesian government. Diphtheria immunization combined with pertussis (whooping cough) and tetanus is called DPT (Diphtheria-Tetanus-Pertussis) immunization [6]. This disease can be prevented by giving DPT 1, DPT 2, and DPT 3 immunizations. Efforts to reduce diphtheria cases are to carry out basic immunization for infants with Diphtheria-Pertussis-Tetanus and Hepatitis B (DPTHB) vaccines. Immunization is the most dominant factor, where children who do not receive DPT immunization are five times more likely to be infected with diphtheria compared to children who are immunized.

The spatial analysis provides information on patterns and spread of infectious diseases, as well as trends in spatial areas at high risk over time. Governments can use it to enhance disease surveillance, build more detailed early warning systems, and more effectively target preventive measures to mitigate disease effects and reduce morbidity and mortality [7]. Spatial analysis is also used to see the diphtheria risk level so that it can detect spatial changes in an area from year to year [3, 7]. Immunization is the most dominant factor in preventing diphtheria risk [3, 5]. Besides, demographic factors [3, 4, 7], environment [3, 4], and nutrition [8] are associated with diphtheria outbreaks. Diphtheria risk analysis involves numerous criteria, so it is necessary to design multiple criteria decisions making (MCDM) modeling. One approach to solving MCDM is to use a technique of grouping data sets with several criteria based on pattern similarities [9]. The clustering algorithm is an unsupervised algorithm that is effective in grouping unlabeled data. The hierarchical clustering algorithm is one of the efficient clustering algorithms in clustering time and implementation [10]. Singh et al. [11] used a hierarchical clustering algorithm to find clusters within the patient population. This technique succeeds in providing a quantitative exploratory analysis based on cluster results.

This paper proposes a new approach to diphtheria risk analysis in Surabaya based on DPT immunization, the number of diphtheria sufferers, and population density using the hierarchical clustering algorithm. Information is presented in the form of spatial mapping of each urban village in Surabaya, thus, it can present information in a smaller scope. The results of the knowledge shown in this application can be used as a decision support analysis for early vigilance in diphtheria in efforts to prevent and monitor diphtheria in Surabaya.

2 Related Works

The spatial analysis of the risk of diphtheria provides an overview of the spread of diphtheria so that it can be identified areas that have a high risk of overtime. The main factor affecting the risk of diphtheria is the provision of DPT 1, DPT 2, and DPT 3 immunizations [5]. However, demographic and environmental factors also affect the diphtheria risk level of vulnerability. Some studies use statistical methods such as correlation and regression to analyze diphtheria risk. Izza and Soenarnatalin [3] studied diphtheria on the basis of spatial data linked to risk factors in East Java in 2010–2011 using a geographic information system. Risk factors suggest population density, sex, schooling, per capita spending and a healthy home are not all risk factors for diphtheria outbreaks.

DPT3 and DT immunization revealed a link between diphtheria and statistically moderate intensity ($r = 0.424$ and $r = 0.348$) using Spearman correlation and Pearson Moment correlation. Saito et al. [7] conducted a spatial mapping of the distribution of clinical, microbiological, and epidemiological factors in diphtheria patients compared to population densities in Metro Manila, Philippines, between 2006 and 2017. Case mapping shows that the distribution of diphtheria sufferers is higher in densely populated areas. Husada et al. [4] analyzed the risk factors for children becoming diphtheria careers with a case-control observation approach carried out from 2011 and 2015 in East Java Province. The results showed that from the demographic and environmental risk factors, the significant risk factor was the father's education (odds ratio = 5.5, 95% confidence interval: 1.6–19.4). Muhammad et al. [8] examined risk factors for diphtheria outbreaks in children 1–10 years of age in Southern Kalimantan using chi-square and multiple logistic regression. The study revealed that the nutritional status of toddlers ($p = 0.049$), mobility ($p = 0.000$) and the source of infection ($p = 0.020$) were correlated with diphtheria.

The clustering algorithm is an unsupervised algorithm that is effective in grouping unlabelled data to solve MCDM. The hierarchical clustering algorithm is one of the efficient clustering algorithms in clustering time [10]. The hierarchical clustering algorithm is primarily composed of agglomerative and divisive methods [9]. The agglomerative clustering approach begins by considering each entity as a cluster and recursively combining the most appropriate clusters. A divisive clustering approach begins with the whole data set as a single cluster and recursively breaks down the most relevant clusters. The procedure will continue until the termination conditions have been met. Chimwayi et al. [12] predicted individuals at risk for Chronic Kidney Disease (CKD) using neuro-fuzzy and hierarchical clustering techniques. A neuro-fuzzy algorithm is used to assess the risk of CKD in patients. The findings of the CKD risk prediction were grouped together by hierarchical clustering of three clusters and showed a close association between chronic kidney disease and diabetes. Singh et al. [11] used agglomerative hierarchical clustering to locate clusters in a patient population. The clustering findings indicated the presence of nine distinct and clinically significant cohort/multi-morbidity groups in the patient population.

This paper implements diphtheria risk analysis in Surabaya based multiple criteria consist of DPT immunization, the number of diphtheria sufferers, and population density using the hierarchical clustering algorithm. Information is presented in the form of spatial mapping of each village in Surabaya so that it can present information in a smaller scope. In Indonesia, disaster risk assessment is governed by the National Agency for Disaster Risk Management, including the disease risk. The area risk index is divided into three categories, namely low, medium, and high [13].

3 Methodology

In general, the diphtheria risk system diagram consists of the clustering and prediction process using hierarchical clustering as shown in Fig. 1.

In Fig. 1, the development of the system begins with data collection consisting of Surabaya map data and some data for diphtheria risk analysis consisting of

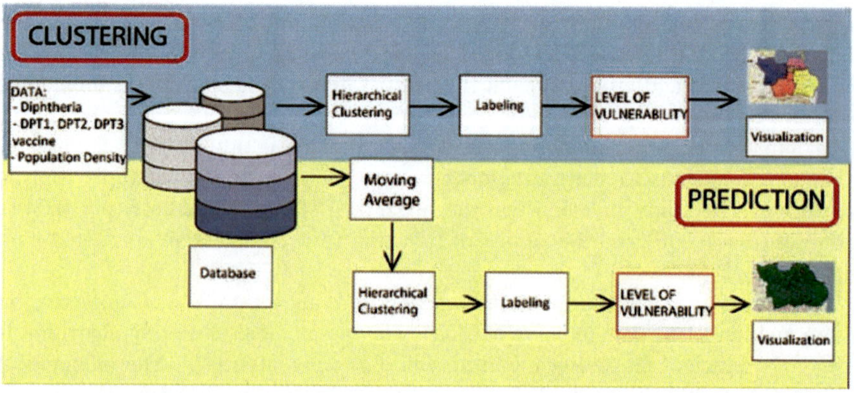

Fig. 1 System diagram of diphtheria risk

diphtheria sufferers, the number of people who have received DPT 1, DPT 2 and DPT 3 vaccines, and population density. The data were obtained from the Surabaya City Health Service and the Central Statistics Agency with the time range of 2016, 2017, and 2018. The spatial data and attributes were processed and stored in the PostgreSQL database. Hierarchical clustering is an approach to grouping the data based on similarities. The method used consists of a single linkage, average linkage, and complete linkage with the Euclidean distance approach. The results of clustering consist of 3 clusters that represent different groups. The labeling process is used to differentiate between getting diphtheria risk clusters based on an average per cluster consisting of low, medium, and high levels of vulnerability. The diphtheria risk level of a vulnerability is visualized in spatial terms by giving different colors, they are green for low, yellow for medium, and red for high.

The prediction process is used to predict the level of diphtheria vulnerability in 2019 using the moving average method using data from the previous 2 years, namely 2017 and 2018. The results of the moving average analysis are hierarchical clustering and labeling to get the diphtheria risk level of vulnerability in 2019. The results of this prediction are visualized in spatial form based on low, medium, and high levels of vulnerability.

3.1 Data Collection

Surabaya is the second-largest city in Indonesia. Administratively, the city of Surabaya has 31 sub-districts and 154 urban villages. In 2017, the total population was 2,827,892 and an area of 350.54 km^2 and a population density of 8067 people/km^2. Surabaya base map was obtained in 2014 in vector form per urban village in Indonesia in shapefile format. The data used in this paper are in the per urban village coverage as shown in Fig. 2.

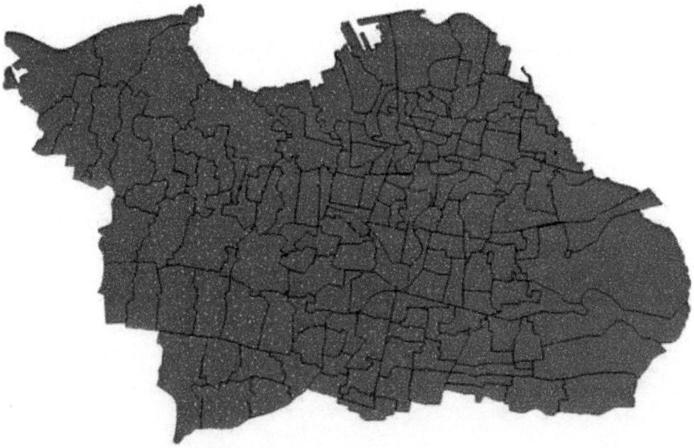

Fig. 2 Surabaya city vector base map in per urban village coverage

The attribute data used to perform the analysis consisted of diphtheria sufferer data, data on the number of DPT 1, DPT 2, DPT 3 vaccinations, and population density data are collected from the Surabaya City Health Service and the Central Statistics Agency. The data obtained is from 2016 to 2018. Spatial data and attributes are saved into the PostgreSQL database for clustering and prediction processes.

3.2 *Hierarchical Clustering Algorithm for Diphtheria Risk*

Hierarchical methods are clustering techniques to form a hierarchy or based on certain levels so that they resemble a tree structure. Thus, the process of grouping is carried out in stages or gradually. Usually, this method is used for not too much data and the number of clusters to be formed is unknown [14]. The agglomerative method is a hierarchical grouping strategy that starts with each object in a separate cluster then forms a growing cluster. That is, the number of initial clusters is the same as the number of objects [15]. In the agglomerative method, clustering techniques are:

a. Single linkage: a technique that combines clusters according to the distance between the closest members between two clusters.
b. Average linkage: a technique that combines clusters according to the average distance of each member pair on the set between two clusters.
c. Complete linkage: a technique that combines clusters according to the distance between the farthest members of the two clusters.

The steps taken to form a cluster with a hierarchical clustering algorithm are as follows [16]:

1. Initialize the proximity cluster matrix from diphtheria sufferer data, data on the number of DPT 1, DPT 2, DPT 3 vaccinations, and population density data.
2. Calculate the minimum distance with the Euclidean distance in the matrix with the equation [16]

$$D(a,b) = \sqrt{\sum\nolimits_{i=1}^{n} (b_i - a_i)^2} \tag{1}$$

   $D(a, b)$ is the distance between points (urban village) a and b, starts from $i = 1$ to the nth data until all points are counted.
3. Merge the two clusters with minimal spacing.
4. Updating the proximity matrix by calculating the distance between the new cluster and other clusters according to agglomerative techniques.
   Single linkage uses equations [16]

$$d_{uv} = \min\{d_{uv}\}, d_{uv} \in D \quad (2)$$

$\min\{d_{uv}\}$ is the distance between U and V data from clusters U and V and chooses the smallest cluster distance of D.
Average linkage uses equations [16]

$$d_{uv} = \frac{1}{|U| * |V|}\sum U \in D \sum V \in D d_{uv} \quad (3)$$

$|U|$ and $|V|$ are the amount of data in clusters U and V from distance d_{uv} of D.
Complete linkage uses equations [16]

$$d_{uv} = \max\{d_{uv}\}, d_{uv} \in D \quad (4)$$

$\max\{d_{uv}\}$ is the distance between U and V data from clusters U and V and chooses the biggest cluster distance of D.
5. Repeat the previous three steps if three clusters are left (low, medium, and high risk of vulnerability).

3.3 *Labeling*

Labeling is used to name the clusters that have been separated according to the cluster formed based on the centroid value. Labeling is based on the average score of all members in the cluster concerned. The largest average value indicates a high level of diphtheria risk and the smallest average value indicates a low level of risk, while between the largest and the smallest values will have a medium level of risk.

3.4 *Prediction*

The prediction process is used to estimate the diphtheria risk level for the next year. In this paper, a prediction of the 2019 diphtheria risk level is carried out based on data for 2017 and 2018. Analysis of the time series moving average (MA) is used to obtain a prediction of the value of diphtheria sufferer data, data on the number of DPT 1, DPT 2, DPT 3 vaccinations, and population density data in 2019 based on these data in 2017 and 2018. Moving Average is commonly used in time series analysis and time series forecasting. Calculation of the moving average requires the formation of a new sequence, the sum of which is the average of the raw observations in the original time series.

The results of the moving average analysis obtained the predicted value of diphtheria sufferer data, data on the number of DPT 1, DPT 2, DPT 3 vaccinations, and population density data in 2019. The prediction data is grouped by hierarchical clustering and labeling to get diphtheria risk level of vulnerability. consisting of low, medium, and high levels.

3.5 Spatial Visualization

The results of the calculation of the diphtheria risk level of vulnerability are displayed in the form of a spatial web-based on a geographical information system (GIS). The applications used are GeoServer, PostgreSQL, and JavaScript Leaflet library. The Surabaya base vector map stored in the PostgreSQL database is connected to GeoServer. GeoServer invokes links in GeoJson format into the GIS web compiler script.

4 Result and Discussion

In this section, testing and evaluation of the results of grouping are carried out using a hierarchical clustering algorithm and prediction results.

4.1 Clustering Result

To find out the results of clustering using the hierarchical clustering algorithm, observations of differences in spatial visualization were carried out using the agglomerative single linkage, average linkage, and complete linkage methods in 2016, 2017, and 2018 as shown in Figs. 3, 4, 5. Visualization is carried out based on looking at the diphtheria risk level of vulnerability per urban village. The green color represents the urban village with a low-risk level, the yellow color indicates a medium risk level, and the red color indicates a high-risk level. As shown in Figs. 3, 4, 5, visually, it can be seen that there are quite significant differences in the results of clustering using single linkage agglomerative, average linkage, and complete linkage.

Figure 6 shows a graph of the comparison of the number of urban villages for each low, medium, and high diphtheria risk level of vulnerability in 2016, 2017, and 2018 using agglomerative hierarchical clustering single linkage, average linkage, and complete linkage. Figure 6a is a single linkage graph, there is no significant change in the number of urban villages with low, medium, and high diphtheria risk level vulnerability in every year after grouping. There are 2 urban villages with high diphtheria risk, 4 urban villages with medium risk, and 148 urban villages with low risk. In Fig. 6b is the average linkage graph, it shows that in 2016, there are 2 urban villages with high diphtheria risk, 23 urban villages with medium

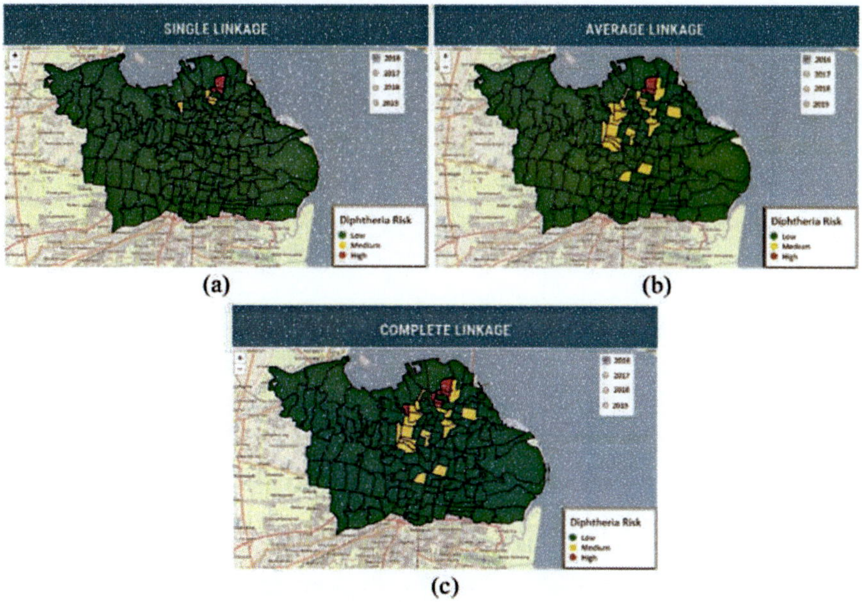

Fig. 3 Spatial analysis of diphtheria risk level of vulnerability results in 2016 using **a** single linkage; **b** average linkage; **c** complete linkage

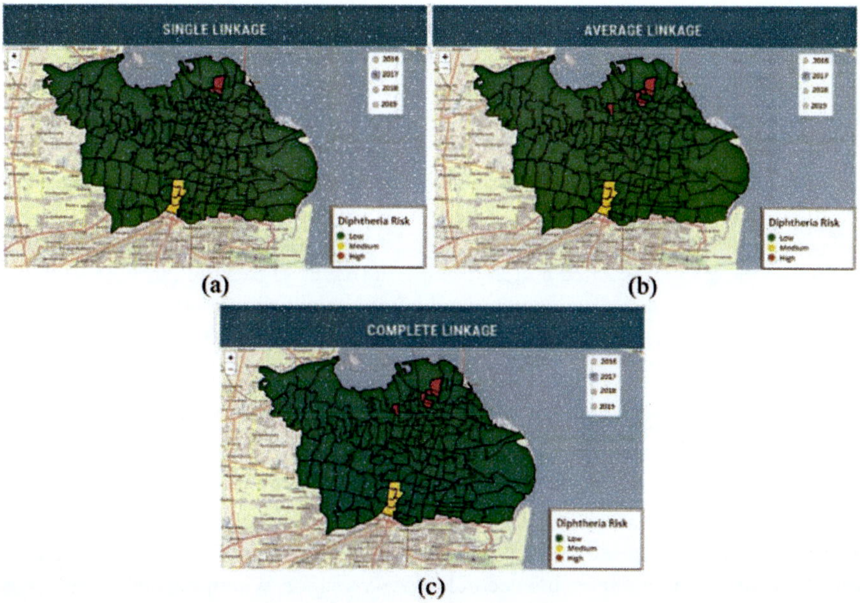

Fig. 4 Spatial analysis of diphtheria risk level of vulnerability results in 2017 using **a** single linkage; **b** average linkage; **c** complete linkage

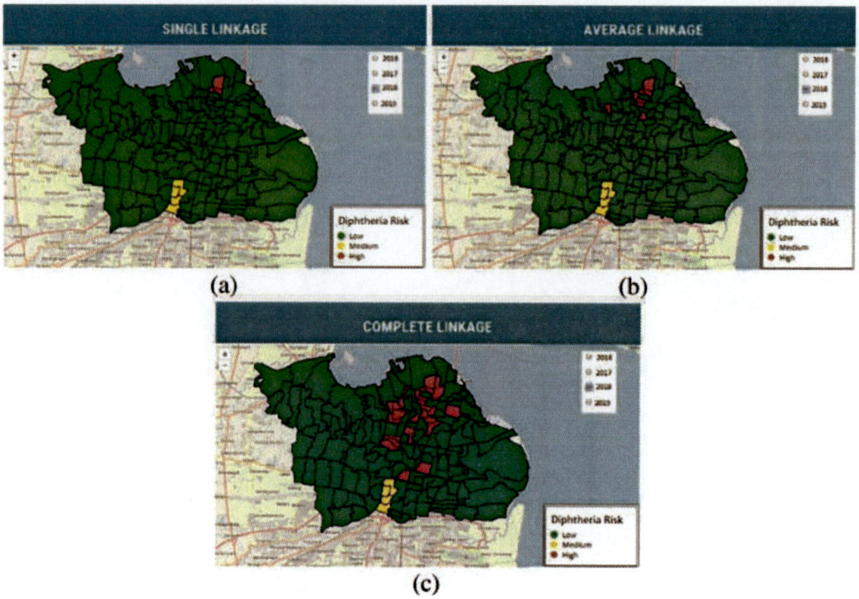

Fig. 5 Spatial analysis of diphtheria risk level of vulnerability results in 2018 using **a** single linkage; **b** average linkage; **c** complete linkage

risk, and 129 urban villages with low risk. In 2017 and 2018 there was a decreasing number of existing urban villages with diphtheria risk level vulnerability. They are 6 urban villages with high diphtheria risk level vulnerability, 4 urban villages with medium risk, and 144 urban villages with low risk. Figure 6c is a graph of complete linkage and there is a different diphtheria risk level of vulnerability each year. But, in 2016 and 2017 there is not a very significant change, only changing the high diphtheria risk level of vulnerability from 2 urban villages increase to 6 urban villages with the number of 4 villages. In 2018 there was an increase in the number of urban villages that reached a high diphtheria risk level to 27 urban villages. This mapping and graphical visualization can be used as a decision support analysis for the prevention and control of diphtheria outbreaks in Surabaya.

4.2 *Clustering Analysis*

Cluster Analysis is used to calculate the resulting value from the clustering effects distribution [17]. There are two types of variance in clustering, variance within-cluster and variance between-cluster. Variance within-cluster (VW) is a variant form that refers to the distance between members of the same cluster that is

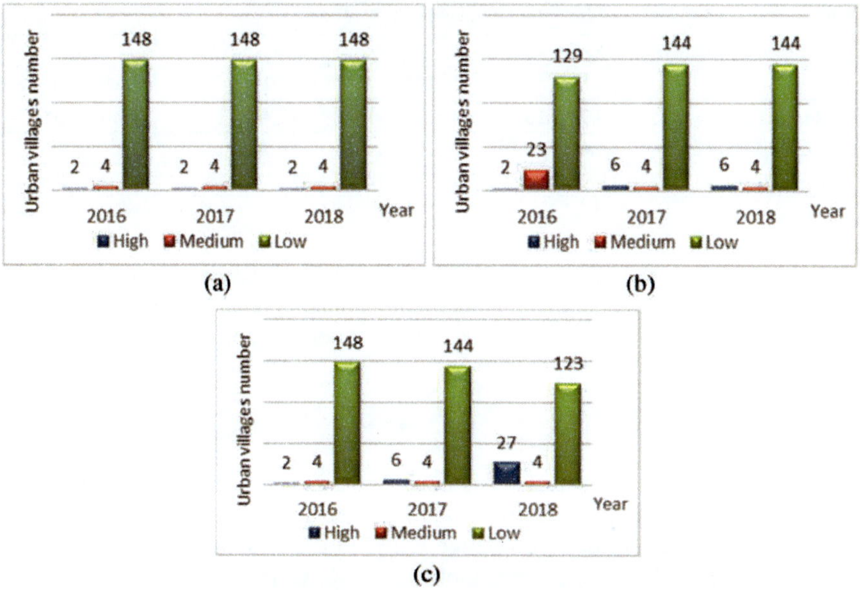

Fig. 6 Graph of the urban villages number comparison with low, medium, and high level of diphtheria risk per year using **a** single linkage; **b** average linkage; **c** complete linkage

included in the internal homogeneity of the cluster. VW of N data, k clusters, n_i data in cluster i, and V_i variance in cluster i is calculated using equation [17].

$$V_w = \frac{1}{N-k}\sum_{i=1}^{k}(n_i - 1).V_i^2 \tag{5}$$

The variance of the cluster (V_c) in cluster c, i-data d_i in a cluster, and average data $\overline{d_i}$ in cluster i is calculated using equation

$$V_c = \frac{1}{n_c}\sum_{i=1}^{c}\left(d_i - \overline{d_i}\right)^2 \tag{6}$$

Variance between-cluster (V_B) is a type of variant that refers to the distance between clusters [17]. V_B of k clusters, n_i data in cluster i, i-data d_i in a cluster, and average of $\overline{d_i}$ ($\overline{d}$) is calculated using equation

$$V_B = \frac{1}{k-1}\sum_{i=1}^{k}n_i\left(d_i - \overline{d}\right)^2 \tag{7}$$

Table 1 Variance analysis of hierarchical clustering result

Agglomerative method	Year			
	2016	2017	2018	Average
Single linkage	8.9×10^{-05}	5.6×10^{-05}	5.6×10^{-05}	5.0×10^{-5}
Average linkage	$\mathbf{4.6 \times 10^{-05}}$	$\mathbf{3.1 \times 10^{-11}}$	5.4×10^{-05}	$\mathbf{3.3 \times 10^{-5}}$
Complete linkage	8.9×10^{-05}	4.9×10^{-05}	$\mathbf{3.7 \times 10^{-05}}$	4.2×10^{-5}

The variance score is considered by comparing the variance within-cluster and the variance between-clusters. The smaller the variance value, the more optimal the product of the cluster. The variance value of V is determined using the equation [17]

$$V = \frac{V_W}{V_B} \tag{8}$$

The results of the variance analysis of the results of the 2016, 2017, and 2018 hierarchical cluster grouping can be found in Table 1.

In Table 1, the agglomerative average linkage method shows a smaller average variance than a single linkage and complete linkage, which is 3.3×10^{-5}. In 2016 and 2017, the smallest variance results were the average linkage method, namely 4.6×10^{-05} and 3.1×10^{-11}. However, in 2018 the smallest variance was the complete linkage method, namely 3.7×10^{-05}. The results of this analysis of variance indicate that average linkage achieves a better clustering scheme than a single linkage and complete linkage.

Changes in the diphtheria risk level of vulnerability from 2016 to 2018 using the results of the average linkage grouping can be seen in Table 2. 38 urban villages experienced a change in diphtheria risk, while the remaining 116 urban villages did not change.

In Table 2, using the hierarchical clustering average linkage method shows an increase and decrease in the status of diphtheria risk levels in several urban villages. 10 urban villages have increased their status from low to high or from low to medium. 20 urban villages have decreased their status from high to low or from medium to low. The remaining 8 urban villages experienced an increasing and decreasing in status for 3 years. Also, 6 urban villages have a significant increase from low to high status, consist of Sonokwijen, Tandes, Genting Kalianak, Sememi, Kandangan, and Lontar. With the analysis of changes in the level of vulnerability, it can be used as a basis for controlling diphtheria outbreaks, especially in providing DPT 1, DPT 2, and DPT 3 immunizations.

Evaluation of the diphtheria risk results is also carried out by comparing the distribution pattern of diphtheria cases in Surabaya in several sub-districts in 2017 [18]. The distribution of cases in several sub-districts in 2017 is shown in Fig. 7 with different color, white color indicates no cases, yellow color indicates 1 case occurred, orange color indicates 2 cases occurred, and red color indicates ≥ 3 cases. Based on the diphtheria risk clustering results with average linkage in 2017

Table 2 Diphtheria risk level changes of 38 urban villages using average linkage

No.	Urban village	Year		
		2016	2017	2018
1	Sonokwijen	Low	Low	High
2	Tandes	Low	Low	High
3	Genting Kalianak	Low	Low	High
4	Sememi	Low	Low	High
5	Kandangan	Low	Low	High
6	Lontar	Low	Low	High
7	Sambikerep	Low	Low	Medium
8	Peneleh	Low	Low	Medium
9	Kapasari	Low	Low	Medium
10	Kedungdoro	Low	Low	Medium
11	Tegalsari	Medium	Low	Low
12	Wonorejo	Medium	Low	Low
13	Tembok Dukuh	Medium	Low	Low
14	Jepara	Medium	Low	Low
15	Gundih	Medium	Low	Low
16	Tambakrejo	Medium	Low	Low
17	Kapasan	Medium	Low	Low
18	Simolawang	Medium	Low	Low
19	Sidodadi	Medium	High	Low
20	Perak Timur	Medium	High	Low
21	Pegirian	Medium	Low	Low
22	Ampel	High	High	Low
23	Wonokusumo	Medium	High	Low
24	Kemayoran	High	High	Low
25	Dupak	Medium	Low	Low
26	Sidotopo Wetan	Medium	High	Low
27	Tambaksari	Medium	Low	Low
28	Pacar Keling	Medium	Low	Low
29	Gading	Medium	Low	Low
30	Petemon	Medium	Low	Low
31	Putat Jaya	Medium	Low	Low
32	Banyu Urip	Medium	Low	Low
33	Kupang Krajan	Medium	Low	Low
34	Kebonsari	Medium	Low	Low
35	Pagesangan	Low	Medium	Low
36	Jambangan	Low	Medium	Low
37	Karah	Low	Medium	Low
38	Sememi	Low	Medium	Low

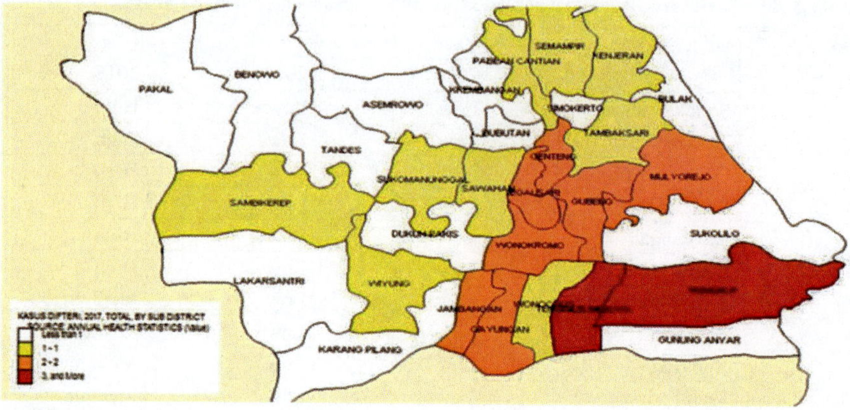

Fig. 7 Distribution of diphtheria cases in Surabaya in several sub-districts in 2017 [18]. The white color indicates there are no cases, the yellow color indicates 1 case occurred, the orange color indicates 2 cases occurred, and the red color indicates ≥ 3 cases

(the best one), there are some similar results, for example, some urban villages in Jambangan sub-district showed medium risk results (number of cases = 2), some urban villages in Pabean Cantika and Semampir sub-districts showed high-risk results (number of cases = 1). However, there are some differences, for example, the Tenggilis Mejoyo and Rungkut sub-districts which have a high number of cases (≥ 3 cases). It is because, in the developed diphtheria risk model, the data is used per urban village and takes into 3 criteria, the number of cases, DPT vaccine administration, and the population density. The ratio of vaccines and the population ratio affected the formation of clusters per village in addition to the number of cases. The data in small scope (urban villages) show more representative to the real conditions.

4.3 Prediction Result

The prediction process can be used to estimate the diphtheria risk level of vulnerability in the following year. In the prediction test, the process of moving average data for diphtheria sufferer data was carried out, data on the number of DPT 1, DPT 2, DPT 3 vaccinations, and population density using time series moving average analysis in 2017 and 2018 is used to estimate those value in 2019. The predicted values for 2019 are grouped unsupervised using a hierarchical clustering algorithm and labeling to obtain predictions of the diphtheria risk level of vulnerability. The results of the diphtheria risk level prediction can be seen in Fig. 8 which is visualized in spatial and graphic form.

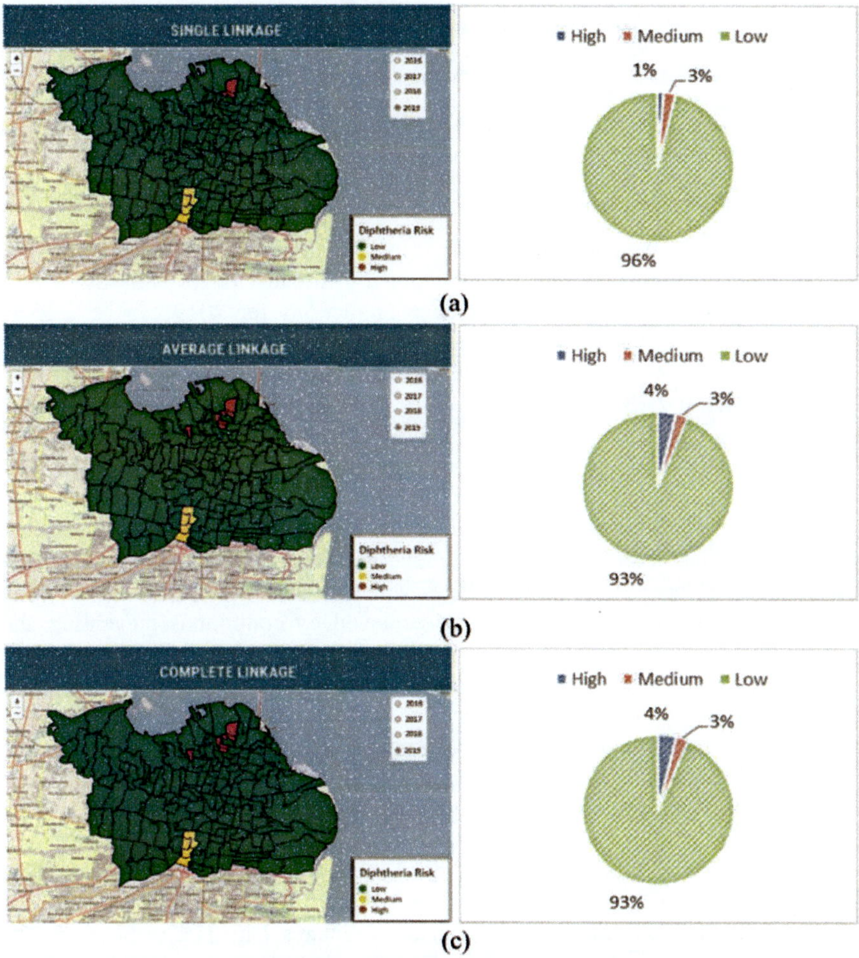

Fig. 8 Visualization and percentage of urban village number of the prediction result in 2019 using **a** single linkage; **b** average linkage; **c** complete linkage

This research compares the results of the prediction of status diphtheria risk level using the single linkage, average linkage, and complete linkage in 2019. Figure 8a is the result of spatial and graphical analysis using a single linkage. There are 2 urban villages with a high risk of diphtheria, 4 urban villages with medium risk, and the remaining 148 urban villages with low risk. Spatial analysis and graphs Fig. 8b with average linkage shows the number of urban villages at risk of high and medium diphtheria is more than a single linkage. There are 6 urban villages with a high risk of diphtheria and 4 urban villages with medium risk, the remaining 144 urban villages have low risk. Figure 8c is a spatial and graphic visualization using

Table 3 Variance analysis of hierarchical clustering result

Agglomerative method	Year
	2019
Single linkage	**4.43×10^{-5}**
Average linkage	4.61×10^{-5}
Complete linkage	4.61×10^{-5}

complete linkage. There are 6 urban villages with a high risk of diphtheria, 4 urban villages with medium risk, and the remaining 144 urban villages with low risk.

Analysis of the results of the variance predictions for 2019 can be seen in Table 3. In general, the variance value is not much difference between the single linkage, average linkage, and complete linkage. The single linkage method produces the smallest variance value, 4.43×10^{-5}, achieving better cluster results than average linkage, and complete linkage. This analysis shows that in 2019 there is a decrease in the number of urban villages that have a high and low level of diphtheria risk compared to 2018. With the average linkage method (best result), in 2018 there were 6 urban villages with high diphtheria risk and 4 urban villages with medium risk. The prediction results of diphtheria risk level with single-linkage (best result) in 2019, there are 2 urban villages with a high risk of diphtheria, 4 urban villages with medium risk. This can be achieved by continuous preventing and monitoring.

Agglomerative hierarchical clustering is an unsupervised bottom-up clustering method were combining the closest pair of clusters that have the same thing until all the data are in one cluster. It can generate informative object sequences for easy-to-implement data display. The limitation of this method is that the determination of the distance matrix and linkage criteria greatly affects the cluster results. Therefore, the use of this type of linkage can affect arbitrary cluster results.

Surabaya City Health Service does not have a spatial analysis that describes diphtheria risk based on the relevant criteria, so this application is very useful. This developed application has been tested at the Surabaya City Health Service. The results of interviews and questionnaires show that this application can be used as a decision support system for preventing and controlling diphtheria outbreaks in Surabaya because it can show the analysis in a small scope, urban villages in Surabaya.

5 Conclusion

This application displays the spatial visualization of the Diphtheria risk level of vulnerability villages in Surabaya based on the influencing factors, diphtheria sufferer data, data on the number of DPT 1, DPT 2, DPT 3 vaccinations, and population density in urban areas. Multi-criteria analysis using the unsupervised hierarchical clustering method can classify the diphtheria risk level well based on the analysis of variance values. The results of clustering using average linkage against data for 2016, 2017 and 2018 achieve the smallest average variance value 3.3×10^{-5} and better than single linkage and complete linkage. This developed application also provides a prediction of the next year's diphtheria risk level. The results of the 2019 predictions show a better diphtheria risk level of vulnerability using a single linkage rather than average linkage and complete linkage with the smallest variance 4.43×10^{-5}. This developed application can be used as a decision support anaysis for preventing and monitoring diphtheria outbreaks in small environmental spaces, namely urban villages. Future work, research on the diphtheria risk level of vulnerability will be developed by developing more detailed influencing factors and developing algorithms for optimal results.

References

1. Center for Disease Control and Prevention, Diphtheria, U.S. Department of Health & Human Services. Last accessed 4 Aug 2020
2. World Health Organization (2019) Diphtheria. https://www.who.int/immunization/monitoring_surveillance/burden/vpd/surveillance_type/passive/diphtheria/en/. Last accessed 4 Aug 2020
3. Izza N, Soenarnatalina S (2015) Analysis of spatial data of Diphtheria disease in East Java Province during the year 2010 and 2011. Buletin Penelitian Sistem Kesehatan 18(2):20946
4. Husada D, Primayani D, Marbun K, Kartina L, Puspitasari D, Tirthaningsih NW, Basuki PS (2018) Risk factors of Diphtheria carriers in Indonesian children. Southeast Asian J Trop Med Public Health 49(4):660–669
5. World Health Organization (2020) Diphtheria reported cases. https://apps.who.int/immunization_monitoring/globalsummary/timeseries/tsincidencediphtheria.html. Last accessed 4 Aug 2020
6. East Java Provincial Health Service (2018) East Java Province health profile, 2018. https://dinkes.jatimprov.go.id/userfile/dokumen/BUKU%20PROFIL%20KESEHATAN%20JATIM%202018.pdf. Last accessed 4 Aug 2020
7. Saito N, Dimapilis VO, Fujii H, Suzuki M, Telan EFO, Umipig DV, Solante RM, Dimapilis AQ, De Guzman F, Salva EP, Nakayama F (2020)Diphtheria in Metro Manila, the Philippines 2006–2017: a clinical, molecular, and spatial characterization. Clin Infect Dis
8. Muhamad IR, Susanti R, Ifroh RH, Noviasty R (2018) Risk factors for diphtheria outbreak in children aged 1–10 years in East Kalimantan Province, Indonesia. F1000Research 7
9. Barak S, Mokfi T (2019) Evaluation and selection of clustering methods using a hybrid group MCDM. Expert Syst Appl 138:112817
10. Chormunge S, Jena S (2015) Efficiency and effectiveness of clustering algorithms for high dimensional data. Int J Comput Appl 125
11. Singh SP, Karkare S, Baswan SM, Singh VP (2018) Agglomerative hierarchical clustering analysis of co/multi-morbidities. arXiv preprint arXiv:1807.04325
12. Chimwayi KB, Haris N, Caytiles RD, Iyengar NCS (2017) Risk level prediction of chronic kidney disease using neuro-fuzzy and hierarchical clustering algorithm(s)
13. National Disaster Management Agency (2012) Head of national disaster management agency regulation number 02 of 2012 on general guidelines for assessment of disaster risk, Jakarta
14. Jain AK, Murty MN, Flynn PJ (1999) Data clustering: a review. ACM Comput Surv 31 (3):264–323

15. Davidson I, Ravi SS (2005) Agglomerative hierarchical clustering with constraints: theoretical and empirical results. In: European conference on principles of data mining and knowledge discovery. Springer, Berlin, Heidelberg, pp 59–70
16. Bouguettaya A, Yu Q, Liu X, Zhou X, Song A (2015) Efficient agglomerative hierarchical clustering. Expert Syst Appl 42(5):2785–2797
17. Dini SK, Fauzan A (2020) Clustering provinces in indonesia based on community welfare indicators. EKSAKTA J Sci Data Anal 20(1):56–63
18. Fitriansyah A (2018) The description of Diphtheria immunization history to Diphtheria patients in Surabaya at 2017. Jurnal Berkala Epidemiologi 6(2):103–111

Internet of Things in Flood Warning System: An Overview on the Hardware Implementation

Nor Hana Mamat, Mohd Hafiz Othman, Wan Zulkarnain Othman, and Mohamad Fadhil Md Noor

Abstract Early warning in flood event can save property and life. The advancement of Internet of Things (IoT) technology along with cheap sensors makes IoT based flood warning system an attractive choice for disaster management. Various methods of IoT implementation have been used for the purpose of flood monitoring and warning. This paper presents an overview of literature related to the hardware implementation of IoT and the corresponding method of installation in flood warning system. The paper contributes by highlighting the sensors, microcontroller and wireless communication, IoT platform and method of installation employed in the literature adopting IoT in flood monitoring and flood warning systems. The paper further contributes by providing recommendations for the most suitable IoT hardware for a practical, cost effective and reliable flood warning system. Ultrasonic sensor that is largely used for water level detection needs to be waterproof to withstand the environmental elements. It is useful to include other sensors for measurement of various hydrological, meteorological and geological data for further use in flood prediction employing artificial intelligence and machine learning methods. NodeMCU ESP8266 is mostly used as it is a combination of microcontroller and Wi-Fi microchip. An update of NodeMCU ESP8266, the NodeMCU ESP32 is recommended as it is more flexible, more energy efficient and provides extra input output connectivity. LoRa which is a low power communication module that provides long range low data rate transmission, can be used for sensor nodes placed far apart providing a larger area coverage of flood warning system. As for IoT platforms, it is beneficial to use a combination of multiple platforms for widespread dissemination of flood alerts to ensure effectiveness of flood warning systems.

Keywords Internet of things · Flood warning · Sensors

N. H. Mamat (✉) · M. H. Othman · W. Z. Othman · M. F. M. Noor
Faculty of Engineering Technology, University College TATI, Teluk Kalong, 24000 Kemaman, Terengganu, Malaysia
e-mail: norhana@uctati.edu.my

H. Triwiyanto et al. (eds.), *Proceedings of the 1st International Conference on Electronics, Biomedical Engineering, and Health Informatics*, Lecture Notes in Electrical Engineering 746, https://doi.org/10.1007/978-981-33-6926-9_23

1 Introduction

Flood is one of the most common natural disaster that devastatingly affect many countries around the world and accounts for almost half of the global natural peril. Flooding usually happens when there is unusual amount of extra water in the river stream due to heavy rainfall causing a rise in water level that subsequently overflows the river banks inundating nearby area [1].

Among all the natural disasters that occur globally in the year 2019, flood occur most frequently, caused highest fatality and second highest in terms of human impact in terms of injury, displaced from home or suffer economic losses. Meanwhile in 2018, although flood recorded less percentage of death among all the natural disasters, it has the highest occurrence and human impact loss. These data are extracted and analyzed from natural disaster reports compiled by Centre for Research on the Epidemiology of Disasters(CRED) [2, 3] as illustrated in charts of Figs. 1, 2 and 3.

Due to significant negative impact of flood events, many researches are devoted to assist mitigating the effect of flood or to prevent future occurrence. Figure 4 shows the tasks involved before a flood warning can be produced, including sensing the environment for danger followed by flood prediction or forecasting [4].

In sensing the environment stage, data are collected from hydrological stations along the rivers, weather stations, Geographic Information System (GIS) data as well as various sensor nodes in a wireless sensor network. Next these data are processed and analyzed into hydrological data, meteorological data and geological data. The three types of data are used to perform flood forecasting or prediction using either hydrodynamic model, artificial intelligence, machine learning methods or any combination of these methods. IoT hardware are being used mostly in the

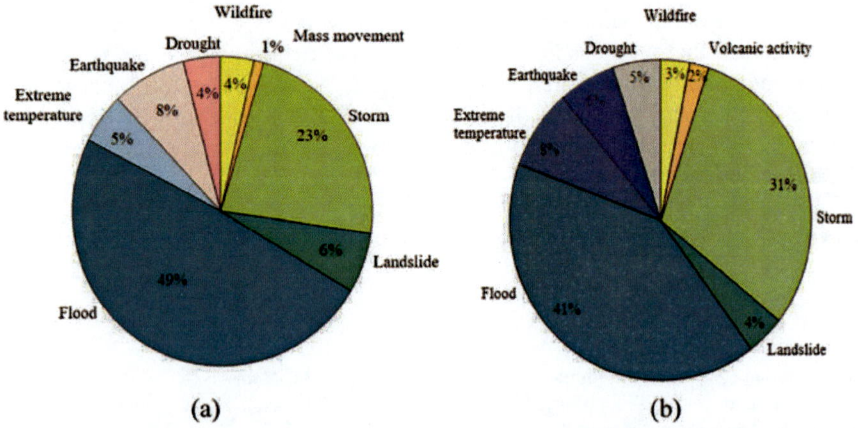

Fig. 1 Comparison of different disaster types in terms of disaster occurrence for the year **a** 2019 and **b** 2018

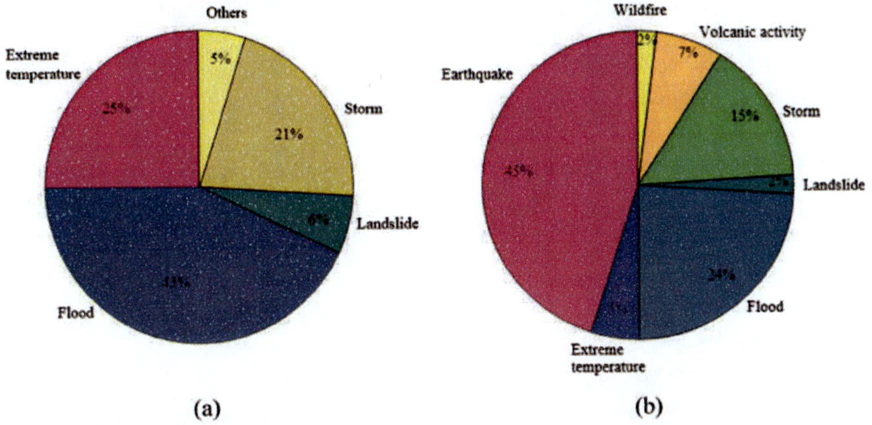

Fig. 2 Comparison of different disaster types in terms of total death for the year **a** 2019 and **b** 2018

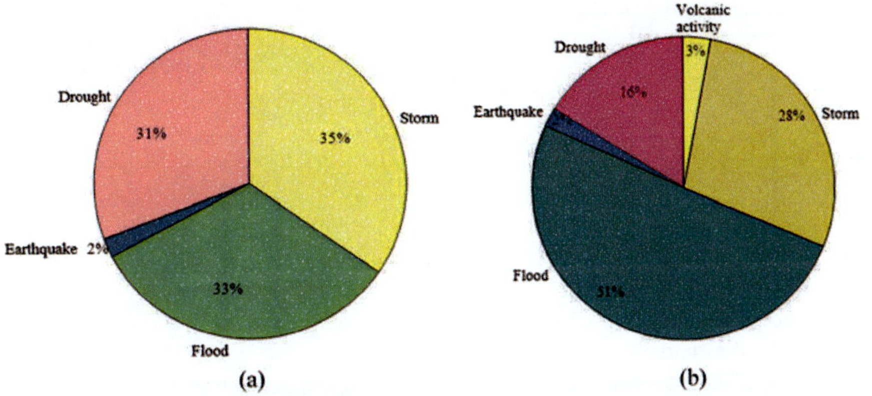

Fig. 3 Comparison of different disaster types in terms of human impact total affected (millions) for the year **a** 2019 and **b** 2018

sensing environment stage and flood warning stage. During sensing the environment stage sensors, microcontrollers and communication modules are involved in data collection and monitoring the hydrological, meteorological and geological parameters. In flood warning stage microcontrollers, communication modules and IoT platforms are used to disseminate warning to the authority or general users based on the outcome of previous flood prediction stage.

Flood warning system is one of the non-structural measures of flood disaster management that can minimize the impact of flood on the community providing early warning giving more time for necessary preparation and arrangement to be made before the flood [4]. Efficient flood warning could prevent loss of property,

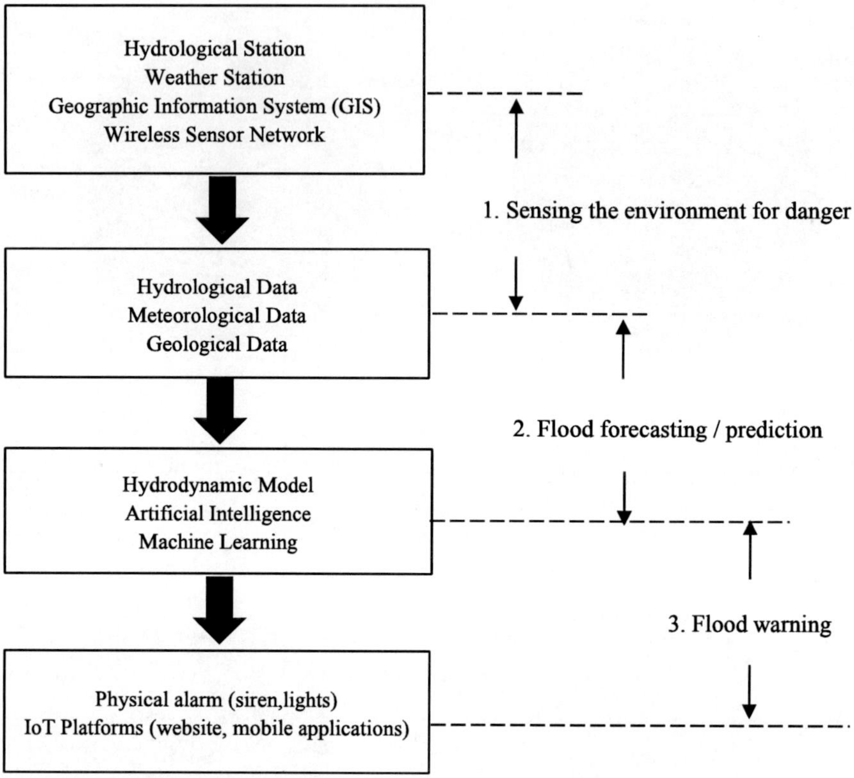

Fig. 4 Stages of flood management and the methods involved

infrastructures and even life especially in flood prone region such as residential area adjacent to the river.

In this overview, emphasis is given on the implementation of flood warning system in terms of hardware, comprising of the first and the last stages. Flood forecasting involves the use of various modelling or prediction methods, thus is not in the scope of this work. An overview of the interconnection of sensors to the Internet of Things (IoT) technology platforms and installation of these systems are provided in this paper.

2 Materials and Methods

This paper focuses on the hardware implementation of Internet of Things (IoT) in flood warning systems. To find detailed information of the most recent IoT development in flood warning, reference materials are obtained from journals and proceedings for the past 5 years. Papers are searched and accessed through

SCOPUS database and Google Scholar using the keywords "IoT" AND "flood warning".

The selection of sensors, microcontroller, wireless communication module, and the IoT platform used are presented. Other more advanced hardware used for IoT application in areas other with similar requirements as flood monitoring are also discussed. Some future considerations and possible adaptations of IoT hardware suitable for flood monitoring system in residential areas are proposed.

3 Review and Discussion

3.1 Internet of Things (IoT) for Flood Warning

Recently IoT received widespread attention with sensors expected to be attached on every objects due to the advancement of sensor technology in terms of hardware and reduced cost for sensors [5]. Automated IoT based monitoring system has been used in many areas such as agriculture [6–8], fall detection [9], and electrical device monitoring [10]. Various type of sensors and communication devices seamlessly interconnected to the internet opens a large probability for a reliable, more precise risk assessment and specific warning being deployed in favors of disaster management [11].

There are a few requirements for IoT devices for used in outdoor, remote areas where sensor nodes for a flood warning system are normally positioned, specifically along the riverbank, over a bridge or in monsoon drains for systems installed in residential areas. To ensure widespread and cost-effective applications of IoT solutions, IoT based unit comprising of a microcontroller and wireless communication module need to have powerful, low powered, low cost, small size and lightweight devices [12]. Smaller size and weight results in a more compact physical appearance of the system hardware, thus provides an advantage for ease of installation. Low cost and low powered devices enable more sensor nodes to be installed in many areas, providing a wider area coverage of the flood warning system.

Current works involving implementation of IoT in flood monitoring and warning system are summarized in Table 1 in terms of type of sensors, controller and wireless connection, IoT platform to display the data and the area of installation of the system.

3.2 Sensors and Installation

A smart flood prediction and warning systems using FDC1004 water level sensor among a few other sensors including LM35 for temperature, BME280 to measure humidity and air pressure as well as a rainfall sensor [13]. FDC1004 is a contactless

Table 1 Implementation of IoT in flood warning system

Reference	Sensor	Microcontroller/ wireless connection	IoT platform	Area
[13]	Temperature (LM35), humidity and air pressure (BME280), water level (FDC1004), rainfall	Raspberry Pi 3	ThingSpeak, ThingTweet	Riverbank
[14]	Ultrasonic (HC-SR04), rain	Arduino Uno	Webpage	–
[15]	Ultrasonic (HC-SR04), rain	ESP 8266	Blynk	High flash flood prone area
[16]	Ultrasonic (HC-SR04), 3 units flow sensor (YF-S201), temperature and humidity (DHT11)	Arduino Mega + Wifi Module (ESP-01)	Blynk	Dam gates
[17]	Ultrasonic (HC-SR04),	ESP8266	Thinger.io	River
[18]	Ultrasonic (HC-SR04)	ESP8266, XBee, LoRa	ThingSpeak	Dam
[19]	Ultrasonic (HC-SR04)	ESP8266	Blynk	Water container
[20]	Water sensor (SEN113104)	Raspberry Pi, GSM Module (USB 3G broadband modem Huawei E173)	SMS	Water container
[21]	Ultrasonic (HC-SR04), rainfall, temperature and humidity (DHT11), pressure (BMP180)	ESP8266	Android App	River
[22]	Ultrasonic (HC-SR04)	ESP8266	Blynk	Vehicle parking
[23]	Ultrasonic (MB7066)	MCU (AT91SAM3X8E)	RiverCore Web platform	River
[24]	Ultrasonic (HC-SR04), atmospheric temperature, pressure, humidity, vibration	Arduino Uno, GSM Module	SMS	Torrential flood

capacitive sensor that requires proper shielding as it is prone to stray capacitance and must be considered in the installation method, which is not described in this work.

Ultrasonic sensor HC-SR04 is used for water level measurement in most of the developed IoT based flood warning systems [14–19, 21, 22, 24]. HC-SR04 measures distance based on ultrasonic waves radiated and then received by the ultrasonic receiver, a principle like the ultrasonic radar [25]. In measurement of water level, the ultrasonic sensors are exposed to water from the environment. Ultrasonic sensor MB7066 used in a river flood monitoring system is a waterproof ultrasonic sensor with PVC casing in a PVC support mount [23].

In most of these works, the ultrasonic sensor is positioned at the bottom to measure the height of flood from the place of installation. Flood height detection was done by placing ultrasonic sensor and rain sensor in the upper part of a paralon pipe, a cork in the cross section acts as a buoy that indicates the level of flood [14]. The use of water sensor SEN113104 indicates whether the sensor is dry, damp or completely immersed by measuring conductivity by placing the sensors at two different levels, as indication of low and high flood levels, respectively [20]. This method does not allow continuous monitoring of the water level, hence suitable for use with SMS notification where alerts are deployed once the critical water level is reached.

Automatic meteorological station (AMS) offers a compact and portable installation of IoT devices. A box with external connectors at the front and sides provides easy attachment of ultrasonic and temperature sensors, GSM antenna for communication module, main power switch and Arduino/PC connector [24].

RiverCore system designed for flood warning in a river where a waterproof ultrasonic sensor is fixed to the cliff with a wire and tied using a cable to a box containing electronic components sealed using a lightweight rubber-like plastic material [23]. The use of waterproof sensor and sealing of electronics components offer adequate protection from the harsh environmental element near the river where the hardware for flood warning system is installed.

3.3 Controller and Wireless Connection

In agricultural IoT implementations, embedded system platforms such as Arduino, Raspberry Pi and ESP-based devices that use system-on chip (SoC) modules are mainly used [26]. This is due to their cost-effectiveness and compatibility with different network protocols making them suitable as sensor nodes or communication gateways. The same trend is observed in IoT applications in flood warning systems.

A smart flood prediction system [13] and an experimental system for flood warning [20] use Raspberry Pi and Raspberry Pi 3 which are single board computer systems based on Wi-Fi communication protocol that operates on a lower, energy efficient voltage level of 3.3 V for input and output. It is programmed using Phyton, an open source programming language. Raspberry Pi provides the capability of a small computer; thus it is a powerful device for IoT application.

NodeMCU ESP8266 is a popular controller for Wireless Sensor Network application in flood monitoring and warning system, used in most of the current literature reviewed [15, 17–19, 21, 22]. NodeMCU ESP8266 module served the purpose of controller and communication as it combines microcontroller and a Wi-Fi microchip [18]. It is a small size and cheap low power IoT device with operating voltage in the range of 3.0–3.6 V and operating current of 80 mA. It has 17 GPIO for input/output connections and can be programmed using Arduino IDE.

NodeMCU ESP8266 requires a multiplexer when more than one analog sensors are used as only one analog to digital converter (ADC) is available.

An updated version of NodeMCU ESP8266, NodeMCU ESP32 is low-cost and low-powered with a wide voltage range of 2.2–3.6 V. This gives the flexibility to power up using USB power supply or external battery [27]. NodeMCU ESP32 has an obvious advantage for remote water level monitoring and data collection over NodeMCU ESP8266 in terms of energy efficiency. It has 18 ADC pins for connection of more analog sensors as opposed to only one in NodeMCU ESP8266. It can be set to operate in several different modes with varying power consumption levels, the most efficient mode being deep sleep mode with only 0.8 mAh of current used [28]. The sensors collecting water level data can be programmed to record data only at specific intervals while at other times deep sleep mode can be used to save energy. This allows more sensor nodes to be deployed in remote area with the use of small solar panel as the source of energy. In terms of performance properties, price and availability in various form-factor, NodeMCU ESP32 is an excellent choice of embedded system for IoT devices [12].

Bluetooth, Zigbee, and Wireless fidelity (Wi-Fi) allow high data rate transmission for short distance communication while LoRa and Sigfox enable long distance communication at low data transmission rate [29]. Wi-Fi microchip in Raspberry Pi and ESP-based controller is sufficient for short range communication between sensor nodes and IoT platform when connected to existing Wi-Fi connection or using a GSM module as access point. In some area of application when water level needs to be monitored in a few different places, combination of short range and long-range communication is needed. In a warning system for dam, for short range communication, XBee modules are used for communication between sensor node and base station and LoRa (Long Range) module enables low data rate transmission for long range connection between base station and command center [18]. This enables wider coverage of flood warning system especially in remote areas as more sensor nodes can be placed further apart.

3.4 IoT Platform

SMS is a preferred and most effective method of choice to spread flood alerts due to the widespread use of mobile phones in many countries [20]. Experimental flood warning system [20] and torrential flood warning system [24] make use of this readily available technology. Flood warning can be promptly communicated to mass public as SMS is available to all mobile phone users as it does not require an application to be installed.

The Blynk application can be installed by the user to their mobile phone via Android Operating System or IOS Operating System and can be used to display the sensor reading as well as flood alerts. Most of the reviewed flood warning system [15, 16, 19, 22] utilized Blynk operation as it is a user-friendly application and accessible using mobile phones.

ThingSpeak platform are used for real-time display of data collected by the IoT flood monitoring system developed for flood warning system in riverbank [13] and dam [18]. Using ThingSpeak display of sensor data is on website and can be further processed and analysed using MATLAB, making it suitable for flood prediction using neural network and machine learning. It uses Message Queuing Telemetry Transport (MQTT) protocol, specifically designed for IoT solution and implementation. MQTT protocol allows open machine-to-machine (M2M) connection utilizing low bandwidth dan data consumption [30].

A river flood warning system uses Thinger IoT platform for real-time display and monitoring of a water level sensor data in multiple locations along the river [17]. IoT platforms such as website [14, 23] and Android application [21] also allow for easy monitoring of sensor data and flood alerts as it is easily accessible by the users.

4 Conclusion

Internet of Things (IoT) technology offers many solutions for flood monitoring and warning system. The hardware components involved in an IoT based flood warning system consists of sensors, microcontroller and wireless communication module, as well as the IoT platform. Ultrasonic sensor is an excellent choice for water level measurement as it is used in almost all flood warning system reviewed in this paper. Other types of sensors are also commonly used namely temperature sensor, rain sensor, pressure sensor, humidity sensor, water flow sensor and GPS sensors. These additional sensors collect hydrological, meteorological and geographical data that are useful for further manipulation in the flood prediction stage using intelligent methods such as neural network and machine learning.

Proper design for casing of the sensor and waterproof seal of the electronic components is needed to protect the hardware from the harsh outdoor environmental elements, especially water. The use of widely available 3D printing technology is recommended in this sense as it is cheap, and the casing can be designed to be compact and durable. The method of installation should consider environmental condition in the area of application and must be positioned carefully so that the sensor is able to provide reliable measurement.

As sensor node and network gateway, system on chip (SoC) devices such as Raspberry Pi and NodeMCU ESP8266 are preferred as the Wi-Fi microchip is integrated is integrated with microcontroller on the same device. These devices are low-powered, low cost and has powerful processing capability. NodeMCU ESP8266 is the most used microcontroller and wireless communication among the works reviewed in this paper. An update of NodeMCU ESP8266 is NodeMCU ESP32 that provides the same capability but with advantages of a larger voltage range, more input output, and a lot more ADC connection. LoRa offers long distance communication capability using low data rate transmission, suitable for sensor nodes positioned far distance apart.

Blynk application is the IoT platform of choice as it can be easily installed on any Android and IOS mobile phones. Thingspeak allows real-time display of sensor data on website and as it is integrated with MATLAB, it permits further analysis and use of data for flood prediction using intelligent methods such as neural network and machine learning. SMS alert may benefit a large section of the community as it can reach many mobile phone users that are registered to receive the flood alert. A combination of different IoT platforms can also be used to ensure the sensor data can be collected for flood prediction, displayed real-time on the website and mobile application as well as send flood warning alerts.

Each IoT solution and method is suitable for different needs based on the requirement of the system. It is crucial to choose the best methods to guarantee the flood warning system works as intended and benefits the community in mitigating the effects of flood.

Acknowledgements This research is fully supported by UCTATI Short Term Grant, 9001-2008. The authors fully acknowledged University College TATI (UCTATI) for the facilities and instrumentations that makes this important research viable and effective.

References

1. Kumari D, Mahato L, Kumar G, Kumar G, Abhinab K (2020) Study on IoT based early flood detection & avoidance. In: International conference on recent trends in artificial intelligence, iot, smart cities & applications, pp 1–3
2. CRED Centre for Research on the Epidemiology of Disasters (CRED) (2019) Natural disasters report 2018. Brussels
3. CRED Centre for Research on the Epidemiology of Disasters (CRED) (2020) Natural disasters report 2019. Brussels
4. Ghapar AA, Yussof S, Bakar AA (2018) Internet of things (IoT) architecture for flood data management. Int J Futur Gener Commun Netw 11(1):55–62
5. Noymanee J, San-Um W, Theeramunkong T (2016) A conceptual framework for the design of an urban flood early-warning system using a context-awareness approach in internet-of-things platform. In: Kim K, Joukov N (eds) Information science and applications 2016, Lecture Notes in Electrical Engineering, vol 376, pp 1295–1305
6. Jisha R, Vignesh G, Deekshit D (2019) IOT based water level monitoring and implementation on both agriculture and domestic areas. In: 2nd International conference on intelligent computing, instrumentation and control technologies (ICICICT), pp 1119–1123
7. Yanes AR, Martinez P, Ahmad R (2020) Towards automated aquaponics : a review on monitoring, IoT, and smart systems. J Clean Prod 263:121571
8. Bin Ismail MIH, Thamrin NM (2017) IoT implementation for indoor vertical farming watering system. In: International conference on electrical, electronics and system engineering (ICEESE), pp 89–94
9. Mozaffari N, Rezazadeh J, Farahbakhsh R, Yazdani S (2019) Practical fall detection based on IoT technologies : a survey. In: Internet of things, vol 8, pp 1–16
10. Gupta AK, Johari R (2019) IOT based electrical device surveillance and control system. In: 4th International conference on internet of things: smart innovation and usages (IoT-SIU), pp 1–5

11. Saha HN, Auddy S, Pal S, Kumar S, Pandey S, Singh R (2017) Disaster management using internet of things. In: 8th Annual industrial automation and electromechanical engineering conference (IEMECON), pp 81–85
12. Maier A, Sharp A, Vagapov Y (2017) Comparative analysis and practical implementation of the ESP32 microcontroller module for the internet of things. In: Internet technologies and applications (ITA), pp 143–148
13. Bande S, Shete VV (2017) Smart flood disaster prediction system using IoT & neural networks. In: International conference on smart technologies for smart nation (SmartTechCon), pp 189–194
14. Satria D, Yana S, Munadi R, Syahreza S (2018) Design of information monitoring system flood based internet of things (IoT). In: Proceedings of MICoMS 20, pp 337–342
15. Mohd Sabre A, Abdullah MS, Faruq SS (2019) Flood warning and monitoring system utilizing internet of things technology. Kinet Game Technol Inf Syst Comput Netw Comput Electron Control 4(4)
16. Patil PS, Jain SN (2019) IoT based flood monitoring and alerting system. Int J Control Autom 12(6):633–641
17. Prafanto A, Budiman E (2018) A water level detection: IoT platform based on wireless sensor network. In: 2nd East Indonesia conference on computer and information technology (EIConCIT), pp 46–49
18. Siddula SS, Jain PC, Upadhayay MD (2018) Real time monitoring and controlling of water level in dams using IoT. In: IEEE 8th international advance computing conference (IACC), pp 14–19
19. Sachio S, Noertjahyana A, Lim R (2018) IoT based water level control system. In: 3rd Technology innovation management and engineering science international conference (TIMES-iCON), pp 1–5
20. Shah W, Arif F, Shahrin AA, Hassan A (2018) The implementation of an IoT-based flood alert system. Int J Adv Comput Sci Appl 9(11):620–623
21. Patil S, Pisal J, Patil A, Ingavale S, Ayarekar P, Mulla PS (2019) A real time solution to flood monitoring system using IoT and wireless sensor networks. Int Res J Eng Technol 6(2):1807–1811
22. Hasbullah A, Rahimi AH, Ikram A, Amrimunawar H (2020) Flood and notification monitoring system using ultrasonic sensor integrated with IoT and Blynk applications: designed for vehicle parking. J Phys Conf Ser 1529:1–11
23. Moreno C et al (2019) RiverCore: IoT device for river water level monitoring over cellular communications. Sensors 19(127):1–21
24. Šarak E, Sedmak SA (2020) IoT based early warning system for torrential floods. FME Trans 48:511–515
25. Jeswin CJ, Marimuthu B, Chithra K (2017) Ultrasonic water level indicator and controller using AVR microcontroller. In: International conference on information communication and embedded systems (ICICES), pp 1–6
26. Navarro E, Costa N, Pereira A (2020) A systematic review of IoT solutions for smart farming emerson. Sensors 20:1–29
27. Study AC, Quang H, Ngo T, Nguyen TP, Nguyen H (2020) Research on a low-cost, open-source, and remote monitoring data collector to predict livestock's habits based on location and auditory information: a case study from Vietnam. Agriculture 10(180):1–26
28. Gatial E, Balogh Z, Hluchy L (2020) Concept of energy efficient ESP32 chip for industrial wireless sensor network. In: 24th International conference on intelligent engineering systems, pp 179–184
29. Fernández-Ahumada LM, Ramírez-Faz J, Torres-Romero M, López-Luque R (2019) Proposal for the design of monitoring and operating irrigation networks based on IoT, cloud computing and free hardware technologies. Sensors 19(2318):1–20
30. MQTT The Standard for IoT messaging. http://mqtt.org

IoT-Based Solar Photovoltaic (PV) Real Time Monitoring System for Power Consumption on Maahad Tahfiz School

Abdul Rahim Pazikadin, Kharudin Ali, Damhuji Rifai, Nur Amalina Awang, Ruzlaini Ghoni, and Nor Hana Mamat

Abstract Electricity resource is one of importance thing needs in daily life, especially for urban and rural residents. Currently, the rural faces a big problem due to insufficient electricity resources which are completely dependent on the use of generators and thus affect the daily usage of electricity. To preventing on this problem, the Solar energy garners attention for its clean nature and renewability with regards to electricity generation. This paper presents an Internet of Things (IoT) monitoring system for real time power consumption on rural area especially at Maahad Tahfiz school in Terengganu. Some essential parameters on PV real time system include Temperature, Power, Anemometer and Irradiance which are sensed using the sensors. The system consists of Thinger cloud, data gateway, and smartphone with Android OS application display for actual value monitoring, indicating the relationship between irradiant and power produced of solar PV. The results demonstrated the sampling data collection stored in Thinger cloud in higher sampling data per hour (15 min/data) yielded higher data accuracy up to 80% as compared to the lower sampling data per hour (60 min/data), with 70% accuracy. the irradiant measurement is directly proportional to the power produced based on the data analysis on Response Surface Methodology (RSM). Henceforth, the total power produced per day for solar panel (PV) will be known accurately based on the online system development and at the same, the estimation time for power will be predicted based on the total capacity of power used in Maahad Tahfiz school in Terengganu.

Keywords Solar PV · Irradiances · Power consumption · Temperature · Anemometer · RSM · IoT

A. R. Pazikadin (✉) · K. Ali · D. Rifai · R. Ghoni · N. H. Mamat
Faculty of Electrical and Automation Engineering Technology, UCTATI, 24000 Kemaman, Terengganu, Malaysia
e-mail: abdul.rahim@zsrvortices.com

N. A. Awang
Akademi Pengajian Bahasa, UiTM, Cawangan Kelantan, Bukit Ilmu, 18500 Machang, Kelantan, Malaysia

H. Triwiyanto et al. (eds.), *Proceedings of the 1st International Conference on Electronics, Biomedical Engineering, and Health Informatics*, Lecture Notes in Electrical Engineering 746, https://doi.org/10.1007/978-981-33-6926-9_24

1 Introduction

The demand for renewable energy resources is currently very high due to its ability to generate electricity in rural areas and far from urban areas [1]. The development and industrialization of an area is closely related to the source of electricity where optimal use is required in carrying out daily activities [2, 3]. The high demand for electricity leads to exposure to smart grid systems for home energy management system (HEMS) aimed at reducing the dependence on current electricity consumption [4]. Thus reforms to large centralized power plants have shifted to smaller and more renewable power stations [5]. The renewable energy sources are sustainable sources taken from environmental benefits such as daylight, wind, rain, tides, waves, and geothermal warmth and non-renewable energy sources are sources of energy that will be depleted and cannot be recycled [6–8].

The benefits of solar energy can be seen based on the generating of electricity through photovoltaic (PV) systems and will show the capability of solar panels to convert sunlight directly into electrical energy [9]. However, the predictions on the electricity produce are difficult to make because of the nature factor that interfere the electricity produce on solar PV [10]. Therefore, several factors that contribute to the generation of electricity for solar PV are identified including temperature, angle and duration of sunlight, intensity and also some environmental conditions such as weather, wind and dust [11].

Looking on the contributing factors on electricity generation for solar PV then the adequate steps need to be taken during its installation. However, since a PV system is usually located in a remote or high location, there still be chances of failures or maintenance problem during its operation. Therefore, remote monitoring is important to ensure that the efficiency of electricity generation for the solar PV system can be maintained.

Conventional methods of monitoring system mainly include manual investigation and remote wired monitoring. This method has several disadvantages such as time consuming and complexity of wiring [12]. The emerging technique of communication technology called Internet of Things (IoT) is offering a new solution to overcome this problem. IoT is a set of physical objects that are included with electronics, software, sensors, and network connections. It allows objects to be perceived and controlled remotely across the existing network infrastructure resulting in increased efficiency, accuracy and economic welfare [13].

Therefore, this paper presents an analysis of off-grid systems in which a connected photovoltaic system (1000 W/m^2) was installed at Maahad Tahfiz Al-Asyraf school in Terengganu. To obtain an efficient all-time energy management for the institutional premises, the parameters of total load and power generation of the institution were monitored by providing a remote and real-time monitoring facilities through IoT-based ESP8266 controller with Internet of Thing for Photo Voltage system (IoTPV). During the study, the energy yielded from the installed PV solar power system was evaluated (2018–2020) along with CO^2 level reduction and diesel fuel savings from diesel supported generator units.

2 Materials and Method

2.1 Electrical Wiring and System Architecture of IoTPV

The solar panel system development included two main parts, namely, the electrical wiring for solar panel and IoTPV system architecture. The electrical solar panel wiring as shown in Fig. 1a consisted of solar panel (1000 W/m2) for fixed angle position (10°), DC breaker, charger controller, battery for voltage storage, and lastly, inverter module. In this system, the maximum inverter in use for AC voltage produced was 5 KW, for each inverter. Meanwhile, the solar panel wiring had four inverter modules of equal maximum power produced, and the separation was made according to the sections lamp, ceiling fan, washing machine, PA system and refrigeration system.

On the other hand, the IoTPV architecture development as seen in Fig. 1b consisted of four important parts within—application or monitoring devices, internet, gateway and lastly, the network sensors connection. This system enabled the monitoring of data to be done either on PC or hand phone using the direct link on the IoTPV system of the user. At this stage, only the authorised user has the access to add or modify the IoT platform based on the data or graph needed and the analysis of the total power produced according to the sensors' measurement (irradiance, temperature and anemometer value). The second part is the internet within which include the cloud storage, analytics pre-processing, server and intelligent processing. The data on the system development were stored in this IoTPV architecture. The IoT Platform was also processed here for data display and collection. The third part is the gateway or router, in which the telco provider lines were used for the interconnection of the IoTPV system development to the internet. The gateway is an important part on this system to ensuring the continuous data measurement to be collected and sent to the internet at a high speed. The last part is the system for network sensor. Here, this system (IoTPV) is the main device for measuring the condition of the weather surrounding with reference to the power produced on solar panel PV. Figure 1 showed the system architecture of IoTPV at Maahad Tahfiz Al-Asyraf school in Terengganu.

2.2 Solar Panel Wiring Setup

The solar panel installation had around 20 pieces of PV panel in use, with high capacity of power (around 3000 W). The type of solar PV used was the monocrystalline solar panel. Each PV panel could produce around 150 W of power and the connection of each PV panel was parallel to the solar controller for high current to be obtained as well as ensuring consistent voltage generation on the solar panel. The maximum voltage produced on this solar PV was 18.2 V and the

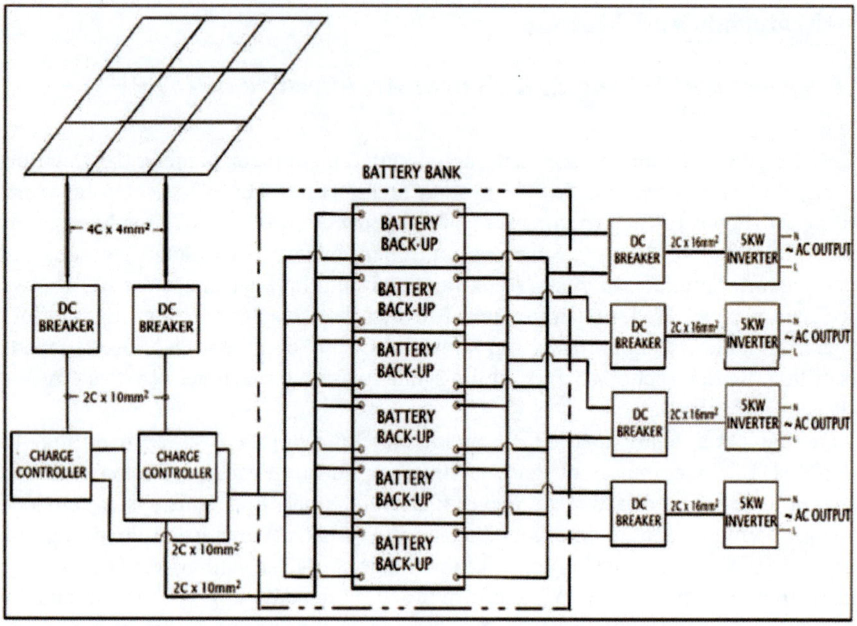

(a)

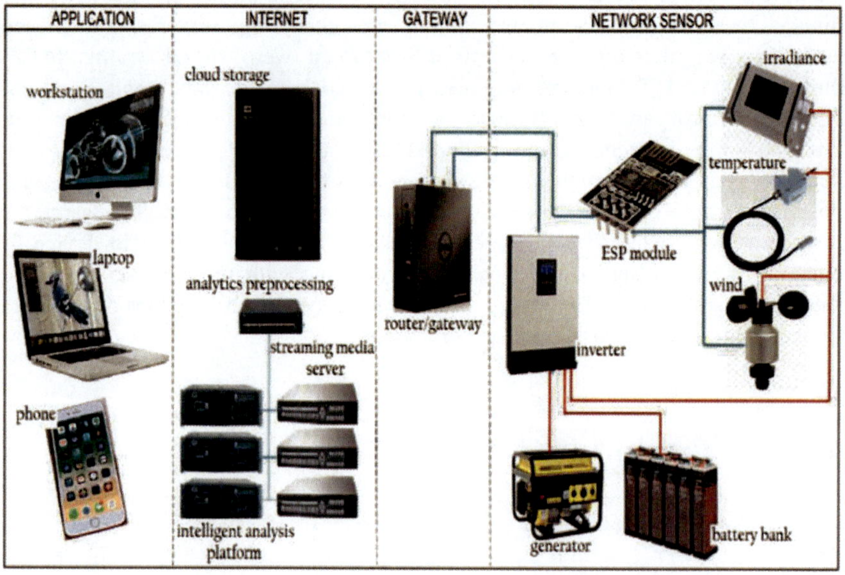

(b)

Fig. 1 **a** PV solar system wiring diagram. **b** architecture of IoTPV based wireless network system

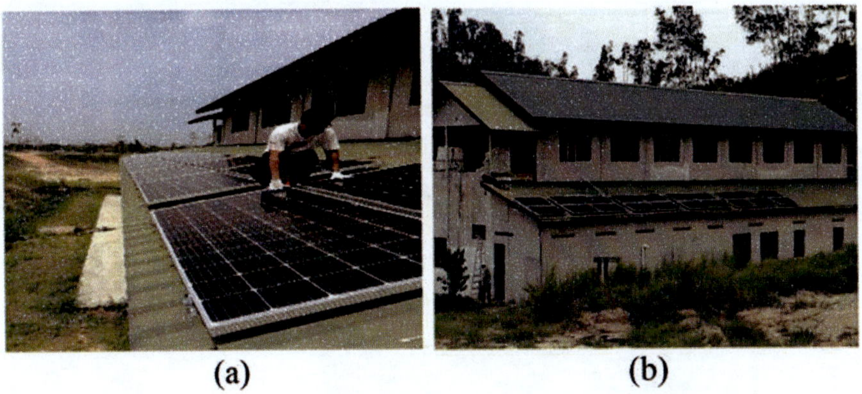

Fig. 2 Solar PV setup

maximum current was 7.69 A. Figure 2 showed the solar panel setup on the rooftop of the Maahad Tahfiz Al-Asyraf school

2.3 Schematic Design and IoT System Platform

The schematic circuit consisted of three important parts which were vital in ensuring the system to function properly. The first part was sensor network applications which include the irradiant sensor, temperature and anemometer. Each of the sensor gave the values to the controller based on the actual weather condition and these readings affect the power produced at solar panel PV. Meanwhile, the second part was the controller. Two types of controllers were used, namely, ATMega 2560 and ESP8266. ATMega 2560 functioned to collect and process all analogue data from sensors network reading and these data were sent serially to ESP8266 for IoT module interfacing. ESP8266 then proceeded to send these data to Thinger IoT Platform to display the value of the sensor measurement. Figure 3 showed the design of the driver circuit for probes connection, microcontroller, and PC interface. Lastly, the data were displayed at Thinger Platform and each of the parameter measurement was shown in value and graphs. The data were recorded for 30 days, then removed on the Thinger system in order for the new measurements to take place. These processes occurred continuously for data measurement purposes.

2.4 IoTPV System Setup

Figure 4 showed the actual circuit development, consisting of three main parts—the power supply, controller, and sensor connection. The power supply used was 12 V

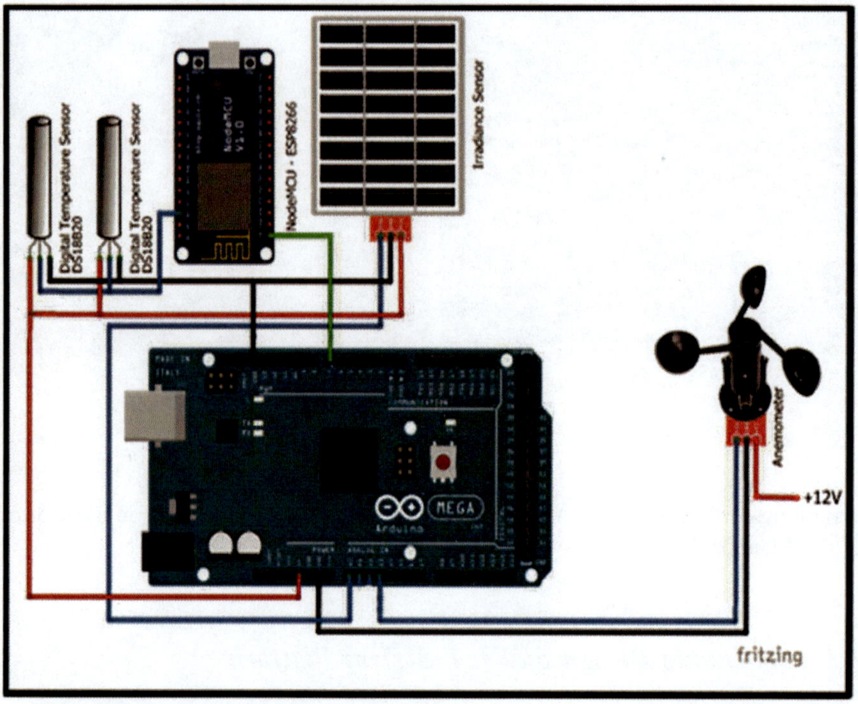

(a)

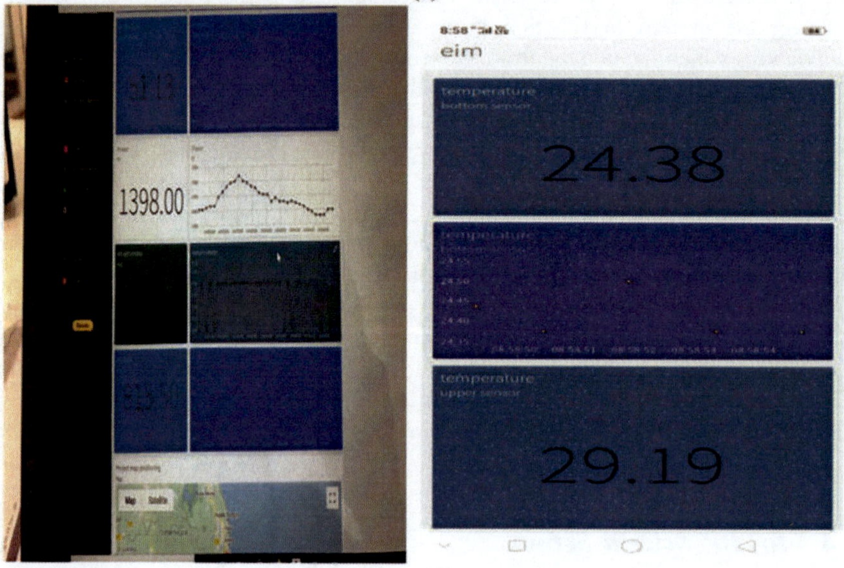

(b)

Fig. 3 IoTPV system. **a** Schematic diagram, **b** Thinger platform

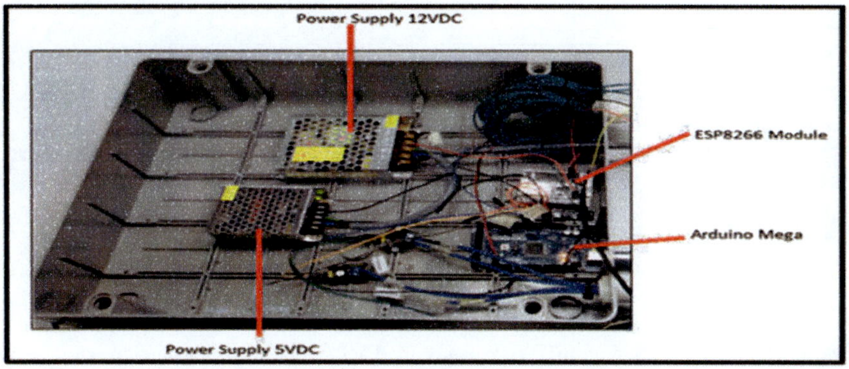

(a)

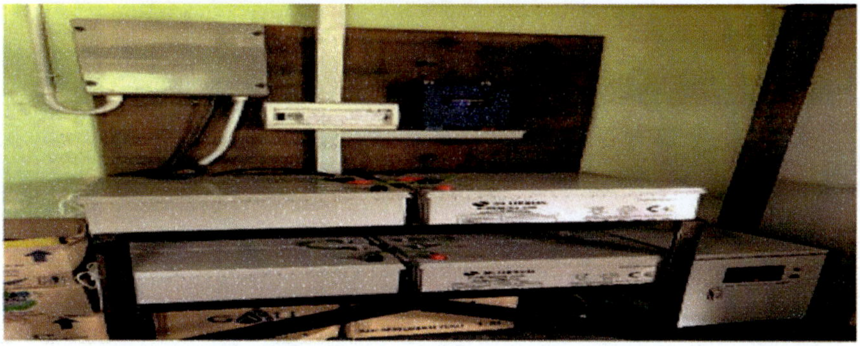

(b)

Fig. 4 IoTPV system setup on Mahadd Tahfiz Al-Asyraf control room. **a** IoTPV circuit, **b** control room for PV inverter and IoTPV system

DC and 5 V DC. The 12 V DC was used for irradiance and anemometer sensors while the 5 V DC was used for controller and temperature sensors. This system included the telco provider for IoT system—the Celcom line was used to transfer the data from the controller to the internet and these data were accessible online. The IoTPV system was placed in the control room together with the battery storage for solar panel, inverter and DC breaker. Then, this IoTPV system monitoring was activated for 24 h daily and the pattern of the data changes were observed in real time.

2.5 Sensor Setup

In order to obtain the actual measurement of irradiance, temperature and anemometer value, the sensors were placed behind the solar panel. The angle of sensor was fixed to be the same as the solar panel to ensure the maximum

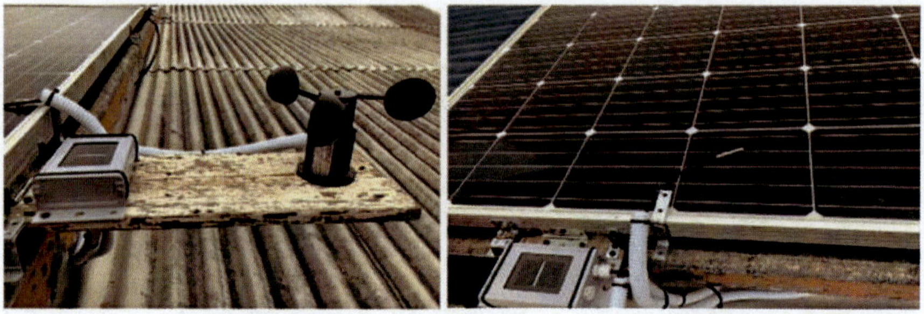

(a) (b)

Fig. 5 Sensors installation on IoTPV system. **a** Irradiant and anemometer, **b** temperature sensor

measurement value of each sensor to also be correctly recorded. Figure 5 showed the sensor setup on the rooftop of Maahad Tahfiz Al-Asyraf school. The limitation of wind speed measured on the anemometer was 35 m/s while the maximum temperature sensor measured was up until 150 °C. The temperature sensor was placed at the solar PV panel to ensure the actual temperature at solar PV panel to be measured. For irradiance sensor, the limitation of solar irradiance measured was until 1400 W/m^2.

3 Result and Discussion

3.1 Data Sampling

Based on Fig. 6 presented the comparison between the data sampling which were taken in 15 and 60 min/data. The blue line represented the power measurement for 15 min' data sampling while the orange colour indicated the measurement of the 60 min' data sampling. Based on the figure below, the maximum power measurement for the 15 min' data sampling was approximately 2000 W, as compared to the 60 min' data sampling which was 1750 W. Thus, the maximum power produced on solar PV was 2500 W. The 15 min' data sampling gave 80% of accuracy whilst the 60 min' data sampling had 70% of accuracy. It could be deduced that the data accuracy increased when the sampling data/minute was high and the data should be taken on a broad daylight only (efficient time for power producing on solar panel). From the discussion on sampling data for Fig. 6 show the maximum power can be produces at data 21 until 29 with the range time 12.00 p.m. until 2.00 p.m. and it will reduce consistently until data 35 at 3.30 p.m. On here the peak power for solar PV can be produce around 2 h only from morning until evening based on IoTPV system monitoring.

The arrangement of the central composite design, responses and values obtained from the experimental results of IoTPV system design parameters were tabulated by

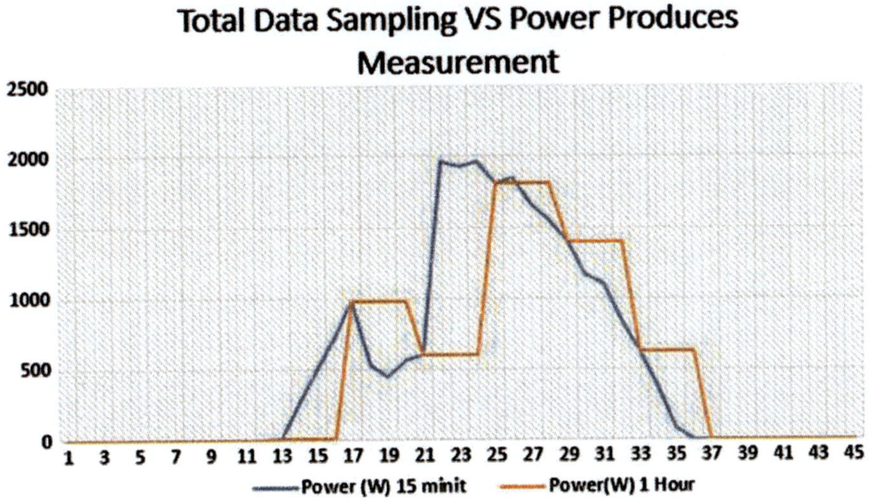

Fig. 6 Data sampling comparing for 15 min/data and 60 min/data

the Solar Irradiance, Temperature and Anemometer value as shown in Table 1. A total number of fourth-five data collection starting from 6.30 a.m. until 6.00 p.m. were conducted. Then, the responses were listed in Table 1. The table below showed that the irradiance value contributed to the effect on the amplitude of power produced on solar PV, in which the temperature recorded the lowest value of 21 °C while the highest values was 49.38 °C. With regards to the increasing of Power (W) amplitude, its efficiency could be reached up to 80% based on the increasing irradiance value. It was observed that the pattern of the Power growth doubled with each 30-min, starting from 7.30 a.m. until 1.00 p.m. Therefore, on the data in Table 1 will be discuss that the Power amplitude was directly proportional to irradiance value.

3.2 *Relation of Temperature, Irradiant and Power Was Produce on IoTPV*

The Analysis of Variance (ANOVA) was employed in the current research for the purpose of investigating the effect of independent parameters in the responses. The experimental results reflected that the number of wind, irradiance and temperature value detection varied in the range of 1–45 as shown in Table 2. Meanwhile, the Analysis of Variance (ANOVA) of Power (W) presented in Table 2 shows that all of the independent variables, the number of wind, irradiant and temperature value were significant ($p < 0.05$). Additionally, the interaction impact of the irradiant and power were found to be insignificant because the p-value was equal to <0.0001 and

Table 1 Data sampling for 1 days

C:\Program Files (x86)\DX7Trial\rahim.dx7 - Design-Expert 7.0.0

File Edit View Display Options Design Tools Help

Notes for rahim
- Design (Actual)
  - Summary
  - Graph Columns
  - Evaluation
- Analysis
  - Power (Analyzed)
- Optimization
  - Numerical
  - Graphical
  - Point Prediction

Std	Run	Block	Factor 1 A:Wind m/s	Factor 2 B:Irradiant W/m2	Factor 3 C:Temperature C	Response 1 Power W
5	11	Block 1	0.00	0.00	21.88	0
16	12	Block 1	0.00	0.00	21.31	0
7	13	Block 1	0.00	3.50	21.88	6
19	14	Block 1	0.00	157.50	23.64	270
10	15	Block 1	1.00	287.00	27.06	492
18	16	Block 1	0.00	427.00	32.50	732
2	17	Block 1	2.00	574.00	36.38	984
8	18	Block 1	1.00	311.50	41.13	534
15	19	Block 1	1.00	259.00	39.75	444
12	20	Block 1	1.00	329.00	44.69	564
20	21	Block 1	3.00	350.00	43.44	600
21	22	Block 1	3.00	1148.00	43.94	1968
22	23	Block 1	3.00	1123.50	48.82	1926
23	24	Block 1	3.00	1144.00	49.06	1962
24	25	Block 1	2.00	1057.00	50.13	1812
25	26	Block 1	1.00	1078.00	52.12	1848
26	27	Block 1	1.00	966.00	49.38	1656
27	28	Block 1	1.00	906.60	45.25	1554
28	29	Block 1	2.00	815.50	47.63	1398
42	30	Block 1	1.00	682.00	43.06	1170
43	31	Block 1	1.00	640.00	43.94	1098
44	32	Block 1	1.00	479.50	44.50	822
41	33	Block 1	2.00	360.50	43.69	618
40	34	Block 1	1.00	213.00	28.94	366
39	35	Block 1	1.00	42.00	31.31	72
38	36	Block 1	0.00	0.00	27.25	0

<0.0408. Hence, this led to the removal of any insignificant term, followed by the repetition of the optimisation process until all of the terms became significant. The *p*-value served as a tool to inspect the significance of each coefficient. In this case, the values of "Prob > F" were less than 0.05 which indicated that the model terms were significant. Meanwhile, A, B, C, AB, AC, BC, A^2, B^2, C^2, ABC, A^2B, A^2C, AB^2, AC^2, B^2C, BC^2, A^3, $B^3$and C^3 were significant factors included in the mathematical model.

The mathematical modelling in Eqs. 1 and 2 was used to identify the power produced based on three parameters input of this paper. The parameters design also predicted the normal condition of weather in Malaysia. In the case of system design validation, the experimental result under the optimum input parameter design was compared to the value of the predicted power produced on solar PV. The residual plots for the number of irradiance value were deemed essential in evaluating the validity of a model. Figure 7 displayed the normal probability plot for the residual distributions which acted as additional validation for the Response Surface Methodology model. The results from the figure clearly showed that the normal

Table 2 Power of solar PV value in surface quadratic model

Source	Sum of Squares	df	Mean Square	F Value	p-value Prob > F	
Model	2.034E+007	19	1.071E+006	3.554E+007	< 0.0001	significant
A-Wind	0.017	1	0.017	0.57	0.04592	
B-Irradiant	37488.67	1	37488.67	1.245E+006	< 0.0001	
C-Temperature	0.55	1	0.55	18.30	0.0002	
AB	0.37	1	0.37	12.20	0.0018	
AC	0.14	1	0.14	4.52	0.0435	
BC	0.68	1	0.68	22.42	< 0.0001	
A^2	0.012	1	0.012	0.39	0.0435	
B^2	0.53	1	0.53	17.72	0.0003	
C^2	0.59	1	0.59	19.52	0.0002	
ABC	0.32	1	0.32	10.51	0.0034	
A^2B	6.821E-003	1	6.821E-003	0.23	0.0438	
A^2C	4.153E-004	1	4.153E-004	0.014	0.0407	
AB^2	0.40	1	0.40	13.18	0.0013	
AC^2	0.061	1	0.061	2.03	0.0166	
B^2C	0.30	1	0.30	10.03	0.0040	
BC^2	0.34	1	0.34	11.18	0.0026	
A^3	7.134E-003	1	7.134E-003	0.24	0.0430	
B^3	0.20	1	0.20	6.64	0.0162	
C^3	0.21	1	0.21	6.99	0.0140	
Residual		0.75	25	0.030		
Lack of Fit		0.75	22	0.034		
Pure Error		0.000	3	0.000		
Cor Total		2.034E+007	44			

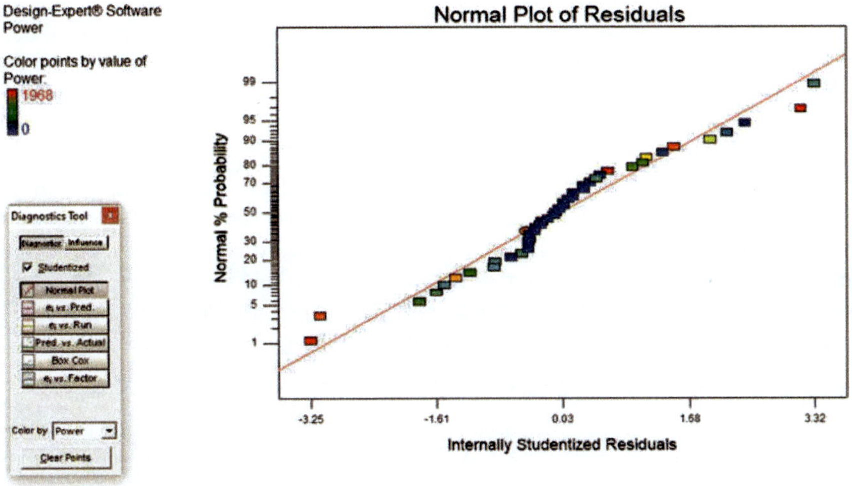

Fig. 7 Normal probability plot for power produces on solar PV

probability diagram for power produced was very close to a straight-line with no evidence of an outlier. Therefore, this indicated that the errors were normally distributed while the full quadratic regression equation exceedingly fitted the observed data.

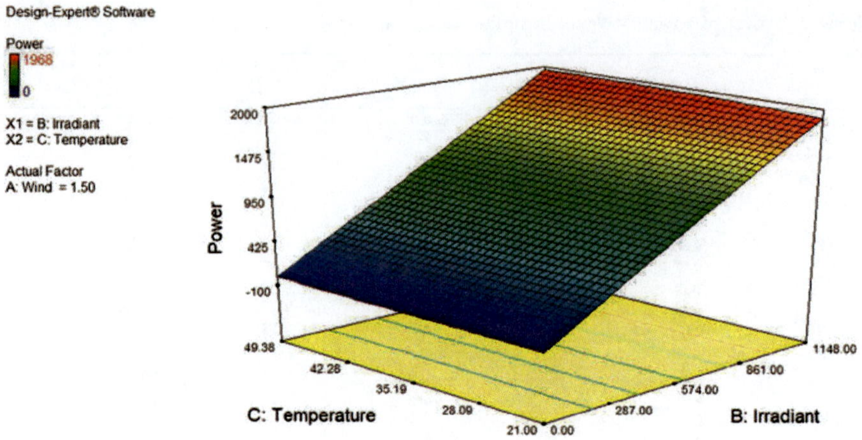

Fig. 8 The 3-d surface plot for influence of temperature and irradiant in power produce on solar PV

Figure 8 illustrated a 3-D surface which explains the effect of the irradiant and temperature values in the sensor network related to the Power value effectiveness for the Power amplitude and Power produced at Maahad Tahfiz Al-Asyraf school in Terengganu. The value of irradiance of 1148 W/m^2 provided a high amplitude of power with the temperature of 21 until 49.38 °C. Figure 8 also demonstrated that low amplitude of power caused by irradiance value which was lower than 574 W/m^2. Overall, the irradiance value was directly proportional to the power produces on IoTPV system.

The significance of each variable was evaluated ($p < 0.05$) using the p-value. The estimated yield regression coefficients for axial defect detection for the quadratic equation with "Pred. R-Squared" of 1.0000 was found to be in a good relationship with the "Adj. R-Squared" of 1.0000 with a difference of <0.05. More importantly, the implementation of RSM produced the following regression equation which described the empirical relationship between the Power of solar panel recording (W) and the independent parameters as shown in Eqs. 1 and 2.

Final Equation in Terms of Coded Factors:

$$\begin{aligned}\text{Power} = & (+984.11) - (0.27 * A) + (980.49 * B) + (2.91 * C) + (5.70 * A * B) \\ & - (4.28 * A * C) + (14.76 * B * C) - (0.68 * A^2) - (9.38 * B^2) \\ & - (6.04 * C^2) - (10.62 * A * B * C) - (0.73 * A^2 * B) \\ & - (0.33 * A^2 * C) + (8.25 * A * B^2) + (3.85 * A * C^2) \\ & + (15.15 * B^2 * C) - (11.13 * B * C^2) + (0.57 * A^3) \\ & - (6.46 * B^3) + (2.61 * C^3)\end{aligned} \tag{1}$$

Final Equation in Terms of Actual Factors:

$$\begin{aligned}
\text{Power} =& (-25.85709) + (6.77540 * \text{Wind}) + (1.62668 * \text{Irradiant}) \\
&+ (2.71803 * \text{Temperature}) + (0.019754 * \text{Wind} * \text{Irradiant}) \\
&- (0.56702 * \text{Wind} * \text{Temperature}) + (6.17050\text{E} - 003 * \text{Irradiant} \\
&* \text{Temperature}) - \left(0.37230 * \text{Wind}^2\right) - (1.08711\text{E} - 004 \\
&* \text{Irradiant}^2\big) - \left(0.090161 * \text{Temperature}^2\right) - (8.69425\text{E} - 004 \\
&* \text{Wind} * \text{Irradiant} * \text{Temperature}) - (5.68336\text{E} - 004 \\
&* \text{Wind}^2 * \text{Irradiant}\big) - \left(0.010441 * \text{Wind}^2 * \text{Temperature}\right) \\
&+ \left(1.66996\text{E} - 005 * \text{Wind} * \text{Irradiant}^2\right) + (0.012735 * \text{Wind} \\
&* \text{Temperature}^2\big) + \left(3.24043\text{E} - 006 * \text{Irradiant}^2 * \text{Temperature}\right) \\
&- \left(9.62579\text{E} - 005 * \text{Irradiant} * \text{Temperature}^2\right) + \left(0.16934 * \text{Wind}^3\right) \\
&- \left(3.41646\text{E} - 008 * \text{Irradiant}^3\right) + \left(9.12428\text{E} - 004 * \text{Temperature}^3\right)
\end{aligned} \tag{2}$$

4 Conclusion

The IoT system is a current technology and it is listed in IR4.0. IoT system is applicable in solar measuring system to getting the online data for sensor measurement, especially to know the power produced on solar panel and to identify the factor that affects the energy production for solar panel. The results showed that the higher sampling data will produce higher accuracy of power storage for IoTPV system. This was proven based on the comparison of two types of sampling—within 15 and 60 min of interval data sampling. Thus, it can be deduced that the 15 min data sampling increased the accuracy until 80% and the 60 min data sampling reduced the accuracy of total power produced, until 70%. Therefore, the relation between irradiance value, temperature and anemometer can be identified based on Eq. 1 and 2. To summaries, the major effect of power produced on solar panel is irradiance value, wherein the irradiance value is directly proportional to the power produced. Meanwhile, the temperature gave a minimal effect on the power produced and the anemometer parameter can be ignored on this system as it did not give much effect to the power measurement. Lastly, this system is capable of predicting the power produced and it can also be used for the forecast in yearly data measurement. Furthermore, this system is also very suitable to use in many places, especially in rural areas for the purpose of livestock and agriculture, settlement development, tourism development and many more. In addition, the analysis of big data can be collected for the analysis of energy use in a settlement and at the same time will develop the field of solar hybrid energy use for mutual benefit.

Acknowledgements We would like to express our gratitude to University College TATI for the facilities, expertise and equipment provided in this experiment work for lab equipment supported through Electrical Lab, Sensor Technology Lab, Electronic Lab, and Microcontroller Lab.

References

1. Kazmierkowski MP, Jasinski M, Wrona G (2011) DSP-based control of grid-connected power converters operating under grid distortions. IEEE Trans Ind Informat 7(2):204–211
2. Elhadidy MA, Shaahid SM (1999) Optimal sizing of battery storage for hybrid (windCdiesel) power systems. Renew Energy 18(1):77–86
3. Elhadidy MA, Shaahid SM (2004) Promoting applications of hybrid (wind photovoltaic diesel battery power) systems in hot regions. Renew Energy 29(4):517–528
4. Shareef H, Ahmed MS, Mohamed A, Hassan EA (2018) Review on home energy management system considering demand responses, smart technologies, and intelligent controllers. IEEE Acc 6:24498–24509
5. Kennel F, Gorges D, Liu S (2013) Energy management for smart grids with electric vehicles based on hierarchical MPC. IEEE Trans Ind Informat 9(3):1528–1537
6. Chakrabarti S, Chakrabarti S (2002) Rural electrification programme with solar energy in remote region: a case study in an island. Energy Policy 30(1):33–42
7. Wagh MM, Kulkarni VV (2016) Modeling and optimization of integration of renewable energy resources (RER) for minimum energy cost, minimum CO_2 emissions and sustainable development, in recent years: a review. Energy Power Eng 3(6):868–875
8. Pazikadin AR, Rifai D, Ali K, Malik MZ, Abdalla AN, Faraj MA (2020) Solar irradiance measurement instrumentation and power solar generation forecasting based on artificial neural networks (ANN): a review of five years research trend. Sci Total Environ 715:136848. https://doi.org/10.1016/j.scitotenv.136848
9. Irvine S (2017) Solar cells and photovoltaics. In: Kasap S, Capper P (eds) Springer handbook of electronic and photonic materials. Springer, Canada
10. Tricahyono RW, Kholis N (2018) Sistem monitoring intensitas cahaya dan daya pada dual axis solar tracking system berbasis IoT J Teknik Elektro Universitas Surabaya 7, p 233
11. Suryawinata H, Purwanti D, Sunardiyo S (2017) Sistem monitoring pada panel surya menggunakan data logger berbasis ATMega 328 dan real time clock DS1307. J Teknik Elektro 9:30
12. Raza A, Ikram AA, Amin A, Ikram AJ (2016) A review of low cost and power efficient development boards for IoT applications. In: Future technologies conference, p 786. IEEE
13. Apurva L (2016) IoT based solar monitoring system. Int J Sci Technol Eng 3:1

Auto Tracking Mobile Robot Navigation Based on HUE Color of Image Pattern

M. Z. Muhammad Luqman, W. T. Wan Faizura, R. A. R. S. Nur Adiimah, A. R. Nazry, A. M. A. Hasib, and A. G. A. Shahrizan

Abstract In industrial, a mobile robot is often used to move an object from its initial location to the final location. To perform the task, the robot needs to move forward following the path provided. The problem has been countered from movement the robot is to find a path that moves the robot from start position to goal while never touch any obstacle. For an auto-tracking mobile robot, the most critical part is the target identification and tracking of the moving object. Although the motion planning problem is defined in the regular world, it lives in another space. In this project, a combination of the HUE-based color of the pattern was used as a tracking object and the mobile robot can only identify the color of that image pattern for the auto-tracking navigation. Therefore, a study was carried out to make a path planning for mobile robot navigation using a vision system which is Pixy CMUcam5 as a sensory point to detect the color of the image pattern of the object for the auto-tracking purpose. Arduino Mega is the main control unit that controls all input and output of the mobile robot. The results of the work presented suggest that the color of image pattern identification used for the mobile robot navigation should be a combination should be at least two combinations so that, the mobile robot could differentiate between the tracking object and the environment.

Keywords Mobile robot navigation · Image processing · Pattern recognition · Color tracking · Pixy camera · Auto tracking robot

M. Z. Muhammad Luqman · W. T. Wan Faizura (✉) · R. A. R. S. Nur Adiimah · A. R. Nazry · A. M. A. Hasib
Faculty of Engineering Technology, University College TATI, Kemaman, Terengganu, Malaysia
e-mail: wanfaizura@uctati.edu.my

A. G. A. Shahrizan
Faculty of Manufacturing Engineering, Universiti Malaysia Pahang, Pekan, Malaysia

H. Triwiyanto et al. (eds.), *Proceedings of the 1st International Conference on Electronics, Biomedical Engineering, and Health Informatics*, Lecture Notes in Electrical Engineering 746, https://doi.org/10.1007/978-981-33-6926-9_25

1 Introduction

Nowadays, the involvement between human and robot is easily seen around the globe either in industries or in everyday life at home. The robot can do a task that would be impossible for a human being to do and sometimes it would be easier to use a robot to solve certain tasks. Thus, robots make human's work easier and more productive. By giving a vision to the robot, it would be further increasing the function of the robot. Luo et al. [1] has proposed a mobile robot path tracking based on color vision. Luo's proposed method is based on the data extracted from HSI (Hue, Saturation, Intensity) color model using fuzzy control. All the images captured will be converted into the HSI color model and using the segmentation method. In addition, the robot path tracking control used fuzzy control.

Sundarajoo et al. [2] used improved the auto-tracking mobile robot based on the HSI color model. The experimental result demonstrates that when HSI color-based filtering algorithm is applied to the visual tracking, it improves the accuracy and stability of color tracking under the condition of varying brightness or even in the low-contrast environment.

Autonomous robot navigation based on pattern recognition techniques and artificial neural networks was proposed by Quinonez et al. [3]. They used four different patterns which are an image of an arrow, a stop signage image, an additional symbol, and a triangle image for the pattern recognition purpose and the TurtleBot 2 as a mobile robot platform. The finding from the research was the robot able to recognize all patterns successfully. It has been verified that the algorithm is not affected by changes of scale and image rotation due to pre-processing performed, an important factor to obtain a better learning performance of the network is enlightenment, because when improving lighting conditions, the coefficients generated by the DCT are more consistent.

For mobile robot following an object, Ahmad et al. [4] has come out with a project, wheelchair luggage follower based on color tracking technique by using Pixy CMUcam5. The Pixy CMUcam5 was used as the vision sensor for the color tracking purpose attached to the luggage and also the project used an ultrasonic sensor for the obstacle avoidance purpose as the additional feature. The outcome from the experiment found that the luggage able to follow the wheelchair from behind without the help of human control.

The method of people detection and tracking based on real-time RGB-D for the mobile robot was proposed by Fang et al. [5] by implementing an open-source robot operating system (ROS) to a mobile robot to track a target. The feature of the target is extracted before the depth information is collected and used to track the target based on the nearest point position information. Then, the implementation of the CAM-Shift algorithm which is based on RGB information is applied to improve the anti-interference ability.

Another method of the people-following mobile robot was proposed by Shih and Li [6]. Kinect camera sensor additional with laser scanner used by Ching as a visionary sensor attached to the mobile robot. It is found that the robot is able to follow the target person. It is also used the range information obtained from a laser scanner to plan its motion and to re-recognize the target person at the same time. The experimental robot system recognizes the target to follow successfully on more than 95% of the trials and the target person recognition time is less than 0.1 s.

In this project, the Pixy camera is attached to the mobile robot as a visionary sensor which is used to move the mobile robot from one location to another location. Meanwhile, the color image pattern will be attached to the human body as a recognition object for the mobile robot auto-tracking.

Next, a microcontroller is also an essential part of auto-tracking to work properly. It is acts as the brain to process all data acquired. Once the image has been captured by the camera, the image will be decomposed into its individual color channel. Based on these color channels, the total intensity and the maximum intensity values of each color channel are calculated. The maximum intensity values between these color channels will determine the dominant color of the object for the purpose of the mobile robot to identify it. Besides that, the microcontroller also sends an electrical signal to the mobile robot's actuators to react to the motion of the tracked image pattern.

The scope of this project is to fabricate a mobile robot that is able to detect an image pattern and navigate the mobile robot based on the area and position of the detected image pattern. As mention earlier, the color for the image pattern is based on HUE color and the mobile robot will test indoor within the lab.

Firstly, the image pattern color must be taught so that, it could recognize the pattern and differentiate it from background noise. Then, the Pixy camera will capture the image and the microcontroller will process the information and monitor the behavior of the image pattern. The smaller the area of image pattern, the far that image pattern from the mobile robot. The bigger the area of the image pattern, the closer the image pattern to the mobile robot.

Next, when the image pattern starts to move, this mobile robot also will follow and tracks the image pattern. At the same time, the mobile robot always maintains distance with the image pattern to prevent from a collision. Besides that, the vision of the robot is up to 180° on the x-axis and y-axis as the camera is attached to a pan-tilt which is able to rotate. The rotation of the camera is control by two servo motors whereas one servo motor is used to control the x-axis movement and another servo motor is used for the y-axis movement.

2 Materials and Methodology

Based on the literature review, suitable components for the project were selected. The schematic circuit for the project is design, drawn and assemble. Then, followed by software and coding development of the project. At the final stage, the mobile robot will be test with auto tracking of color image pattern in lab. Figure 1 shows the methodology flowchart for the project of auto tracking mobile robot.

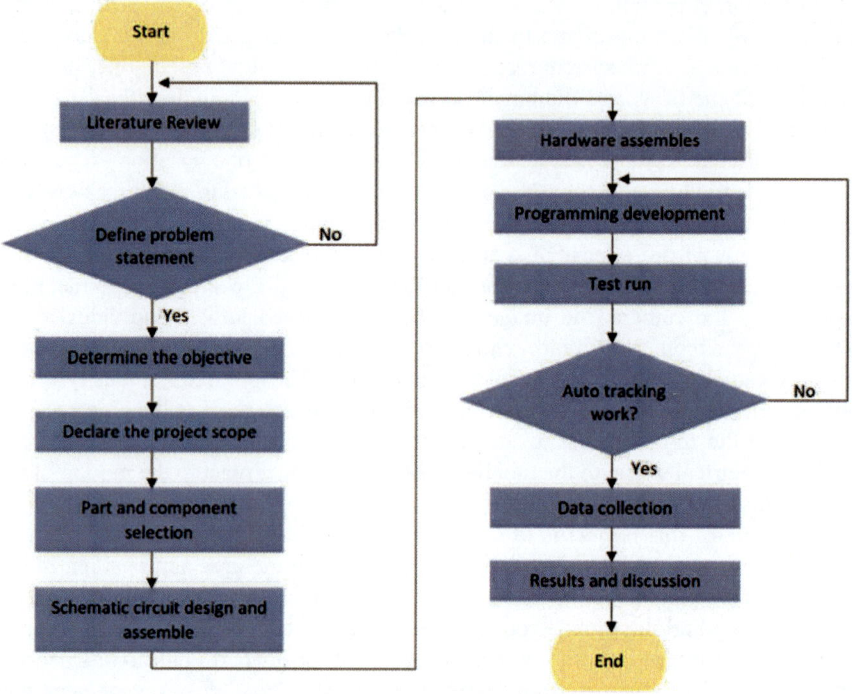

Fig. 1 Methodology flowchart for auto tracking mobile robot navigation

2.1 Pixy CMUcam5

The Pixy2 CMUcam5 is smaller, faster and more capable than the original Pixy. Like its predecessor, the Pixy2 can learn to detect objects that teach to it, just by pressing a button. Additionally, the Pixy2 has new algorithms that detect and track lines for use with line-following robots. With these new algorithms, it can detect intersections and "road signs" as well. The road signs can tell the robot what to do, such as turn left, turn right, slow down, etc. The best part is that the Pixy2 does all of this at 60 frames-per-second, so the robot can be fast, too.

The Pixy2 uses a color-based filtering algorithm to detect objects. Color-based filtering methods are popular because they are fast, efficient, and relatively robust. Pixy2 calculates hue and saturation of each RGB pixel from the image sensor and uses these as the primary filtering parameters. The hue of an object remains largely unchanged with changes in lighting and exposure. Changes in lighting and exposure can have a frustrating effect on color filtering algorithms, causing them to break. Pixy2's filtering algorithm is robust when it comes to lighting and exposure changes [7].

2.2 *Arduino Mega 2560*

Arduino Mega 2560 was selected as the controller for the mobile robot. The Arduino Mega is a microcontroller board based on the ATmega2560. It has 54 digital input/output pins (of which 14 can be used as PWM outputs), 16 analog inputs, 4 UARTs (hardware serial ports), a 16 MHz crystal oscillator, a USB connection, a power jack, an ICSP header, and a reset button. It contains everything needed to support the microcontroller; simply connect it to a computer with a USB cable or power it with an AC-to-DC adapter or battery to get started [8].

2.3 *MDD10A Motor Driver*

This kind of motor driver are selected due to it support maximum 10A of current. MDD10A is the dual-channel version of MD10C which is designed to drive 2 brushed DC motors with high current up to 10A continuously. Like MD10C, MDD10A also supports locked-antiphase and sign-magnitude PWM signal. It uses full solid-state components that offers faster response time and eliminates the wear and tear of the mechanical relay. Nonetheless, it is compatible with Arduino or any microcontroller that can output logic signal at 3.3 or 5.0 V, and that includes Arduino Zero and Arduino Micro. And not to forget the famous Raspberry Pi SBC too [9].

2.4 *Electronic Block Diagram*

The main electronic component and part used for the building an auto tracking mobile robot for navigation are the Arduino Mega 2560 as the controller unit, Pixy CMUcam5 camera as the visionary sensory device, motor driver to drive the robot wheel, DC motor and servo motor. All component is connected as shown in block diagram (see Fig. 2). The block diagram shows the representation of principal part that were used in mobile robot which represented by blocks and connected lines to show the relation to all component and also for input and output in the mobile robot.

Pixy CMUcam5 acquire the data of the tracked image pattern including the size of area and position in the pixel location and send it to Arduino Mega 2560. Arduino processes the received data and make a decision for the DC motor movement to keep tracking the image pattern. Besides that, the servo motor is directly controlled by Pixy CMUcam5 itself.

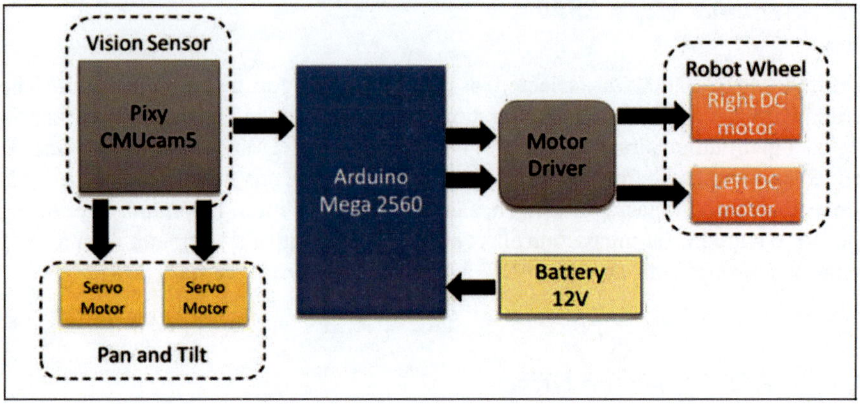

Fig. 2 Block diagram for auto tracking mobile robot

2.5 *Hardware Design*

Figure 3 shows the complete mobile robot base equipped with Pixy CMUcam5 for the color image pattern detection and tracking purpose. In addition to the camera, the mobile robot also equipped with two DC motor including rubber wheel, Arduino Mega 2560, motor driver and servo motor.

The mobile robot base is built up by using hollow metal rod and aluminum plate. Overall weight of the mobile robot is approximately 7 kg.

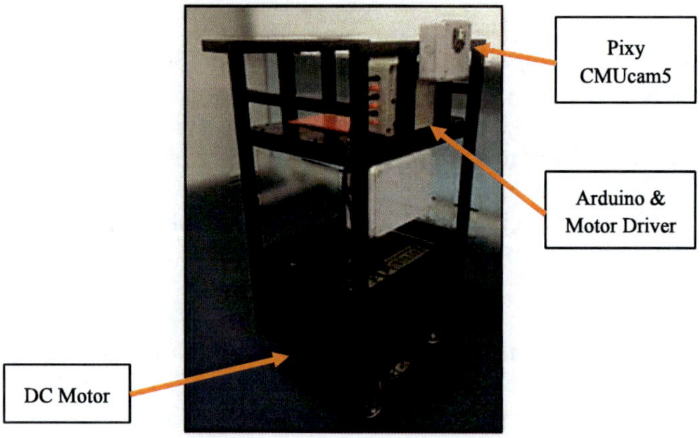

Fig. 3 Mobile robot hardware design

2.6 *Color Code Image Pattern*

For the color image pattern detection, two combination of color code based on HUE color were used which is red and yellow and the image pattern shows in Fig. 4. The combination of two color or more is important so that, Pixy CMUcam5 could recognize the pattern as a special symbol. Controller used will be program to recognize and response only if the Pixy CMUcam5 detect the image pattern. The color code also used as a medium to differentiate the detected pattern and the unnecessary background.

3 Results and Discussion

The mobile robot able to track the color image pattern effectively as proposed at normal condition. Several experiments were carried out on to ensure the consistency of the image pattern detection and for the mobile robot navigation purpose. First experiment was to determine the target locking consistency. Second experiment is to evaluate the navigation consistency of mobile robot while maintaining it distance around 2 ft from the image pattern plate and track the image pattern plate wherever it goes. Both experiments were conducted in lab with a moderate lighting. The distance between mobile robot and the target couldn't get far more than 7 ft due to mobile robot always catch up the target.

3.1 *Target Locking Consistency*

The objective of this experiment is to determine the target locking consistency and the target for the experiment is the color code image pattern plate. The Pixy CMUcam5 able to lock the target up to 240 cm for the object dimension around 6 cm in diameter [2]. However, the distance for the detection could be increase if the size of the object uses to detect is larger. The larger the target size, the farther the distance of the target can go [7].

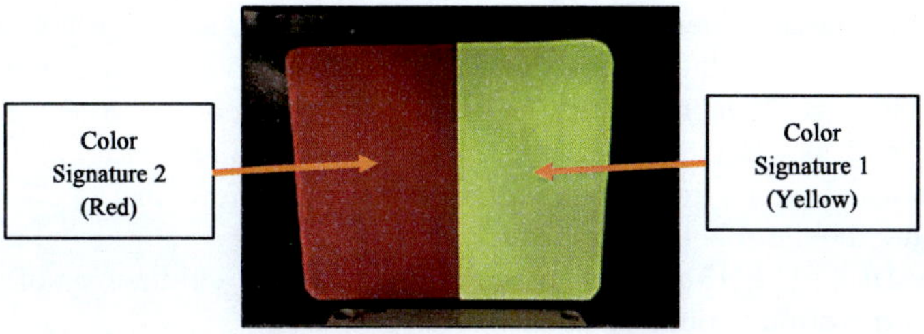

Fig. 4 Color code of image pattern used

Table 1 Result for the first experiment

Signature range (ft)	Noise level	Target lock stability
1.0	None	High
2.0	None	High
3.0	None	High
4.0	None	High
5.0	None	High
6.0	None	High
1.0	None	High

The tabulated result from the experiment conducted shows in Table 1. The sample image captured from the experiment shows that there is no noise level appear in the background and the target locked consistently (see Fig. 5). Other image sample for detection and target locking also shown in Figs. 10, 11, 12, 13, 14, 15. The target locking is improved when use more than 1 color signature and make it as color code detection and it will get a noise level at zero.

3.2 *Auto Tracking Navigation Consistency of Mobile Robot*

The combination of color signature known as color code also become an important criterion for the auto tracking to work smoothly and consistently. The Pixy CMUcam5 will use this information to differentiate between color code image pattern and the background. The way detection work and the tracking response explain in the Figs. 6, 7, 8 and 9. The box represented the full of view (FOV) area of Pixy CMUcam5. The number in each block represented the zone for the detection. The coordinate initial position for both x-axis and y-axis is at the center of the box. The initial position for the detection is at zone 5 and in actual condition, it's about 2 ft from the mobile robot to the target. Two color signatures used which is color signature 1 as yellow and color signature 2 as red.

Figure 6 shows the detection at zone 1 with small area which means the target is far ahead and the mobile robot will track the color image pattern with forward motion together with turning left motion. Meanwhile, the detection area in Fig. 7 shows that the target is nearer but it's slightly to the right. Mobile robot will move forward motion a little bit together with turning right motion until it reach initial position. There is no motion occur of mobile robot when the target detected as occur in Fig. 8. For Fig. 9, the mobile robot motion is same as Fig. 6.

The tabulated results from the experiment conducted shows in Table 2. It can be seen that the mobile robot can track the target consistently.

Figures 10, 11, 12, 13, 14 and 15 shows the detection and tracking of the color image pattern with a various position.

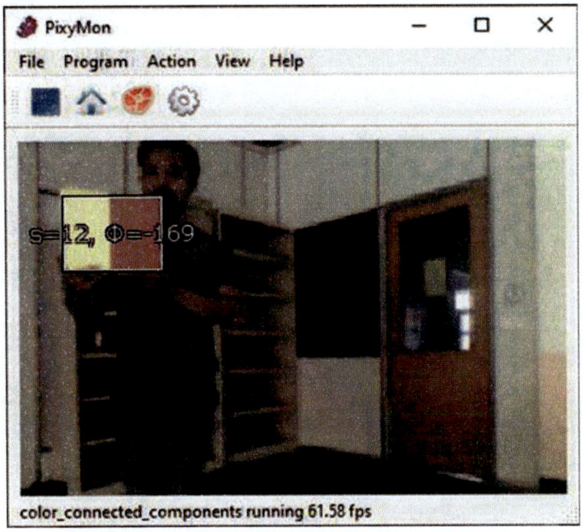

Fig. 5 Locked target consistently without any noise for both color signature

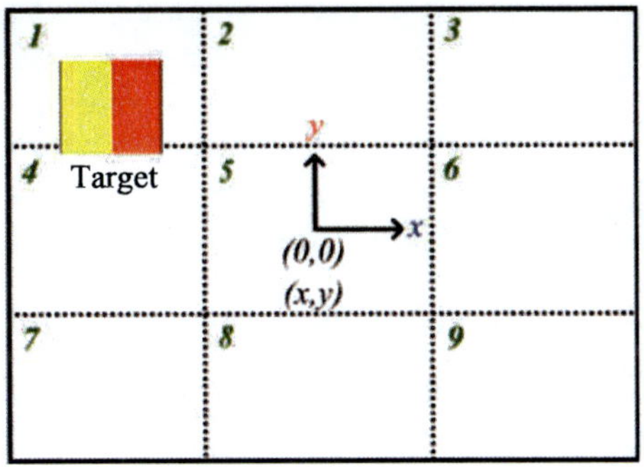

Fig. 6 Detection at zone 1 with small area

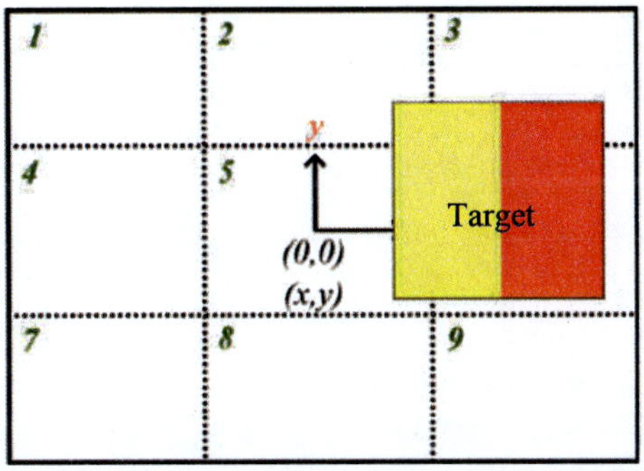

Fig. 7 Detection at zone 6 with large area

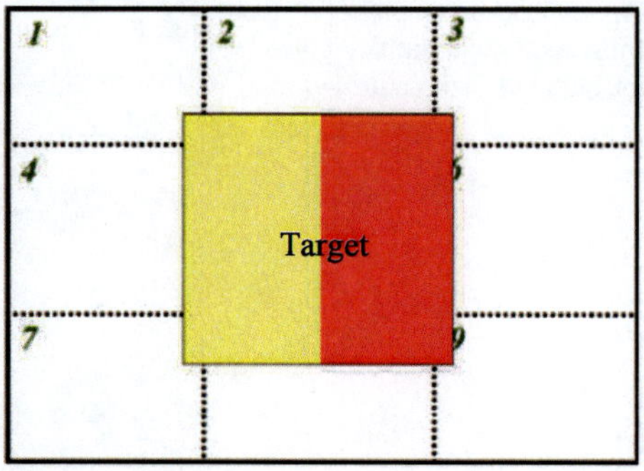

Fig. 8 Detect at zone 5 with large area

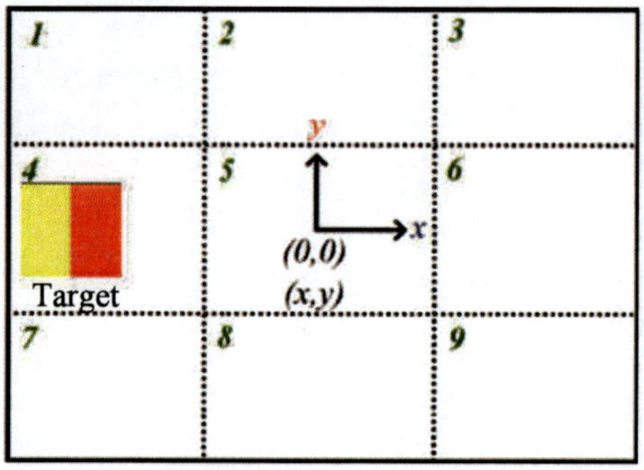

Fig. 9 Detection at zone 4 with small area

Table 2 Result for the second experiment

Signature range from the robot (ft)	Image pattern position (*x*, *y*)	Mobile robot motion	Target lock stability
1.0	0, 0	Reverse	High
2.0	0, 0	Stop	High
3.0	3, 1	Forward + Turn Right	High
4.0	0, 0	Forward	High
5.0	−9, 3	Forward + Turn Left	High
6.0	12, −1	Forward + Turn Right	High
7.0	0, 3	Forward	High

Fig. 10 Detected at 1.5 ft

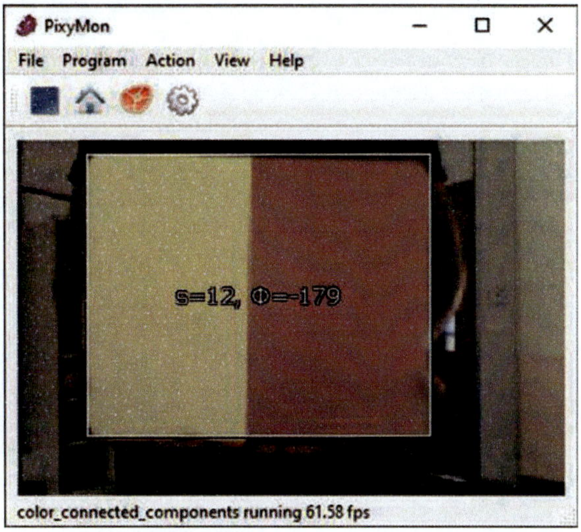

Fig. 11 Detected at 7 ft

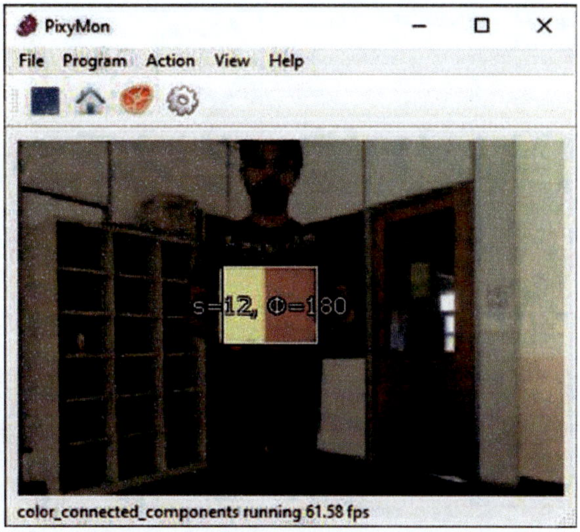

4 Conclusion

From the research conducted, it is found that the mobile robot able to detect and track the target which is image pattern consistently. There factor that make it successfully occur are the use of color code at the target in order to reduce the noise level that come with the background. The other factor for the successful of auto

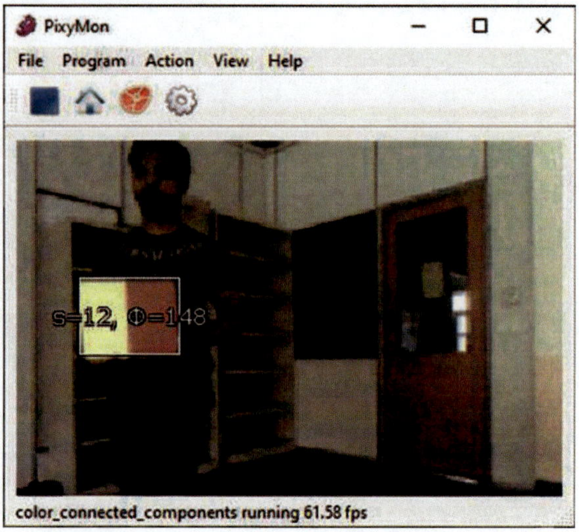

Fig. 12 Detected at 7 ft to the left

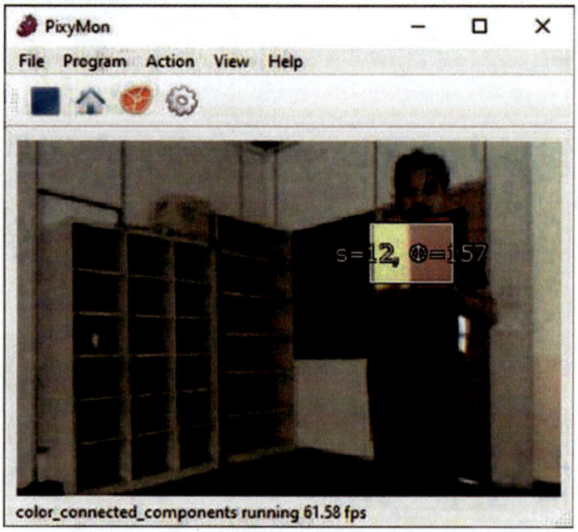

Fig. 13 Detected at 7 ft to the right

tracking of mobile robot navigation is the target itself. The target size is big enough so that, the Pixy CMUcam5 could recognize it even it is far ahead. The chosen of color code also play as the main role. It should be the combination of HUE color that have big different of dark and light color. The other factor is the environment lighting that have enough light so that, Pixy CMUcam5 can work efficiently. Overall, the use of color code of target surface for detection and tracking in order to

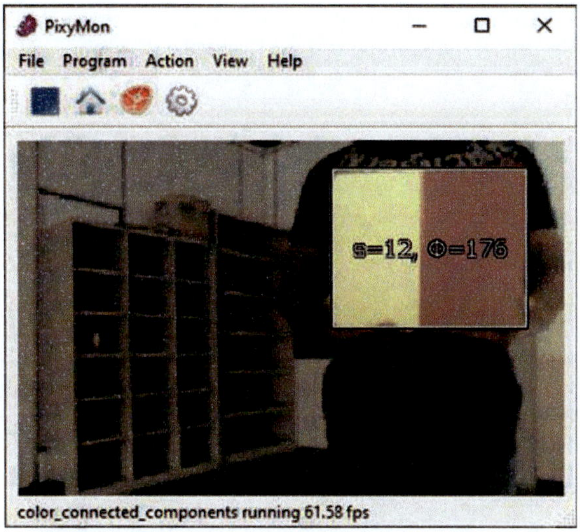

Fig. 14 Detected at 2 ft to the right

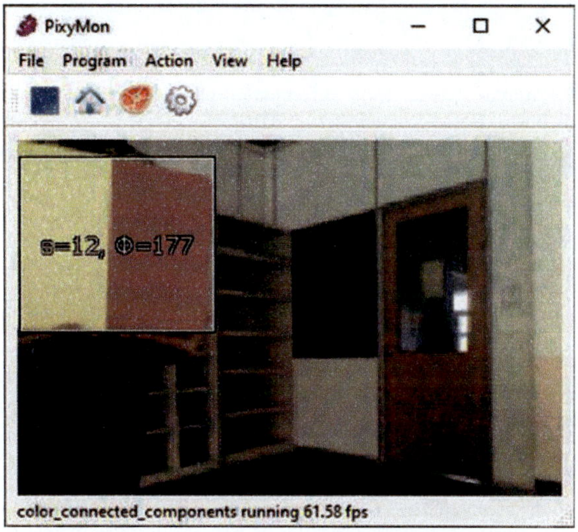

Fig. 15 Detected at 2 ft to the left

stabilize the target lock stability and mobile robot navigation is recommended. For future work, the research should consider the environment lighting for the mobile robot navigation in a dark area by using contrast enhancement method or dark area elimination.

Acknowledgements This research is fully supported by UCTATI Short Term Grant, 9001-1812. The author fully acknowledged University College TATI (UCTATI) for the facilities and instrumentations that makes this important research viable and effective.

References

1. Luo B, Ding Y, Hao K, Liu J (2015) Research on mobile robot path tracking based on color vision. In: Chinese automation congress, Wuhan, China
2. Sundarajoo S, Shahrizan A, Ghani A (2018) Improvement of auto-tracking mobile robot based on HIS color model. Indonesian J Electr Eng Comput Sci 12(3):1349–1357
3. Quinonez Y, Ramirez M (2015) Autonomous robot navigation based on pattern recognition techniques and artificial neural networks. In: IWINAC, Part II, LNCS 9108, pp 320–329
4. Ahmad MF, Rong HJ (2017) Colour tracking technique by using pixy CMUcam5 for wheelchair luggage follower. In: 7th IEEE international conference on control system, computing and engineering (ICCSCE 2017), pp 187–192
5. Fang F, Qian K, Zhou B, Ma X (2017) Real-time RGB-D based people detection and tracking system for mobile robots. In: Proceedings of 2017 IEEE international conference on mechatronics and automation, 6–9 Aug, Takamatsu, Japan
6. C-L Shih, C-C Li (2018) A people-following mobile robot using kinect and a laser scanner. Robot Autom Eng J:1–8
7. Pixy CMUcam5 information page. https://my.cytron.io/p-pixy-2-cmucam5-image-sensor. Last accessed 9 Aug 2020
8. Arduino Mega 2560 information page. https://my.cytron.io/p-arduino-mega-2560-r3-main-board. Last accessed 9 Aug 2020
9. MDD10A motor driver information page. https://my.cytron.io/p-10amp-5v-30v-dc-motor-driver-2-channels. Last accessed 9 Aug 2020

Implementation of EC and PH Value Monitoring for NFT-Based Hydroponic System Applying Internet of Things (IoT)

Lia Safiyah, Raja Siti Nur Adiimah, Farah Hanan, Suzanna, and Khairul Irwan

Abstract Nutrient Film Technique (NFT) is introduced as an uplifted technique in conventional hydroponics system. This soil free farming method offers an option to solve the global soil salinity issue. This technique is using fertilized water known as nutrient solution which flows through the plant roots. The nutrient concentration is indicated by the value of electrical conductivity (EC) and pH. An optimum value of EC is very important in producing healthy growing plants. Using conventional method, the reading of these two parameters manually. Thus, this will yield to ineffective data records and consume more time since the person need to attend at the plant area to take the readings. Therefore, through this research, an EC and pH sensor are incorporated in the NFT system to detect the parameter values. These values can be monitored and recorded in continuous real-time (online) using internet of things (IoT) through an android application-Blynk app. With less than 10% of data irregularities recorded, the research resulted that this system is reliable in monitoring real time data monitoring and recording used in NFT.

Keywords IoT monitoring · pH sensor · EC sensor · NFT · Hydroponic

1 Introduction

1.1 Background

An overwhelmed phenomenon of global scarcity of water resources, environmental pollution and salinity of soil and water beginning of twenty-first century [1]. These phenomena occurred due to many factors including increment of human population and soil salinity thus resulted in reduction of land available for cultivation, crop productivity and quality. The flooding, over-irrigation, seepage, silting and a rising water level have been reported as the main cause of soil salinization [2]. A wide

L. Safiyah (✉) · R. S. N. Adiimah · F. Hanan · Suzanna · K. Irwan
University College TATI, Kemaman, Terengganu, Malaysia
e-mail: liasafiyah@uctati.edu.my

H. Triwiyanto et al. (eds.), *Proceedings of the 1st International Conference on Electronics, Biomedical Engineering, and Health Informatics*, Lecture Notes in Electrical Engineering 746, https://doi.org/10.1007/978-981-33-6926-9_26

range of adaptations and mitigation strategies are required to cope with such impacts. Efficient resource management and crop/livestock improvement for evolving better breeds can help to overcome salinity stress. However, such strategies being long drawn and cost intensive, there is a need to develop simple and low-cost biological methods for salinity stress management, which can be used on short term basis [3]. This has led to grow plants in nutrient solution as an alternative method called Nutrient Film Technique (NFT). This technique is an uplifted technique from a conventional hydroponic system introduced early 19s.

The advantages of NFT include low running costs, adequate maintenance of oxygen level and high yields, while disadvantages include high installation costs, high disease incidence and loss of nutrient balance [4]. Commercially NFT technique has been used throughout the world for successful production of leafy as well as other vegetables with 70–90% savings of water [5].

NFT is one of the soil free method in growing plant. The plant is supplied with a flowing nutrient solution (mixture of fertilizer and water) along the pipes circulated through root of the plant. An optimum nutrient solution is very crucial to ensure development and growth rate of the plant. The two crucial parameters need to be taken care of are EC and pH values. EC of nutrient can determine the amount of salt in the nutrient and also to indicate the amount of ions to the plants [6]. The ideal EC and pH are specific for each crop and dependent on environmental conditions. Higher EC hinders nutrient uptake by increasing osmotic pressure and lower EC may severely affect plant health and yield. A study has been done proving that too high or too low EC would induce nutrient stress, enhance plant antioxidant enzyme activities, and suppress growth and quality [7]. Other findings suggest that through experimentation and proper testing of pH and EC the nutrient content can be administered adequately in order to produce maximum plant growth [8]. Series of experiments of lettuce grown in summer conditions found evidence in proper EC and pH management for optimum yield and tip burn control [9].

Thus, checking and monitoring the value of these two parameters is very important to ensure that the solution is in an optimum condition. Analyzing massive amount of data can be done by accessing and connecting various devices with the help of IOT [10]. A conventional method is done by manually check and record the values for future reference. Apparently, this method is ineffective and provide a non-stable performance of taking and recording the data and inefficient data record management. Thus, this paper is focusing on monitoring the EC and pH value in real time using IOT.

An Android application, (BLYNK) is used as the interface. Blynk helps businesses get connected to the Internet of Things taking care of mobile app building, cloud services and embedded solutions [11]. A research results indicated that the developed method (smart capsules) and Blynk application can effectively work together and are deemed suitable for use in smart farming [12]. Also, BLYNK apps give advantage for the user to monitor and control the system with less effort and requires no presence at the farmed area [13].

2 Materials and Method

2.1 EC and PH Sensor

In this paper, an EC and pH sensors are quite similar to each other in terms of its practical features. Both sensors are partially immersed in the solution tank (see Fig. 1) for taking the readings of the nutrient solution. With a built-in meter board designed for both EC and pH sensors, (see Figs. 2 and 3) these sensors are simple and convenient to the system. In terms of liquid, the reciprocal of resistance is used for measuring EC, which is conductance, as a measurement. The conductivity of water can reflect the level of electrolytes present in the water. Depending on the concentration of the electrolyte, the conductivity of the aqueous solution is different. The higher the electrical conductivity detected means the higher the concentration of nutrient solution. Thus, water has to be added as counteract to lower the concentration of nutrient solutions. The reading is sent to the controller to execute the program and display the value through the apps.

The total pH scale ranges from 1 to 14, with 7 considered to be neutral. A pH less than 7 is said to be acidic and solutions with a pH greater than 7 are basic or alkaline. It can accurately be quantified by a sensor that measures the potential difference between two electrodes: a reference electrode (silver/silver chloride) and a glass electrode that is sensitive to hydrogen ion. The sensors are not a stand alone

Fig. 1 Solution tank where the sensors are located

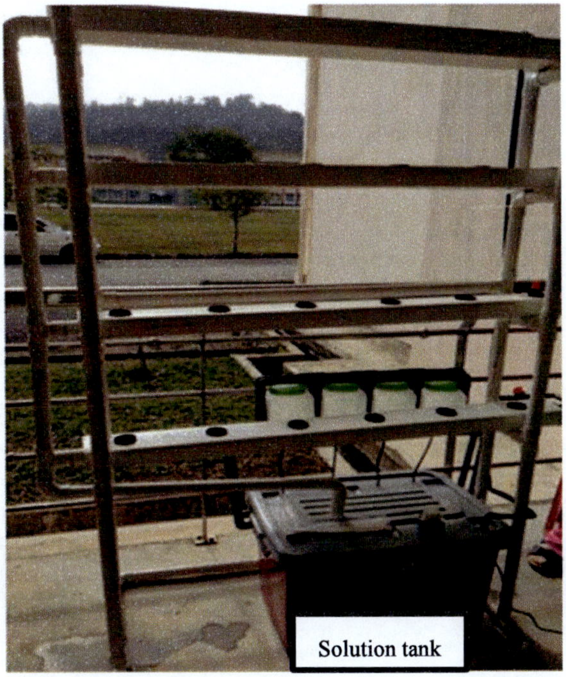

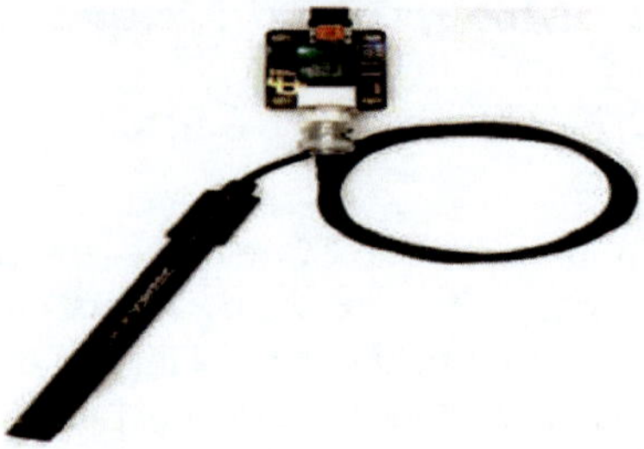

Fig. 2 Analog EC sensor

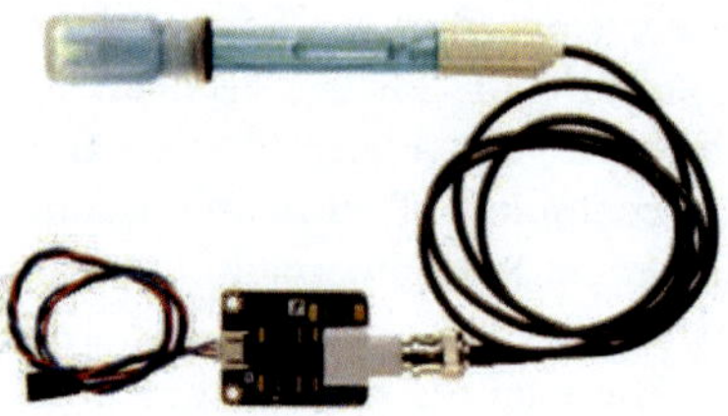

Fig. 3 Analog pH sensor

type an electronic circuit is developed to condition the signal appropriately. A well-conditioned and amplified signal is sent to a micro-controller, ESP32 to execute further output actuation.

2.2 *Espressif ESP32*

This board has dual processed microprocessor, Tensilica Xtensa 32-bit as the main processor and an ultralow-power co-processor. Practically, the features of two processors are so helpful because when one processor is used to handle "communication", the other one is in charge of I/O control. For example, this feature will prevent some issues that happen with others such as ESP8266, where the sole CPU needs to stop controlling input and output when handling signal communication. It is vital in this project to keeps projecting continuous real-time measurement of the nutrient solution and at the same time, conducting automatic control of the nutrient's concentration and pH value.

ESP323 is used to provide continuous real-time measurement of the nutrient solution. The signal from the sensors are processed in a built program in this microcontroller. The values are displayed in the apps for monitoring purposes. The function of recording and recollecting the data also incorporated in this project to ensure better data managements and recordings. This is very important as the reference for any future improvements. Table 1 shows the input pins connections to ESP32 used in this project.

Table 1 Input pins for sensors

Input	Pin address
EC sensor	GPIO34
pH sensor	GPIO35

2.3 *Arduino IDE*

Arduino is an open source electronics platform based on easy-to-use hardware and software. Arduino boards are able to read input—finger on a button, button on the virtual site and turn it into an output—light on or off, switch on or off the circuit and many others output type based on desired project. Board on Arduino performs an output of the circuit based on the instruction that can be program that can be set on microcontroller. To make instruction, it can be perform using Arduino Programming Language (based on Wiring) and the Arduino Software (IDE) based on processing.

ESP32 microcontroller used in this project is programmed using this platform. The program is written using C language and encoded with several function, to control the actuation of both automation and monitoring system. Furthermore, this software is needed to be installed with special ESP library to support the connection of ESP32 board.

2.4 *Blynk Apps*

Blynk is an Internet of Things Platform aimed to simplify building mobile and web applications for the Internet of Things. It is a Platform with iOS and Android apps to control Arduino, Raspberry Pi and the likes over the Internet. For this project, it is used to control the ESP32 and projecting all required data from sensors to the internet by using Wi-Fi communication. It's a digital dashboard where the graphical interface for this project was created by simply dragging and dropping widgets.

3 Results and Discussions

3.1 *Data Recording*

All data acquired were graphically transformed into line charts where the data could be easily read and understood with a volume or organized and interpreted numbers. The purpose of this part is to provide an effective and convincing presentation of result where the results are analyzed by its line chart in terms of its pattern and consistency. The results for this experimental research were arranged in topics of the sensor itself. Each sensors measurement was compared between the two data acquisition design of weekly average data and an hour data of every minute

3.2 Findings

The tabulation of data (Fig. 4) in line chart presenting the average value of EC measurements for a day, during a whole week data acquisition. The graphical presentation shows a variety of data tabulation ranging from 1.05 to 1.25 of electrical conductivity. The highest average of EC recorded in a day was 1.22 (mS/cm) at 12.00 a.m. In contrary, the lowest value of EC was 1.06 (mS/cm) at both 1.00 p.m. and 2.00 p.m. In selection of changes in EC, the graph shows that the EC value measurement was in decrement from night until 2 p.m. in the evening. Then, the EC value starts to increase in average until in the middle of the night.

Both graphical data above are presented to make comparison of 2 different hours taken from 2 random days in a week, (see Fig. 4), EC value for day 2 in overall was higher than day 1 data (Fig. 5). The highest EC recorded in day 1 was at 1.22 (mS/cm) and lowest at 0.98 (mS/cm) consecutively at 12.30 p.m. and 13.06 p.m. For day 2 collected data, the highest EC was 1.26 (mS/cm) at 13.25 p.m. In contrary, the lowest was 1.12 (mS/cm) at 12.32 p.m. and 12.52 p.m. Similar pattern was shown (see Fig. 5.) where the overall EC value of day 2 is higher than day 1. Significantly Fig. 6 shows that the highest EC of day 1 was 1.72 (mS/cm) at 10.46 p.m. and with big gaps, the lowest EC was 1.02 (mS/cm) at 3 different times; 10.15 p.m., 10.36 p.m., and 10.56 p.m. Meanwhile, the EC values taken in day 2 from 10 to 11 p.m. show a very stable pattern of measurement. The highest of its EC was 1.19 (mS/cm) at 6 different times and slightly different value as the lowest was 1.14 (mS/cm) at 10.55 p.m. in the evening.

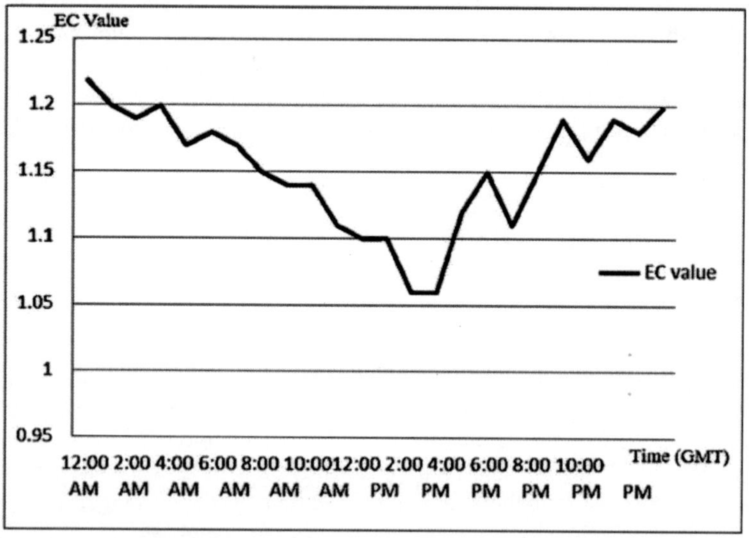

Fig. 4 Weekly average EC values

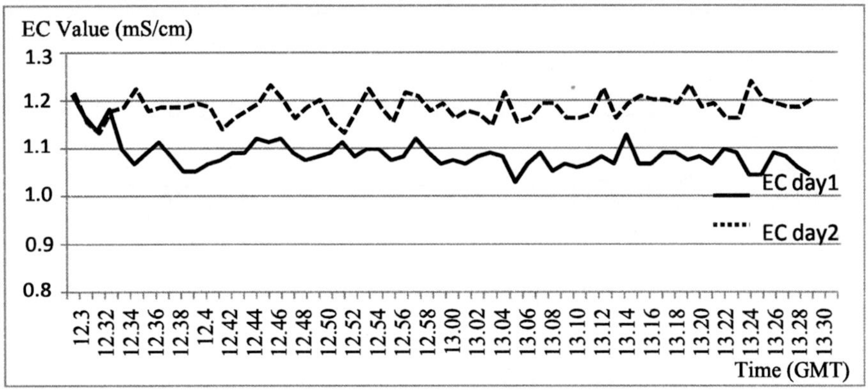

Fig. 5 EC value (12.30–13.30 p.m.)

This automatic NFT system with online monitoring system was primarily set with certain value of EC and pH. A pre-defined value is set to 6, in range of 5.5–6.5. Weekly average value of pH (see Fig. 8) is in range of from 6 to 7. The graph also illustrates that the pH value was gradually decrease from 12 a.m. to 12 p.m. and oppositely starts to gradually increase from 12.00 p.m. to 11 p.m. (Fig. 7). In selection of the significant values, the figure shows that the highest value was 6.94 in pH at 12 a.m. in the morning and the lowest data recorded was 6.29 in pH at 12.00 p.m. in the afternoon.

By comparing both data (see Figs. 8 and 9), a quite similar pattern is produced, with only slight differences in the initial data acquisition. Highest value of pH is at 7.94 for day 1 and 7.36 for day 2 at 13.01 p.m. and 13.19 p.m., consecutively (see Fig. 8). Significantly, the figure also compares the lowest pH measurement for

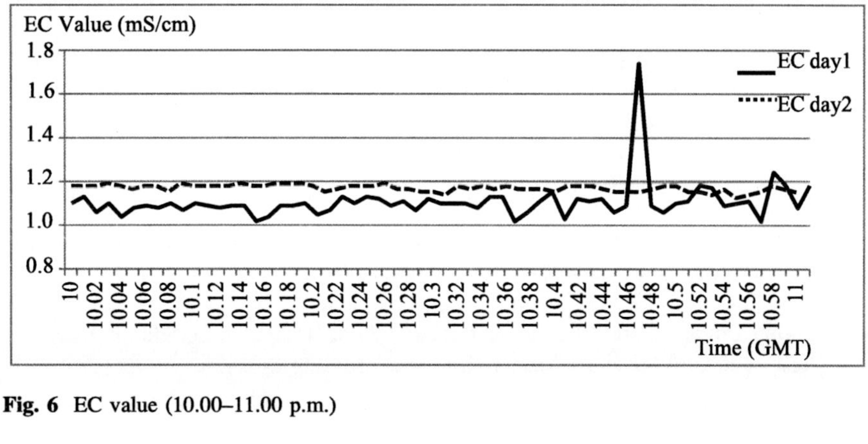

Fig. 6 EC value (10.00–11.00 p.m.)

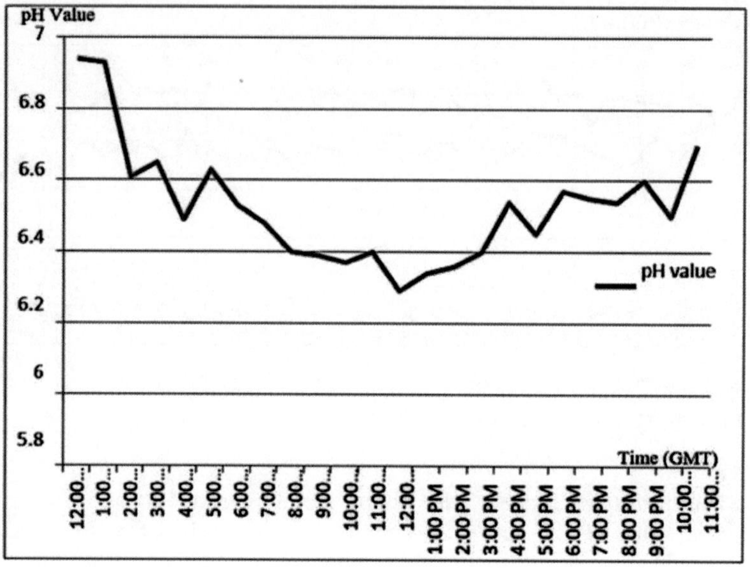

Fig. 7 Average pH value

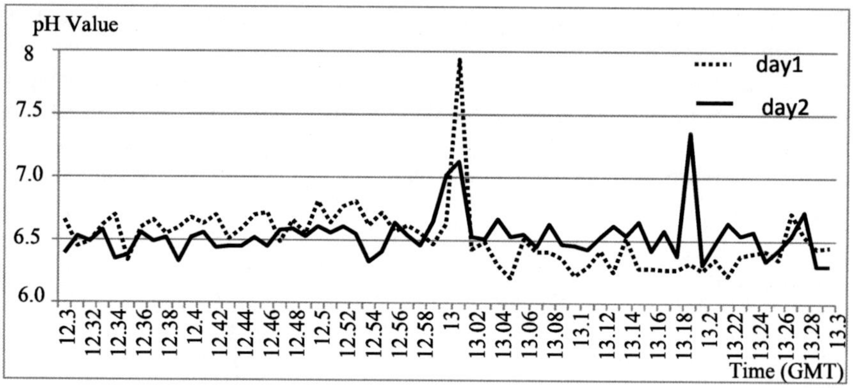

Fig. 8 pH value (12.30–1.30 p.m.)

both days at 6.20 for day 1 and 6.30 for day 2. The lowest measurement for day 1 was taken at 13.05 p.m. and same lowest measurement taken at 13.29 p.m. and 13.30 p.m. for day 2. The highest pH is measured at day 1 with 7.06 pH value. Data acquisition from day 2 start with lowest pH at 5.97 at 10.02 p.m., gradually increase to highest peak of 6.99 at 10.24 p.m. before decreasing again.

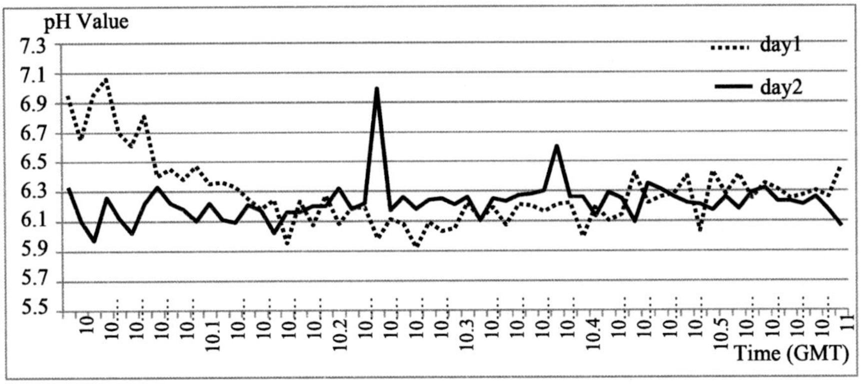

Fig. 9 pH value (10.00–11.00 p.m.)

3.3 *Stability of Data Acquisition*

All the measured data from the sensors are transferred to the BLYNK cloud server. In case of any delay, data transferred through Wi-Fi communication and data acquired by users from smartphone interface might be ended with some irregularities within the range of data acquired. Across all 240 data acquired from all sensors during 2 different hours in two different days are recorded. Irregularities are defined in this analysis as deviation of data from normal or expected value, ranging from either clearly out of range data or drastically changes in data from high to low or in opposite.

Based on results on previous section, in terms of consistency, all graphs show great display of data acquisition where users could always monitor the parameters of nutrient solution in every minute. In case irregularities, the total accumulation of irregularities of data sent by the sensors is shown in the following Table 2.

In this paper, data analysis is done to determine the percentage of any irregularities happened while recording the data. A quite similar system developed by [14] and [15] but no percentage of irregularities is tabulated. The purpose of this improvement is to indicate system reliability and stability.

Table 2 Data accumulation and irregularities

Parameter	Total data	Total irregularities	Percentage of irregularities (%)
EC	120	4	3.33
pH	120	11	9.17

4 Conclusion

The limitation of this paper is only two parameters are measured without considering any effects on temperature and other factors affecting the system. From this paper, it is clearly stated that one of the methods that can be used in NFT monitoring is by using Blynk Apps with ESP32 as programming platform. This also supported by percentage of irregularities occurred is only 3.33% for EC data and 9.17% for pH data. Both contribute to less than 10% of irregularities of the total data collected. Thus, this paper has proved that this IOT monitoring system is reliable in real time data monitoring and recording used specifically for NFT EC and pH value monitoring.

Future works should be carried out with integration of more parameters or sensors such as temperature sensor and flow sensor to ensure a better monitoring purposely for optimum plant growth.

References

1. Shahbaz M, Ashraf M (2013) Improving salinity tolerance in cereals. Crit Rev Plant Sci. https://doi.org/10.1080/07352689.2013.758544
2. Zaman M, Shahid SA, Heng L, Shahid SA, Zaman M, Heng L (2018) Soil salinity: historical perspectives and a world overview of the problem. In: Guideline for salinity assessment, mitigation and adaptation using nuclear and related techniques
3. Shrivastava P, Kumar R (2015) Soil salinity: a serious environmental issue and plant growth promoting bacteria as one of the tools for its alleviation. Saudi J Biol Sci. https://doi.org/10.1016/j.sjbs.2014.12.001
4. Resh H (2012) Nutrient film technique. In: Hydroponic food production
5. Sharma N, Acharya S, Kumar K, Singh N, Chaurasia OP (2018) Hydroponics as an advanced technique for vegetable production: an overview. J Soil Water Conserv. https://doi.org/10.5958/2455-7145.2018.00056.5
6. Ibrahim MNR, Solahudin M, Widodo S (2015) Control system for nutrient solution of nutrient film technique using fuzzy logic. Telkomnika (Telecommunication Comput Electron Control). https://doi.org/10.12928/telkomnika.v13i4.2113
7. Ding X et al (2018) Electrical conductivity of nutrient solution influenced photosynthesis, quality, and antioxidant enzyme activity of pakchoi (*Brassica campestris* L. Ssp. Chinensis) in a hydroponic system. PLoS One. https://doi.org/10.1371/journal.pone.0202090
8. Mohammed SB, Sookoo R (2016) Nutrient film technique for commercial production. Agric Sci Res J
9. Samarakoon U, Palmer J, Ling P, Altland J (2020) Effects of electrical conductivity, pH, and foliar application of calcium chloride on yield and tipburn of *Lactuca sativa* grown using the nutrient–film technique. HortScience. https://doi.org/10.21273/hortsci15070-20
10. Alipio MI, Dela Cruz AEM, Doria JDA, Fruto RMS (2019) On the design of Nutrient Film Technique hydroponics farm for smart agriculture. Eng Agric Environ Food. https://doi.org/10.1016/j.eaef.2019.02.008
11. Blynk (2015) Blynk: Startups—IEEE Internet of Things: 1–17. Startups—IEEE Internet of Things. Web
12. Serikul P, Nakpong N, Nakjuatong N (2019) International conference on ICT and knowledge engineering (IEEE computer society), vols 2018-November, pp 70–75

13. Aris RSNAR, Bin Mohammad KI, Safiyahbintisyafie L, Bintiazimi FH, Aw SB (2020) Front-end development of nutrient film technique for hydroponic plant with IoT monitoring system. Int J Adv Trends Comput Sci Eng. https://doi.org/10.30534/ijatcse/2020/0291.32020
14. Helmy, Mahaidayu MG, Nursyahid A, Setyawan TA, Hasan A (2017) Nutrient film technique (NFT) hydroponic monitoring system based on wireless sensor network. In: 2017 IEEE international conference on communication, networks and satellite, COMNETSAT 2017—Proceedings 2018-January, Institute of Electrical and Electronics Engineers Inc., pp 81–84
15. Filho AFM, de Azevedo CAV, de Azevedo MRQA, Fernandes JD, da Silva CR, Fernandes PD (2018) Monitoring, calibration and maintenance of optimized nutrient solutions in curly lettuce (*Lactuca sativa* L.) hydroponic cultivation. Aust J Crop Sci. https://doi.org/10.21475/ajcs.18.12.04.pne858

State-of-the-Art Method to Detect R-Peak on Electrocardiogram Signal: A Review

Anita Miftahul Maghfiroh, Syevana Dita Musvika, Levana Forra Wakidi, Lamidi Lamidi, Sumber Sumber, Muhmmad Ridha Mak'ruf, Andjar Pudji, and Dyah Titisari

Abstract The detection of the R peak on the ECG signal is very important to use to see the amount of variability in the heart rate. So that a person's vital signs can be known if there are heart defects including arrhythmias. Besides, several recent studies suggest that the detection of the R peak in the ECG signal can also be used to detect respiratory rate signals. Therefore, an appropriate algorithm is needed to detect the R peak in the ECG signal so that there is no mistake in diagnosing a person's physiological state. Several researchers have developed methods for detecting the R peak in the ECG signal with advantages and disadvantages. Therefore, this paper aims to provide a specific description of the R peak detection method to facilitate other authors in developing R peak detection methods in ECG signals. References in this paper are gathered from several journals and procurements regarding the definition of peak R. The results showed that some researchers used an adaptive threshold system with an accuracy rate of 99.41%, while some other researchers used the 99.5% decomposition method, some researchers used the convoluted neural network (CNN) method with an accuracy level of 99.7%. The benefit for the next researcher is to develop a real-time R peak detection tool to use to see the amount of variability in the heart rate by using one of these methods.

Keywords R-peak detection · Review

1 Introduction

The detection of the R peak on the ECG signal is very important to use to see the amount of variability in the heart rate. So that a person's vital signs can be known if there are heart defects including arrhythmias. Besides, several recent studies

A. M. Maghfiroh (✉) · S. D. Musvika · L. F. Wakidi · L. Lamidi · S. Sumber ·
M. R. Mak'ruf · A. Pudji · D. Titisari
Department of Electromedical Engineering, Politeknik Kesehatan Kementerian Kesehatan Surabaya, Jl. Pucang Jajar Timur no. 10, Surabaya 60283, Indonesia
e-mail: anitamiftah@poltekkesdepkes-sby.ac.id

H. Triwiyanto et al. (eds.), *Proceedings of the 1st International Conference on Electronics, Biomedical Engineering, and Health Informatics*, Lecture Notes in Electrical Engineering 746, https://doi.org/10.1007/978-981-33-6926-9_27

suggest that the detection of the R peak in the ECG signal can also be used for the detection of an aspiration rate signal [1, 2]. Therefore, the detection of the R peak in the ECG signal is necessary. The R peak detection algorithm has been developed by many researchers with its advantages and disadvantages, but the main problem in R peak detection is noise interference. The basic principle is that all methods used for R peak detection involve transforming the ECG signal carried out by different transformation techniques including Fourier transform, Hilbert transforms, wavelet, etc. [3]. Sadhukhan and Mitra [4] used double difference and RR interval processing for detection of R peaks by sorting and thresholding squared double-difference signals from ECG data to find estimates of R peak detection, This algorithm has low computation but is not sensitive to low frequencies such as noise and baseline wander. The complete ensemble empirical mode decomposition with the adaptive noise (CEEMDAN) method has also been carried out by Hossain et al. [5]. Noise can be reduced well using this method, but the P signal detection still uses an approximate signal so that the P wave detection is sometimes read as the R peak wave. The decomposition method is also carried out by Mabrouki et al. [6], by combining empirical mode decomposition (EMD) and Hilbert transform. Several researchers have successfully used the wavelet method for the detection of the R peak [7–9]. Goodfellow et al. [8], who stated that discrete wavelet transform (DWT) is considered capable and effective to be used for detection of the peak Aqil et al. [9], used continuous wavelet transform (CWT) to analyze the R peak using a selective scale. There is also Thiamchoo and Phukpattaranont [10], who uses the wavelet method for detection of R peaks by utilizing CWT to eliminate sound interference and the energy of Shanon is used to determine the peak of the R wave. The convolution neural network (CNN) method is also used for the detection of R peaks consisting of level and sub-level objects to extract QRS waves automatically [11–13]. The detection of the R peak using the second derivative algorithm was done by Arteaga-Falconi et al. [14] by using a threshold based on the sampling frequency. R wave grouping is done for the detection of R peaks based on the Hierarchical Clustering method [15]. The adaptive threshold is also reported to be able to detect R peaks well and is easy to apply to portable systems [16, 17].

From these studies, it is shown that there have been many studies explaining the R peak detection algorithm in ECG signals which has excess and flaws. So that a special review is needed to be related to the R peak detection method to facilitate other authors in developing the R peak detection method in the ECG signal. A summary of the latest methods in the development of R peak detection on ECG is described in Table 1.

Table 1 State of the art method to detect R-peak

Author	Method	Result
Sadhukhan and Mitra [4]	The detection of the R peak in the ECG signal uses a simple algorithm based on double derivatives with 3 steps, namely: 1. A double squared difference. 2. By comparison. 3. Interval of RR	The results of this algorithm produce a detection sensitivity value of 99.8%
Hossain et al. [5]	Complete ensemble empirical mode decomposition with adaptive noise (CEEMDAN). The method used is the detection of the P signal wave on the ECG signal. This method identifies the P wave automatically without getting any prior information	The results of this method produce a sensitivity value of 99.96%, a positive predictive value of 99.9%, and an error of 0.13%
Arteaga-Falconi et al. [14]	The detection of the R peak using the second derivative algorithm was carried out by Arteaga-Falconi et al. by using a threshold based on the sampling frequency	The test results obtained positive sensitivity and predictive value, with a sensitivity value of 99.43% and a positive predictive value of 99.22%
Chen et al. [15]	R wave grouping is done for detection of R peaks based on the Hierarchical Clustering method	The results of the algorithm evaluation reached an average detection accuracy of 99.83%, sensitivity 99.89%, and positive prediction of 99.94% from the validation database
Goodfellow et al. [8]	In this paper, the DWT method was chosen for the detection of the R peak using the mother wavelet doubecies	The results of this method are a sensitivity of 99.61%, a positive prediction of 99.88%, and an accuracy of 99.50%
Aqil et al. [9]	The continuous wavelet transform (CWT) method is used to analyze the R peak using a selective scale	From the test results yielded an average of 99.16% and in terms of recognition, an average of 1.09 s was obtained
Ramazan Özgür Do˘gan et al. [11]	In this paper, the method used is Convolutional Network Network (CNN)	The results of the study obtained automatic detection with an accuracy value of 99.6%
Lu et al. [16]	R peak detection using an adaptive threshold	The results obtained were a detection rate of 99.41%, sensitivity (Se) 99.72%, and specificity (Sp) of 99.69% in the MIT-BIH arrhythmia database
Mabrouki et al. [6]	The detection of the R peak of the ECG signal is carried out by a combination of the empirical Mode Decomposition (EMD) approach and the Hilbert transformation	The resulting performance result is a sensitivity value of 94.71%, compared to the sensitivity of other techniques, namely 91.71%

(continued)

Table 1 (continued)

Author	Method	Result
Thiamchoo and Phukpattaranont [10]	Wavelet method for detection of R peaks by utilizing CWT to eliminate sound interference and Shanon energy is used to determine the peak of the R wave	The results with this method have resulted in a better detection error rate (EDR), namely 0.79–0.85%
Xiang et al. [12]	Segmentation of the ECG signal to look for QRS waves then perform feature extraction using CNN	The proposed technique reaches Sen = 99.86%, PPR = 99.89%, DER = 0.25%, and Acc = 99.75%

2 State-of-the-Art

2.1 Pre-processing Signal

In this section, we will discuss the ECG signal pre-processing before the detection of the R peak is carried out because in general, the ECG signal frequency is in the 0.05–100 Hz range, to get the frequency in this range, a filtering process is required both analog and digitally. Meanwhile, to eliminate interference from the 50 Hz frequency originating from PLN, a notch filter is needed to ward it off. The ECG signal output still has some interference from both noise and power lines, so some researchers pre-process the signal to eliminate the interference before the detection of the R peak. The Pan-TOMKIN band-pass filter method is used by Mohanty et al. [3], for pre-processing ECG signal with a bandwidth frequency between 5 and15 Hz. Deboleena Sadhukhan and Mitra [4], perform smoothing and filtering to remove power frequencies and high frequencies such as noise. Whereas Swathi et al. [7], ECG signal pre-processing is done using wavelets, it is explained that wavelets are capable of deconstructing complex signals into signals that have limited bandwidth and then reconstructing them again with little information loss. A band-pass filter consisting of a low pass filter and a high pass filter has been designed by Lu et al. [16], with a predetermined frequency ranging from 5 to 12 Hz to reduce noise. To maintain all major frequencies of the ECG signal components Tsai et al. [17], use a band-pass filter with a frequency bandwidth between 0.5 and100 Hz. As an illustration, Fig. 1 shows the ECG signal before signal pre-processing. The signal still has noise interference, so filtering is necessary to eliminate the interference. While the ECG signal output after signal pre-processing is shown in Fig. 2.

2.2 R-Peak Detection

In this section the author will discuss several methods in more detail, the methods discussed are the discrete wavelet transform (DWT) decomposition [7, 8],

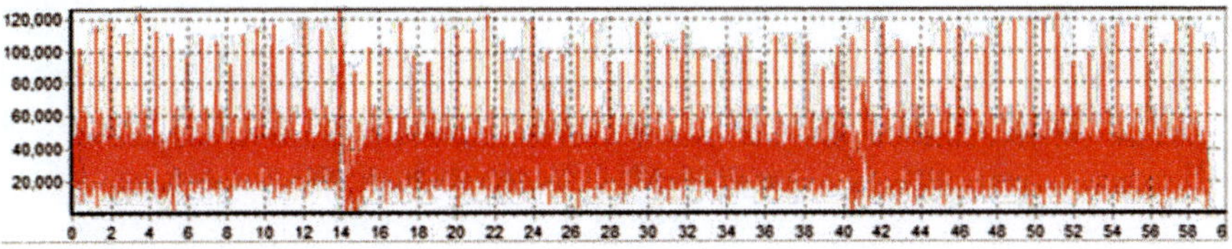

Fig. 1 ECG signal before signal pre-processing

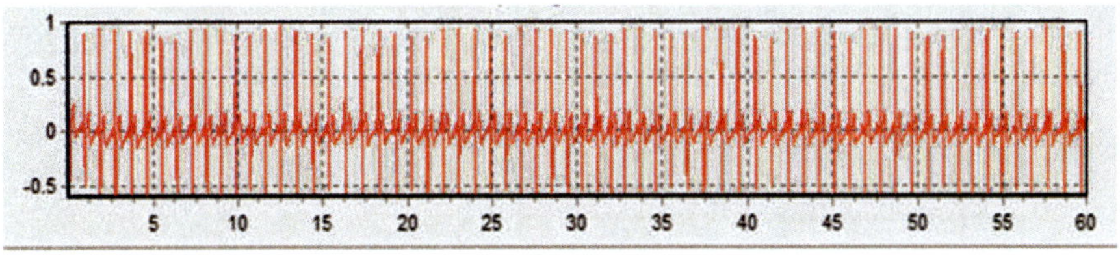

Fig. 2 ECG signal output after signal pre-processing

R definition based on adaptive threshold [16], and searching for QRS waves using CNN [12].

DWT Based R-peak Detection

DWT is a decomposition process consisting of a low pass filter and a high pass filter. DWT analyzes signals at different frequency bands and the signals are decomposed using different resolutions into approximate coefficient (y_{low}) and detailed information (y_{high}), as described in Eq. 1.

$$\begin{aligned} yhigh[k] &= \sum_n x[n].g[2k-n] \\ ylow[k] &= \sum_n x[n].h[2k-n] \end{aligned} \tag{1}$$

The complex signal is deconstructed into the basic signal of the limited bandwidth and then reconstructed at a piece of slight loss information. To obtain the R-peak, the first step is to pre-process the ECG signal based on DWT denoising. In several studies, the Daubechies mother wavelet was used for the decomposition process [7, 8]. The decomposition process is carried out up to the 5th level, then the decomposed signal is subjected to soft thresholding to obtain the R-peak. The threshold used for R peak detection is 50% of the maximum value of the ECG signal. To determine the effectiveness of R detection from the DWT method it is carried out based on Eqs. 2–4.

$$Se = \frac{TP}{TP + FN} \times 100 \quad (2)$$

$$Sp = \frac{TP}{TP + FP} \times 100 \quad (3)$$

$$Acc = \frac{TP}{TP + FN + FP} \times 100 \quad (4)$$

where Se is Sensitivity, Pp is Positive Predictivity and Acc is Accuracy. In general, the diagram block of the DWT method is described in Fig. 3.

The results of this method are a sensitivity of 99.61%, a positive prediction of 99.88%, and an accuracy of 99.50%.

Adaptive Threshold Based R-peak Detection

In this method, ECG signal pre-processing is carried out using the pan-TOMKIN method. To reduce signal noise, it passes through the low pass and high pass filters with a bandwidth of 5–12 Hz [16]. The detection of the R peak then determines the maximum value as a QRS wave candidate. In detecting the R peak, the signal is compared with a value that moves following the R signal peak, if the maximum value drops to more than half the value, it will also be detected as a peak and will follow the peak value until it finds a new peak (either up or down). Threshold detection is done by initializing the threshold by taking the first point sample at the maximum value found. There are identified signal peaks and noise peaks. The peak detection for R is based on Eq. 5 [16].

$$\begin{aligned} \text{M\_VAL} &= \max(\text{INPUT}(1:300)), \\ \text{SPK} &= 0.13 * \text{M\_VAL}, \\ \text{NPK} &= 0.1 * \text{SPK}, \\ \text{Threshold} &= 0.25 * \text{SPK} * 0.75 * \text{NPK}, \end{aligned} \quad (5)$$

where input is the result of the preprocessing signal while M_VAL is the value maximum of the first 300 sampling points, the SPK is an estimate of peak signal, NPK is peak noise, and THRESHOLD is the threshold applied. As an illustration of the R peak detection process with the adaptive threshold method, it is described in the block diagram in Fig. 4.

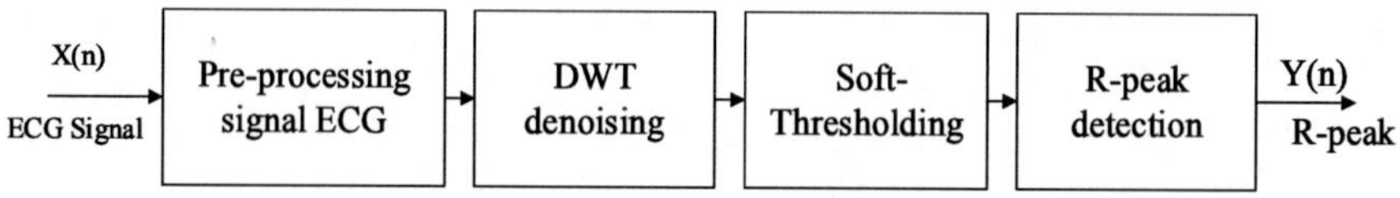

Fig. 3 Diagram block of R-peak detection using the DWT method

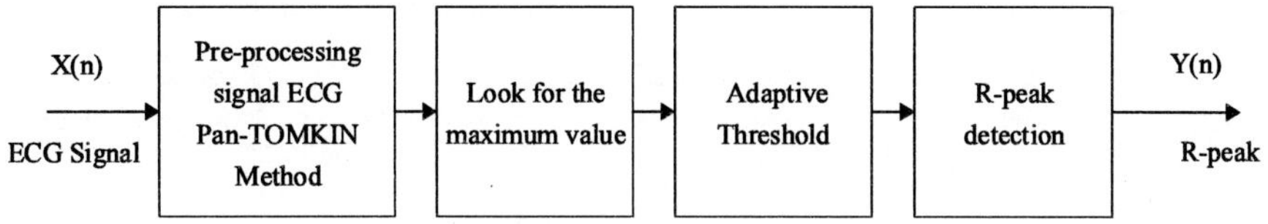

Fig. 4 Diagram block of R-peak detection using the adaptive threshold method

The results obtained were a detection rate of 99.41%, sensitivity (Se) 99.72%, and specificity (Sp) of 99.69% in the MIT-BIH arrhythmia database.

Convolutional Neural Network Based R-peak Detection

Detection of the R peak on the CNN method, the first step taken is preprocessing the ECG signal to highlight the QRS complex wave [12]. Next is to segment the ECG signal covering the entire heart rate cycle and the QRS complex when the current detection point is the R-peak. segmented the ECG signal to look for QRS waves then performed feature extraction using a combined two-tier CNN then sent it to the MLP for the detection of the final QRS wave complex. The output value of neurons in the CNN layer is calculated by Eqs. 6 and 7 and the CNN output in the MLP layer is calculated by Eq. 8 [12].

$$a_k^l = f\left(\sum_{i=1}^{N_{l-1}} 1Dconv\left(w_{ki}^{l-1}, s_i^{l-1}\right) + b_k^l\right) \tag{6}$$

$$s_k^l = 1Dusbs\left(a_k^l\right) \tag{7}$$

$$s_k^l = f\left(\sum_{k=1}^{N_l} w_{jk}^l s_k^l + b_j^m\right) \tag{8}$$

The process of determining the QRS wave complex consists of a learning and decision-making process. The learning process is used for weight and bias optimization, while the configured decision making of the neural network with weights and bias is used for the detection of R wave crests. To evaluate CNN's performance, it is calculated using Eqs. 9–12.

$$\text{Sen }(\%) = \frac{\text{TP}}{\text{TP} + \text{FN}} \times 100 \tag{9}$$

$$\text{PPR }(\%) = \frac{\text{TP}}{\text{TP} + \text{FN}} \times 100 \tag{10}$$

$$\text{DER }(\%) = \frac{\text{FN} + \text{FP}}{\text{TP} + \text{FN}} \times 100 \tag{11}$$

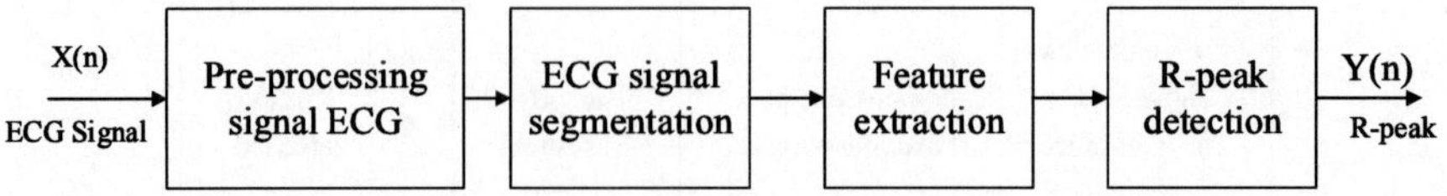

Fig. 5 Diagram block of R-peak detection using the CNN method

$$\text{Acc}\ (\%) = \frac{\text{TP}}{\text{TP} + \text{FP} + \text{FN}} \times 100 \tag{12}$$

where Sen is Sensitivity, PPR is Positive Predictivity, DER is detection error rate and Acc is Accuracy. As an illustration of the R peak detection process with the CNN method, it is described in the block diagram in Fig. 5.

The CNN method in the detection of the R peak yields an accuracy value of 99.7%.

3 Conclusion

This article aims to review the development of the R peak detection algorithm method on ECG signals from several researchers with advantages and disadvantages. As in the decomposition method, in this method, the resulting accuracy reaches 99.8% but the computation used is quite heavy, while in the adaptive threshold method the computation is lighter but is very vulnerable to noise. The CNN method was also developed by several researchers with excellent results. CNN is described as being able to reduce noise and be accurate in predicting the R peak, but the computation used is quite heavy. However, several things can be improved by further researchers, namely detection of R peaks carried out online and finding new algorithms to minimize noise interference which is the main problem in the detection of R-peaks.

References

1. Sarkar S, Bhattacherjee S, Pal S (2015) Extraction of respiration signal from ECG for respiratory rate estimation. In: Michael Faraday IET international summit, pp 336–340. https://doi.org/10.1049/cp.2015.1654
2. Maghfiroh AM, Arifin A, Sardjono TA (2019) Wavelet-based respiratory rate estimation using electrocardiogram. In: Proceedings of international seminar on intelligent technology and its applications ISITIA 2019, pp 354–359. https://doi.org/10.1109/isitia.2019.8937201

3. Mohanty MD, Mohanty B, Mohanty MN (2017) R-peak detection using efficient technique for tachycardia detection. In: Proceedings of 2nd international conference on man and machine interfacing MAMI 2017, vol 2018-March, pp 1–5. https://doi.org/10.1109/mami.2017.8307877
4. Sadhukhan D, Mitra M (2012) R-peak detection algorithm for ECG using double difference and RR interval processing. Procedia Technol 4:873–877. https://doi.org/10.1016/j.protcy.2012.05.143
5. Hossain MB, Bashar SK, Walkey AJ, McManus DD, Chon KH (2019) An accurate QRS complex and p wave detection in ECG signals using complete ensemble empirical mode decomposition with adaptive noise approach. IEEE Acc 7:128869–128880. https://doi.org/10.1109/access.2019.2939943
6. Mabrouki R, Khaddoumi B, Sayadi M (2014) R peak detection in electrocardiogram signal based on a combination between empirical mode decomposition and Hilbert transform. In: 1st International conference on advanced technologies for signal and image processing ATSIP 2014, pp 183–187. https://doi.org/10.1109/atsip.2014.6834603
7. Swathi ON, Ganesan M, Lavanya R (2017) R peak detection and feature extraction for the Diagnosis of heart diseases. In: International conference on advances in computing, communications and informatics ICACCI 2017, vol 2017-Janua, pp 2388–2391. https://doi.org/10.1109/icacci.2017.8126204
8. Goodfellow J, Escalona OJ, Kodoth V, Manoharan G, Bosnjak A (2010) Denoising and automated R-peak detection in the ECG using discrete wavelet transform. In: 2016 computing in cardiology conference, vol 43, pp 1045–1048. https://doi.org/10.22489/cinc.2016.301-506
9. Aqil M, Jbari A, Bourouhou A (2016) Adaptive ECG wavelet analysis for R-peaks detection. In: Proceedings of 2016 international conference on electrical and information technologies ICEIT 2016, pp 164–167. https://doi.org/10.1109/eitech.2016.7519582
10. Thiamchoo N, Phukpattaranont P (2016) Application of wavelet transform and Shannon energy on R peak detection algorithm. In: 13th International conference onelectrical engineering/electronics, computer, telecommunications and information technology ECTI-CON 2016. https://doi.org/10.1109/ecticon.2016.7561280
11. Bölümü BT Evri ¸ simsel Sinir A glan ile Elektrokardiogram Sinyalinde R-tepelerinin Tespiti R-peaks Detection with Convolutional Neural Network in Electrocardiogram Signal, no 2, pp 1–4
12. Xiang Y, Lin Z, Meng J (2018) Automatic QRS complex detection using two-level convolutional neural network. Biomed Eng Online 17(1):1–17. https://doi.org/10.1186/s12938-018-0441-4
13. Cai W, Hu D (2020) QRS complex detection using novel deep learning neural networks. IEEE Acc 8:97082–97089. https://doi.org/10.1109/access.2020.2997473
14. Arteaga-Falconi J, Al Osman H, El Saddik A (2015) R-peak detection algorithm based on differentiation. In: IEEE international symposium on intelligent signal processing (WISP) proceedings. https://doi.org/10.1109/wisp.2015.7139157
15. Chen H, Maharatna K (2019) An automatic R-peak detection method based on hierarchical clustering. In: Proceedings of IEEE biomedical circuits and systems conference (BioCAS), pp 1–4. https://doi.org/10.1109/biocas.2019.8919208
16. Lu X, Pan M, Yu Y (2018) QRS detection based on improved adaptive threshold. J Healthc Eng. https://doi.org/10.1155/2018/5694595
17. Tsai YR, Chang ZY, Huang CW (2019) Time-domain multi-level R-peak detection algorithm for ECG signal processing. In: Proceedings of IEEE Eurasia conference on biomedical engineering healthcare and sustainability ECBIOS, pp 35–38. https://doi.org/10.1109/ecbios.2019.8807887

A Review on Robotic Hand Exoskeleton Devices: State-of-the-Art Method

T. Triwiyanto, Endro Yulianto, Muhammad Ridha Mak'ruf, Dyah Titisari, Triana Rahmawati, Sari Luthfiyah, Torib Hamzah, Syaifudin Syaifudin, and I. Dewa Gede Hari Wisana

Abstract An exoskeleton is a device that helps the process of medical rehabilitation for people who have disorders in using their limbs. A low cost, effective sensor, control system, and an actuator are still the central issue in developing exoskeleton devices. This study aims to review an exoskeleton device, development, and recent technologies. The contribution of this study is that the paper can be used as a guideline to design an exoskeleton device. Specifically, the focus of this review discusses hand exoskeleton design. This review discusses three things, namely control signal, control mechanism, and exoskeleton actuator. In terms of the control signal, it addresses several techniques to control the exoskeleton by utilizing EMG, EEG, voice, and FSR (forced sensor) signals. In terms of control mechanism, several studies utilize pattern recognition based on machine learning and virtual reality to assist in using the exoskeleton. In terms of the actuator, the exoskeleton that was designed still has some shortcomings, namely weight and ergonomic design. The review results show that EMG signals are more often used in controlling exoskeleton devices. In the method section, pattern recognition using machine learning is still a significant part of the development of exoskeleton. In the actuator section, DC motors and linear actuators are more widely used than other types of motors. So, overall, the exoskeleton can still be improved from various aspects to make the subject more comfortable in use.

Keywords Exoskeleton · EMG signal · FSR sensor · Control system

T. Triwiyanto (✉) · E. Yulianto · M. R. Mak'ruf · D. Titisari · T. Rahmawati · S. Luthfiyah · T. Hamzah · S. Syaifudin · I. D. G. H. Wisana
Department of Electromedical Engineering, Politeknik Kesehatan Kemenkes Surabaya, Jl. Pucang Jajar Timur no. 10, Surabaya 60283, Indonesia
e-mail: Triwiyanto123@gmail.com

H. Triwiyanto et al. (eds.), *Proceedings of the 1st International Conference on Electronics, Biomedical Engineering, and Health Informatics*, Lecture Notes in Electrical Engineering 746, https://doi.org/10.1007/978-981-33-6926-9_28

1 Introduction

Hands have a vital role in daily life [1]. Losing some abilities of a hand, especially moving the fingers, can hamper the activities of daily living, and also reduce the quality of our lives [2]. Previously, in order to overcome the loss of the ability of the hand, many approaches have been developed to restore its function, such as orthosis, functional electrical stimulation, and physical therapy. The positive results of physical rehabilitation are very dependent on the physical condition, duration, intensity, and orientation of the training [3]. In the world, stroke is one of the third leading causes of paralysis and the likelihood of paralysis in the extremities is very high [4]. In order to overcome this problem, there have been many studies specifically developed devices to assist physical rehabilitation [5]. Li et al. have conducted research and made an exoskeleton in which the device is controlled using an EEG signal. This signal is used to measure the level of attention or concentration of subjects [6]. However, EEG signals require specific conditions in the data acquisition process and are susceptible to noise.

On the other hand, Diez et al. have designed an exoskeleton that is controlled using a 5DT glove or a glove equipped with an optical force sensor that is useful for detecting hand movements. Moreover, the device is also equipped with virtual reality to see the feedback when the subject's hands make movements [7].

Several studies used EMG signals to control the upper limb exoskeleton [8, 9]. Lu et al. have made a hand exoskeleton that is controlled using EMG signals with a pattern recognition method [10]. Similarly, research conducted by Gearhart et al. utilized EMG signals to control the exoskeleton to increase grip strength [11]. In a study conducted by Kiguchi and Hayashi in which the exoskeleton was controlled using a 16 channel EMG signal that had processed through a neuro-fuzzy modifier to perform seven different movements [12]. In the study, they used a lot of EMG channels to control a complex motion of exoskeleton. Besides of EMG signal, Wang et al. have also conducted research and made an exoskeleton that is controlled through voice [13]. Oppus et al. conducted similar research based on voice control. This study has two control modes, namely based sound and brain signals (mindwave) [14]. Likewise, Kandalaft et al. also conducted a study using voice signals and 5DT glove on a normal hand to control the robotic arm [15].

From those studies, it can be shown that there have been many studies on exoskeleton hand robots with strengths and weaknesses. The sensory system, frame materials, actuator, low cost, wearable, and low power consumption are still the main issue reported in the development of exoskeleton. Therefore, a specific review related to the hand exoskeleton design is needed. Find out more detail the results of previous studies are essential in order to contribute the researcher in developing a hand exoskeleton. Hence, the study aims to review the hand exoskeleton, specifically related to the state-of-the-art method.

2 State-of-the-Art Method

This section will describe various methods in the development of the upper limb exoskeleton, especially on the hands. Various kinds of exoskeleton hand device development will be discussed in detail, especially for the sensor and control systems. In this review paper, the references were collected from journal and proceeding for the last ten years. Moreover, we classified the state-of-the-art method by grouping into method, sensor, muscle location, and actuator (Table 1).

Table 1 State of the art method to control the hand exoskeleton

Authors	Method	Sensor	Muscle location	Actuator
Wang et al. [13]	Voice recognition; Bluetooth	Mic sensor	N/A	Five motor DC
Badesa et al. [16]	PID controller	5DT glove; Potentiometer	N/A	Five linear actuators
Lu et al. [10]	Mean absolute value (MAV); Support vector machine (SVM)	Bipolar electrode (Delsys)	Dorsal interossei; flexor digitorum superficialis; flexor digitorum profundus; Extensor digitorum; abductor pollicis longus; Extensor digiti minimi, and extensor pollicis longus muscles	Five linear actuators
Gearhart et al. [11]	10% of the average maximum force	FSR sensor; Ag (Ag/Cl); Three electrodes	Forearm muscles; Right anterior forearm; proximal to elbow	Five DC motor
Oppus et al. [14]	NeuroSky API	MainWave EEG headset; Voice recognition module	Head band	Five servo motor
Leonardis et al. [17]	Full wave; rectification; Lowpass filtering; Multi layer neural network	Ag (Ag/Cl); Three electrodes; Pressure sensor	Flexor digitorum; Extensor digitorum; Adductor policis	Two motor
Fajardo et al. [18]	Voice controller; EMG signal processing; Feature extraction; Machine learning	Ag (Ag/Cl); Two electrodes	Extensor digitorum; Palmaris longus	One motor

(continued)

Table 1 (continued)

Authors	Method	Sensor	Muscle location	Actuator
Ho et al. [1]	20% maximum voluntary contraction (MVC)	Ag (Ag/Cl); Two electrodes	Abductor pollicis brevis; Extensor digitorum	Five linear actuators
Takahashi et al. [2]	Root mean square (RMS)	Joint angle sensor; Ag (Ag/Cl); MRI images	Right wrist extensor; Left wrist extensor; Biceps	Pneumatic

2.1 Control Signal

This section will reveal the source of the signal used to control the exoskeleton. Several studies have succeeded in developing an exoskeleton device based on EMG signal control. This signal is more preferred than others because it has a good response in motion. As an example, Tong et al. used the EMG signal to control the hand exoskeleton. In this case, the EMG signal is recorded on the hands that are experiencing paralysis. This was done by placing electrodes on the abductor pollicis brevis (ABD) and extensor digitorum (ED) muscle where the ABD muscle was used to control hand closing, and ED used to control hand open (Fig. 1). Besides managing the EMG signals, directly, by connecting the electrode through cables to amplifier terminals, others used a wireless EMG module to control the hand exoskeleton, whether close or open [1]. In this case, Lu et al. utilized EMG signals to control the exoskeleton. Correctly, a Bagnoli-8 EMG system was used to collect the EMG signals from subjects, wirelessly. Furthermore, seven electrodes were attached to the dorsal interossei muscle, flexor digitorum superficialis, flexor digitorum profundus, extensor digitorum, abductor pollicis longus, extensor digiti minimi, and extensor pollicis longusel. Also, the electrode reference was mounted on the olecranon muscle as ground or reference [10]. In a similar project, Kiguchi and Hayashi also used EMG signals to control the exoskeleton that was developed. In this case, there are sixteen EMG channels installed on the user to control the exoskeleton [12]. Besides using a single sensory system, a multi-modal sensory system was proposed by Fajardo et al. In this case, they also used EMG signals as the primary signal control. Additionally, a TFT touchscreen and voice activation are used to control the designed exoskeleton. In the study, there are two muscles, namely extensor digitorum and palmaris longus [18], which involved in the study.

In addition, there are self rehabilitation exoskeleton which has been proposed by several studies. For example, Leonardis et al. designed an exoskeleton which used an EMG signal as a control signal. In their study, the EMG signal that is located on a non-paretic (normal) hand will control the exoskeleton attached to the paretic hand (disturbed). In more detail, there are three muscles used in this study, namely extensor digitorum longus (EDL), flexor digitorum longus (FDL), and abductor

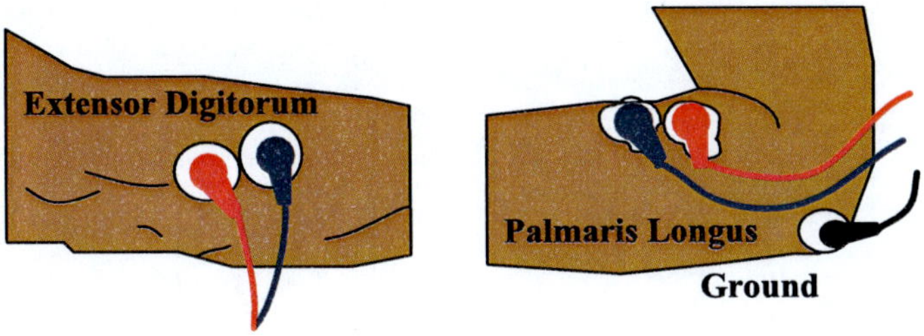

Fig. 1 Electrode placement

pollicis brevis (APB) [17]. Still in exoskeleton development, Li et al. also proposed two sessions rehabilitation mode, namely active and passive training. Where in passive training, the system uses an EEG sensor that is Neurosky to control the exoskeleton. In this selection, the user will be presented with a motion illustration as an image in MATLAB, and when the user focuses on what is displayed, it will produce a concentration that will be used to control the exoskeleton. Meanwhile, for active training, the system utilized force sensors to measure the strength of the grip. Furthermore, in operation, the forced sensor is placed at the fingertips of the exoskeleton [6]. Such that any movement of the finger will be detected and activated the exoskeleton unit.

Witkowski et al. also utilizes EEG and EOG signals to control the exoskeleton. This study uses conventional EEG (Acti-cap and Brain-Amp, Brain Products, Gilching Germany). EOG electrode placement according to the standard on the left and right outer canthus (LOC/ROC) [19]. In addition to the use of EMG signals, Diez et al. made an exoskeleton with a control process using a glove called 5DT glove, where the glove was equipped with forced sensors [7] (Fig. 2). In the same case, Gearhart et al. designed a hand exoskeleton using a forced sensor (FSR) which installed on the exoskeleton. This sensor is used to detect the pressure exerted by the hand so that it would move the motor on the hand exoskeleton [11]. In addition to the EMG signal, Wang et al. developed an exoskeleton based on voice control. This proposed method is used as an alternative in controlling the exoskeleton device. Furthermore, this research utilized the voice recognition application on smartphones [13] so that the design can be simple and low cost. In addition to the EMG signal, Oppus et al. have studied an exoskeleton that can be controlled using EEG signals by utilizing the Neurosky Mindwave module. Furthermore, the exoskeleton can also be controlled using a recorded human voice [14].

2.2 Control Mechanism

A control mechanism is an essential part of designing exoskeleton devices. Thus the device could run effectively. In a study conducted by Tong et al., the hand exoskeleton activation system was regulated by adjusting the threshold value of

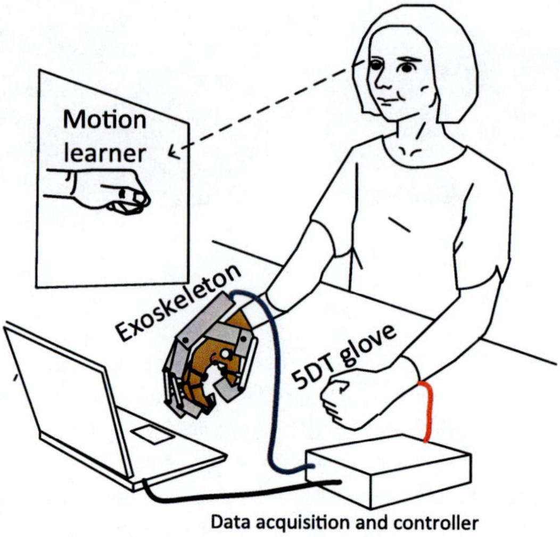

Fig. 2 Diez's exoskeleton [7]

20% of the maximum voluntary contraction (MVC) EMG signal. This threshold was detected whenever the arms were open and closed. When the system was running for hand close, then it will wait for the EMG signal from the APB to exceed 20% of its MVC value and to do hand open, it will wait until the EMG signal from the ED exceeds 20% of its MVC [1]. In the study of Zhiyuan et al. which the EMG signal was collected by using the Bagnoli-8 EMG system (Fig. 3). Furthermore, the signal will be displayed on the desktop computer with a resolution of 16 ADC bits. This EMG signal will be recognized by applying a pattern recognition based on machine learning to train the system. After the training process, the system is then tested to see that the model can recognize the motion [10].

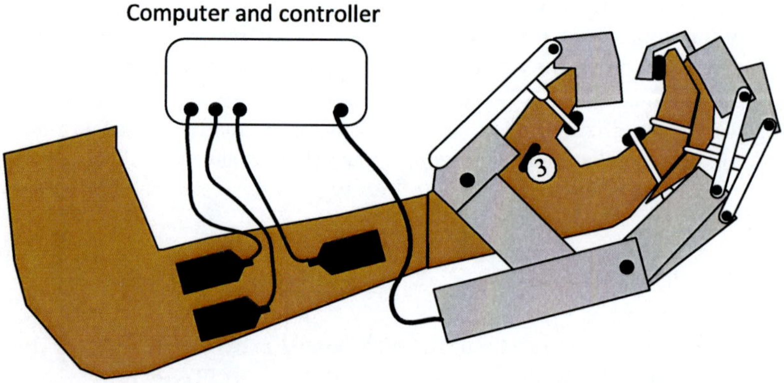

Fig. 3 Hand exoskeleton with Bagnoli EMG sensor

Kiguchi and Hayashi designed a controlled exoskeleton using 16 EMG channels and proposed Neuro-fuzzy to process and recognize the EMG signals from each channel. First of all, the EMG signal from each channel will extract the EMG feature, and then the neuro-fuzzy will train into a model. Moreover, the model will be tested on the subject directly to evaluated the model accuracy [12]. To complement this study, Fajardo et al. designed an exoskeleton device that has three control modes. These modes have a hybrid activate exoskeleton in which can use LCD TFT, human voice, or EMG signal. Based on LCD TFT, the operator directly able to move the exoskeleton unit according to a trajectory. Moreover, the user also able to activate exoskeleton based on voice control. The third mode is exoskeleton based on EMG pattern recognition. In this case, the user must first perform offline training before being able to use the exoskeleton [18]. Similarly, the research conducted by Leonardis et al., the electrodes connected to the EMG circuit will be filtered using a BPF filter of 20–500 Hz. Furthermore, subsequently, the EMG features will be used as input for artificial neural networks (ANN) to predict the movements made when an EMG signal is detected. ANN is used to map muscle activity to grip strength. For this reason, the initial dataset was obtained from 6 healthy subjects. In the experiment stage, every subject is asked to hold objects that are given a pressure sensor. For feedback from grasping pressure, a bar is provided on the LCD screen display, then subjects are told to match the pressure level provided with various references [17].

In the study of Li et al. to be able to use the tool that has been designed, the user needs to go through stages to get the threshold value of the user's concentration using Neurosky. In the proposed method, the system is divided into three stages, specifically, resting conditions, concentration with visual image guidance, and without visual guidance, and with distractions? It aims to get the threshold value from the user so that later it can be used to control the exoskeleton [6]. In Matthias Witkowski's study, in order for the user able to use the designed exoskeleton. The user must follow the stages of calibration or training data in advance to get the threshold value at rest or to think a grasping motion according to the visual cues provided. In the second part, the user must also calibrate the commands from the EOG, where the user will be given a command to move the eye left or right to get the threshold value for exoskeleton activation. [19]. In addition to the EMG signal, Diez et al. designed an exoskeleton with a 5DT glove control. In the experiment setup, a 5DT glove would be attached to a non-paretic hand, and when it detected a motion such as grasping, then the exoskeleton attached to the paretic hand would follow the position of the hand with glove sensor. In the study, a monitor unit also was provided to display a virtual reality movement that was used for training or testing [7].

In the study of Gearhart et al., the mechanism of the exoskeleton movement was controlled by a forced sensor (FSR). Any pressure change in the finger will change the FSR resistance. Further, this resistance changing could be used by Arduino into proportional commands, which simultaneously drived the three linear actuators [11].

In the research conducted by Wang et al., in order to operate the exo-tendon gloves, the user gives a voice command to the application, which interprets the input and sends a signal to the microcontroller for motor activation [13]. On the other hand, an exoskeleton designed by Oppus et al. can be controlled through activation of EEG signals. In the study, the EEG signal was recorded using a neurosky mindwave. Moreover, every signal received or captured by neurosky will map what commands are given and used to control the servo that was mounted on the hand exoskeleton. This was in order to make an exoskeleton movement according to the obtained activation command. In addition to the EEG signal, the device can also be activated using a voice signal. The voice signal is recognized using a voice recognition module so that when a voice command was given, then this module will read to find out what commands are given, and the command is used to move the hand exoskeleton [14].

2.3 Exoskeleton Actuator

The use of linear actuators has been found in several hand exoskeleton studies. One such study was conducted by Tong et al. In the study, after the device intercepts the EMG signal from the patient, it will make the hand exoskeleton move according to the input given, which is hand open or hand close, where this exoskeleton hand uses a linear mini actuator to drive the exoskeleton [1]. Likewise, Lu et al. have developed a hand exoskeleton that uses five linear mini actuators to move the device so that it can perform hand closing movements; hand opening; thumb, index, and fingers closing; thumb, index and middle fingers opening; middle, ring, and little fingers opening [10]. Some researchers have only developed an exoskeleton for finger rehabilitation needs. Gearhart et al. made a hand exoskeleton where the design was made only for three fingers, namely the index, middle finger, and ring finger only, where to move mounted three linear mini actuators on each finger [11]. In comparison, Witkowski developed for the use of the thumb and index finger [19]. Some other researchers also use linear actuators to move the hand exoskeleton [6, 7].

Some studies used open-source hand based on 3D printing as an exoskeleton unit. Fajardo designed the hand exoskeleton unit based on Galileo bionic hand. A linear actuator was used to move the fingers, which embedded in it [18]. In the study of Leonardis et al., the hand exoskeleton he designed was named BRAVO, which has 2 degrees of freedom (DOF), one for the fingers one for the thumb. In the study, the exoskeleton is equipped with two motors to push and pull the fingers. The weight of this exoskeleton is around 950 g [17]. In addition to the hardware design, some researchers developed exoskeleton devices at a simulation level, which the user cannot directly use [13, 14].

3 Potential Development

Based on the literature review, which considered three-section, namely control signal, control mechanism, and exoskeleton actuator. It showed that there are advantages and disadvantages of previous research in the design of exoskeleton. Therefore, to obtain a better design, there must be some development from previous studies. In terms of signal control, it is known that the most widely used method to control the exoskeleton is to utilize EMG signals. EMG signals are very effective to be used to control the exoskeleton, but there are still weaknesses, namely, the dependency on the subject, electrode location, and muscle fatigue [20, 21]. In addition to using the EMG signal, there are also those who use EEG signals to control the exoskeleton, but it requires the right concentration so that it can work well in the implementation. So that in terms of the control signal, the EMG signal still preferred to be used. There is also another alternative control signal to control the exoskeleton, which is by using voice as a control signal. This technique can be applied by utilizing speech recognition that has been built on smartphones. Even so, development can still be done by utilizing voice signals and combined with EMG signals so that they can control the exoskeleton better.

In the control mechanism section, some studies applied pattern recognition based on machine learning to recognize the signal control pattern. This technique is very effective for classifying more specific movements. Possible development is to improve the model of pattern recognition such that the accuracy of machine learning can be improved. In the actuator section, several studies have succeeded in developing a hand exoskeleton that used a mini linear actuator. Therefore, the subject can wear the exoskeleton directly. In order to reduce the weight of the exoskeleton, most researchers use a linear actuator because it is easy to control and lightweight. Another important factor that needs to be considered in the design of this exoskeleton is ergonomics, which must provide comfort to the subject.

In this review paper, various methods of developing exoskeleton hand devices have been disclosed. The sensor system, process control mechanism and actuator used have been revealed in sufficient detail. However, this article has not revealed details about the signal pattern recognition process using either an EMG signal or other control signals.

4 Conclusion

This article aims to review matters related to the development of exoskeleton devices in terms of control signals, control mechanisms, and actuators. Although the EMG signal requires some special treatment, the results of the review revealed that the EMG signal was widely used to control the exoskeleton of the hand compared to other control signals. Force sensors also have the potential to develop hand exoskeleton hands because they are not susceptible to noise. In the control mechanism, the use of machine learning is still recommended by several researchers. In order to get a lightweight exoskeleton, as a driving force, linear actuators are more widely used compared to DC motors. There have been many studies in the medical rehabilitation field. But there are still a number of things that can be improved, including integrating clinical parameters and cloud server-based information systems so that medical doctors in a long-distance can access the rehabilitation process.

References

1. Ho NSK, Tong KY, Hu XL, Fung KL, Wei XJ, Rong W et al (2011) An EMG-driven exoskeleton hand robotic training device on chronic stroke subjects: task training system for stroke rehabilitation. In: IEEE international conference on rehabilitation robotics, p 1–5. IEEE
2. Takahashi CD, Der-Yeghiaian L, Le V, Motiwala RR, Cramer SC (2008) Robot-based hand motor therapy after stroke. Brain 131(2):425–437
3. Feys H, De Weerdt W, Verbeke G, Steck GC, Capiau C, Kiekens C et al (2004) Early and repetitive stimulation of the arm can substantially improve the long-term outcome after stroke: a 5-year follow-up study of a randomized trial. Stroke 35(4):924–929
4. Johnson W, Onuma O, Owolabi M, Sachdev S (2019) WHO Stroke a global response is needed. In: Bulletin of the World Health Organization, p 633–708
5. Patton J, Small SL, Zev Rymer W (2008) Functional restoration for the stroke survivor: informing the efforts of engineers. Top Stroke Rehabil 15(6):521–541
6. Li M, He B, Liang Z, Zhao C, Chen J, Zhuo Y (2019) An attention-controlled hand exoskeleton for the rehabilitation of finger extension and flexion using a rigid-soft combined mechanism. Front Neurorobot 13(May):0–13
7. Diez JA, Blanco A, Catalán JM, Badesa FJ, Lledó LD, Garcia-Aracil N (2018) Hand exoskeleton for rehabilitation therapies with integrated optical force sensor. Adv Mech Eng 10(2):1–11
8. Triwiyanto T, Pawana IPA, Irianto BG, Indrato TB, Wisana IDGH (2019) Embedded system for upper-limb exoskeleton based on electromyography control. Telkomnika (Telecommunication Comput Electron Control) 17(6):2992–3002
9. Triwiyanto, Wahyunggoro O, Nugroho HA, Herianto (2016) String actuated upper limb exoskeleton based on surface electromyography control. In: Proceedings of 6th international annual engineering seminar (InaES), pp 176–181
10. Lu Z, Tong K, Shin H, Li S, Zhou P (2017) Advanced myoelectric control for robotic hand-assisted training: outcome from a stroke patient. Front Neurol 8(March):107
11. Gearhart CJ, Varone B, Stella MH, Busha BF, Member S (2016) An effective 3-fingered augmenting exoskeleton for the human hand. In: 38th Annual international conference of the IEEE engineering in medicine and biology society (EMBC), p 590–593. IEEE
12. Kiguchi K, Hayashi Y (2012) An EMG-based control for an upper-limb. IEEE Trans Syst Man, Cybern Part B 42(4):1064–1071
13. Wang X, Tran P, Callahan SM, Wolf SL, Desai JP (2019) Towards the development of a voice-controlled exoskeleton system for restoring hand function. In: 2019 International symposium on medical robotics ISMR 1, pp 1–7
14. Oppus CM, Prado JRR, Marinas AG, Reyes RSJ, Escobar JC, Mariñas JAG et al (2016) Brain-computer interface and voice-controlled 3d printed prosthetic hand. In: IEEE region 10 conference (TENCON), p 2689–2693. IEEE

15. Kandalaft N, Kalidindi PS, Narra S, Saha HN (2018) Robotic arm using voice and Gesture recognition. 2018 9th annual IEEE information technology; electronics and mobile communication conference, pp 1060–1064
16. Badesa FJ, Blanco A, Garcı N, Lledo LD, Diez JA, Blanco A et al (2018) Hand exoskeleton for rehabilitation therapies with integrated optical force sensor. Adv Mech Eng 10 (2):1687814017753881
17. Leonardis D, Barsotti M, Loconsole C, Solazzi M, Troncossi M, Mazzotti C et al (2015) An EMG-controlled robotic hand exoskeleton for bilateral rehabilitation. IEEE Trans Haptics 1412(c):1–12
18. Fajardo J, Lemus A, Rohmer E (2015) Galileo bionic hand: sEMG activated approaches for a multifunction upper-limb prosthetic. In: IEEE thirty fifth central american and panama convention (CONCAPAN XXXV), p 1–6. IEEE
19. Witkowski M, Cortese M, Cempini M, Mellinger J, Vitiello N, Soekadar SR (2014) Enhancing brain-machine interface (BMI) control of a hand exoskeleton using electrooculography (EOG). J Neuroeng Rehabil 11(1):1–6
20. Triwiyanto T, Wahyunggoro O, Nugroho HA, Herianto H (2018) Muscle fatigue compensation of the electromyography signal for elbow joint angle estimation using adaptive feature. Comput Electr Eng Oct 71(July):284–293
21. Triwiyanto T, Wahyunggoro O, Nugroho HA, Herianto H (2016) DWT analysis of sEMG for muscle fatigue assessment of dynamic motion flexion-extension of elbow joint. In: 8th International conference on information technology and electrical engineering (ICITEE) [Internet], p 1–6. IEEE Conference Publications, Yogyakarta

Experimental Validation of the Multifunctional Device for Measuring Forces and Torques on Spine Phantoms

Mikhail A. Solovyev, Andrei A. Vorotnikov, Andrey A. Grin, Daniil D. Klimov, Yuri V. Poduraev, and Vladimir V. Krylov

Abstract In modern spinal surgery, minimally invasive procedures using mechatronic and robotic systems are actively developing. Moreover, for the development of optimal designs of such systems, information is needed on the range of forces arising from the interaction of medical instruments and patient tissues at all stages of surgical intervention. The authors have developed and manufactured a prototype of a multifunctional device for measuring forces and torques during operations. The purpose of this article is to describe the laboratory validation of this prototype. Two experiments of the multifunctional device were carried out on medical phantoms in conditions close to real medical practice. In particular, an imitation of the retraction of the back muscles was carried out, and the screw was screwed into a vertebral pedicle phantom. The data obtained made it possible to confirm the correspondence of the characteristics of the sensor elements of the device to the required measurement ranges. The operability of the device was proved, and the possibility of using the device in medical practice was confirmed. The results obtained will allow the transition to clinical trials of the prototype.

Keywords Surgical instrument · Medical robotics · Multifunctional device · Force and torque measurement · Soft tissue

---

M. A. Solovyev (✉) · A. A. Vorotnikov · Y. V. Poduraev
Moscow State University of Technology "STANKIN", Moscow, Russia
e-mail: mikke2@yandex.ru

A. A. Grin · V. V. Krylov
Sklifosovsky Research Institute of Emergency Medicine, Moscow, Russia

A. A. Grin · D. D. Klimov · V. V. Krylov
A. I. Evdokimov, Moscow State University of Medicine and Dentistry, Moscow, Russia

A. A. Grin
Moscow Healthcare Department, Moscow, Russia

V. V. Krylov
Ministry of Health of the Russian Federation, Moscow, Russia

H. Triwiyanto et al. (eds.), *Proceedings of the 1st International Conference on Electronics, Biomedical Engineering, and Health Informatics*, Lecture Notes in Electrical Engineering 746, https://doi.org/10.1007/978-981-33-6926-9_29

1 Introduction

The medical equipment market is characterized by a huge variety of appliances and devices that vary based on the purpose of the function. Over the past forty years, it has seen a shift towards a significant increase in the share of robot-assisted surgery appliances [1]. Such trends are due to the transition to a qualitatively new type of surgical interference called minimally invasive surgery. This type's basis is the principle of downsizing an injury caused to a patient, thus reducing the risk of post-surgery complications and providing a qualitatively higher safety level [2–5]. Due to the high requirements imposed on the movement's accuracy, which often exceed a surgeon's capabilities, the need for robotic and mechatronic devices for performing minimally invasive surgeries arises [6]. However, today, there are a large number of medical robots for performing operations in neurosurgery [7]. However, there is still a high need for upgrading existing solutions and fundamentally developing new appliances for back neurosurgery. In this regard, developers of such kind of equipment face plenty of scientific problems. One of the problems is determining the initial design parameters, which include forces and torques that occur during the interaction of surgical tools with a patient's tissues, depending on a surgery type. The wrong comprehension of these parameters results in the development of oversized structures or systems that are unsafe for patients.

As of now, the methods already exist that make it possible to determine the initial parameters for cutting tissues. For example, Sorouri et al. [8] describes a robotic system for measuring forces when cutting soft tissues of a palate at different angles using a scalpel. The method in question involves applying specific tissue samples and is not suitable for researching conditions of real surgeries. A similar mechanical system for determining forces and torques for introducing medical instruments into a liver "in vitro" is described in [9]. Another approach to obtaining the required characteristics is to use models of the tissues that have already been explored. Mendoza and Laugier [10] presents a simulation model of soft tissue cutting that uses the finite element technique. However, to obtain such models, a specialized experimental unit is required as well. The application of simulation models is a convenient way to determine the force limits. But since different tools feature different sizes of the surface contacting the tissues, as well as different force directions, there are chances to get the values that are not always correct. Therefore, the development of robotic and mechatronic systems used for spinal neurosurgery, with some of them being presented in the report [11], requires a new solution for the preliminary force determination. Such a requirement is predicated on peculiarities of manipulations performed by a surgeon during the interference, namely, the interaction not only with soft tissues but with bone tissues as well, which requires larger forces to be applied to the tools. Additionally, a surgeon is needed to operate a large number of different surgical instruments within a single surgery. In terms of these difficulties, the authors of this article have developed a multifunctional device (MFD) for measuring forces and torques for performing neurosurgical operations [12].

2 Materials and Methods

2.1 *Construction of MDF*

Figure 1 shows the elements of MFD construction. The instruments used in real surgical practice of transpedicular fixation operation were taken as a basis. The device includes a set of interchangeable surgical instruments, (5) mated with a handle (1) through unified mechanical structural joints. These joints are adapter flanges (2, 4). These joints allow a multi-component force/torque sensor (3) to be integrated inside the device.

2.2 *Data Processing System*

A data processing system from a multi-component sensor was also implemented to measure the forces and torques using the MFD. The diagram of the resulting system is presented in Fig. 2. Its main component is an analog signal processing module, which uses a six-channel amplifier for GSV6 bridge circuits. Through the analog-to-digital conversion of signals from the MFD sensor. The control of the processing module is realized using a single-board computer raspberry pi 3. Following the control program of the data controller via the UART interface, the command module is received and transmitted to control the conversion and processing processes. Two power converters supply voltages to the processing module and the controller. The first AC–DC converter is used to convert the AC input from an external source to DC with an output voltage of 24 V. The assumed voltage is transmitted to the second linear, low-noise S-USV converter, which is the power source for all the system elements.

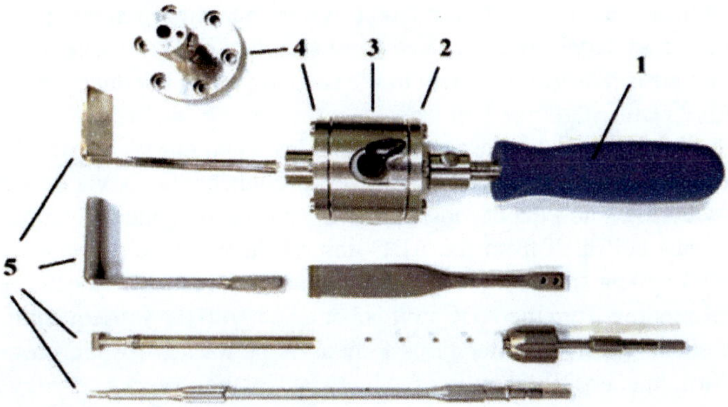

Fig. 1 The elements of MFD construction

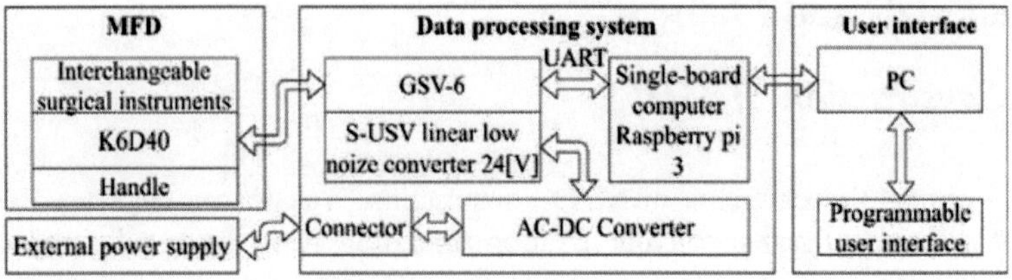

Fig. 2 Structural scheme of the data processing system

2.3 Software Algorithms

A user interface was developed to interact with the data processing system. This interface is a software that allows a surgeon to send control commands using a personal computer, display in a graphical form the data coming from the MFD sensor in real-time, as well as record or additionally process the obtained measurements. The interface between the data processing system and a computer with a human-machine interface was implemented using an Ethernet local network. The system controller is connected via a twisted pair cable to the computer. This interface includes the ability to warn of approaching the working range of the measured values of the forces and torques of the sensor, as well as to warn of the approach of a critical situation in which rupture and breakdown of tissues with which removable surgical instruments interact during the operation are possible. The limit of the measured force is set by the surgeon in the software, based on his experience and data obtained through numerous experimental studies [13]. The user interface operates by the following algorithm presented in Fig. 3.

At the first stage of the program, the application's graphical interface is initialized. Next, an attempt is made to connect the data processing system's server from the sensor. In case of a successful connection, a polling cycle of the data processing system starts, during which the data packet is received, the data is checked for exceeding the limit thresholds; the information is displayed in a graphical environment and written to a text file. In the case when the device cannot connect to the host server, it is checked for a software error. A negative test result for a software error returns the system to the stage of trying to connect to the server, and a positive result starts the software error processing mode.

The algorithm of the data processing system is shown in Fig. 4. After turning on the power, the controller initializes the server to connect clients via data exchange protocols with the subsequent possibility of receiving control commands and transferring data collected from the ADC unit. If there are no software errors, the server goes into client standby mode. At the moment the client connects, an endless cycle of data reading from the ADC unit is launched with the subsequent transfer of data to the client. After each iteration, a check is performed for the presence of a software error, the positive result of which, as in the case of a software error detected at the server initialization stage, switches to the software error processing mode.

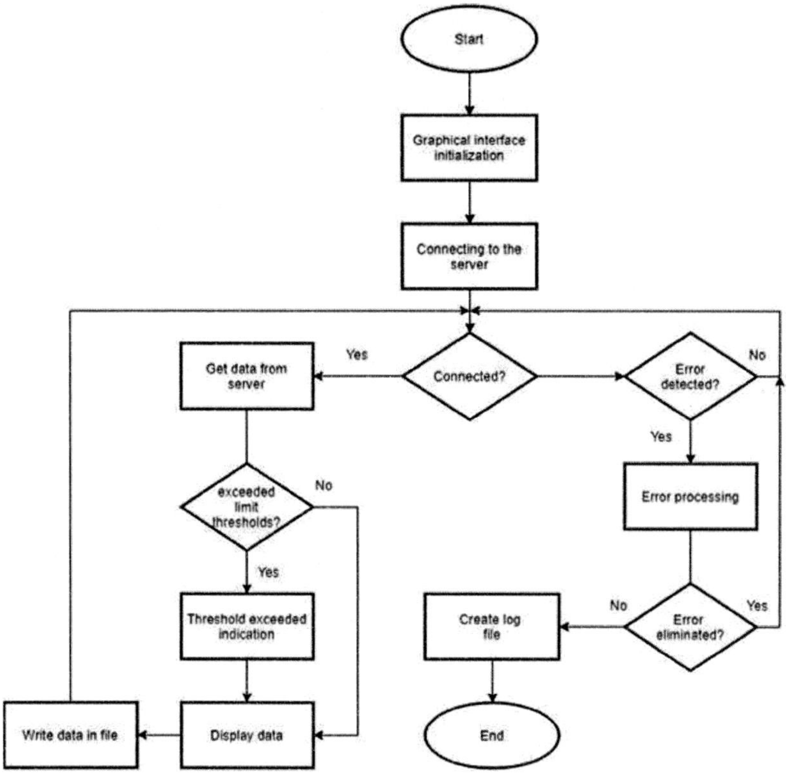

Fig. 3 User interfaces operating algorithm

2.4 Laboratory Experiments

By receiving data from the sensor, it becomes possible to determine the values of the surgeon's forces and torques to various instruments during the operation. However, before using the developed multifunctional device in clinical practice, it was necessary to verify its ability to perform its functions. Therefore, the authors of the article carried out laboratory experiments on the MFD on the back phantom.

Verification of the operability of the device was carried out by conducting experiments in laboratory conditions, including two surgical procedures. These manipulations were adopted from the most common spinal surgery—transpedicular fixation. The first is a retraction of the back muscles aimed at getting access to the spinal column. Conducting laboratory experiments with this surgical manipulation will make it possible to test the device efficiency during interaction with soft tissues. The second surgical manipulation is twisting the axial screw directly into the vertebra pedicle. This type of surgery involves forcing on the vertebral tissue (cortical plate). Having simulated this interference with the MFD, it will become

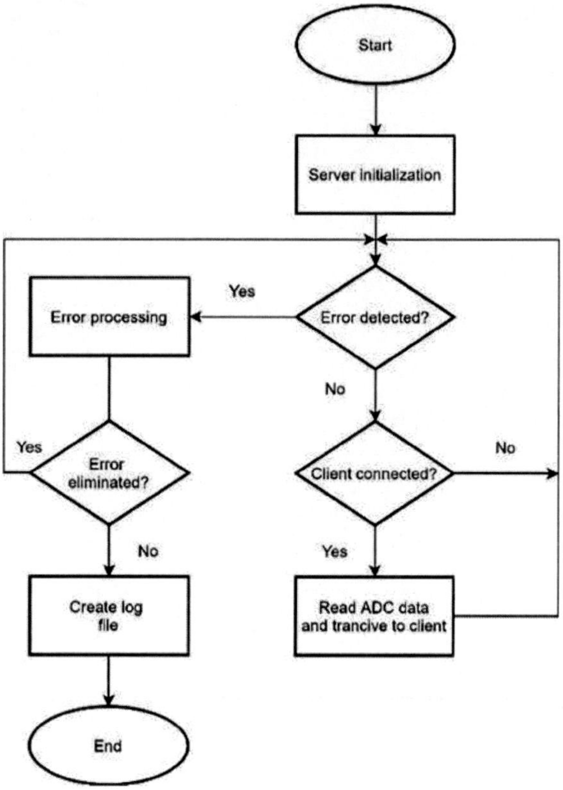

Fig. 4 Data processing system algorithm

possible to confirm the possibility of using it to interact with the bone tissue. Moreover, the analysis of the determined torques and forces will give an idea of the compliance of the multi-component force-torque sensor's characteristics with the required measurement ranges.

For performing laboratory experiments, specialized back phantoms produced by the Sawbones company were used. During the first experiment, a model representing the silicone-filled sacral part of the vertebral column was used to simulate the retraction of the back muscles. The back muscles were simulated by the silicone featuring specially selected mechanical parameters. A tool with an L-shaped retractor tip was inserted into the silicone cut. Then, the instrument was used to retract the silicone (12 mm) sideways from the cut until access to the spinal column could be obtained. The second MFD-related experiment was performed on a phantom of the sacral part of the vertebral column. A replaceable MFD tool was used to twist axial screws into pedicles of this phantom, set on a special silicone bed.

For data collection, the multifunctional device used a built-in multi-component force-torque sensor. At any specific time, a six-component vector $\overrightarrow{F_i}$ was read off from it.

This vector can be conceived of as:

$$F_i = \left(F_{xi}, F_{yi}, F_{zi}, M_{xi}, M_{yi}, M_{zi}\right)^T \quad (1)$$

where: F_{xi}, F_{yi}, F_{zi}—components of the force vector in the Cartesian coordinate system M_{xi}, M_{yi}, M_{zi}—components of the torque vector in the Cartesian coordinate system.

By using the values received from the multi-component sensor, it becomes possible to measure the forces produced by tools during surgical manipulations by different components. As well as converting these forces into resulting vectors of force and torque, these values were determined as modules obtained from components of the corresponding vectors:

$$F_{i\sum} = \sqrt{F_{xi}^2 + F_{yi}^2 + F_{zi}^2} \quad (2)$$

$$M_{i\sum} = \sqrt{M_{xi}^2 + M_{yi}^2 + M_{zi}^2} \quad (3)$$

3 Results

When testing to determine the force of interaction with soft tissues, five retractions of the silicone cut edge were performed. The graphs for each of the sensor's vector components are shown in Fig. 5.

Two force impacts were performed on the left part of the cut and three—on the right one. The graphs show it with a corresponding increase in values along the axis F_Z for the force vector and components M_X and M_Y for torque. The maximum force obtained for each of the vector components equate to 13.3 N, 2.88 N, 38.06 N for components F_X, F_Y, F_Z и 0.613 N m, 2.25 N m, 0.175 N m for the components M_X, M_Y, M_Z, respectively. Based on these values, it also becomes possible to determine the maximum values of the force and torque vectors applied to the tools that equate to 39.2 N, 2.29 N m. The graph also demonstrates minor zero-based fluctuations of values at the beginning of measurements and between the impacts on tissues. These fluctuations are due to the gravity influence on the tool when being moved since it had no supporting point in the form of soft tissues. Based on the data on the marginal values measured by the force-torque sensor (200 N for the force components and 5 N m for the torque components), it can be argued that there is a large margin for the measurement range of the multifunctional tool for this type of surgical intervention.

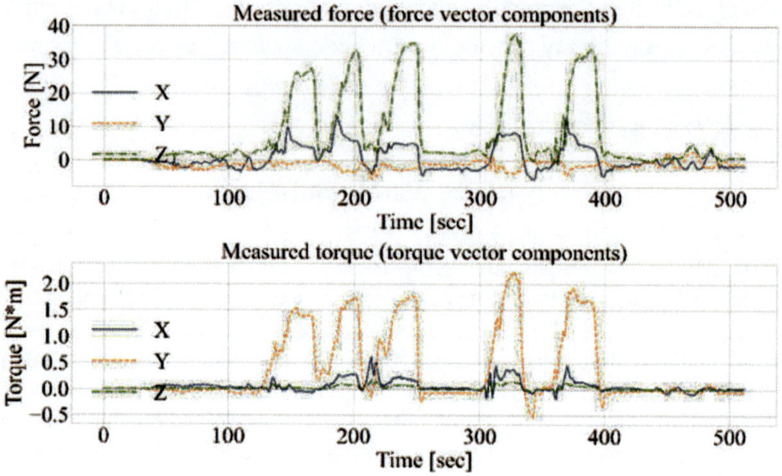

Fig. 5 Forces during lateral expansion of the silicone layer by the L-shaped retractor

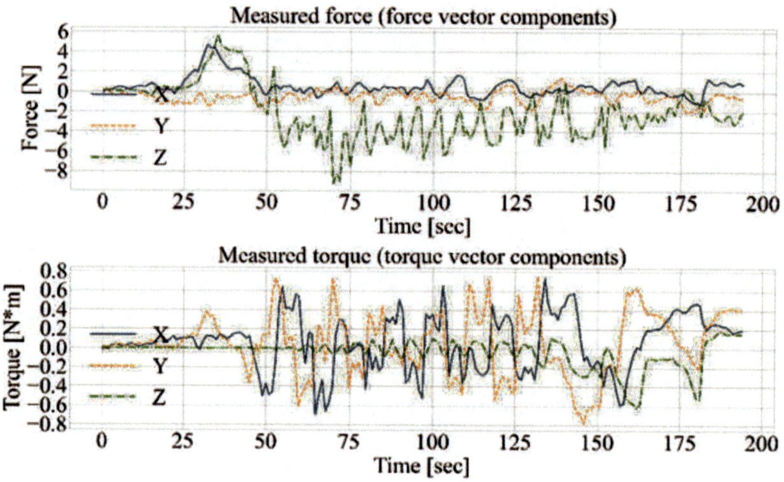

Fig. 6 Obtained force and momentum data for twisting in the axial screw

Fundamentally different data is generated when using the MFD for bone tissue. Figure 6 shows graphs of the obtained force and torque values for twisting the axial screw in the spine phantom. They demonstrate major zero-based fluctuations in the values at the beginning of measurements. These fluctuations are caused by the application of a longer tool, which results in the stronger gravity influence when the tool is moved. The average value of these fluctuations equates to 0.8 N for the force vector and 0.1 N m for the torque vector.

Moreover, it can be seen that when screwing in, the nature of the application of force and torque by the surgeon is periodical. This feature of the graph is caused by the need to change the position of the hand on the handle when screwing in. Thus, the maximum values of the force and torque vectors in question equal to 9.201 N and 0.885 N m make it possible to argue that the multifunction tool features the margin for the force measurement range for this type of surgical interference. These values, as well as the values 4.71, 2.01, 9.16 N for the components F_X, F_Y, F_Z and 0.73, 0.77, 0.61 N m for the components M_X, M_Y, M_Z make it possible to argue that the multifunction tool features the margin for the force measurement range for this type of surgical interference. Thus, it has been confirmed that it can be applied for measuring forces and torque when contacting a patient's bone tissue.

4 Discussion

In this study, we validate the performance of a prototype MFD through two laboratory experiments. The experiments carried out made it possible to check the device in conditions close to real surgical practice. The primary task was to test the data processing system and the ability of the surgeon to interact with the user interface. The resulting graphs demonstrate the possibility of receiving and subsequent processing of data. The interface algorithms related to the indication in exceeding the threshold values were also tested and showed positive results. An essential feature of these experiments was the verification of the operability of the design of interchangeable instruments. In all the other works considered above, strictly, one type of instrument is used as a tool based on which the measuring system is built. In [8, 9] used scalpels to cut tissue. There are also known examples where the sensor elements of the measuring system are installed directly on the tool body. For example, Hanna et al. [14] describes forceps on the handles of which strain gauges were installed to track the force of pressing by the surgeon. Compared with these instruments, the resulting prototype has greater versatility since it is not based on one type of tool. Also, the prototype has a wider range of force and torque measurement due to selecting the sensor element. These features make it possible to obtain data on efforts not only from soft but also from hard tissues for various types of surgical interventions.

However, when building a universal solution, it was important to make sure that the tool could be changed. Also, it was necessary to confirm the compliance of the characteristics of the multi-component force-torque sensor with the required measurement ranges. It was in connection with these that two experiments were carried out reflecting different types of effects on the patient's tissues. The values obtained for various types of phantoms prove the possibility of using interchangeable instruments in one system, thereby confirming the versatility of the proposed device.

The limitations of this study are related to the fact that phantoms were used for the research. Although the characteristics of phantoms are close to the real physical properties of human tissues, however, practical values may differ. Also, according to the data obtained, it can be argued that there is a large margin of the measurement range of a multifunctional instrument for this type of surgical intervention. As a result, the device's ability to perform the assigned tasks was confirmed. During the tests, one design feature of the MFD was also discovered. When screwing in the axial screw, the surgeon must continuously rotate the instrument in one direction. With many turns, the wire used to receive data from the force-torque sensor begins to twist, which can cause inconvenience for the surgeon when working with this instrument for a long time. In this regard, when forming a solution based on a prototype for implementation in clinical practice, it is planned to replace data transmission via a wire to a radio channel.

The future clinical implication of this solution will make it possible to obtain information at a qualitatively new level about what forces arise when the surgeon acts on the patient's tissues. This information will allow the surgeon to receive feedback on the force and moment during the surgical intervention. Besides, it becomes possible to design more optimal medical robotic systems and analyze the properties of patient tissues.

5 Conclusion

This article aimed to validate the MFD by conducting laboratory tests on medical phantoms. The results obtained for two different operations using one device confirmed the possibility of constructing a multifunctional measuring device based on a surgical instrument. The operability of the sensor data processing system was also approved. The obtained maximum values of the components of forces and moments do not exceed the measuring range of the sensor, which confirms the correct choice of the sensor element of the system. Thus, the performance of the MFD prototype was demonstrated.

Our future work will focus on two goals. The first goal is to form the final solution based on the prototype, further integrated into medical practice. The main work will focus on the ergonomics and mobility of the device. The second goal is to test the device in clinical practice. A multifunctional instrument in real surgical operations will allow collecting statistical data on the forces and torques applied by the surgeon to the instrument. The data obtained will make it possible to carry out the design of medical-robotic systems and complexes at a higher quality level.

Acknowledgements This study was supported by the Ministry of Health of the Russian Federation in the framework of the State Contract No. 056-00149-18-02 of July 3, 2018.

References

1. Abitbol J, Munir A, How J, Lau S, Salvador S, Kogan L, Kessous R, Breitner L, Frank R, Kucukyazici B, Gotlieb W (2020) The shifting trends towards a robotically-assisted surgical interface: clinical and financial implications. Health Policy Technol 9(2):157–165
2. Krylov V, Grin A, Timerbaev V, Genov P, Efremenko S, Grigorieva E, Nikitin S, Kurenkov A, Khit M (2014) Spine and spinal cord injury. OOO Print-Studio, Moscow, Russian Federation, Moscow
3. Chunikhin A, Bazikyan E, Poduraev Y, Vorotnikov A, Klimov D (2019) Comparative experimental assessment of the accuracy of nanosecond laser surgery of the oral cavity when the instrument is moved by a robotic complex and a surgeon. Russian Open Med J 8(3)
4. Chunikhin A, Poduraev Yu, Vorotnikov A, Klimov D, Sahakyan M, Bazikyan E (2017) Efficiency assessment of nanosecond laser robotic maxillofacial area surgery in experiment. Sovremennye Tehnologii V Med 9(4):123–128
5. Vorotnikov A, Klimov D, Romash E, Bashevskaya O, Poduraev Yu, Bazykyan E, Chunihin A (2017) Cutting velocity accuracy as a criterion for comparing robot trajectories and manual movements for medical industry. Mech Ind 18:712
6. Vorotnikov A, Poduraev Y, Romash E (2015) Estimation of error in determining the centers of rotation of links in a kinematic chain for industrial robot calibration techniques. Meas Tech 58(8):864–871
7. Klimov D, Vorotnikov A, Solovyov M, Poduraev Y, Grin A, Krylov V (2019) Medical robotics for neurosurgery. Bull MSTU Stankin 48(1):81–87
8. Sorouri K, Podolsky D, Wang AM, Fisher D, Wong K, Looi T, Drake J, Forrest C (2018) Utilization of a robotic mount to determine the force required to cut palatal tissue. J Mech Behav Biomed Mater 86:433–439
9. Chanthasopeephan T, Desai J, Lau AC (2003) Measuring forces in liver cutting: new equipment and experimental results. Ann Biomed Eng 31:1372–1382
10. Mendoza C, Laugier C (2003) Simulating soft tissue cutting using finite element models. IEEE Int Conf Robot Autom 1:1109–1114
11. Solovyev M, Vorotnikov A, Klimov D, Kovalskii V, Poduraev Y (2017) Control system of the articulated arm braking mechatronic machine (AABMM). In: Proceedings of the 28th DAAAM international symposium 28(1):1002– (2017)
12. Soloviev M, Vorotnikov A, Grin A, Klimov D, Poduraev Yu, Krylov V (2020) The concept of building a multifunctional device for measuring forces and moments during neurosurgical operations. Med ment 58(3):28–32
13. Prokhorenko L, Klimov D, Mishchenkov D, Poduraev Y (2020) Surgeon-robot interface development framework. Comput Biol Med 120
14. Hanna G, Drew T, Arnold G, Fakhry M, Cuschieri A (2008) Development of force measurement system for clinical use in minimal access surgery. Surg Endosc 22(2):467–471

Advanced Biomechanical Systems: Development and Design of an Accelerometer-Based Prosthetic Sensorimotor Platform

Peter Anto Johnson, John Christy Johnson, and Austin Mardon

Abstract Following stroke, injury, or exposure to physically limiting conditions, limbs can become physiologically compromised. In particular, motor and fine-dexterity tasks involving the arm, particularly in locomotion, grasp and release, can be influenced becoming either delayed and having to deal with greater force demands. Current prosthetic systems use electromyography (EMG)-based techniques for creating functional sensorimotor platforms. However, several limitations in practical use and signal detection have been identified in these systems. Accelerometer-based sensorimotor systems have been suggested to overcome these limitations but only proof-of-concept has been demonstrated. Here, we explore design specifications for accelerometers being developed for prosthetic integration. We have developed optimizations for the current model, evaluated system properties to enhance sensitivity and reduce signal noise, and performed a pilot test using simulation to test this model. The data suggest these novel design parameters can enhance signal detection, when compared to conventional accelerometers. Future avenues should focus on validation of this design prototype in a full prosthetic system.

Keywords Biomechanical model · Accelerometer design · Signal simulation

1 Introduction

Currently, approximately 35–40 million people globally require prosthetic or orthotic support after stroke, injury, and/or other conditions affecting limb function [1]. With the growing incidence of musculoskeletal conditions and non-communicable diseases including stroke and diabetes however, this number is

P. A. Johnson (✉) · J. C. Johnson · A. Mardon
Faculty of Medicine & Dentistry, University of Alberta, Edmonton, AB T6G 2R3, Canada
e-mail: paj1@ualberta.ca

J. C. Johnson
Faculty of Engineering, University of Alberta, Edmonton, AB T6G 2R3, Canada

H. Triwiyanto et al. (eds.), *Proceedings of the 1st International Conference on Electronics, Biomedical Engineering, and Health Informatics*, Lecture Notes in Electrical Engineering 746, https://doi.org/10.1007/978-981-33-6926-9_30

expected to double by the middle of this century. Movement and range of motion is significantly reduced and limited for these individuals. As a result, there is an emerging and exponentially increasing need for supporting prosthetic and orthotic support devices.

For affected individuals, performance of motor and fine-dexterity tasks, particularly those involving upper limbs, in locomotion, grasp and release, can be influenced significantly, becoming both delayed and requiring greater force demands. Applied and external acceleration are crucial determinants of these force demands, especially for systems requiring sensory integration and output generation, such as robotic prosthetic limbs. For many of these tasks, appropriate input and output command signals must be determined. Currently, such biomechanical systems have placed a focus on providing both sensory and motor feedback platforms to the user through electromyography (EMG)-controlled prosthesis [2]. EMG utilizes electrical activity between muscle fibers during contraction and relaxation phases to quantify the neuromuscular signaling patterns of the innervating motor units.

While it is possible to perform invasive or non-invasive sensing, non-invasive is virtually always preferred, as it would allow surface EMG signal detection from the skin surface alone. However, this technique has several limitations including higher levels of difficulty in identifying signal acquisition sites, high sensitivity for motion and motion artifacts, and overall lower dexterity [2, 3]. Compared to this, intramuscular EMG signals using implantable sensors provide enhanced access for signal detection and additionally enable multiple degrees of control to the prosthetic.

Many current prosthetics, including myoelectric prosthetic upper and lower limbs, employ EMG-based methods for sensing, detection, and feedback processing of motor control signals. Over the recent years, there has been a growing body of evidence establishing the utilization of tri-axial MEMs (Micro Electro-Mechanical System) sensor accelerometers as an alternative or composite sensorimotor feedback platform for use in rehabilitation [4–7]. Here, we suggest a novel design for accelerometers for the implementation of this model, which could allow multiple degrees of freedom (DOF) sensors built into prosthetic and orthotic wearable.

2 Prosthesis Model

Clinical prosthetic require the use of compact elements that include drive systems, cells, and microprocessors for functional motion adjustment and response. Within drive systems, servomotors enable continuous monitoring of feedback signals and on-going adjustment of movement for any deviations detected. Additionally, these system elements must have appropriate interfaces and the ability to sustain constant activity for practical prosthesis. Kyberd and Poulton suggest the use of a tri-axial system whereby sensors and controllers are employed to detect and correct for (1) segment orientation, (2) motion compensation, and (3) inertial platform [4]. This basic model represents an intermediate stage prior to full integration with limbs,

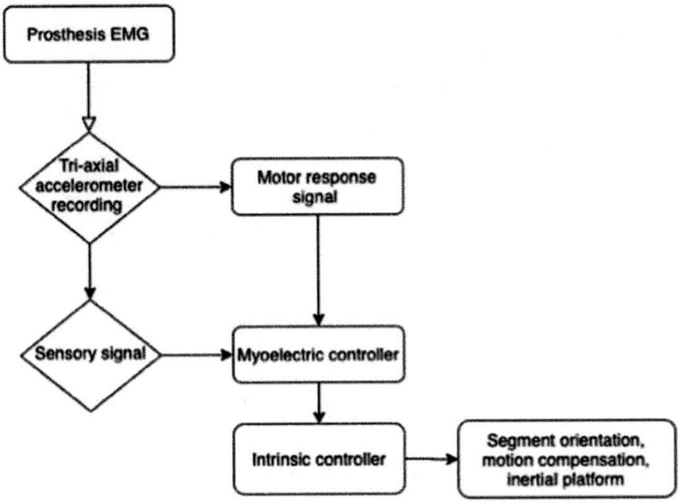

Fig. 1 Block diagram of proposed tri-axial model. EMGs are combined with accelerometer sensors to create a functional system that uses sensory and motor command signals to regulate segment orientation, motion compensation, and inertial platform

where certain actuators and sensors are independently controlled to create a functional system (Fig. 1). Segment orientation is a compensatory mechanism for the accelerometer that takes into consideration the gravitational forces and tri-dimensional, spatial alignments in order to accommodate the motor demand accordingly. Motion compensation adapts for the positioning using the surrounding prosthetic limb segment kinematics. Inertial platform uses holistic, mathematical analysis of prosthesis in interaction with an object of interest.

While a proof-of-concept has been established for the use of accelerometers, this current model has several limitations, which must first be addressed. First, the measurement of motion requires the input signal to be integrated over time, which results in a high signal noise leading to drift. Although the use of inertial sensors has been described as a technique to reduce this effect, several current models have yet to incorporate these within prosthetic designs, while relying exclusively on EMG-based sensing methods. Additionally, sensitivity, which refers to the ratio of change in output to the change in expected input of the sensor, and the bias, which results from the non-zero of the output signal of acceleration generated by the sensor, are both commonly observed limitations of MEMs sensor accelerometers. Both input and output signals could also be influenced by factors such as material, construction, operation conditions (e.g., temperature, pressure, surrounding electrical and/or mechanical prosthesis elements, etc.) It is additionally possible for factors within a biomechanical system to influence the signal, including levels of strain resulting from applied forces. As accelerometer sensing data also depends significantly on the integration, even a subtle acceleration error could have a large effect on detected data (e.g., in a position estimation test, a double integration of an acceleration error of 0.1 g can result in a 350 m position error) [8].

Moreover, several proof-of-concept designs limit their models to a single joint with limited range of motion (i.e., transradial prosthetic wrists with only 2 DOFs). In light of the replacement of such joints, there are often times a functional need to establish more advanced ranges of motion. Many studies also make assumptions regarding idealized trajectories, static conditions, downstream output signaling effects, etc. In most cases, it is additionally challenging to analyze real-time data being collected by sensors. The objective of design and development of this novel prototype model was to provide an improved model that addressed many of these inherent limitations.

3 Prototype Design and Development

Through this prototype model, we made several considerations to update conventional biomechanical prosthetic systems. Design specifications were developed by our team for variable considerations at the accelerometer-level. In this model, we utilized a template Totally Modular Prosthetic Arm with high Workability (ToMPAW) prosthetic arm design [9]. Figure 2 displays this prosthetic arm design and the site of accelerometer incorporation. Although the accelerometer can be employed at numerous sites on the ToMPAW arm, we selected to examine a focused trans-radial segment capacitating motions in multiple DOFs, namely corresponding to the condyloid (between radius and carpal bones of wrist) and saddle (between trapezium carpal bone and first metacarpal bone) joints.

Fig. 2 ToMPAW prosthesis arm and accelerometer site

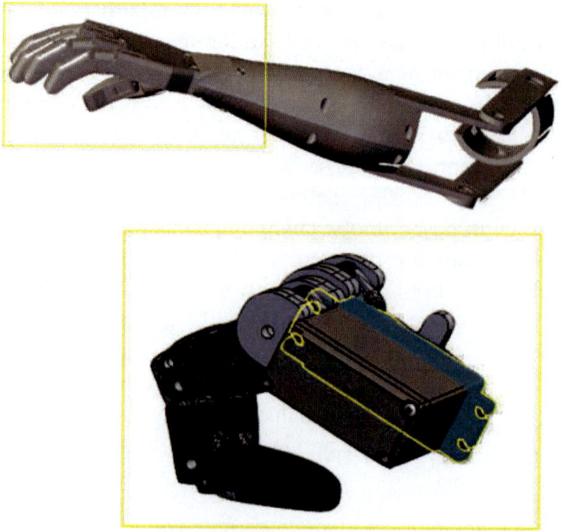

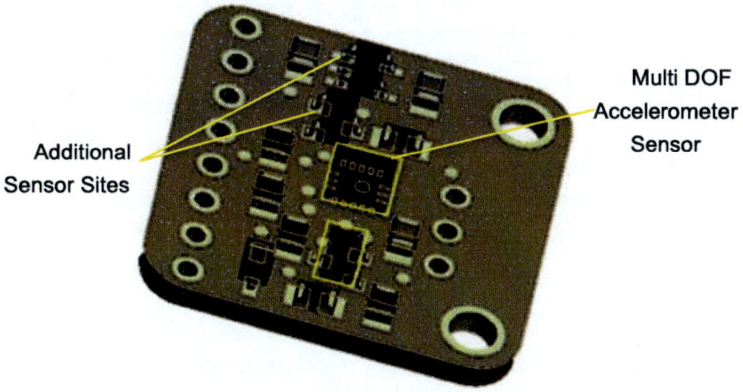

Fig. 3 Tri-axial accelerometer prototype design

As the primary aim of this design was to reduce limitations in noise for signal integration, we focused on (i) determining optimal properties for accelerometer and sensor construction and (ii) evaluating its effects on real-time signal quality improvement and feasibility. First, we incorporated support arrays to enable the implementation of additional sensing devices, such as more accelerometers, gyrometers, and magnetometers as required to the conventional design (Fig. 3). The most commonly utilized accelerometers include capacitive and piezoelectric accelerometers. Capacitive accelerometers uses a capacitive coupling mechanism and is typically preferred for low-frequency tasks, while piezoelectric accelerometers are transducers that use the accumulated electric charge resulting from applied mechanical stress and typically preferred for high-frequency, vibration and high shock measurements. Both of these types of accelerometers offer a good measure of dynamic changes in acceleration within a system. MEMs-based accelerometers are the conventional standard for accelerometers recommended for prosthetic integration and can use either piezoelectric transduction or capacitive sensing to detect acceleration. While several advantages, such as low temperature sensitivity, linearity, and small footprint, relative to other available techniques, have been suggested for capacitive sensing accelerometers [10], practically, piezoelectric MEMs-based accelerometers have been reported to offer higher sensitivity, good linearity, and lower noise [11]. To enhance current specifications, we decided to utilize piezoelectric MEMs-based accelerometers in our model. For the construction of the accelerometer, we used a standard FR-4 PCB, which consists of woven glass-reinforced epoxy laminate material.

While a conventional circuit board unit was utilized, we upgraded the model to incorporate multiple sites for the incorporation of these piezoelectric MEMs-based accelerometer sensors and other elements (e.g., capacitive sensors, gyrometers, magnetometers, thermistor, etc.) We also selected a commercially available, additive piezo-ceramic material for the construction of sensors for long durability and stability, especially under varying temperature ranges, enhancing the sensitivity of current prosthetic accelerometer sensor designs.

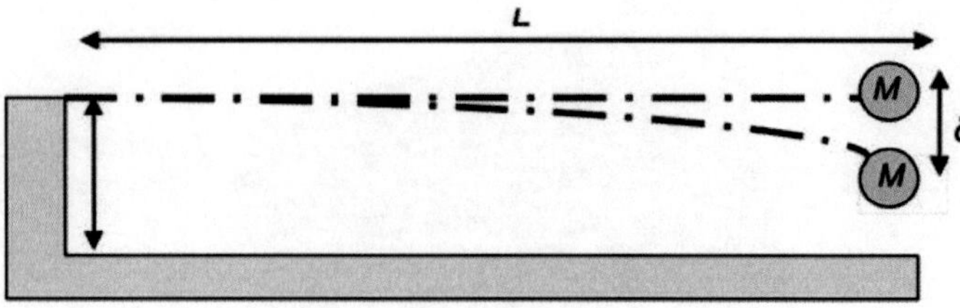

Fig. 4 Accelerometer sensor base-excited cantilever model

In addition to defining specifications for accelerometer construction material, we explored the optimal design considerations for sensor design. A typical MEMS-based piezoelectric accelerometer sensor consists of two basic units, including a cantilever and seismic mass. The physical properties of these sensors determine the sensitivity of measured signals, as well as the level of noise and drift that occurs during movement tasks. In order to account for low sensitivity limitations observed in current models, we designed sensor elements to allow high-resolution measurements. In order to do this, we calculated optimal dimensions, material constants, and sensor properties, including deflection, stress, and strain. Assuming linear constitutive law, the sensor system can be modelled using a mass-spring-damper model where the seismic mass is equivalent to the mass element, M, and the cantilever beam is equivalent to the spring and damper elements in a base-excited configuration of the model (Fig. 4).

This model also assumes both the spring and damper are in mechanical parallel and that motor input is received from the base.

3.1 *Design Considerations*

According to the assumptions made by the above model, it is possible to determine optimal design standards for various material properties for sensor construction including:

- *Q-factor*: a measure of how under-damped an oscillator is. As all materials have a natural frequency of vibration, determining the Q-factor can be utilized to measure the dampening according to the construction material properties. If the Q-factor is too low, damping in the system will result in a reduced sensitivity. The Q-factor can be calculated by:

$$Q = \frac{\sqrt{Mk}}{D} \tag{1}$$

where Q is the Q-factor, M is inertial mass, k is the spring constant, and D is the damping coefficient, where

$$k = \frac{Ewt^3}{4L^3} \tag{2}$$

and

$$D = -\frac{F_{drag}}{v} \tag{3}$$

where E is Young's Modulus, w is cantilever width, t is its thickness, and L is its length. In calculation of the damping coefficient, the drag force, F_{drag}, and velocity, v, and ultimately, the rigidity parameter are largely dependent on material properties. By this proof, a sensor design of higher sensitivity must utilize an optimized higher inertial mass, cantilever construction using a material with a higher spring constant.

- *Deflection*: the degree to which a cantilever is displaced under a load. A higher deflection is typically an indicator of a higher cantilever design sensitivity [12]. The Stony Equation can be utilized to calculate deflection:

$$\delta = \frac{L^2}{t^2}\frac{3\sigma(1-v)}{E} \tag{4}$$

where δ is the cantilever deflection, L is the length of the cantilever beam, t is its thickness, σ represents the uniaxial stress or force per unit square, v is Poisson's ratio, and E is Young's modulus. Deflection is inversely proportional to the spring constant.

- *Stress*: a measure of the internal forces resulting within a material system. Mechanical stress can be classified according to the type of forces acting on the system and include: scalar (tension or compression), bending, and torsional (shear) stress. In a cantilever beam system, the increasing the structural load, M, notably increases levels of bending and shearing stress.
- *Strain*: a measure of stretch or deformation that occur as a result of mechanical stress. Strain occurs when a force is applied to an object and results in a physical change, whereas stress concerns only the forces regardless of any physical changes to the material. The resolution of measurements, quantifiable by the Q-factor, and deflection levels, rely essentially on both of these parameters. This is demonstrated mathematically by the Young's modulus ratio and its presence as a variable in calculations for the spring constant (ultimately, Q-factor) and deflection:

$$E = \frac{\sigma}{\varepsilon} \tag{5}$$

where σ is the uniaxial stress, determined as a pressure or force per square unit, and ε is the strain, which is a dimensionless quantity representing the proportion of deformation. Based on optimization used in the design of multi-DOF robotic

Table 1 Design parameter optimization to enhance signal detection quality

Parameter	Description
Q-factor	Low Q-factors results in damping, which achieves a lower sensitivity within a system. As such, a system with higher Q-factors is favoured in an optimization
Inertial mass	Higher inertial masses are preferred to increase system sensitivity. However, masses must be optimized to ensure the structural stability of the system
Spring constant	Materials with higher spring constants (e.g., piezo-ceramics), which also tend to have associated modulus parameters, favour higher sensitivity systems
Rigidity	Within a system, the sensor's damping coefficient, which is based on the material's resistance to the drag force at a given velocity, should be low to ensure a higher Q-factor
Cantilever dimensions	Length, thickness, and width of the cantilever affect vibrational frequency capacities of the sensor. Higher design sensitivity features an inverse relationship between length and thickness producing higher deflection and Q-factor values. Width also influences the spring constant of the system
Deflection	Higher deflection is an indicator for a higher cantilever design sensitivity and associated with lower signal noise events
Young's Modulus	A material's resistance to applied mechanical stresses and strain capacity are key variables in deflection and Q-factor measurements in the system. Typically, a higher strain capacity and lower stresses are achieved in an ideal system

arms in varying gravitational fields to enhance load bearing [13], it is possible to describe optimal vibration frequencies and strain magnitudes. Both stress and strain therefore influence the overall resolution of measurements and must be considered in the design.

In Table 1, we summarize the changes that are required according to these design parameters in order to enhance the quality of measurement signals.

4 Design Specifications

Based on these properties, design specifications were developed for a novel prototype using fixed accelerometer dimensions. In Table 2, we report the above optimization equations, modelling, and feasibility parameters, which approximated threshold specifications for novel accelerometer design. In Table 3, we compare technical specifications between existing conventional and MEMs accelerometers and the novel design prototype.

Table 2 Threshold specifications for accelerometer parameters calculated according to optimization equations and earlier models for novel design prototype

Parameter	Specification
Accelerometer mass (fixed)	150 μg
Accelerometer dimensions (fixed)	750 × 250 μm
Minimum cantilever length	214 μm
Maximum cantilever thickness	18 μm
Vibration resonance frequency	125 Hz
Average acceleration	2.5 m/s/s
Piezoelectric sensor material	Modified $PbTiO_3$

Table 3 Comparison of novel design prototype to existing accelerometer designs

	Resolution (mg)	Sensitivity (mV/g)	Frequency range (Hz)	Amplitude limit	Linearity
Conventional	3	100	1–2000	±50	<±5%/ 1 kHz
MEMs	2	160	1–6000	±5	±1%/ 1 kHz
Prototype	0.08	256	1–11,250	±3	±0.2%/ 1 kHz

5 Simulation Modeling

To test optimizations, we employed MATLAB to perform simulations using pre-existing prosthetic movement acceleration dynamics data. Modeling was based on crank-slider mechanism optimization, which uses predictive and output data to calculate position, crank velocity, and acceleration over time [14]. We utilized available tracked prosthetic movement data with six DOFs and generated acceleration over time plots to compare the signal-to-noise ratio and drift between conventional accelerometers and our novel design. Figure 5 displays the dynamics data capturing translational movement along an X-axis, translation along a Y-axis, translation along a Z-axis, rotation around a roll axis, rotation around a pitch axis, and rotation around a yaw axis. This data includes movement requiring segment orientation, motion compensation and an inertial platform. In Fig. 6, results of the simulations for a calibrated conventional accelerometer model and our novel prototype design model are shown. It displays the difference in signal quality during segment orientation, motion compensation, and inertial platform. As a result, these algorithms can then used to generate command outputs in a prosthetic system. Of the two, our prototype was determined to reduce signal-noise effects observed in conventional accelerometers. Our modeling and prototype therefore demonstrates it

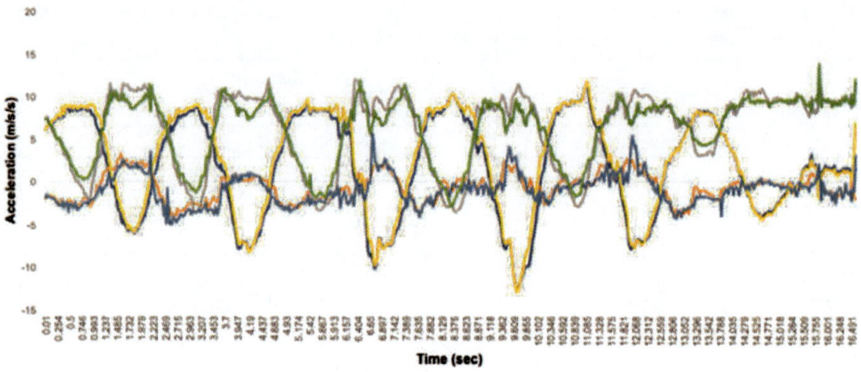

Fig. 5 Raw tracked prosthetic movement acceleration dynamics data

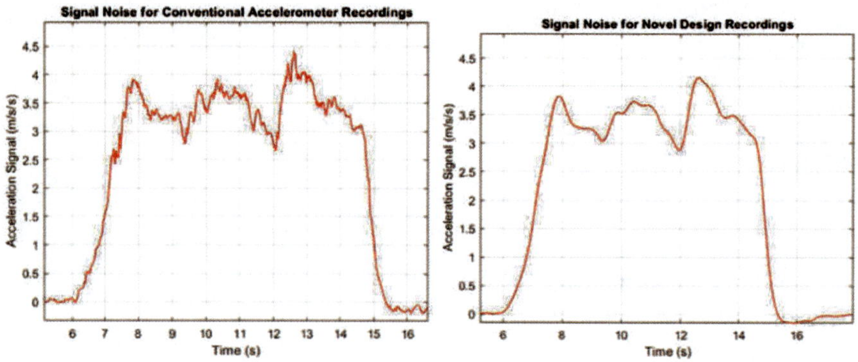

Fig. 6 Signal-noise reduction in novel design prototype. Using acceleration dynamics data for prosthetic arm movement using six degrees of freedom, an integrated acceleration value was generated using a model on MATLAB for a conventional accelerometer sensor design and the design for the novel accelerometer prototype

is not only possible to mechanically dampen a system, but also that we can reduce noise and increase signal sensitivity by upgrading accelerometer design specifications.

6 Limitations and Future Avenues

While promising, this proposed model still has several limitations and integral design considerations must be made before its implementation. First, it is a proof-of-concept having been tested only via simulation and must be evaluated in a prosthetic system. Our simulation also focuses on two main accelerometer subtypes in modelling signal quality and would benefit from examination of other subtypes. It is additionally necessary to validate these results by a comparative analysis with concurrent EMG measurements to ensure the recording is indeed detecting a motor signal within the prosthetic system. While this novel prototype could overcome several limitations with EMG sensorimotor systems in limb prosthesis, extensive work must be done to model movements using six or more DOFs. Thus, future avenues should also focus on exploring multi-DOF sensor application, which may significantly reduce the time and cost required to perform manoeuvres. Another of area of interest should focus on real-time noise filters and integrating previously described strain devices for osseo-integrated prosthesis devices, which can be optimized for bone adaptation.

7 Conclusion

We have proposed a model for optimization, system properties and considerations for its implementation, described a novel piezoelectric MEMS accelerometer prototype design for prosthetic integration, and demonstrated a proof-of-concept using a simulation to show enhanced signal quality detection. Future studies should focus on incorporation of this design and real world testing in complete prosthesis systems.

Acknowledgements We would like to thank the public for donating money to our funding agencies: this project was supported by the Canada Service Corps, TakingITGlobal, and the Government of Canada.

References

1. World Health Organization (2017) Standards for prosthetics and orthotics—part 1: standards. Geneva, Switzerland
2. Sudarsan LS, Sekaran EC (2012) Design and development of EMG controlled prosthetics limb. Procedia Eng 38:3547–3551
3. Geethanjali P (2016) Myoelectric control of prosthetic hands: state-of-the-art review. Med Devices Evid Res 9:247–255
4. Kyberd PJ, Poulton A (2017) Use of accelerometers in the control of practical prosthetic arms. IEEE Trans Neural Syst Rehabil Eng 25:1884–1891
5. Yang J, Kusche R, Ryschka M, Xia C (2018) Wrist movement detection for prosthesis control using surface EMG and triaxial accelerometer. In: Proceedings of 10th international congress on image and signal processing, biomedical engineering and informatics (CISP-BMEI), vol 2018, Jan, pp 1–6. Institute of Electrical and Electronics Engineers Inc., Hokaido, Japan
6. Culhane KM, O'Connor M, Lyons D, O'Laighin G (2005) Accelerometers in rehabilitation medicine for older adults. Age Ageing 34:556–560
7. Klisic D, Kostic M, Dosen S, Popovic D (2009) Control of prehension for the transradial prosthesis: natural-like image recognition system. J Autom Control 19:27–31

8. Kowalczuk Z, Merta T (2014) Modelling an accelerometer for robot position estimation In: Proceedings from 19th international conference on methods and models in automation and robotics (MMAR), pp 909–14. Institute of Electrical and Electronics Engineers Inc., Międzyzdroje, Poland
9. Kyberd PJ, Poulton AS, Sandsjö L, Jönsson S, Jones B, Gow D (2007) The ToMPAW modular prosthesis: a platform for research in upper-limb prosthetics. J Prosthetics Orthot 19:15–21
10. Mohammed Z, Elfadel I, Rasras M (2018) Monolithic multi degree of freedom (MDoF) capacitive MEMS accelerometers. Micromachines 9
11. Albarbar A, Mekid S, Starr A, Pietruszkiewicz R (2008) Suitability of MEMS accelerometers for condition monitoring: an experimental study. Sensors 8:784–799
12. Ansari MZ, Cho C (2009) Deflection, frequency, and stress characteristics of rectangular, triangular, and step profile microcantilevers for biosensors. Sensors 9:6046–6057
13. Johnson JC, Johnson PA, Mardon AA (2020) Development of a mechanical strain device to prevent microgravity-induced bone loss. Pac J Sci Technol 21:274–275
14. Halicioglu R, Dulger LC, Bozdana AT (2014) Modelling and simulation based on matlab/simulink: a press mechanism. J Phys: Conf Ser 490:012053

A Simple Design of Sterilizer Equipment for Infant Incubator Using Ultraviolet Germicidal Lamps

Mamurotun, Indah Nursyamsi Handayani, Nur Hasanah Ahniar, and Catharine Bernadette

Abstract Infant incubator is an electromedical device used to treatment for a newborn which has the possibility to become a place of spread infection. Therefore, this study aims to design a simple infant incubator sterilizer as an effort to reduce the level of nosocomial infection in the neonatal intensive care unit. The simple design of infant incubator sterilizer has been made using UV germicidal lamps, arduino mega, remote control, and equipped with a sterilization time setting. The device was tested under laboratory conditions, with observational parameters consist of sterilization time, a display showing the countdown time of sterilization and the hour meter of the ultraviolet lamp, as well as remote testing, to turn on/off the device. Furthermore, the effectiveness of sterilization was tested on three types of gram-positive bacteria namely *Escherichia coli*, *Staphylococcus aureus*, and *Bacillus cereus* with sterilization time variations of 30, 60, 90 and 120 min. The result of this research is a prototype of sterilizer equipment using an ultraviolet germicidal lamp that can be applied to infant incubators. The effectiveness of sterilization using this equipment showed a trend gradually decrease the number of bacteria.

Keywords Infant incubator · Sterilizer · Ultraviolet germicidal lamp

1 Introduction

Infant incubators are very popular electromedical equipment used for newborn treatment, especially for births with special conditions such as low birth weight, ill newborn and premature. Infant incubators are usually placed in Neonatal Intensive Care Units (NICU) to support the achievement of optimal environment. In order, to preserve optimal conditions, it is necessary to control some parameters such as

Mamurotun · I. N. Handayani (✉) · N. H. Ahniar · C. Bernadette
Department of Electromedical Engineering, Poltekkes Kemenkes Jakarta II, Jakarta, Indonesia
e-mail: indah.nursyamsi@poltekkesjkt2.ac.id

H. Triwiyanto et al. (eds.), *Proceedings of the 1st International Conference on Electronics, Biomedical Engineering, and Health Informatics*, Lecture Notes in Electrical Engineering 746, https://doi.org/10.1007/978-981-33-6926-9_31

temperature, humidity, airflow, and oxygen concentration. Furthermore, the Centers for Disease Control and Prevention (CDC) also regulates procedures for disinfection and sterilization of infant incubators to reduce the risk of infection in newborn [1]. The research that has been reported by Nanou Christina (2015) indicate that nosocomial infections cause an increase in the proportion of infections in the neonatal intensive care unit [2]. Several studies, presented the result of investigation a number of pathogens that are spread on environmental surfaces in neonatal incubator (e.g. *Enterococcus spp.*, *Pseudomonas spp.*, *Staphylococcus saprophyticus*, *Escherichia coli*, *Streptococcus agalactiae,* and other bacteria) which is very possible to be a cause of nosocomial infection [3, 4]. These pathogens can be directly or indirectly transferred to the patients, i.e. the skin patients contact of contaminated surfaces/equipment or via the hands of healthcare workers [5, 6]. In addition, these pathogens grow optimally a temperature of about 37 °C, which is the environment temperature for infant incubators. Therefore, it is recommended to carry out preventive maintenance on periodically and sterilization infant incubators after used for baby care to control nosocomial infections.

Ultraviolet light is a type of electromagnetic radiation has a wavelength range from 10 to 400 nm. Based on the wavelength ranges, ultraviolet radiation can be divided into three categories, the relatively long-wavelength namely UV-A (315–400 nm), medium-wavelength is UV-B (280–315 nm) and short-wavelength UV-C (100–280 nm). Ultraviolet-C radiation has immediate benefit to destructive the DNA molecule of bacteria, viruses and other fungi so that it can reduce replication and proliferation. Therefore ultraviolet-C lamps are also known as ultraviolet germicidal lamps. The sterilization using ultraviolet germicidal lamp is one of the most commonly used methods in the industry of water treatment, food products, medical equipment, etc. Several studies on the effects of germicidal ultraviolet lamps have been widely reported, among others, by Bialka and Demirci (2007) reporting a decrease in the number of *Salmonella* and *E. Coli* bacteria by 4.3 and 2.9 log CFU/g, respectively in the decontamination process of blueberries using UV lights [7]. Levetin et al. [8] analyze the effect of UV germicidal radiation for reducing fungal contamination in the Air Handling Unit. Besides, the design and development of UV sterilizer devices have also been widely carried out, one of them is Welch [9] developed an irradiation chamber using a far UV-C lamp to control the spread of the H1N1 aerosol influenza virus carried in the air. Namala [10] has developed a design of food sterilization systems using UV lamps with manually switches to control the sterilization time and the distance of the lamp to the sample. UV sterilizer devices with remote control using android have also been introduced by Bentancor and Vidal [11] for periodic conditioning of culture rooms.

The process sterilization of infant incubators as far as the results of literacy is done by using disinfectant liquid, then dried using a clean cloth or towel [12]. This method is still considered very conventional with a low level of guarantee. Therefore, as an attempt to increase confidence in the infant incubator sterilization process after manual cleaning, authors study characteristics of ultraviolet germicidal lamps that have long been known to have benefits for killing bacteria and have been used extensively for sterilization such as sterilization in the hospital rooms [13], sterilization of medical equipment [14] and pharmaceutical products. This makes the ultraviolet lamp particularly promising to be applied as a sterilizer for infant incubators. The objective of this study has reported a simple design of sterilizer equipment that can be applied as an infant incubator sterilizer.

2 Materials and Methods

2.1 *Sterilizer Equipment*

Infant incubator sterilizer was designed using an ultraviolet germicidal lamp with a remote control to operate a device from a distance. This equipment has been made using three main components consist of ultraviolet germicidal lamps, the main control unit of Arduino Mega 2560, and IR remote. IR Remote was used as a sterilization time setting and controls the on/off of the sterilization system from distance. The sterilizer equipment is also completed with an hour meter that is displayed on the device it aims to monitor the lifetime of the germicidal ultraviolet lamp. Another advantage of this sterilizer equipment, it has been made by a simple design so that it is easy to carry and available batteries as a substitute for the electric power supply from the state.

2.2 *Irradiation Bacteria by UV Lamps*

The prototype tested under laboratory conditions, with observational parameters consist of sterilization time, a display showing the countdown time of sterilization and the hour meter of the ultraviolet lamp. Sterilization time is set at 4 measurement points for two hours with 30 min intervals, the timing of sterilization is compared to the stopwatch. In order to evaluate the effectiveness of sterilization, a media plate count agar (PCA) is used to count the total bacteria before and after UV light irradiation with 4 treatments of irradiation time, 30, 60, 90, 120 min and accompanied by the control group. The bacteria used are *Escherichia coli*, *Staphylococcus aureus*, and *Bacillus cereus*. Petri dishes containing bacteria are placed on the mattress in an infant incubator.

3 System Design

This research has been carried out in the electronic laboratory of the electromedical engineering department and the microbiology laboratory of the environmental health department, Poltekkes Kemenkes Jakarta II. In general, this research was divided into two main parts, first is hardware design and the second is software design. Hardware and software systems are designed to be integrated, so the system that can work optimally. The two parts of the devices will be discussed further as follows.

3.1 Hardware Design

The hardware design begins by creating a wiring diagram using AutoCAD software as shown in Fig. 1. The hardware had several parts consists of a voltage booster module, a phototransistor, a microcontroller unit, an alarm, an inverter module, an ultraviolet lamp, and a display. Furthermore, after the system design in the software was completed then the prototype of sterilizer equipment can be developed.

1. Voltage Booster Modul
   The voltage booster module is a switching regulator to convert DC to DC power with a large input voltage range and adjustable output voltage. In this study, a voltage booster is used to increase the voltage of the battery by 3.7 V_{DC} to 6 V_{DC}. This is because the electronic circuit requires a minimum voltage power supply of 5 V_{DC}.
2. Phototransistor
   Phototransistor in this electronic circuit is part of remote control that functions as a receiver and detector of infrared light. The remote control is one of an

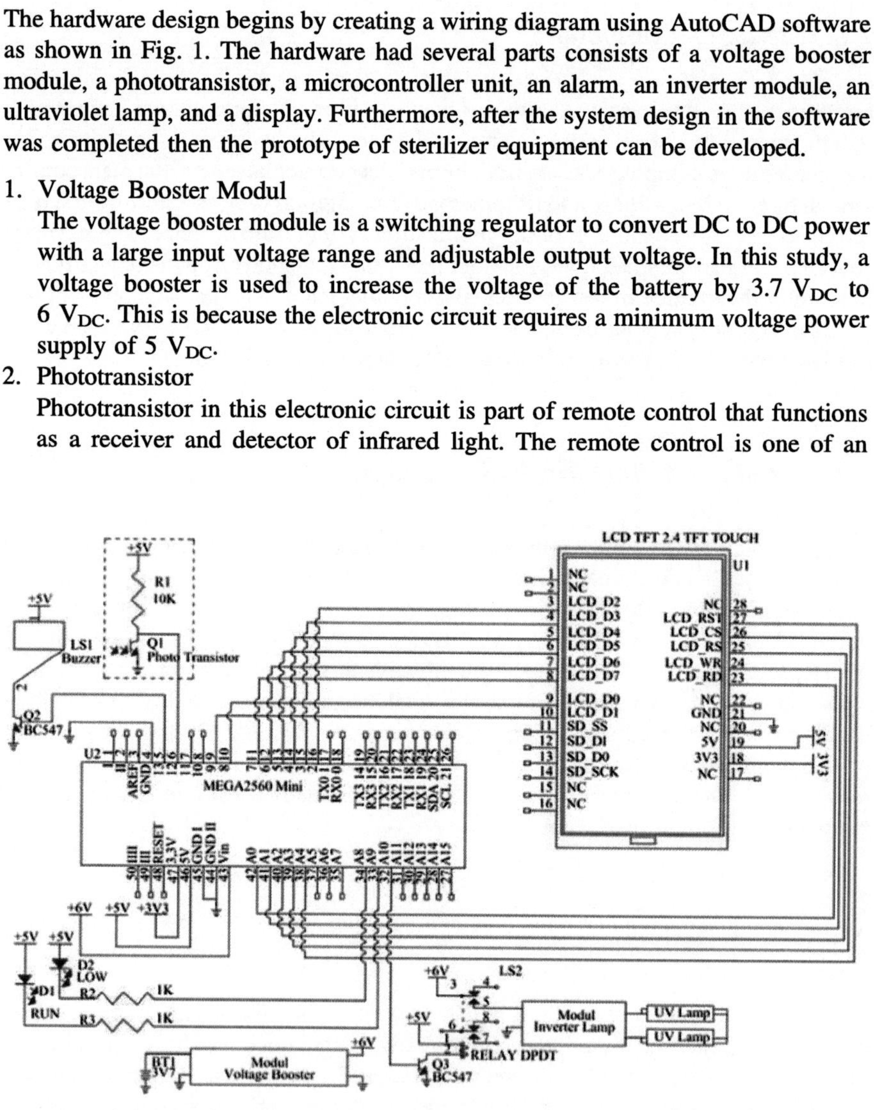

Fig. 1 Wiring diagram of infant incubator sterilizer

alternative wireless long- distance communication that is easy to get, practice and inexpensive. Remote control at this equipment is used to set the time of sterilization and controller active or deactivate the sterilization system.

3. Microcontroller Unit
The Arduino Mega 2560 is a microcontroller board based on the ATmega2560 (datasheet). The technical specification of Arduino Mega 2560 such as 54 digital input/output pins (of which 14 can be used as PWM outputs), 16 analogue inputs, 4 UARTs (hardware serial ports), a 16 MHz crystal oscillator, an USB connection, a power jack, an ICSP header, and a reset button. The ATmega2560 has 256 KB of flash memory for storing code (of which 8 KB is used for the bootloader), 8 KB of SRAM and 4 KB of EEPROM (which can be read and written with the EEPROM library).
The Arduino Mega 2560 has advantages such as resettable poly-fuse that protect the computer's USB ports from shorts circuit and overcurrent. In addition, the device is designed in a way that allows it to be reset by software running on a connected computer.
4. Alarm
An alarm on the device aims as audio signaling if the sterilization time has ended or if the command stops actively. The work of the buzzer is controlled from the microcontroller, because the buzzer draws more current than the maximum current that the Arduino pin can provide, it is necessary to connect the buzzer to the Arduino using a transistor. The alarm used is an active buzzer with an operational voltage of 5 V_{DC}.
5. Ultraviolet Germicidal Lamp
The most important component at this equipment for sterilizing infant incubator enclosures is two ultraviolet germicidal lamps mounted on the sides of the appliance. The ultraviolet germicidal lamp has been obtained from the market with the brand Sankyo Denki type G4T5. This lamp can transmit ultraviolet rays at a wavelength of 253.7 nm and power UV output 0.8 watts.
6. Modul Inverter
The inverter module is one type of electronic ballast used in this study to convert direct voltage (DC) generated by a voltage booster of 6 V_{DC} to an alternating voltage (AC) of 220 V_{AC}. The output of this inverter module is used in principle to provide a voltage source to the ultraviolet germicidal lamp.
7. Display
The display unit that has been used in this study is a 2.4 in. TFT LCD. The display unit is able to display data in the form of text or strings, graphics or images (bitmaps) with a resolution of 320 × 240 pixels. Besides, the 2.4 in. TFT LCD includes a touchpad and able to display 65,000 different colors. The pin configuration used can be seen in the Table 1.
In this study, the display is used to input sterilization time settings and display the time, display the hour meter from the ultraviolet germicidal lamp and also provide a Start menu option to activate the system as an alternative to the start menu found on the remote.

Table 1 2.4" TFT LCD pinout

Pin name	Category
5 V, 3.3 V, GND	Power pins
LCD_RST	LCD command pins
LCD_CS	
LCD_RS	
LCD_WR	
LCD_RD	
LCD_D0–LCD_D7	LCD data pins

3.2 *Software Design*

Software design is a starting point to translate the system becomes a detailed document like a flowchart which states logically step by step system procedures. Figure 2 shows a flowchart of the sterilizer that has been made to allow implement better and easier computer programs. From Fig. 2, it can be seen that the sterilization process will start after the time setting and ends when the sterilization time has finished or when the stop button is pressed. Computer programs are prepared using the Arduino Integrated Development Environment Software (IDE) in assembly C. Furthermore, the computer programs are downloaded onto the Arduino Mega 2560 board.

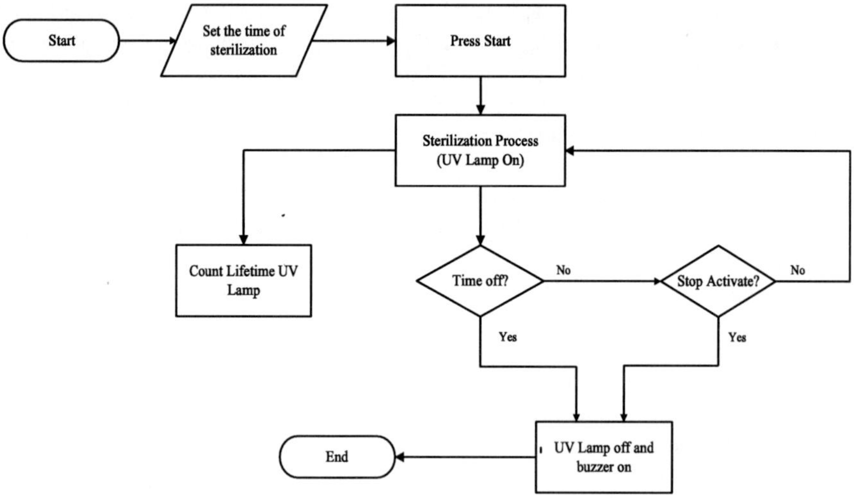

Fig. 2 Incubator sterilizer system flowchart

4 Results and Discussions

The size of the device is one of the observations recorded to ensure the device can be placed properly inside the infant incubator enclosure. The prototype of sterilizer equipment using an ultraviolet germicidal lamp that have been made has a size 200 × 375 × 75 mm (Width × Length × Height) as shown in Fig. 3. This size is good enough to be able to sterilize the infant incubator's surface area. Figure 4 shows the packaging of the device on the hard case as a protection of the lamp from impact, shocks and makes it easier to transport the equipment from one place to another place.

Another observation, the test results of the TFT LCD screen can be seen in Fig. 5, TFT LCD is able to run the sterilization time and display it. In addition, start and stop commands can be Run by touching the START menu on the screen. The LCD is also able to show the hour meter of the ultraviolet lamp.

UV Sterilizer equipment has a precise irradiation time design. This is proven by measuring the irradiation time performance using a digital stopwatch with brand ANYTIME which is presented in the form of data as can be seen in the Table 2. In addition, Fig. 6 shows linear graph of time duration of UV sterilizer equipment and time performance with mighty coefficient correlation R square = 1 which represents the UV sterilizer equipment has a good performance.

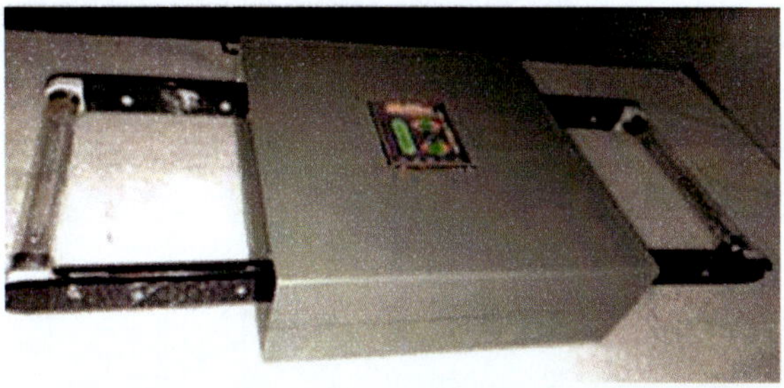

Fig. 3 The infant incubator sterilizer with two ultraviolet germicidal lamps on both sides

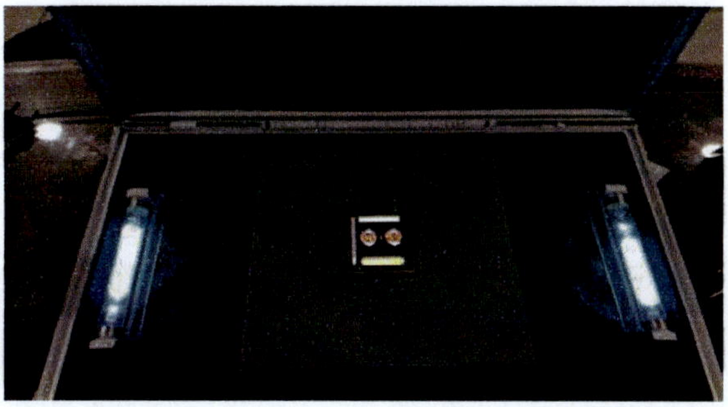

Fig. 4 The infant incubator sterilizer on the hard case box

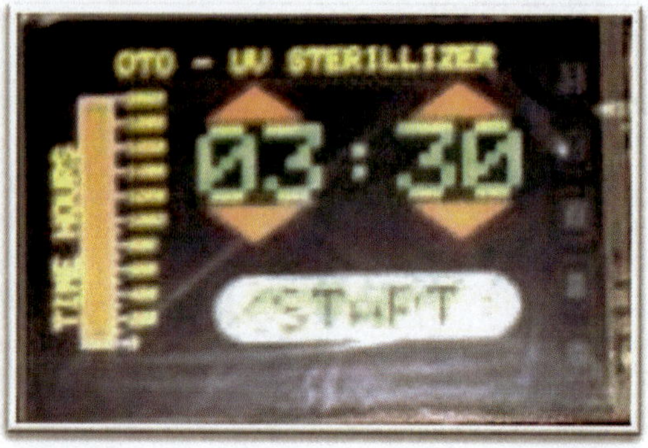

Fig. 5 Touch menu on the display unit

Table 2 Time irradiation data

Time (s)	Time of UV sterilizer (s)										t mean	Time of stopwatch (s)
	1	2	3	4	5	6	7	8	9	10		
1800	1800	1800	1800	1800	1800	1800	1800	1800	1800	1800	1800	1800
3600	3600	3600	3600	3600	3600	3600	3600	3600	3600	3600	3600	3600
5400	5400	5400	5400	5400	5400	5400	5400	5400	5400	5400	5400	5400
7200	7200	7200	7200	7200	7200	7200	7200	7200	7200	7200	7200	7200

Fig. 6 Linear graph of time irradiation of UV sterilizer

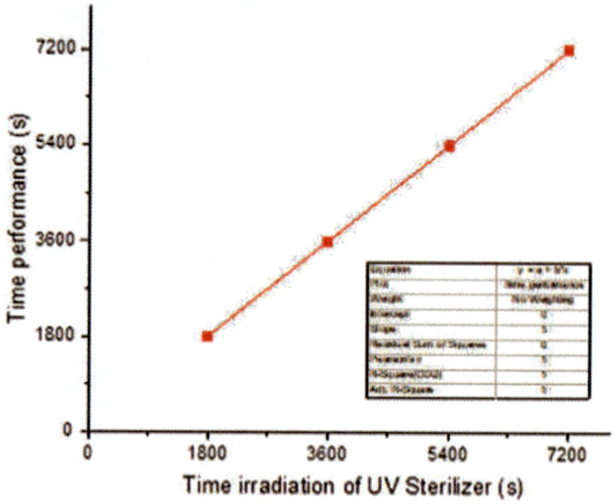

4.1 *UV Light Irradiation*

The effectiveness of UV light irradiation on sterilization of infant incubators has been observed. From the Fig. 7 shows that potentially percentage reduction in the number bacterial colonies of *Bacillus cereus* up to 52% and *Escherichia coli* up to

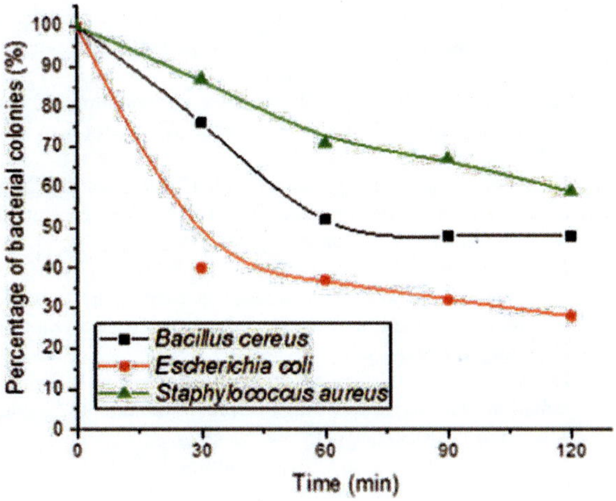

Fig. 7 The graph percentage of bacterial colonies after UV irradiation

37% after 60 min UV light irradiation. The percentage of bacterial colonies *Staphylococcus aureus* reduce significantly up to 59% after 120 min UV light irradiation.

5 Conclusion

The design of an infant incubator sterilizer using germicidal ultraviolet lamps can work following the design that has been done. As briefly described in this article, the research results time sterilization of UV sterilizer equipment has a good performance with coefficient correlation R square = 1 and indicate that UV light irradiation has potentially decreased the number of bacterial colonies of *Bacillus cereus*, *Escherichia coli* and *Staphylococcus aureus* in PCA media placed on the mattress in an infant incubator. The next work is the design of the installation of ultraviolet germicidal lamps which are safer from shocks and impact so as not to require hard box cases.

Acknowledgements This research was supported by Poltekkes Kemenkes Jakarta II through the Penelitian Hibah Bersaing Perguruan Tinggi 2017 (DL.02.021/5374/2017).

References

1. Rutala WA, Weber DJ (2013) Disinfection and sterilization in healthcare facilities. Bennett Brachman's Hosp Infect, 6th edn
2. Christina N, Ioanna P, George L, Konstantinos T, Georgios S (2015) Risk factors for nosocomial infections in neonatal intensive care units (NICU). Heal Sci J 9(2)

3. Fattorini M, Buonocore G, Lenzi D, Burgassi S, Cardaci RMR, Biermann KP et al (2018) Public health since the beginning: neonatal incubators safety in a clinical setting. J Infect Public Health [Internet] 11(6):788–792
4. Alkharasani MFT (2014) Bacterial contamination of new born incubator for delivery in Al-Zahraa teaching hospital in Al-Najaf Al-Ashraf province. Int J Innov Res Sci Eng Technol 3(2):9447–9449
5. Khan HA, Baig FK, Mehboob R (2017) Nosocomial infections: epidemiology, prevention, control and surveillance. Asian Pac J Trop Biomed [Internet] 7(5):478–482
6. Morillo-García Á, Aldana-Espinal JM, Olry de Labry-Lima A, Valencia-Martín R, López-Márquez R, Loscertales-Abril M et al (2015) Hospital costs associated with nosocomial infections in a pediatric intensive care unit. Gac Sanit [Internet] 29(4):282–287
7. Choudhary R, Bandla S (2012) Ultraviolet pasteurization for food industry. Int J Food Sci Nutr Eng 2(1):12–15
8. Levetin E, Shaughnessy R, Rogers CA, Scheir R (2001) Effectiveness of germicidal UV radiation for reducing fungal contamination within air-handling units. Appl Environ Microbiol 67(8):3712–3715
9. Welch D, Buonanno M, Grilj V, Shuryak I, Crickmore C, Bigelow AW et al (2018) Far-UVC light: a new tool to control the spread of airborne-mediated microbial diseases. Sci Rep [Internet] 8(1):1–7
10. Namala B, Shivashankar S, Harikrishna E, Swetha M (2017) Design, development and fabrication of batch type continuous UV-C light system for food products. J Pharmacogn Phytochem JPP 6(4):2078–2081
11. Bentancor M, Vidal S (2018) Programmable and low-cost ultraviolet room disinfection device. HardwareX [Internet]
12. Bokulich NA, Mills DA, Underwood MA (2013) Surface microbes in the neonatal intensive care unit: changes with routine cleaning and over time. J Clin Microbiol 51(8):2617–2624
13. Anderson DJ, Gergen MF, Smathers E, Sexton DJ, Chen LF, Weber DJ et al (2013) Decontamination of targeted pathogens from patient rooms using an automated ultraviolet-C-emitting device. Infect Control Hosp Epidemiol 34(5):466–471
14. Messina G, Burgassi S, Messina D, Montagnani V, Cevenini G (2015) A new UV-LED device for automatic disinfection of stethoscope membranes. Am J Infect Control [Internet] 43(10):e61–e66

Microstructure and Corrosion Behavior of Bioabsorbable Polymer Polylactic Acid-Polycaprolactone Reinforced by Magnesium-Zinc Alloy for Biomedical Application

Aprilia Erryani, Alfiyah Rahmah, Talitha Asmaria, Franciska Pramuji Lestari, and Ika Kartika

Abstract Medical composites have a lot of applications in medicine and orthopedic. Biomedical/orthopedic composites belong to biomaterials (Biomaterial can substitute natural tissues in the body and perform their functions). In this research, PLA (Polylactic Acid) and PCL (Polycaprolactone) polymer matrices filled with Mg6Zn alloy and observed the microstructure and electrochemical impedance spectroscopy. PLA and PCL were combined with a ratio of 7:3, 6:4, and 5:5 then dissolved respectively using chloroform. After that, mixed with Mg6Zn with three separate compositions of 5, 10 and 15%, it was then mould into a petri dish until it was dry. The structure was observed using scanning electron microscopy (SEM JEOL, JSM-6390A Japan). The immersion test examined the corrosion rate by observing the change in the pH, weight loss, and solubility of the composite in the simulation body solution using UV-Vis by looking at the specific functional group wavelength absorption area. Uv-Vis Analysis was conducted using Metrohm auto lab spectroelectrochemistry. The The microstructure found that the PLA-PCL-Mg6Zn biocomposite content is homogeneously mixed and uniformly distributed. Corrosion activity found by the immersion test, the reduced mass is not so large that it will last longer for bioabsorbable biomedical applications. 5PLA5PCL10Mg6Zn is an optimal composition because it decreases with pH most a little from the other, although the weight loss is not the least insignificant.

Keywords Bio-composite material · Poly-lactic acid · Poly-caprolactone · Magnesium · Zinc · Biomedical application

---

A. Erryani (✉) · T. Asmaria · F. P. Lestari · I. Kartika
Research Center for Metallurgy and Materials, Indonesian Institute of Sciences (LIPI), Kawasan Puspiptek Gedung 470 Serpong Tangerang Selatan, Banten 15314, Indonesia
e-mail: apri011@lipi.go.id

A. Rahmah
Departement of Metallurgy, University Technology of Sumbawa, Jl. Olat Maras, Batu Alang, Kec. Moyo Hulu, Kab, Sumbawa, Nusa Tenggara Barat, Indonesia

H. Triwiyanto et al. (eds.), *Proceedings of the 1st International Conference on Electronics, Biomedical Engineering, and Health Informatics*, Lecture Notes in Electrical Engineering 746, https://doi.org/10.1007/978-981-33-6926-9_32

1 Introduction

The perfect biomaterial for promoting medicine should be non-toxic, biocompatible, and has the capacity to stimulating tissue growth with adequate mechanical and physical property [1, 2]. The rate of degradation of biopolymers in biological systems can be exploited by changing the condition of the processing. Biodegradable polymers are desirable for orthopaedic fixation implants, cardiovascular stent, aneurysm clip and drug delivery system [3].

Orthopedic implants play an essential role in restoring daily activities and enhancing the quality of life of millions of people. Orthopedic implants are typically known as reconstructive or fracture management implants. One of the beneficial characteristics is the potential to degrade spontaneously in the physiological setting to prevent a second removal operation and to minimize the risk of local inflammation that may occur after long-term implantation of non-biodegradable implants [4–6].

Biodegradable technology offers the potential to create a vibrant market for peripheral stents, especially in the treatment of lower limb arteries. Biodegradable stents are usually designed to be absorbed in time scales smaller than those associated with metal stent fatigue, so long-term structural stability, strut fracturing, and fatigue stent failure are less concerned [7, 8]. For aneurysm clip, polymer composite be an alternative material for magnetic resonance (MR) susceptibility artifacts caused by metal clips [9, 10].

Most importantly, for the drug delivery system, these therapies are designed to be successful locally when needed. They are expected to monitor the drug release rate to maintain the drug target concentration without reaching a harmful level or falling below the minimum sufficient level. For these purposes, a significant effort has been made to create biodegradable materials capable of releasing drugs through reproducible and predictable kinetics [11–13].

Biocompatibility of materials is of primary importance for the prevention of inflammatory reactions and cytotoxic reactions. Biocompatibility with metallic implants is difficult to achieve due to the corrosive nature of the metals. Also, metals exhibit mechanical properties that are not equivalent to natural tissues, and thus, their mechanical properties need to be modified [14]. This can be achieved through the manufacture of composite materials. When the particles (as flakes or powders) of the reinforcement material are embedded or dispersed in the matrix material, they formed the composite particulates. In contrast, whereas the other forms are reinforced fiber composites and laminar composites [15]. In this article, a particulate reinforced composite was developed by embedding metal particles into a polymeric matrix. PLA (Polylactic Acid) and PCL (Polycaprolactone) are two essential members of the aliphatic polyester class of biodegradable materials.

For the ongoing task of dimensioning the ligament increase device (LAD), we are studying models to simulate the mechanical behavior evolution with the degradation that applies to this biodegradable device design process. Both these thermoplastics are hydrophilic with a slow degradation rate and have, therefore, been chosen for this specific application [16–18].

Magnesium materials have remarkable biodegradable properties and bioactive behavior due to the release of Mg^{2+} ions, which offer a promising potential for their use as biomaterials for tissue regeneration. However, Mg is one of the most reactive metals with a high rate of degradation. In contact with water, H2 is released, associated with the risk of implant failure [19, 20]. One solution to mitigate this draw-back is the use of Mg particles surrounded by biodegradable, biocompatible polymers [21, 22].

Similar to magnesium, zinc is an important trace element of the human body. It is a part of more than 300 enzymes and an even a larger number of other proteins, illustrating its indispensable role in human health. If zinc and magnesium are made as an alloy, the presence of zinc can withstand the reaction rate up to a level of 6% of the zinc composition in the alloy. So that in this study used PLA and PCL polymer matrices filled with Mg6Zn alloy for biomedical application and observed the microstructure and electrochemical impedance spectroscopy.

2 Experimental Method

Magnesium powder with 98.5% purity and particle size 0.06–0.3 mm, and zinc powder (99% purity, particle size <45 μm) were purchased from Merck. Polylactic acid (PLA) and Polycaprolactone (PCL) were purchased from Nature Work. Magnesium and zinc were combined with a ratio of Mg6Zn using a shaker mill for 30 min. PLA and PCL were mixed with a ratio of 7:3, 6:4, and 5:5 then dissolved respectively using chloroform. After dissolving, mixed with Mg6Zn with 3 variations of composition 5, 10, and 15%, then molded into a petri dish until dry. Microstructural analysis was performed by using Scanning electron microscopy (JEOL, JSM-6390A Japan). The corrosion rate was tested by immersion test, then observed changes in pH, weight loss, and solubility of the composite in the simulation body solution were observed using UV-Vis by looking at the absorption area of the wavelength of certain functional groups. Uv-Vis Analysis was performed by using Metrohm auto lab spectroelectrochemistry.

3 Result and Discussion

3.1 Microstructure Analisis

Caracterization of Mg6Zn Alloys

Magnesium and zinc are the main elements needed by the human body. Every day, the human body can absorb Mg and Zn within certain limits without affecting the human body condition. Magnesium is known to have a reasonably high degradation rate. The presence of Zn can help reduce the degradation rate of Mg. The Mg6Zn was used as a comparison because previous studies discussed the effect of adding

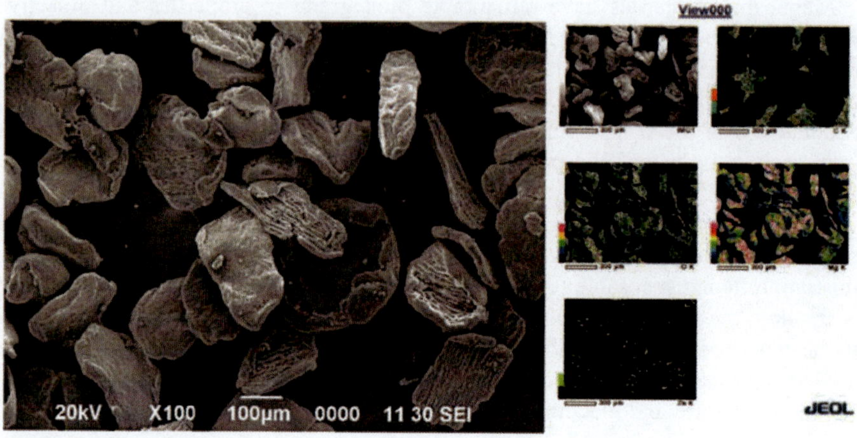

Fig. 1 SEM images and mapping Mg6Zn alloy

Zn to magnesium, where the optimum addition of Zn was at 6%. The addition of Zn to Mg can reduce the Mg maximum degradation rate at a 6%. More than 6%, the degradation rate of Mg will increase [21]. Figure 1 shows the SEM results of the Mg6Zn alloy after the milling process for uniform particle size.

The results of the SEM images of the particle size between Mg and Zn are almost uniform and the mapping results show that the distribution is evenly distributed between Mg and Zn particles. In the mapping results there is also a small amount of oxide. This is because the high-speed mixing process with a steel ball refiner produces heat and causes a reaction that produces oxides.

Optical Microscopy Analysis

Checking images using metallography aims to see the microstructure and distribution of metal alloys in the polymer. In the metallographic image (Fig. 2), there is no visible metal distribution in the biocomposite. In this figure, only the difference in polymer fiber pattern between PLA and PCL is seen, where the fiber owned by PCL is bigger than PLA, although there are differences in fiber patterns, PLA and PCL polymers can be mixed homogeneously using the same solvent. To confirm the distribution of metal alloys in the composite, it can be seen further using SEM with a greater magnification than metallography.

SEM Analysis of Biocomposite

See Fig. 3.

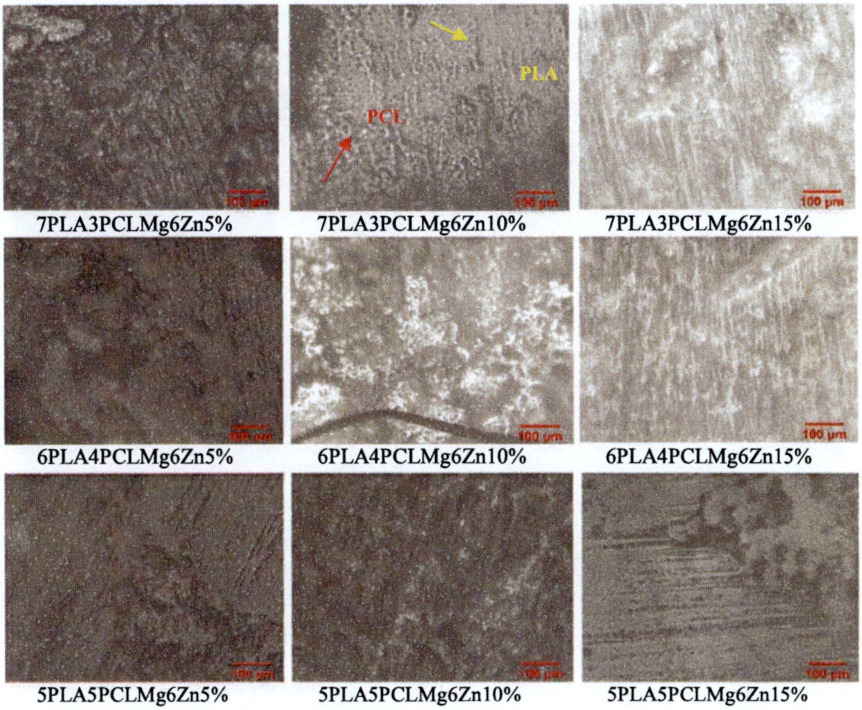

Fig. 2 Optical microscopy images of biocomposite PLA-PCL-Mg6Zn

3.2 Corrosion Evaluation

The corrosion rate was evaluated using the immersion method. Immersion is a real time observation of the rate of degradation of a material which is observed for 30 days. The material was immersed in a simulated human body solution. In this study, the solution used was hanks solution pH 7.4–7.6. During the observation process, what was observed every day was the change in pH and weight lost every 24 h (1 day). Then the material dissolved in the hanks solution will be observed using the UV-Vis spectrum.

pH Analysis of Hanks Solution during immersion Test

pH of the hanks solution, which was originally 7.4, will decrease to become acidic because the PLA and PCL which are acidic dissolve in the solution. In Table 1, the changes in pH in the hanks solution were recorded every 5 days. PLA as the dominant material in the bio composite causes the pH of the hanks solution to become increasingly acidic. PLA as an implant material that is biodegradable experiences degradation or corrosion as indicated by a decrease in the pH value to around 5–6 on the 30th day.

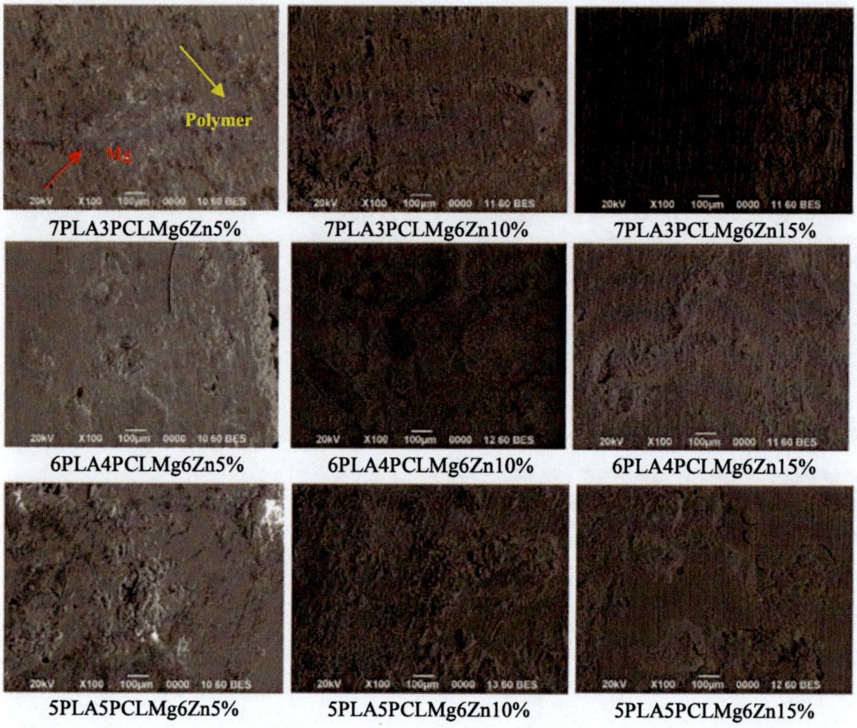

Fig. 3 SEM images of biocomposite PLA-PCL-Mg6Zn

Table 1 pH of hanks *level* solution during immersion test

Speciment composition(gram)	Days to -					
	5	10	15	20	25	30
5PLA5PCL5Mg6Zn	7.2	6.9	6.5	5.9	5.7	5.2
5PLA5PCL10Mg6Zn	7.5	7.4	7.3	6.9	6.7	6.5
5PLA5PCL15Mg6Zn	7.4	7.0	6.8	6.0	5.4	5.0
6PLA4PCL5Mg6Zn	7.0	6.0	5.7	5.7	5.0	5.0
6PLA4PCL10Mg6Zn	7.3	6.6	6.0	5.5	5.4	5.0
6PLA4PCL15Mg6Zn	6.0	6.7	6.2	5.7	5.0	5.0
7PLA3PCL5Mg6Zn	7.0	6.6	5.8	5.6	5.4	5.0
7PLA3PCL10Mg6Zn	6.5	6.1	5.8	5.6	5.3	5.1
7PLA3PCL15Mg6Zn	7.3	6.8	6.4	6.0	5.9	5.5

Table 2 Weight loss of Bio composite during immersion test

Specimen composition (gram)	Days to -						
	0	5	10	15	20	25	30
5PLA5PCL5Mg6Zn	0.695	0.693	0.685	0.682	0.684	0.674	0.656
5PLA5PCL10Mg6Zn	0.930	0.926	0.916	0.912	0.902	0.884	0.857
5PLA5PCL15Mg6Zn	0.250	0.248	0.237	0.233	0.220	0.209	0.203
6PLA4PCL5Mg6Zn	0.517	0.516	0.516	0.515	0.508	0.481	0.456
6PLA4PCL10Mg6Zn	0.522	0.520	0.516	0.508	0.522	0.509	0.485
6PLA4PCL15Mg6Zn	0.908	0.906	0.902	0.889	0.891	0.843	0.784
7PLA3PCL5Mg6Zn	0.467	0.463	0.453	0.450	0.418	0.328	0.306
7PLA3PCL10Mg6Zn	0.626	0.625	0.625	0.611	0.618	0.580	0.551
7PLA3PCL15Mg6Zn	1.155	1.153	1.145	1.130	1.118	1.113	1.056

Weight Loss Analysis

Because it has biodegradable and bioabsorbable properties, PLA/PCL/Mg6Zn composites will certainly experience corrosion or degradation during immersion in the simulated body solution. The weight loss in the sample was recorded every 5 days and its multiples up to day 30:

The weight loss that occurs during the immersion test also shows the occurrence of corrosion or degradation of the biocomposite material every immersion day. From the figures listed in the Table 2, the decline that occurs is not too significant when viewed every 5 days. The speed of weight loss that occurs will be faster with the length of the immersion time. From 0.002 to 0.02 every 5 days for up to 30 days. When compared to metal-based biodegradable implant materials such as Magnesium alloy, the corrosion rate is very fast so that additional treatment is needed to reduce the corrosion rate of Mg. The use of metal-polymer biocomposites is one solution that can be used to regulate the corrosion rate of implant materials. Of the weight loss observed for 30 days. The reduced mass is not so significant that it can last longer in its use.

UV-Vis Analysis of Hanks Solution after immersion process

The UV-Vis absorption test of the simulated body fluid, which in this experiment is a hanks solution, aims to determine the solubility of biocomposites that occurs on the fifth day and its multiples. For UV-Vis absorption data, it can be seen in one of the compositions of the biocomposite.

The UV-Vis absorption results support the results of the previous immersion test, the decrease in pH and mass loss that occurs during the immersion test. From the UV-Vis absorption data in Fig. 4, it can be seen that the absorption peak is getting bigger and bigger. The absorption peak height indicates the amount of material contained in the solution. In this observation, what is clearly visible is the absorption peak of the carboxyl group (RCOOR) at a wavelength of 204 nm which is the PLA functional group. The absorption peak of the PLA building blocks was the most visible because the PLA composition was most dominant in the

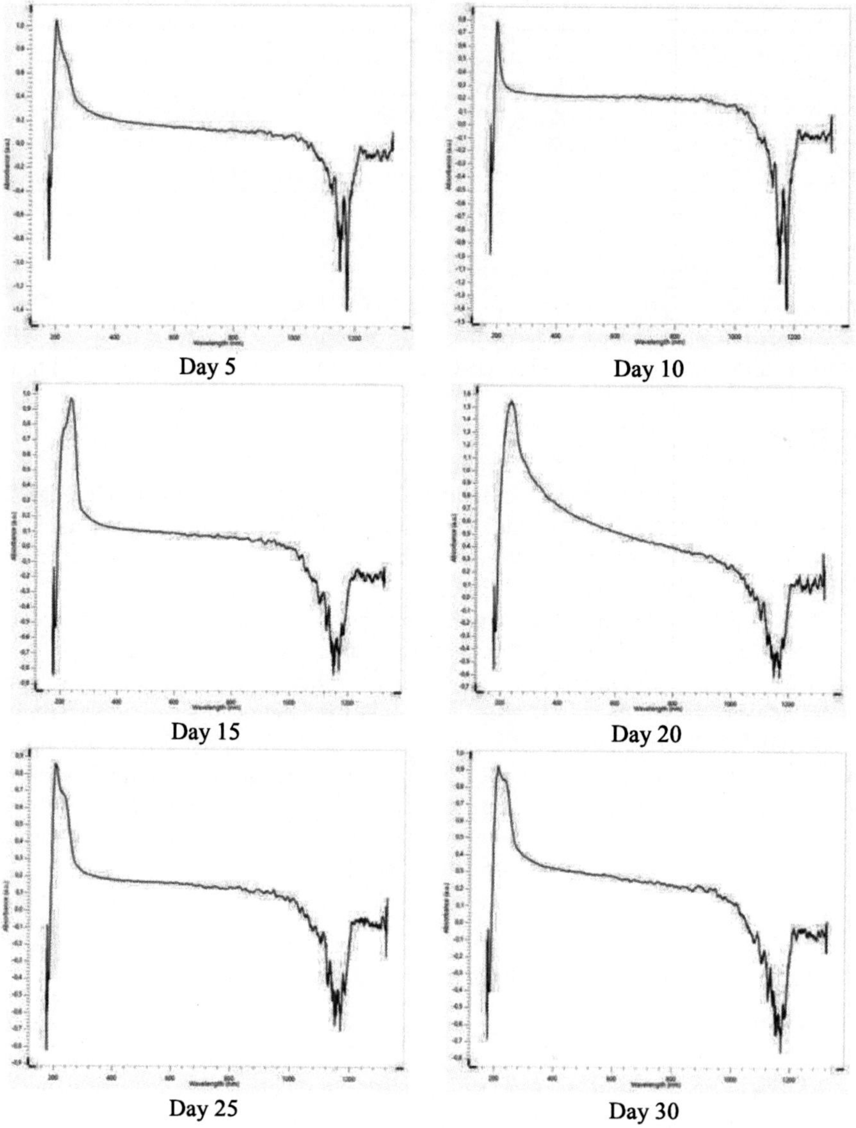

Fig. 4 UV-Vis absorption of hanks solution after immersion test

biocomposite material. Meanwhile, the functional groups possessed by PCL or metal alloys have not been seen due to the very few numbers and observations were only carried out for 30 days. From the result of pH and weight loss analysis, 5PLA5PCL10Mg6Zn is optimum composition because decreases of pH most a little from the other, although the weight loss not the least but the difference is insignificant.

4 Conclusion

Biocomposite PLA-PCL-Mg6Zn has been successfully prepared by solvent casting method. From microstructure analysis, the results of both optical microscopy and SEM can confirm that the PLA-PCL-Mg6Zn biocomposite material is homogeneously mixed and evenly distributed. Corrosion behaviour observed by immersion test, the reduced mass is not so significant that it can last longer in its use for bioarbsorbable biomedical application. But there are still improvements that need to be made to changes in pH. To keep the pH stable at 7.4–7.6, you can modify the composition or the process of making the material. 5PLA5PCL10Mg6Zn is optimum composition because decreases of pH most a little from the other, although the weight loss not the least but the difference is insignificant.

Acknowledgements This research was funded by riset and development, Health Ministry of Republic Indonesia. Special thanks to biocompatible & Biomedic research group for support and teamwork. First author of this paper is Aprilia Erryani.

References

1. Park S, Lih E, Park K, Ki Y, Keun D (2017) Progress in polymer science biopolymer-based functional composites for medical applications. Prog Polym Sci 77–105
2. Mohan S, Oluwafemi OS, Kalarikkal N, Thomas S, Songca SP (2016) Biopolymers application in nanoscience and nanotechnology. Recent Adv Biopoly 1(1):47–66
3. Praven Kumar A, Jackson Irudhayam S, Naviin D (2012) A Review on importance and recent applications of polymer composites in orthopaedics. Int J Eng Res Devel 5(2):40–43
4. Manivasagam G, Suwas S (2014) Biodegradable Mg and Mg based alloys for biomedical implants. Mater Sci Technol 30(5):515–520
5. Moutos FT, Guilak F (2008) Composite scaffolds for cartilage tissue engineering. Biorheology 45(3–4):501–512
6. Jin Sing Y, Jason LG, Antonious GM, Chunyan H, Guang C (2018) Material processing and design of biodegradable metal matrix composites for biomedical applications. Ann Biomed Eng 46(9):1229–1240
7. Peuster M, Wohlsein P, Brügmann M, Ehlerding M, Seidler K, Fink C, Brauer H, Fischer A, Hausdo G (2001) A novel approach to temporary stenting: degradable cardiovascular stents produced from corrodible metal—results 6–18 months after implantation into New Zealand white rabbits, pp 563–569

8. Zhu Y, Yang K, Cheng R, Xiang Y, Yuan T, Cheng Y, Sarmento B, Cui W (2017) The current status of biodegradable stent to treat benign luminal disease. Mater Today 20(9):516–529
9. Teping F, Fischer G, Huelser M et al (2019) A new clip generation for microsurgical treatment of intracranial aneurysms-the first case series. World Neurosurg 1–6
10. Won Sang C, Kyung il C, Jeong Eun K, Tae Sik J, Eun Jin H, Hyun Seung K, Young Je S, Seung Hong C, Seung hyun L, Chong Chan K, Jeong Yun S, Hyoun Ee K (2018) Zirconia-polyurethane aneurysm clip. World Neurosurg 155, 14–23
11. Aoki K, Saito N (2020) Biodegradable polymers as drug delivery systems for bone regeneration, pp 1–19
12. Najabat Ali M, Ansari U, Sami J, Qayyum F, Mir M (2016) To develop a biocompatible and biodegradable polymer-metal composite with good, mechanical and drug release properties. J Mater Sci Eng 5(5)
13. Nigmatullin R, Thomas P, Lukasiewicz B, Puthussery H, Roy I (2015) Polyhydroxyalkanoates, a family of natural polymers, and their applications in drug delivery. J Chem Technol Biotechnol 1209–1221
14. Vieira AC, Vieira JC, Ferra JM, Magalhães FD, Guedes RM, Marques AT (2011) Mechanical study of PLA—PCL fibers during in vitro degradation. J Mech Behav Biomed Mater 4 (3):451–460
15. Stanislav E, Pavel D, Mikhail T, Sarkis D, Sergey R, Anastasia S, Mikhail K, Stepan K, Ivan S, Petr T, Iskander A (2019) Flexible polycaprolactone and polycaprolactone/graphene scaffolds for tissue engineering. Materials
16. Zhao C, Wu H, Ni J, Zhang S, Zhang X (2017) Development of PLA/Mg composite for orthopedic implant: tunable degradation and enhanced mineralization. Compos Sci Technol
17. Yongjun C, Zhigang X, Christopher S, Jag S (2014) Recent advances on the development of Magnesium alloys for biodegradable implants. Acta Biomaterialia
18. Zivić F, Grujović N, Manivasagam G, Richard C, Landoulsi J, Petrović V (2014) The potential of magnesium alloys as bioabsorbable/biodegradable implants for biomedical applications. Tribol Ind 36(1):67–73
19. Lei B, Guo B, Rambhia KJ, Ma PX (2018) Hybrid polymer biomaterials for bone tissue regeneration
20. Ferrández Montero A, Lieblich M, González Carrasco JL, Benavente R, Lorenzo V, Detsch R, Boccaccini AR, Ferrari B (2019) Development of biocompatible and fully bioabsorbable PLA/Mg films for tissue regeneration applications. Acta Biomater 98:114–124
21. Levy GK, Goldman J, Aghion E (2017) The prospects of Zinc as a structural material for biodegradable implants—a review paper, pp 1–18
22. Walsh CT, Sandstead HH, Prasad AS, Newberne PM, Fraker PJ. Zinc (1994) Health effects and research priorities for the 1990s, pp 5–46

Seizure Classification on Epileptic EEG Using IMF-Entropy and Support Vector Machine

Achmad Rizal, Inung Wijayanto, and Sugondo Hadiyoso

Abstract Various methods have been developed by researchers to recognize brain abnormalities through EEG signals. One of the diseases or disorders of the brain is seizures in epilepsy. EEG signals in seizure conditions display a different pattern compared to EEG signals in normal conditions. Researchers analyzed the EEG signal using a variety of observed approaches. One phenomenon used to analyze EEG signals is signal complexity. Signal complexity captures fluctuating patterns of EEG signals quantizing them to distinguish normal and seizure signal conditions. In this study, we propose the proper feature extraction method based on the basic characteristic of the signal. We extract the EEG signal's information using entropy calculation from the intrinsic mode function (IMF entropy). Our main goal is to distinguish normal and seizure EEG signals. The entropy is calculated from the IMF resulted from empirical mode decomposition (EMD), then entropy from the relative energy of each IMF. To test the performance of the proposed feature extraction method, the support vector machine (SVM) is used as a classifier. The highest accuracy is 86.3%, sensitivity is 86.33%, and the specificity is 93.17% for three data classes: normal, interictal, and seizure. The proposed method has the potential to improve its performance, considering there are still many variations of EMD methods and decomposition levels that can be evaluated. Furthermore, testing on more massive datasets is interesting to do in future research.

Keywords Epilepsy · EEG · Entropy · IMF · SVM

A. Rizal (✉) · I. Wijayanto
School of Electrical Engineering, Telkom University, Bandung, Indonesia
e-mail: achmadrizal@telkomuniversity.ac.id

S. Hadiyoso
School of Applied Science, Telkom University, Bandung, Indonesia

H. Triwiyanto et al. (eds.), *Proceedings of the 1st International Conference on Electronics, Biomedical Engineering, and Health Informatics*, Lecture Notes in Electrical Engineering 746, https://doi.org/10.1007/978-981-33-6926-9_33

1 Introduction

Some abnormalities in the brain and nervous system produce different patterns of signal electroencephalogram (EEG). This difference can be seen from the shape of the signal, signal dynamics, or frequency content of the signal [1]. Various methods have been developed to help doctors automatically analyze abnormalities in EEG signals due to the nonstationary nature of EEG signals. The method used usually consists of a transformation process and a feature extraction method. The example of signal transformation methods are wavelet transform [2], empirical mode decomposition (EMD) [3] or short-term Fourier transform (STFT) [4]. Meanwhile, feature extraction methods used are such as entropy [5], fractal [6], or statistical parameter [7].

EMD is quite widely used in EEG signal analysis. EMD for seizure detection in EEG signals is reported in [8]. The statistical features on the IMF are used for the classification of EEG signals. The proposed method was resulting in an accuracy of up to 96%. Meanwhile, EMD and fuzzy entropy produced 99.8% accuracy for the classification of normal and seizure EEG [9]. Liu et al. used the coefficient of variation and fluctuation index from the results of EMD and SVM decomposition for the Ictal EEG classification [10]. In other studies, EMD combined with entropy yielded an accuracy of up to 97.3% for three data classes [11].

In the aforementioned studies, the features are calculated from the IMF as the result of the EMD. The number of features produced depends on the features calculated from each IMF. Another approach for calculating the characteristics of EMD results is proposed by Yu et al. [12]. The relative energy is calculated in the IMF to get the entropy value based on EMD energy. This method was tested for roller bearing fault diagnoses. This study proposes the use of EMD energy entropy by using several IMF. As we know, the most significant signal energy is spread in the early IMF. By using different IMF, we can see the energy distribution of the original signal.

2 Materials and Methods

2.1 EEG Dataset

This study uses a public dataset made by Andrzejak et al. [13] from Bonn University, Germany. The dataset is recorded from scalp EEG following the 10–20 international electrode placement. An average common reference and 128 channel amplifier system are used in the recording process. This dataset consists of five different classes, normal, interictal, and ictal conditions. The normal condition is recorded from volunteers with eyes open (set Z) and eyes closed (set O) conditions. The interictal condition is recorded by using intracranial electrodes from the hippocampal formation of the brain (set N) and from the epileptogenic zone (set F).

The last class is the ictal condition (set S), which recorded in the seizure activity. The example of each class from Bonn University dataset is shown in Fig. 1.

2.2 Empirical Mode Decomposition

A biological signal is known as a non-stationary signal. A proper method is needed to analyze such a signal. Empirical mode decomposition (EMD) is a well-known method to analyze a non-stationary signal. Decomposing a biological signal into several levels can give better information. The use of EMD to decompose biological signals such as EEG has done by other studies such as in [14–16]. EMD decomposes the EEG signal into a number of intrinsic mode functions (IMF)s. The IMFs is a band-limited function that has two main criteria. The first one is the number of extrema and zero-crossings of the whole IMFs must be equal with one, but at some case can be differed at most one. The local minima and maxima's mean values must be zero for any data location is the next IMF's criteria that need to be fulfilled [17]. The representation of EMD is shown in (1).

$$s(t) = \sum_{m=1}^{M} h_m(t) + r_m(t) \tag{1}$$

Here, the $s(t)$ is the signal, $h_m(t)$ is the IMF, and $r_m(t)$ is the last number of IMF, or the signal's residue.

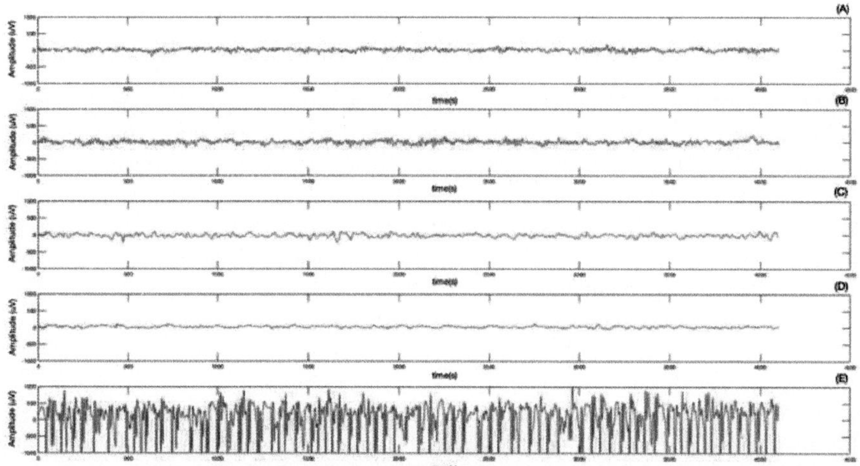

Fig. 1 Example of each class from Bonn University dataset

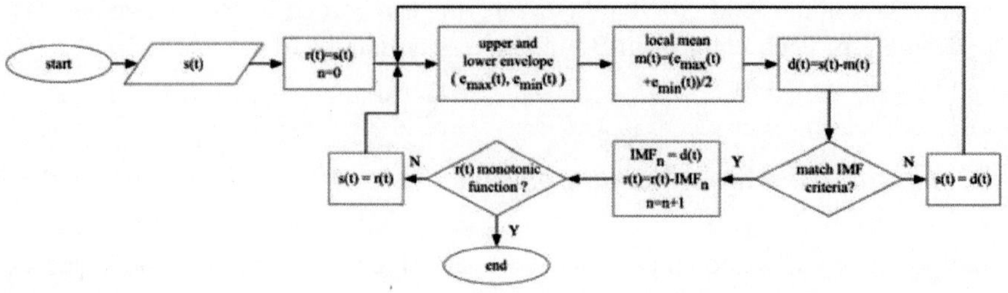

Fig. 2 EMD process

Figure 2 describe the process of EMD in generating IMFs. First is calculating the lower $(e_{\min}(t))$ and upper envelope $(e_{\max}(t))$ followed by calculating the local mean using (2).

$$m(t) = \frac{e_{\min}(t) + e_{\max}(t)}{2} \tag{2}$$

The $m(t)$ is then used to calculate the detail using (3).

$$d(t) = s(t) - m(t) \tag{3}$$

Here, the detail then checked whether it is matched with the IMF's criteria or not. If it does not match, then the detail is used as the new input, while if it does match, then the detail is selected as the IMF $(h_m(t))$. The process is continued by removing the IMF from the signal using (4).

$$r(t) = r(t) - h_m(t) \tag{4}$$

The process is repeated until the $r(t)$ becomes a monotonic function.

IMF that produced by the EMD, has some limitations. One of them is the mode mixing caused by the abnormal distribution of the local extrema. Mode mixing made the IMFs have multiple intrinsic time scales at different frequencies. This condition made two adjacent IMFs face an aliasing condition. Thus, it made them hard to discern [18, 19]. However, this study does not focus on resolving the mode mixing problem, but to assess the nonstationary feature of the IMF's energy by analyzing the entropy feature.

2.3 *IMF Entropy*

The IMF entropy was first proposed by Yu et al. [12]. In IMF entropy, entropy is calculated from the energy in each IMF $(IMF(n))$ resulting from EMD. As in the previous subsection the signal $s(n)$ is stated as in (5).

$$s(n) = IMF(n)_1 + IMF(n)_2 + \ldots + IMF(n)_k + R_s(n) \quad (5)$$

With $R_s(n)$ is the residue. The energy of IMF (E_i) is calculated using (6) and (7), while the relative energy of each IMF (P_i) is expressed as in (8).

$$E_i = \sum (IMF_i)^2 \quad (6)$$

$$E_t = \sum_{i=1}^{k} E_i \quad (7)$$

$$P_i = E_i / E_t \quad (8)$$

Thus, the IMF entropy can be calculated as (9).

$$IMF_{ent} = -\sum P_L . \ln P_l \quad (9)$$

The number of IMF used in this study was changed from 2 to 5. The number of IMF = 5 was determined based on previous research, which proved that IMF = 5 produced the highest accuracy [14]. For this reason, in this study, we used four features that correspond to the number of IMF = 2, 3, 4, and 5.

2.4 Classification

In this stage the proposed feature extraction method is validated by classifying the measured feature vectors. We use support vector machine (SVM) with several kernels to test the performance of the proposed method. SVM was chosen in this study because it has been reported to have a good performance in the application of classification cases, especially biomedical signals [14, 20, 21]. Since it was first introduced by Vapnik, the concept of SVM is to find the best separation line between two classes [22]. This separation line is then called a hyperplane with supporting vectors [23]. SVM was initially implemented in linear cases, but then there were many cases of non-linear classification so that a non-linear kernel was developed to deal with the problem. In this study, feature vectors are having linear characteristics so that performance validation is performed using the linear kernel. SVM with linear kernel is expressed in (10).

$$K(X, Y) = X^T Y \quad (10)$$

Since the SVM is a supervised learning method, cross validation is required to separate the training data and the test data. It is also used to avoid overfitting. In this study, ten-fold cross validation is used to run the performance test simulation of the proposed method.

3 Results

Figure 3a–d shows the value of IMF entropy for IMF2 to IMF5. IMF2 entropy had 2 IMFs used to calculate entropy, while at IMF5, it means there were 5 IMFs used to calculate entropy. It can be seen that some IMF entropy values overlap, giving rise to potential errors in the classification process. The performance of the use of IMF entropy was tested using SVM with several test scenarios.

Table 1 displays the classification accuracy using three data classes, normal (set Z and O), interictal (set N and F), and ictal/seizure (set S). The highest accuracy reached 86.3% for class Z-N-S with a sensitivity of 86.33% and specificity 93.17%.

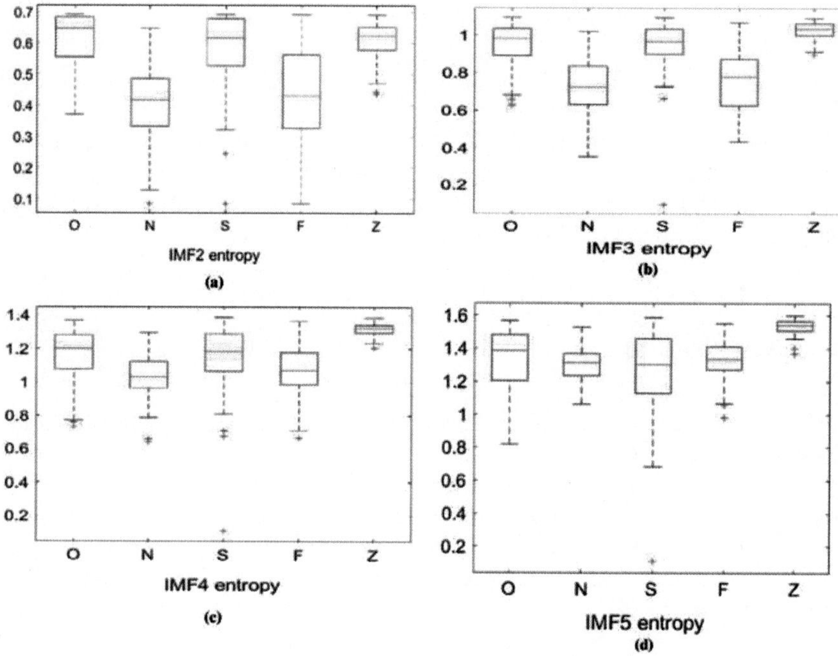

Fig. 3 **a** IMF2 Entropy; **b** IMF3 Entropy; **c** IMF4 Entropy; **d** IMF5 Entropy

Table 1 Classification result using Linear SVM

Scenario for 3 classes	Number of data	Acc (%)	Sens (%)	Spe (%)
Z-N-S	100-100-100	86.3	86.33	93.17
Z-F-S	100-100-100	85.3	95.33	92.67
O-N-S	100-100-100	82.67	82.67	91.33
O-F-S	100-100-100	84.67	84.67	92.33
ZO-NF-S	200-200-100	82.6	80.17	90.72

If sensitivity is the primary performance metric, the best classification result was achieved for Z-F-S with a sensitivity of 95.33%. This result was achieved using five IMF entropy values because the use of only one entropy value would result in lower accuracy. In general, IMF entropy produced relatively the same value in each class because IMF entropy was calculated from the relative energy value of each IMF. Figure 3a–d show that there are similar values in each category. As in Fig. 3a, the entropy values of set Z, set O, and set S are intersect with each other, so does with set N and set F. Thus, a combination between the five IMF entropy is used to give a better characteristic of the signal.

Meanwhile, the total energy from the EMD was not much different for each EEG signal. This caused the IMF entropy value not to change too much for each class of data. As in Table 1, the classification results are quite moderate, considering the small number of features. The accuracy produced by the proposed method is not as good as reported in previous studies using other entropies [8–11] However, this method provides a new alternative to the calculation of entropy in biomedical signals. One of the advantages of EMD is that the ability to display fundamental fluctuations of signals independent of any kernel can be strengthened by calculating the entropy from the generated IMF. Some possible developments of the proposed method include the calculation of involving more number of IMF, calculation by involving residual EMD results, or the use of other variations of EMD.

4 Conclusion

This research proposes the feature extraction method using IMF entropy for the classification of EEG seizures. The proposed method used the IMF of EMD results to calculate the EEG signal's entropy as a characteristic to distinguish the EEG signal. The IMF entropy value for each data class looks not too different, so it looks overlap between data classes. The use of several IMF entropy values was proven to produce accuracy up to 86.3% for three classes of data. This value was quite high compared to using only one entropy value. Even though the accuracy produced was not as high as other methods, this method can still be developed by exploring several EMD parameters and entropy. The proposed method can also be used in other biological signals such as ECG and EMG.

References

1. Yuvaraj R, Murugappan M, Mohamed Ibrahim N, Sundaraj K, Omar MI, Mohamad K, Palaniappan R (2014) Detection of emotions in Parkinson's disease using higher order spectral features from brain's electrical activity. Biomed Signal Process Control 14:108–116
2. Malar E, Gauthaam M (2020) Wavelet analysis of EEG for the identification of alcoholics using probabilistic classifiers and neural networks. Int J Intell Sustain Comput 1:3

3. Djemili R, Bourouba H, Amara Korba MC (2016) Application of empirical mode decomposition and artificial neural network for the classification of normal and epileptic EEG signals. Biocybern Biomed Eng 36:285–291
4. Patil A, Deshmukh C, Panat AR (2016) Feature extraction of EEG for emotion recognition using Hjorth features and higher order crossings. In: IEEE on 2016 Conference on advances in signal processing (CASP), pp 429–434
5. Wijayanto I, Rizal A, Hadiyoso S (2018) Multilevel wavelet packet entropy and support vector machine for epileptic EEG classification. In: Proceedings—2018 4th international conference on science and technology, ICST 2018
6. Ferenets R, Lipping T, Anier A, Jantti V, Melto S, Hovilehto S (2006) Comparison of entropy and complexity measures for the assessment of depth of sedation. IEEE Trans Biomed Eng 53:1067–1077
7. Padma Shri TK, Sriraam N (2016) Spectral entropy feature subset selection using SEPCOR to detect alcoholic impact on gamma sub band visual event related potentials of multichannel electroencephalograms (EEG). Appl Soft Comput 46:441–451
8. Shaikh, MHN, Farooq O, Chandel G (2019) EMD analysis of EEG signals for seizure detection. In: Lecture notes in electrical engineering, pp 189–196
9. Tripathi D, Agrawal N (2019) Epileptic seizure detection using empirical mode decomposition based fuzzy entropy and support vector machine. In: Lecture notes in electrical engineering, pp 109–118
10. Li S, Zhou W, Yuan Q, Geng S, Cai D (2013) Feature extraction and recognition of ictal EEG using EMD and SVM. Comput Biol Med 43:807–816
11. Wijayanto I (2019) Epileptic seizure detection in EEG signal using EMD and entropy. In: The international conference on advancement in data science, E-learning and information systems 2019 ICADEIS2019)
12. Yu Y, YuDejie Junsheng C (2006) A roller bearing fault diagnosis method based on EMD energy entropy and ANN. J Sound Vib 294:269–277
13. Andrzejak RG, Lehnertz K, Mormann F, Rieke C, David P, Elger CE (2001) Indications of nonlinear deterministic and finite-dimensional structures in time series of brain electrical activity: dependence on recording region and brain state. Phys Rev E 64:061907
14. Wijayanto I, Hartanto R, Nugroho HA (2020) Comparison of empirical mode decomposition and coarse-grained procedure for detecting pre-ictal and ictal condition in electroencephalography signal. Inf Med Unlocked 19:100325
15. Sharma R, Pachori R, Acharya U (2015) Application of entropy measures on intrinsic mode functions for the automated identification of focal electroencephalogram signals. Entropy 17:669–691
16. Muralidhar Bairy, G., Hagiwara, Y.: Empirical Mode Decomposition-Based Processing For Automated Detection Of Epilepsy. J. Mech. Med. Biol. 19, (2019)
17. Huang NE, Shen Z, Long SR, Wu MC, Shih HH, Zheng Q, Yen NC, Tung CC, Liu HH (1998) The empirical mode decomposition and the Hilbert spectrum for nonlinear and non-stationary time series analysis. Proc R Soc London Ser A Math Phys Eng Sci 454:903–995
18. Xue Y, Cao J, Du H, Zhang G, Yao Y (2016) Does mode mixing matter in EMD-based highlight volume methods for hydrocarbon detection? Experimental evidence. J Appl Geophys 132:193–210
19. Tao R, Ren H, Peng X (2017) Modeling, design and simulation of systems. Asian Simul Conf 752:249–260
20. Mohammadpour M, Hashemi SMR, Houshmand N (2017) Classification of EEG-based emotion for BCI applications. In: IEEE on 2017 Artificial intelligence and robotics (IRANOPEN), pp 127–131

21. Bradbury JH, Jenkins GA (1984) Determination of the structures of trisaccharides by 13C-n.m.r. spectroscopy. Carbohydr Res 126:125–156
22. Boser BE, Guyon IM, Vapnik VN (1992) A training algorithm for optimal margin classifiers. In: Proceedings of the fifth annual workshop on Computational learning theory—COLT '92, pp 144–152. ACM Press, New York, USA
23. Cevikalp H (2017) Best fitting hyperplanes for classification. IEEE Trans Pattern Anal Mach Intell 39:1076–1088

Influence of Thermo-Mechanical Processing on Microstructure, Mechanical Properties and Corrosion Behavior of Ti-6Al-6Mo Implant Alloy

Ika Kartika, Fendy Rokhmanto, Yudi Nugraha Thaha, Ibrahim Purawiardi, I. Nyoman Gede Putrayasa Astawa, Aprilia Erryani, and Talitha Asmaria

Abstract In this work, titanium alloy with additional aluminum and molybdenum is expected to be used as a clip aneurysm material. Thermo-mechanical processing (TMP) is required to achieve excellent workability in this alloy. The TMP of Ti-6Al-6Mo alloy composition has been successfully prepared. The alloy was homogenized at 1100 °C–12 h. The method is then continued to solution treatment with T = 1100 °C–30 min and hot-rolled by 80% deformation. The last method is heat-treated with T = 1100 °C–1 h followed by quenching in different media of air, water, and ice. The corrosion behavior of this alloy was investigated using Hank's solution by polarization method. In the Ti-6Al-6Mo alloy with a hardness value of 44.4 HRc, the TMP and the quenching in water obtained various nucleations of the α-phases, less of the lamellar α-phase and less of the α-colony. The water-quenched Ti-6Al-6Mo alloy has excellent passive film stability and is more likely to increase the alloy corrosion efficiency.

Keywords Ti-6Al-6Mo alloy · Thermo-mechanical processing · Alpha-colony

1 Introduction

These Ti-6Al-6Mo alloy categorizes as (α + β) titanium alloy, where 6 wt% Al as a stabilizer of α-phase and 6 wt% of Mo as a stabilizer for β [1]. The successfully developing (α + β) titanium alloys can be controlled by the heat treatment and its parameters. In addition, an increasing number of substituting elements would have

I. Kartika (✉) · F. Rokhmanto · Y. N. Thaha · I. Purawiardi · I. N. G. P. Astawa · A. Erryani · T. Asmaria
Research Center for Metallurgy and Materials, Indonesian Institute of Sciences (LIPI), Kawasan Puspiptek Serpong, Tangerang Selatan 15310, Indonesia
e-mail: ikak061001@gmail.com

H. Triwiyanto et al. (eds.), *Proceedings of the 1st International Conference on Electronics, Biomedical Engineering, and Health Informatics*, Lecture Notes in Electrical Engineering 746, https://doi.org/10.1007/978-981-33-6926-9_34

an effect on mechanical strength and ductility. The mechanical properties are highly affected by the microstructure and will also affect the corrosion resistance of this alloy.

In the ($\alpha + \beta$) titanium alloy, the structure has been characterized into several types, specifically grain boundary allotriomorph α, globular of primary α, widmanstatten, basketweave, and martensitic which depending on cooling rate and previous of heat treatment process. The change of β-phase will mention according to heat-treated or final temperature of hot forming process and also have a heterogeneous morphology mainly based on the cooling rate and the composition of the Ti alloy. At rapid cooling, the β-phase can change to α martensitically, but it alters to Widmanstatten plates of α by nucleation and growth at lower cooling rates [2].

Besides that, Ti alloy corrosion resistance as implant surgical is very interesting and needs to be studied. The Ti implant alloy is maintained being destructive when reacting in the biological body fluid because of the releasing of prosthesis, inflammation, abrasive corrosion, and metabolism. The TiO_2 passive film in Ti alloys will covering the surface making its alloy has good corrosion resistance [3]. The atmosphere, chemical composition and the applied potential are the parameters that will affect the configuration of the passive layer on Titanium based alloys [4]. Guo and Krawiec concluded that the presence of a various passive film and some oxides will improve the protection of the properties of Titanium alloys [5, 6]. The Tafel extrapolation method used to persistence corrosion rates is well-founded by the condition as follow; the anodic and cathodic reactions which demonstrate at the corrosion potential are also the only reactions which reveal during the persistence of the polarization curves; corrosion in general, and localized corrosion does not take place; the polarization curves are hold steady [7].

There has not been much literature on the influence of thermo-mechanical processing on the microstructure, mechanical property, and Ti-6Al-6Mo alloy corrosion resistance. Therefore, this study will give an overview of thermo-mechanical processing and quenching in various media in Ti-6Al-6Mo alloy. From this study, the result will illustrate the characteristics of the Ti alloy and categorize it. Thermo-mechanical processing is supposed to have a uniform structure. Such a condition is suitable for the workability of Ti-6Al-6Mo alloy as a material for the implant.

2 Experimental

2.1 *Alloying Element and Thermo-Mechanical Processing (TMP)*

The metallic elements are 99.9% purity of Ti, Mo, and Al from Merck. The alloy composition target is 6 wt% Al, 6 wt% Mo and 98 wt% of Ti. All metallic elements are dissolved through a vacuum arc furnace in the atmosphere of argon. The as cast alloy after re-melted has a diameter approximately 7.5 mm, and the length is

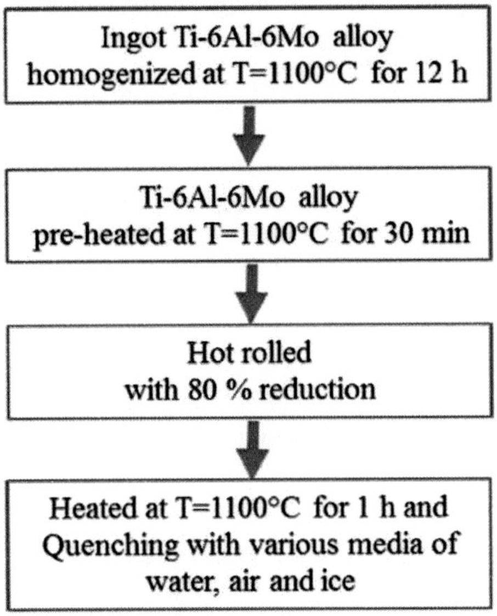

Fig. 1 The flow chart of heating process on the alloy of Ti-6Al-6Mo

80 mm. It was homogenized at vacuum tube furnace at temperature of 1100 °C–12 h and cooling in a furnace with atmosphere of argon. Pre-heating was conducted to the alloy composition at a temperature of 1100 °C–30 min followed by 80% and greater of the heavy hot rolling deformation. The solution treatment at temperature of 1100 °C–1 h was conducted after hot rolling, and quenching at different media of cooling; ice, water, and air. The flow chart of the above heating process was explained in Fig. 1.

2.2 *Microstructure Observation and Mechanical Test*

The alloy samples after heat-treated were observed using optical microscopy (OM) to investigate the phase that was formed after thermo-mechanical processing (TMP) followed by quenching in various media. The surface of the samples corroded by using Kalling's reagent etchant. The alloy mechanical property after heat-treated was measured by Rockwell hardness testing.

2.3 *Corrosion Test*

The solution used to examine the corrosion resistance of the alloy is Hanks' solution. Hanks' solution chemical composition is shown on Table 1. The solution was maintained at human body temperature at 37 °C and the pH was 7.4.

Table 1 Composition of Hanks' solution (g/L) used to investigate the action of corrosion of Ti-6Al-6Mo alloy

NaCl	$MgCl_2$	$CaCl_2$	KCl	KH_2PO_4	NaHCO3	Na_2HPO_4	KH_2PO_4	Glucose
8.0	0.2	0.14	0.4	0.06	0.35	0.06	0.06	1.0

The corrosion rate was conducted to the as-cast, as-hot rolled and the alloy after TMP- quenching in different media. Linear polarization as well as Tafel extrapolation methods were used to assess the corrosion rate. Corrosion testing was conducted using the GIATEC potentiostat potentiodynamic polarization process. This system has variety of electrodes, such as test, counter and reference at a scan rate of 1 mv/s. A potential was maintained in the range of OCP (open circuit potential) ranging from 100 to 300 mV.

3 Results and Discussion

3.1 Thermo-Mechanical Processing and Microstructure Result

The structure of ingot Ti-6Al-6Mo alloy showed a basket weave structure where lamellar α-phase in the interior of β matrix, α + β colony and β-prior grain boundary (Fig. 2). The β grain size is large ($\geq$ 100 μm). The value of the hardness of the ingot alloy is approximately 44 HRc.

Figure 3a–d exhibited optical microscopy of the Ti-6Al-6Mo alloy after thermo-mechanical processing (TMP) and quenching in air, water, and ice. The hot rolled alloy structure showed numerous lamellar α-phases in the β matrix, α + β colony, less of α-colony and β-prior grain boundary (Fig. 3a). Figure 3b obtained nucleation α-phase in β grain interior, less of lamellar α-phase and β-phase as a matrix, while in Fig. 3c showed that α-phase was nucleated along β grain boundaries, nucleation α-phase in the interior β grain and less of lamellar α-phase. The β grain boundary in the ice quenched alloy has not shown fully formed yet. As can be seen in the Fig. 3d, numerous α-phase was nucleated in the interior grain of β matrix. Also, α-phases was formed along the β-prior grain boundary (Fig. 3d).

3.2 Hardness Result

The alloy hardness value after TMP-quenching was obtained in Fig. 4. The hardness value after TMP measured approximately 46 HRc, while after TMP-quenched in air, water, and ice are 45.4; 44.4; and 41.6 HRc, respectively.

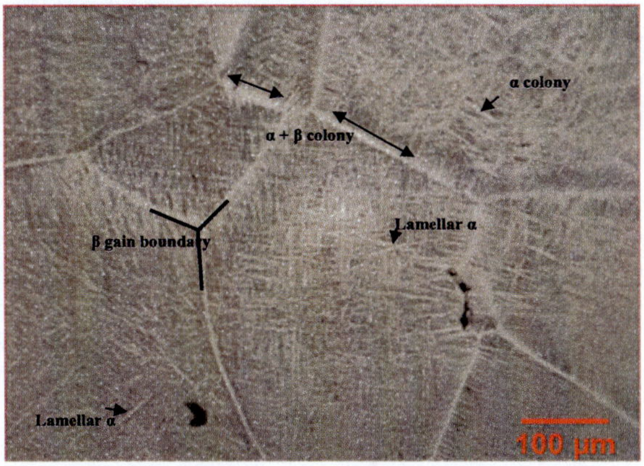

Fig. 2 Optical microscopy of ingot Ti-6Al-6Mo alloy. Etched by Kalling's reagent

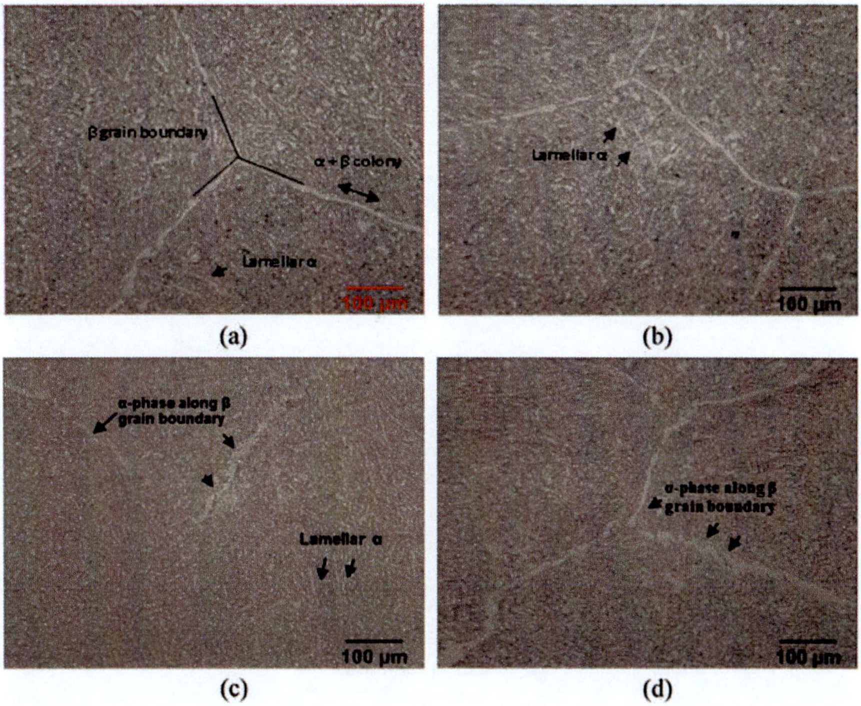

Fig. 3 Optical microscopy of ingot Ti-6Al-6Mo alloy; **a** thermo-mechanical processing (TMP); **b** water quenched; **c** ice quenched; **d** air quenched. Etched by Kalling's reagent

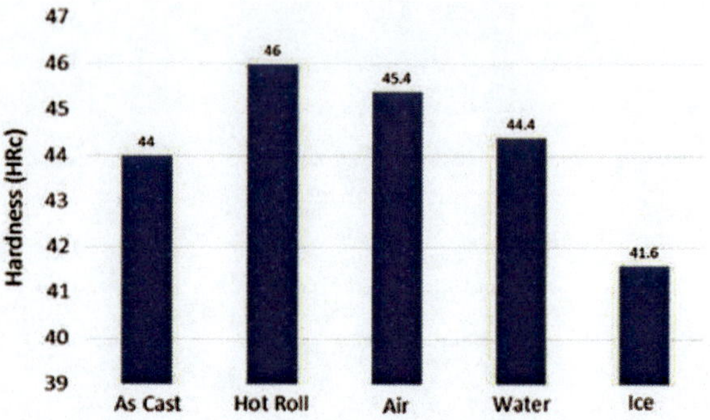

Fig. 4 The Ti-6Al-6Mo alloy hardness value after thermo-mechanical processing (TMP) and quenched in different media

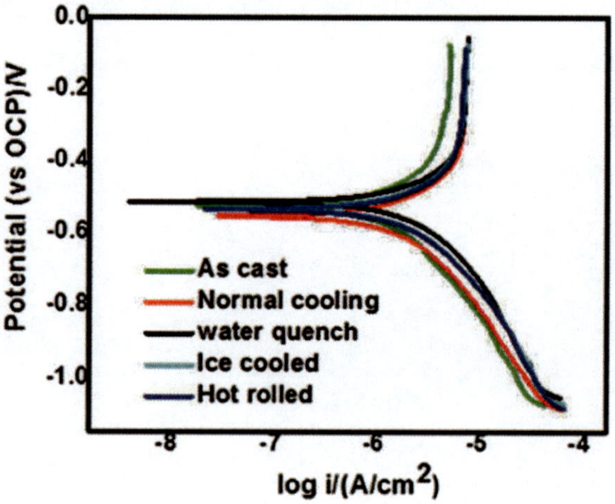

Fig. 5 Potentiodynamic polarization curve recorded at scan rate of 1 mV/sec for as cast, hot rolled and quenching of Ti-6Al-6Mo alloy immersed in Hanks solution

3.3 *Corrosion Test Result*

The cathodic and anodic polarization curves of Ti-6Al-6Mo alloy after immersion in Hanks solution at 37 °C are depicted in Fig. 5. Table 2 is representative value of electrochemical parameters, together with corrosion current density and corrosion potential, determined from potentiodynamic polarization curve of Tafel extrapolation.

It could be seen that air-quenched Ti-6Al-6Mo alloy gives high Icorr and high corrosion rates compared to others. As shown in Fig. 5, the Ecorr is maintained in the cathodic area; the most negative corrosion is normal cooling, followed with hot rolled, ice quenched, as cast, and water quenched.

3.4 *Discussion*

The result of raw material structure proofed that ingot Ti-6Al-6Mo alloy was categorized as ($\alpha + \beta$) titanium alloy (Fig. 2). This categorization was supported by

Table 2 Corrosion rate of Ti-6Al-6Mo alloy immersed in Hanks' solution

Process variable	βa/[V/dec]	βc/[V/dec]	Ecor[Vs OCP]/[V]	Icorr/[A/cm^2]	Corrosion rate [mm/year]
As cast	0.07886	0.080114	−0.52999	3.80E-07	0.006215
Air quench/Normal cooling	0.18882	0.15245	−0.57075	9.45E-07	0.01545
Water quench	0.13183	0.11599	−0.51614	6.41E-07	0.010489
Ice quench	0.16606	0.17424	−0.53599	8.91E-07	0.014566
Hot rolled	0.1272	0.14558	−0.53833	7.38E-07	0.012061

the x-ray diffraction (XRD) analysis result for ingot alloy from another reference [8], which was revealed α-phase and β-phase.

The mechanical property in this alloy can be explored when conducting the thermo-mechanical processing (TMP) as shown in Fig. 3a–d. Lutjering [9] observed in (α + β) titanium alloys that crystallographic textures can arise in the hcp α-phase and in the bcc β-phase during the rolling process. In the deformation step of (α + β) titanium alloy, as observed by Lutjering [9], lamellar α-phase is deformed plastically without separation. The plastic deformation should be enough to dislocation to complete standing the recrystallization step. From this study, conclude to the reference [9] that numerous of nucleation of α-phases was formed and growth, reduce the lamellar α-phase in the TMP-quenched alloy in different media (Fig. 3b–d). Other reference for (α + β) titanium alloy observed lamellar of α-phase fill out at different orientation with grain boundary as perimeter after solution treated at temperature of 1050 °C. The α-phase was created and established in the interior of prior β grain [10].

The optimal hardness value after TMP and quenching in water concluded with the structure that was formed, as shown in Fig. 3a, b, which numerous lamellar phases observed in the interior β matrix and less of α-phase colony was observed. Lutjering [9] added that under conditions of increased cooling rate, yield strength would increase in (α + β) Ti alloys, and a decrease in the α-phase colony. In this study, as shown in Fig. 3a, b, the α-phase colony was observed decreasing, followed with a high hardness value (Fig. 4). Besides that, the mechanical property of the Ti alloy can be illustrated by a lamellar structure. Important parameters of lamellar structures are the size of the β-grain, the size and thickness of the lamellar phase colonies and the morphology of the interlamellar in the β-interface [11, 12].

The Tafel results in Fig. 5 showed that water quenched, and as-cast Ti-6Al-6Mo alloy is positive corrosion compared to air quenched/normal cooling. The corrosion resistance of Ti-6Al-6Mo alloy is attributed to the TiO_2 acts as the barrier layer inhibits the corrosion process on the Ti alloy surface. The passive TiO_2 layer also alters the surface potential and reduces the number of load carriers in the interlayer between the alloy and the electrolyte that successively save the substrate from corrosion damage [13, 14]. When the TiO_2 in the surface layer of Ti alloy brake, corrosion occurred, and the Ti ions are let out sustainably unless the layer is regenerated. The number of Ti ion released is very depending on the regeneration time. In the surgical implant alloy, time of repassivation is designated as regeneration time and depending on the materials that used [15].

4 Summary

This study investigates the thermo-mechanical processing (TMP) effect followed by quenching on structure, mechanical property, and corrosion resistance of Ti-6Al-6Mo alloy. The TMP carried out to Ti-6Al-6Mo alloy after homogenization at 1100 °C–12 h; solution treated at 1100 °C for 30 min followed by hot rolling up to 80% reduction and continuing to solution treated at 1100 °C for one hour followed by quenching in various media of air, water, and ice. The TMP and quenching in water obtained good mechanical property and good corrosion behavior from all the results. The structure after quenching in water is formed nucleation of α-phases in the interior of the β matrix and along β prior grain boundaries, less of the lamellar α-phase, and less of α colony. The optimum hardness value of 44.4 HRc performed after TMP and quenching in the water of Ti-6Al-6Mo alloy is due to less of α colony and numerous lamellar α-phase. The high stability of passive film and good corrosion performance demonstrated in water quenched Ti-6Al-6Mo alloy attributed to the TiO_2 acts as barrier layer inhibits the corrosion process on Ti alloy surface.

Acknowledgements Authors would like to thank for financial support from Health Research and Development Agency, Ministry of Health of the Republic of Indonesia 2020.

References

1. Lutjering G (1940) Chapter 1 microstructure and mechanical properties of titanium alloys general electric aircraft engines, Cincinnati, OH, USA 1
2. Pederson R (2002) Microstructure and phase transformation of Ti-6Al-4V
3. Hsu RWW, Yang CC, Huang CA, Chen YS (2004) Electrochemical corrosion properties of Ti-6Al-4V implant alloy in the biological environment. Mater Sci Eng A 380:100–109
4. Bojinov M, Stancheva M (2014) Coupling between dissolution and passivation revisited—kinetic parameters of anodic oxidation of titanium alloys in a fluoride-containing electrolyte. J Electroanal Chem 737:150–161
5. Guo WY, Sun J, Wu JS (2009) Electrochemical and XPS studies of corrosion behavior of Ti-23Nb-0.7Ta-2Zr-O alloy in Ringer's solution. Mater Chem Phys 113:816–820
6. Krawiec H, Vignal V, Loch J, Erazmus-vignal P (2015) Influence of plastic deformation on the microstructure and corrosion behaviour of Ti-10Mo-4Zr and Ti-6Al-4V alloys in the Ringer' s solution at 37 ° C. Corros Sci 96:160–170
7. Mccafferty E (2005) Validation of corrosion rates measured by the Tafel extrapolation method. Corros Sci 47:3202–3215

8. Kartika I, Werdaningsih R, Alfirano, Rokhmanto F, Thaha YN (209) An investigation of α and α' phases intensity and hardness of Ti-6Al-6Mo implant alloy influenced by temperature of solution treatment and quenching media. In: AIP conference proceedings, vol 2120, p 50009
9. Lutjering G (1998) Influence of processing on microstructure and mechanical properties of (α + β) titanium alloys. Mater Sci Eng A 243:32–45
10. Polytechnic B. Heat Treatment of The Casted Ti6Al4V Titanium Alloy Tepelné Spracovanie Liatej Titánovej Zliatiny Ti6Al4V. vol 1, pp 4–9
11. Sha W, Malinov S (2009) Titanium alloys: modelling of microstructure, properties and applications. Woodhead Publishing Limited and CRC Press LLC
12. Filip R, Kubiak K, Ziaja W, Sieniawski J (2003) The effect of microstructure on the mechanical properties of two-phase titanium alloys. J Mater Proces Technol 133:84–89
13. Yerokhin AL, Nie X, Leyland A, Matthews A (2000) Characterisation of oxide films produced by plasma electrolytic oxidation of a Ti-6Al-4V alloy. Surf Coat Technol 130:195–206
14. Shokouhfar M, Dehghanian C, Montazeri M, Baradaran A (2012) Applied surface science preparation of ceramic coating on Ti substrate by plasma electrolytic oxidation in different electrolytes and evaluation of its corrosion resistance: Part II. Appl Surf Sci 258(7):2416–2423
15. Manivasagam G, Dhinasekaran D, Rajamanickam A (2010) Biomedical implants : corrosion and its prevention—a review. June 2015

Covid-19 and Tuberculosis Classification Based on Chest X-Ray Using Convolutional Neural Network

Suci Aulia, Sugondo Hadiyoso, Tati L. E. R. Mengko, and Andriyan B. Suksmono

Abstract The high rate of patients with tuberculosis (TB) with the graph showing a continual increase requires the research in any sector as the programs to eradicate tuberculosis. One of the applications is the Decision Support System (DSS) that helps the medical experts particularly doctors in diagnosing TB grade 1+. 2+ , and 3+ rapidly. Another problem is related to the imbalance between the number of patients and the number of medical practitioners in the condition of pandemic Corona Virus Disease (Covid-19) today. Hence, DSS is highly required and it can be used for the long-term management of Covid. In this study, the rapid classification of normal lung, tuberculosis lung, and Covid-19 lung based on the Chest X-Ray (CXR) image was proposed as the initial step of DSS implementation. The proposed image processing based CXR classification using Deep Learning Convolutional Neural Network (CNN) obtained the highest accuracy rate of 88.37%. This accuracy was obtained in the second scenario with the 208 CXR datasets. The small number of datasets used was related to the limited number of CXR Covid-19 images with good quality brightness. The proposed system developed is expected to help doctors in diagnose lung disease.

Keywords Chest X-Ray · Corona virus · Tuberculosis · CNN

1 Introduction

Many people suffer from Mycobacterium Tuberculosis (MTB) which causes Tuberculosis (TB) in every year and part of them occur in Indonesia (the country with the third-highest burden of TB after India and China with the number of

S. Aulia (✉) · S. Hadiyoso · T. L. E. R. Mengko · A. B. Suksmono
School of Electrical Engineering and Informatics, Institut Teknologi, Bandung, Indonesia
e-mail: suciaulia@telkomuniversity.ac.id

S. Aulia · S. Hadiyoso
School of Applied Science, Telkom University, Bandung, Indonesia

H. Triwiyanto et al. (eds.), *Proceedings of the 1st International Conference on Electronics, Biomedical Engineering, and Health Informatics*, Lecture Notes in Electrical Engineering 746, https://doi.org/10.1007/978-981-33-6926-9_35

patients around 10% of the total the number of TB patients in the world). Therefore, TB in Indonesia is still viewed as a deadly disease, particularly in the current pandemic Covid-19.

Patients with tuberculosis (TB) should be more aware of the potential transmission of the new type of Covid-19 [1], as compared to the healthy people, the impact caused by the virus will be more fatal [2] for the patients with TB. The modalities of transmission of TB and Covid-19 are closely identical or similar, such as coughing as the main symptom of TB for more than two weeks. This is the same as the early detection for Covid-19. However, Covid-19 shows a very fast reaction in which 2–3 days after coughing accompanied by fever, patients usually experience respiratory problems. To reduce the rate of transmission, the patient must be isolated for 2 weeks. This applies to conditions when the pandemic Covid-19 occurs. Various existing resources in TB service management can also be used to handle Covid-19. Conversely, investing in a variety of current Covid-19 handling resources is very possible to be used for long-term TB management in the future. In addition to services, the implementation research also plays an important role in controlling TB and Covid-19.

The image of the lungs indeed becomes one of the references to observe the happening corona virus infection. This is why, in addition to a throat swab examination, chest X-ray or chest x-ray (CXR) is also used as one of the tests conducted to detect Covid-19. Similarly, in the TB examination, a quick test for early identification of TB patients at the Hospital is commonly through by CXR Rontgen followed by microscopic examination to diagnose TB class 1+. 2+, and 3+. The challenge in diagnosing TB or Covid-19 is the lung imaging of both of them are looking very similar. However, TB and Covid-19 still have different impressions so that it can be thought that deep learning will be able to classify them. As far as we know, there have not been many previous studies discussing the classification of Covid-19 lung and tuberculosis lung. Therefore, this study is proposed a system that can classify normal lungs, positive Covid-19 lungs, and positive TB lungs. In this system, we propose a convolutional neural network (CNN) method for characterization and classification. We have performed several test scenarios to find out, investigate, and obtain the highest detection accuracy.

This proposed study is the initial step to build a DSS or an accurate diagnostic system for TB. Also, DSS can be used as a support system to anticipate the pandemic Covid-19 in the future. According to WHO the research on DSS TB is one of the most urgent implementation studies required today [3–5]. Several studies based on image processing [6–12] have been carried out to detect MTB and so far the CNN method [13–15] shows the best performance among other methods [14, 16, 17].

2 Material and System Design

As a soft organ, the normal lung will show black or dark color on all parts of the X-ray as shown in Fig. 1a. Patients with severe Covid-19 infection will show blurred X-ray images on one or both of their lungs as shown in Fig. 1b, so that they will look different from normal lung X-ray images [18]. Meanwhile, the active TB CXR in Fig. 1c shows the opacification of airspaces within the lung parenchyma. Consolidation can be patchy, dense, irregular, or hazy.

In CXR Covid-19 infection with the moderate severity, the lungs resemble a condensed glass when exposed to hot steam—in medical terms, it is commonly known as ground-glass opacity. In cases of severe Covid-19 infection, the lungs begin to be filled with fluid and debris from cells that have died for being failed to fight the virus, then causing swelling [20]. Such a condition makes it difficult for patients to breathe oxygen or becomes breathless. In this condition, patches or white areas in the lungs have become increasingly clear, no longer blurred. The spots also appear to connect into nodular lesions so that they cover the lung as shown in Fig. 2 [21].

Experiments in this study used the open database of chest x-ray Covid-19 from https://github.com/ieee8023/covid-chestxray-dataset and chest x-ray tuberculosis from https://www.kaggle.com/qyleong13/tb-dataset. The Covid-19 dataset obtained showed a variety of different sources, showing the difference in the process of

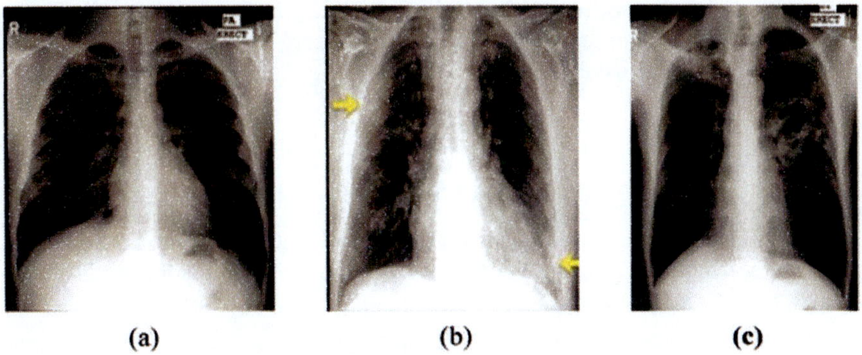

Fig. 1 **a** Normal lung , **b** image of the lung of Corona patient, showing a white layer that covers part of the lung, **c** pulmonary images of TB patients, nodular lesions [19]

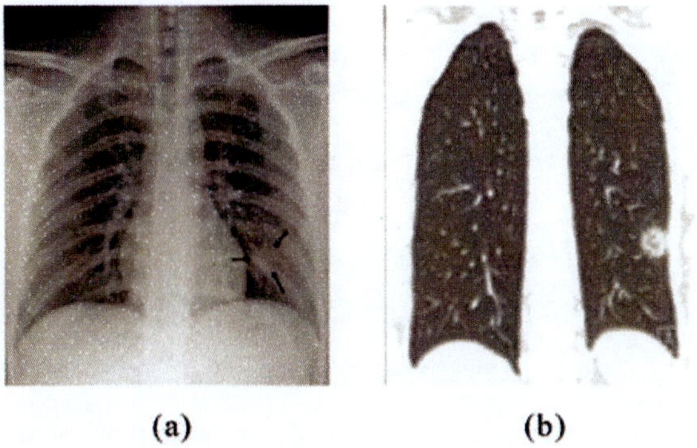

Fig. 2 Covid-19 with the single nodular lesion, **a** CXR imaging, **b** CT scan imaging

acquisition of CXR images carried out. Whereas, the CXR dataset of normal and TB originates from one source. Thus, in this study, there were three test experiments to determine the effect of variations in acquisition on the accuracy of the CXR imaging classification for Normal, Covid-19, and TB lungs.

In this study they are four steps of image processing were carried out to classify CXR images into normal, positive TB, or positive Covid-19. The first stage is image enhancement using median filtering, the second stage is noise removing using thresholding by converting the CXR image to binary, the third stage is segmenting to separate the object and background, then the last stage to classify the lung image using CNN.

2.1 Convolutional Neural Network (CNN)

There are four steps in CNN architecture, they are convolutional, max pooling, flattering, and full connection as shown in Fig. 3 [22]. In the step-1 convolutional process by using detector features [23, 24], many feature maps are created to get the first convolution layer using Eq. 1.

$$(f * g)(t) \cong \int_{-\infty}^{\infty} f(\tau)g(t-\tau)d\tau \tag{1}$$

Where f is input image matrix, g is filter or kernel matrix, t is time domain and τ is shifting convolution. In step-2 pooling process aims to compress feature map data for each layer of CNN that denoted by L. Pooling layer has x_1^j as input, o_1^j as output, and (W_1^j, b_1^j) as parameters, where j is the channel index of filters in the convolutional layer and c_1 is the number of the convolutional filter. The output pooling layer can be written as Eq. 2.

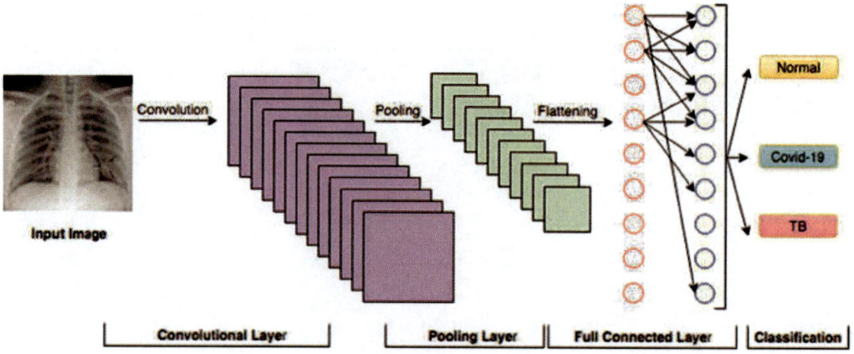

Fig. 3 Deep learning architecture of convolutional neural network

$$o_l^j = \text{pool}\left(\sigma\left(\sum_{j=1}^{c_l-1}\left(W_l^j x_l^j + b_l^j\right)\right)\right), j \in [1, c_l] \quad (2)$$

In step-3, flatten process is convert the 2D vector of pooled feature map become 1D vectors that formulated as Eq. 3.

$$o_L^{\text{flatten}} = \text{flatten}\left(\left[o_L^1, o_L^2, o_L^3, \ldots, o_L^j\right]\right), j = c_l \quad (3)$$

Finally, in step-4 the full connection is transformed into model output $\hat{y}$, thus formulated as Eq. 4. Where W_f and b_f are parameters of the full connection process.

$$\begin{aligned}\hat{y} &= W_f o_L^{flatten} + b_f \\ &= W_f\left(flatten\left(pool\left(\sigma\left(\sum_{j=1}^{c_l-1}(W_l^j x_l^j + b_l^j)\right)\right)\right)\right) + b_f\end{aligned} \quad (4)$$

2.2 Proposed System Architecture

In this study, a digital queue system equipped with an application user interface for registration and monitor of the queue number was implemented using a Latte panda, thermal printing machine, monitor, and an Android smartphone to perform online registration and monitoring functions. Figure 1 displays the system architecture designed in this study. Meanwhile, the design of a queue registration and monitoring system through the internet network is shown in Fig. 2.

Based on Fig. 1, the developed queuing system has the main components, as already explained, namely mini PCs, printing machines, speakers, and displays. In this study, additional features were in the form of a monitoring application designed using the Android platform installed on a smartphone so that it can see the status of the queue in real-time and online. To support the application, the mini-computer was connected to the WiFi Router as a gateway to the internet network. Queue data would be sent to the server so that it could be accessed online through the internet network.

2.3 Hardware Queue Machine and Desktop Applications Implementation

Figure 1 shows the hardware design of the queuing system at the Public Health Center. The central control was carried out by a mini personal computer based on the Windows operating system with QT-Creator as the basis for developing desktop applications. This desktop application performed: reading input from buttons, printing queue ticket numbers, performing digital display the queue status, and calling functions. The workflow of the proposed system can be seen in Fig. 4.

When the queue number button was pressed, the device would retrieve the latest queue number data from the server, and then the printer would print the ticket number. The queue number was obtained from the last queue number +1 in decimal value. If the clerk pressed the call button (either counter 1, counter 2, or counter 3), the device would retrieve the counter number data from the server, then showed it on display and sound the speaker to call the queue number. The counter number

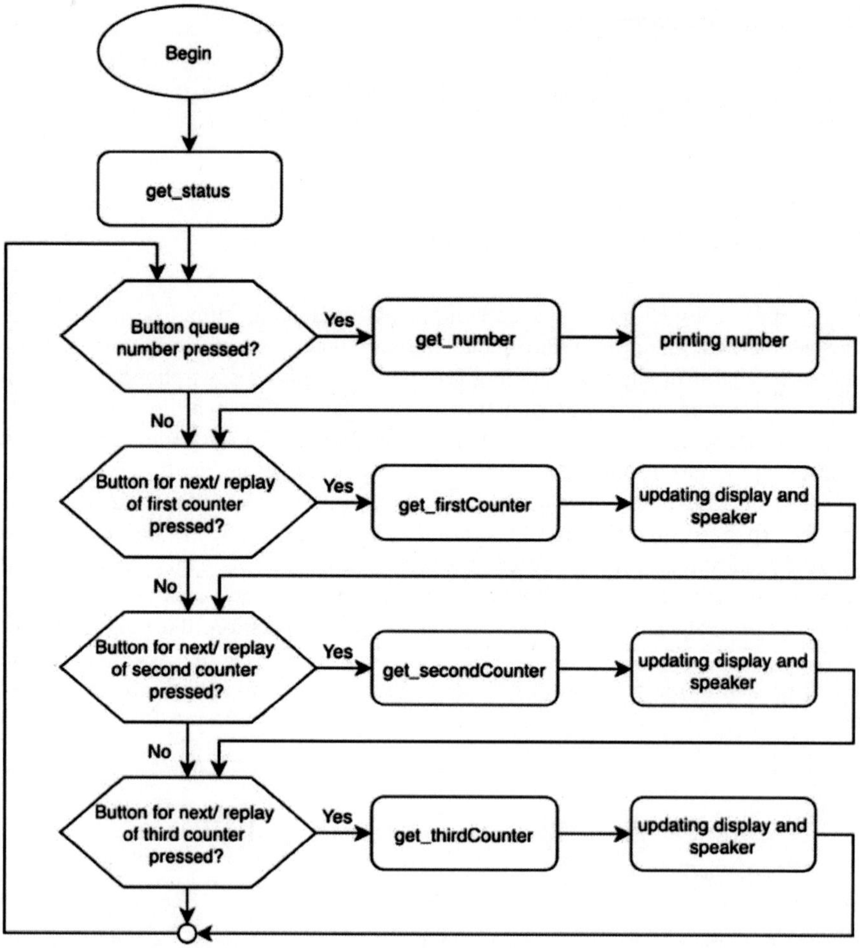

Fig. 4 The workflow of the hardware queue machine

was obtained by finding the highest value from counter-1, counter-2, and counter-3, which then +1 in decimal value.

The desktop application was designed to display queue numbers and counters according to the administrator registration instructions. The system implemented in this study supports calling and displaying queue numbers up to three counters.

3 Results

This first experiment used 243 CXR image datasets consisting of 80 normal pulmonary data, 104 data about the positive Covid-19 pulmonary, and 59 pulmonary data of positive TB. All data which is used in this scenario came from 60 databases. Each CXR image was separated by 80% for the training process and 20% for the testing process. This image classification of normal CXR, Covid-19, and TB used CNN with training cycle parameters (epoch = 100, iteration = 200, and iterations/epoch = 2), validation parameters (frequency = 30 iterations, patience = 5), and 0.01 learning rate was obtained by validation accuracy of 48.98%. The low level of accuracy is also shown by the graph in Fig. 6 in which there was a large gap in both the validation accuracy line with the testing graph (blue line) and the loss line with the testing graph (red line).

With the same parameters as in the first experiment, in the second experiment, a dataset was filtered based on the brightness level as shown in Fig. 5. In Fig. 5a, b, and c in HVS (Human Visual System), it can be seen the difference in brightness degradation that greatly affects the accuracy. Then the experimental-2 dataset was filtered against the distribution of brightness using a histogram as shown in Fig. 6.

From Fig. 6, a minimum threshold (minTh) matrix is generated for each histogram graph. The minTh matrix for Fig. 6a, b, and c shown in Table 1. Then calculate the mean of each of the minTh matrices, this mean value then used as the threshold filtering.

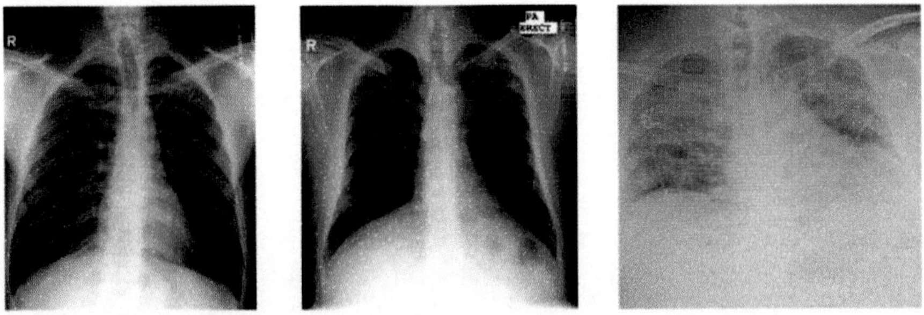

(a) (b) (c)

Fig. 5 Brightness dregradation. **a** dataset125.png, **b** dataset137.png, **c** dataset231.png

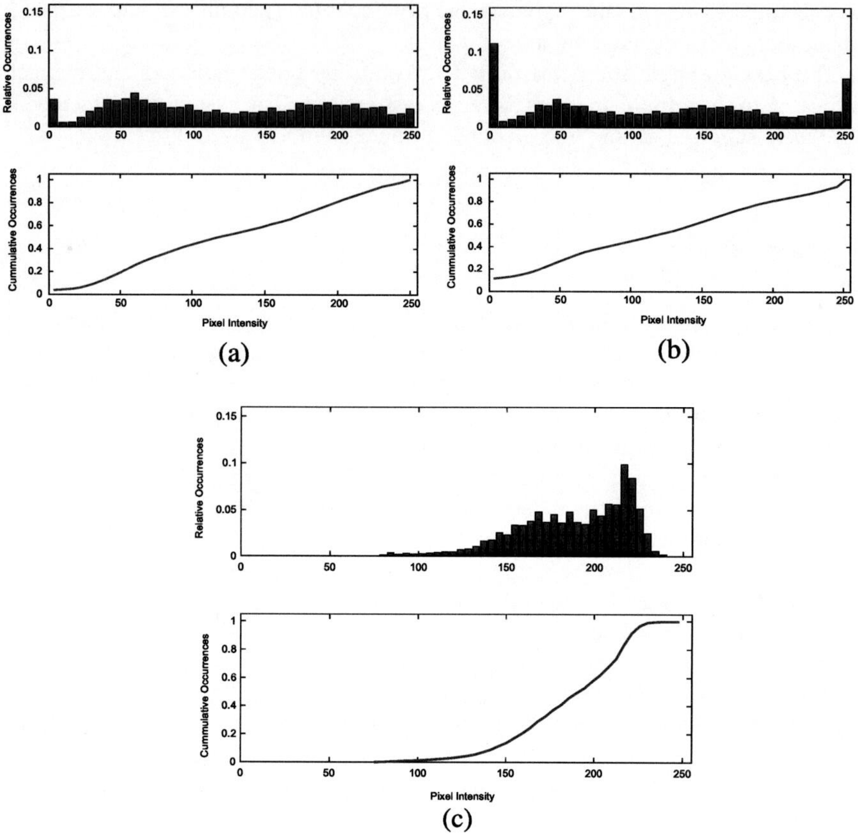

Fig. 6 Histogram of brightness degradation. **a** dataset125.png, **b** dataset137.png, **c** dataset231.png

Table 1 Minimum thresholding matrix and mean value from the histogram

Histogram	minTh matrix	Mean
Figure 6a	[9 47 73 85 111 130 142 161 187 199 218 237]	133.25
Figure 6b	[10 41 61 80 92 105 124 156 182 194 214 245]	125.30
Figure 6c	[75 88 97 150 159 173 181 195 204 212 248]	162

This filtering process aimed to reduce the variation or uniformity of the dataset in the training process. Thus, in experiment-2 several datasets in experiment-1 that have mean histogram >150 have been removed. Then the number of datasets became 208 (70 normal, 84 Covid-19, 54 TB) from 243 datasets. The 208 datasets were separated for the training and testing process (80–20%). As seen in Fig. 8a, the validation accuracy line increased close to the testing graph (blue line) and the declined loss line made it coincided with the testing graph (red line). In experiment-2 the accuracy rate approach of 88.37% that much higher than the experiment-1 (48.98%) (Fig. 7).

Continue to the third experiment, the scenario was adding dataset variations based on the acquisition of CXR images. The variation of acquisition means the variation of tools used during the capture of the X-Ray image. In experiment-3 was used 333 datasets (70 normal, 208 Covid-19, 55 TB) derived from more than 70 variations or database acquisition sources. In this scenario, the dataset was also filtered based on brightness using histogram the same as in experiment-2. The accuracy in this experiment decreased by 61.67% as shown in Fig. 8b. The validation of the accuracy line again decreased away from the blue line-the testing graph as similarly occurred in the loss line again increasing away from the red line the testing graph.

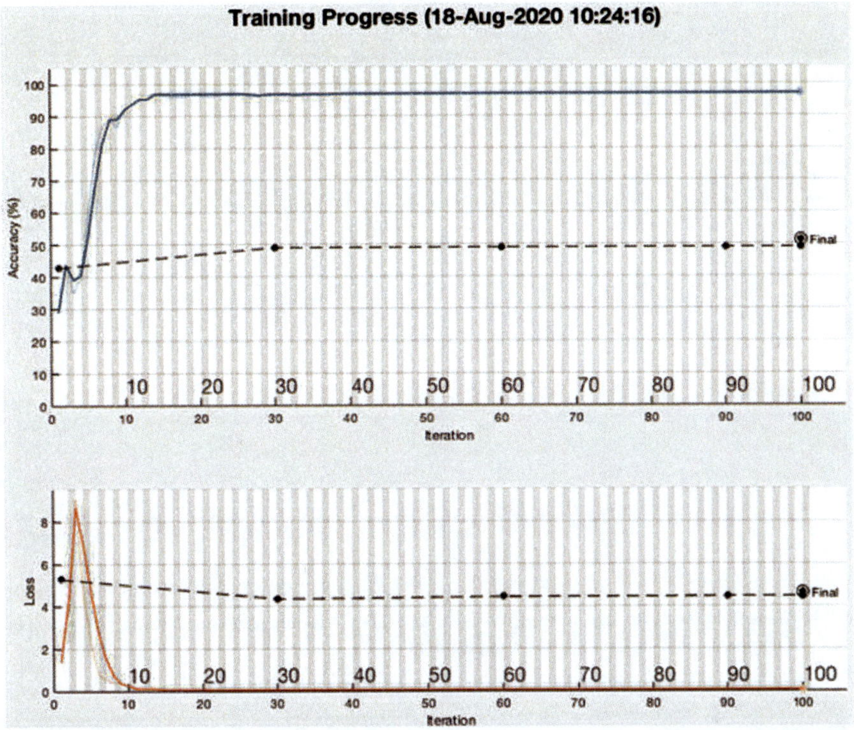

Fig. 7 The results of experimental testing-1: CXR imaging-based classification of normal lung, Covid-19, and TB Discussion

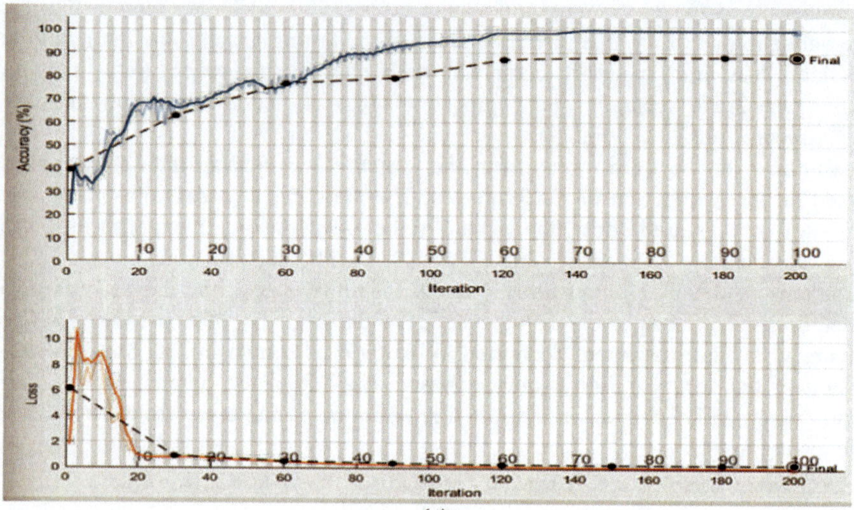

(a)

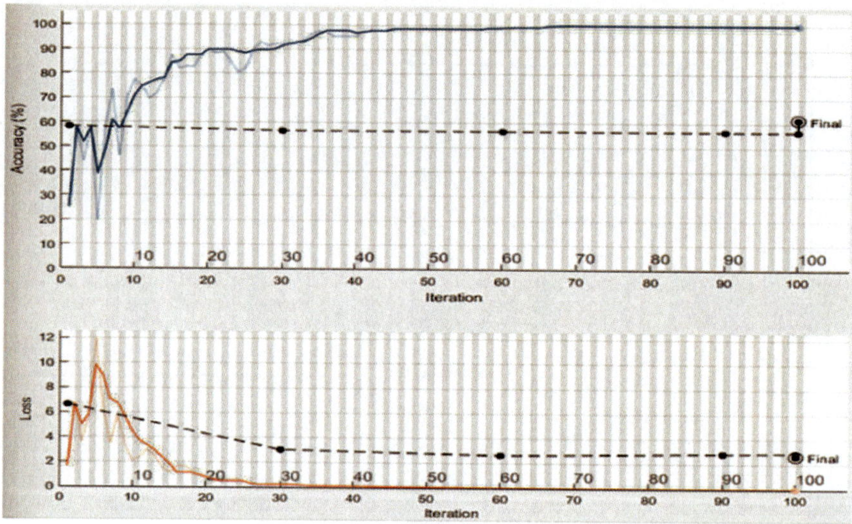

(b)

Fig. 8 Classification of normal lung, Covid-19, and TB CXR imaging-based using CNN. **a** The results of experiment-2, **b** the results of experiment-3

4 Discussion

This study develops a decision support system application for automatic classification of normal lung, Covid-19 lung, and pulmonary TB. The scenarios that were tested in this study included (1) scenario-1 using 243 images, without selection based on brightness, (2) scenario-2 using 208 selected images based on brightness level, and (3) scenario-3 using 333 images selected based on brightness level. In this study the CNN configuration was used as follows: epoch = 100, iteration = 200, and iterations/epoch = 2, meanwhile the validation parameters (frequency = 30 iterations, patience = 5), and 0.01 learning rate. This configuration applies to all scenarios. Test in scenario-1 shows the highest accuracy obtained is 48.98%.

In experiment-2 and experiment-3, pre-processing was performed on the CXR images before performing the feature extraction and classification. This stage aim of increasing the brightness level, separating the objects of the lungs from the background, and denoising the artifact. Also to observe the effect on detection accuracy, the flow process is shown in Fig. 9. The next step was segmentation or masking. The results of this masking were the input images in the classification process with CNN, as shown in Fig. 10. Nodular lesions cover the TB lungs and cover more Covid-19 lungs accompanied by ground-glass opacity showing a significant difference from masking as seen in the intact normal lungs.

The highest accuracy achieved in experiment-2 and experiment-3 was 88.37% and 61.67%, respectively. These two scenarios show an improvement in accuracy compared to experiment-1. This indicates that the image pre-processing stage affects the feature extraction and classification process. The brightness level of the CXR image is very influential in the detection process. In this study, we used a histogram to identify the brightness level of the image. CXR images with brightness below the threshold are not used in experiment-2 and experiment-3. This selection mode is also to minimize variations in the brightness level of the image. Thus the bias in the result of feature extraction can be reduced. This can be thought of as the reason why experiment-2 and experiment-3 produce higher accuracy compared to experiment-1. However, experiment-3 yields lower accuracy than experiment-2. The dataset used in experiment-3 is more numerous and it derived from more than 70 variations or database acquisition sources with different X-ray machines. These results confirm that the consistency and uniformity of CXR images have an impact on the accuracy of detection as reported in the study [25, 26]. The DSS application in this study yields quite a good accuracy (>80%). The DSS which is developed is also able to solve the classification problems in three data classes. This is more advantageous than the previous study by [27, 28] where the proposed system is only for classifying two data groups (Normal and Covid-19). However, the proposed DSS in this study has limitation that histogram-based image selection is still done manually. This is a challenge for future studies to be developed so that the system can generate high accuracy with several brightness variations on the CXR image.

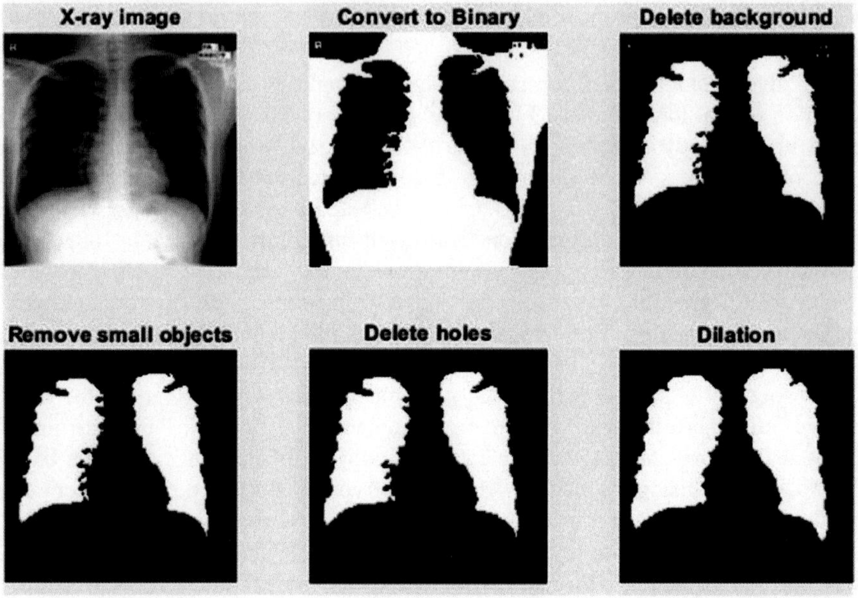

Fig. 9 The results of CXR pre-processing

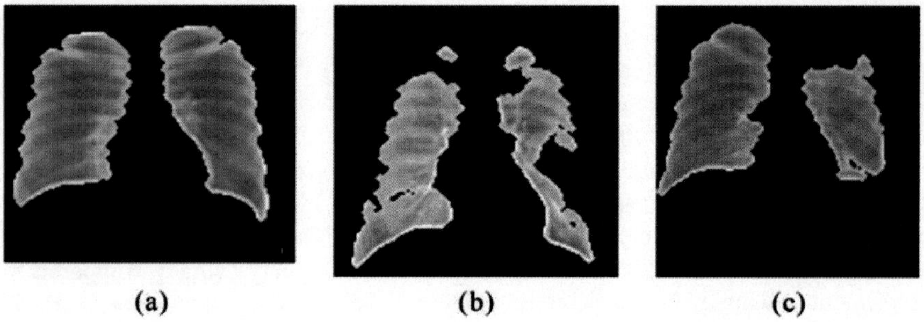

Fig. 10 The segmentation results of CXR, **a** normal lung, **b** Covid-19 lungs, and **c** TB lungs

5 Conclusion

In this study, we have developed a decision support system for the classification of Covid-19 and tuberculosis. Three experimental scenarios were carried out to classify the images of normal lung chest x-ray (CXR), tuberculosis lungs, and Covid-19 lungs. We proposed the CNN Deep Learning method for performed this system. The first scenario resulted in an accuracy rate of 48.98% obtained by using a ratio of 80%: 20% of training data and testing data from 242 variations (brightness levels) of CXR images and the dataset used came from 60 database sources. The second scenario used the same CNN parameters as in the first scenario, and it obtained an accuracy rate of 88.37%. This level of accuracy increased since filtering was done on a dataset from 242 datasets into 208 datasets by removing the CXR images with poor quality. In the third scenario, 208 datasets in the second scenario were added with the qualified CXR images; however, from 10 new database sources, 333 datasets were obtained, but the accuracy rate obtained was reduced to 61.67%. The number of database sources was directly proportional to the variation of CXR image acquisition obtained, hence, it still becomes a challenge for future studies in increasing accuracy and applying to a larger dataset with varying brightness levels.

References

1. Alagna R et al (2020) Celebrating TB day at the time of COVID-19
2. Liu Y et al (2020) Active or latent tuberculosis increases susceptibility to COVID-19 and disease severity. Infect Dis (except HIV/AIDS)
3. Hatherill M, Chaisson RE, Denkinger CM (2019) Addressing critical needs in the fight to end tuberculosis with innovative tools and strategies. PLoS Med 16(4)
4. Anthwal D et al (2019) Development and evaluation of novel bio-safe filter paper-based kits for sputum microscopy and transport to directly detect Mycobacterium tuberculosis and associated drug resistance. PLoS ONE 14(8)
5. Sulis G et al (2016) Recent developments in the diagnosis and management of tuberculosis. NPJ Prim Care Resp Med 26(1):16078
6. Pandey V et al (2019) SeeTB: a novel alternative to sputum smear microscopy to diagnose tuberculosis in high burden countries. Sci Rep 9(1):16371
7. Mithra KS, Sam Emmanuel WR (2019) Automated identification of mycobacterium bacillus from sputum images for tuberculosis diagnosis. SIViP 13(8):1585–1592
8. Zingue D, Weber P, Soltani F, Raoult D, Drancourt M (2019) Automatic microscopic detection of mycobacteria in sputum: a proof-of-concept. Sci Rep 8(1):11308
9. Ayma V, De Lamare R, Castaneda B (2015) An adaptive filtering approach for segmentation of tuberculosis bacteria in Ziehl-Neelsen sputum stained images. Latin America congress on computational intelligence (LA-CCI), pp 1–5
10. Rulaningtyas R, Suksmono AB, Mengko TLR, Saptawati P (2016) Nearest patch matching for color image segmentation supporting neural network classification in pulmonary tuberculosis identification. In: International conference and workshop on basic and applied sciences (ICOWOBAS 2015), p 120002
11. Shah MI, Mishra S, Sarkar M, Sudarshan SK (2016) Automatic detection and classification of tuberculosis bacilli from camera-enabled smartphone microscopic images. In: Fourth international conference on parallel, distributed and grid computing (PDGC) 2016, pp 287–290
12. Rulaningtyas R, Suksmono AB, Mengko TLR, Saptawati P (2017) Colour segmentation of multi variants tuberculosis sputum images using self organizing map. J Phys Conf Ser 853:012012
13. El-Melegy M, Mohamed D, ElMelegy T, Abdelrahman M (2019) Identification of tuberculosis bacilli in ZN-stained sputum smear images: a deep learning approach IEEE/CVF. In: Conference on computer vision and pattern recognition workshops (CVPRW), p 7
14. Bobak CA, Titus AJ, Hill JE (2019) Comparison of common machine learning models for classification of tuberculosis using transcriptional biomarkers from integrated datasets. Appl Soft Comput 74:264–273

15. Panicker RO, Kalmady KS, Rajan J, Sabu MK (2019) Automatic detection of tuberculosis bacilli from microscopic sputum smear images using deep learning methods. Biocybernetics Biomed Eng 38(3):691–699
16. Edafe A, Mumini OO, Oluwarotimi S (2015) A genetic-neuro-fuzzy inferential technique for diagnosis of tuberculosis. In: Proceedings of the 2015 workshop on pervasive wireless healthcare. Mobilehealth, pp 39–44
17. Mithra KS, Sam Emmanuel WR (2018) GFNN: gaussian-fuzzy-neural network for diagnosis of tuberculosis using sputum smear microscopic images. J King Saud Univ—Comput Inf Sci
18. Wang X, Zhang X, He J (2020) Challenges to the system of reserve medical supplies for public health emergencies: reflections on the outbreak of the severe acute respiratory syndrome coronavirus 2 (SARS-CoV-2) epidemic. China Bio Sci Trends 14(1):6
19. Jaeger S, Karargyris A, Antani S, Thoma G (2012) Detecting tuberculosis in radiographs using combined lung masks. In: 2012 Annual International Conference of the IEEE Engineering in Medicine and Biology Society, Aug 2012, pp 4978–4981. https://doi.org/10.1109/EMBC.2012.6347110
20. Shi H et al (2020) Radiological findings from 81 patients with COVID-19 pneumonia in Wuhan, China: a descriptive study. Lancet Infect Dis 20(4):425–434
21. Yoon SH et al (2020) Chest radiographic and CT findings of the 2019 novel coronavirus disease (COVID-19): analysis of nine patients treated. Korea Korean J Radiol 21(4):494
22. Chen F-C, Jahanshahi MR (2018) NB-CNN: deep learning-based crack detection using convolutional neural network and Naïve Bayes Data Fusion. IEEE Trans Ind Electron 65 (5):4392–4400
23. LeCun Y, Kavukcuoglu K, Farabet C (2010) Convolutional networks and applications. In: Vision proceedings of 2010 IEEE international symposium on circuits and systems, pp 253–256
24. Gu J et al (2018) Recent advances in convolutional neural networks. Pattern Recogn 77 (May):234–377
25. Beaulah Jeyavathana R, Balasubramanian R, Pandian AA (2016) A survey: analysis on pre-processing and segmentation techniques for medical images. Int J Res Sci Innov 3 (6):2321–2705
26. Prajakta S, Varsha R (2020) Robust pre-processing module for leaf image analysis. Int J Eng Adv Technol 9(4):2083–2087. https://doi.org/10.35940/ijeat.d9099.049420
27. Aziz MA et al (2020) New machine learning method for imagebased diagnosis of COVID-19. PLoS ONE 15(June):1–18. https://doi.org/10.1371/journal.pone.0235187
28. Saiz F, Barandiaran I (2020) COVID-19 detection in chest X-ray Images using a deep learning approach. Int J Interact Multimedia Artif Intell 6(2):1–4. https://doi.org/10.9781/ijimai.2020.04.003

Control of Wheelchair on the Ramp Trajectory Using Bioelectric Impedance with Fuzzy-PID Controller

Masyitah Aulia, Achmad Arifin, and Djoko Purwanto

Abstract A person who has a severe disability, have difficulty walking, climbing, and descending stairs, so requires assistive devices for daily mobility. in particular, the paralysis of the upper and lower limbs resulted in them being unable to use the wheelchair properly. So that in this study, an electric wheelchair that can be used by persons with disabilities is made, which is able to move based on the bioelectrical impedance signal on the part of the body that can still be moved. The pre-existing research is controlling wheelchairs on flat roads, whereas when the road goes up or down, the wheelchair has an unstable speed. This research was developed by utilizing Fuzzy-PID control, which is able to control the wheelchair speed so that it is more stable. This electric wheelchair with Fuzzy-PID control is able to walk on an up and down ramp at an angle not exceeding 10°, at a stable speed. The trial subjects used were four people with different weights. The error rate at each speed increases as the ramp gets steeper, and the user load gets higher. Success in this trial is at an average success rate of 80%. This occurs because of the change in the width of the bioimpedance signal, which affects the slow and fast commands when given the command to move, and the tilt angle of the track which affects the motor speed when the wheelchair crosses the track.

Keywords Wheelchair · IMU sensor · Fuzzy-PID controller

1 Introduction

The human nervous system is the connection between complex networks in the human body. The coordinate of the nervous system interprets and controls interactions between the individual and the surrounding environment [1]. Failure that occurs when weakness or damage to the nervous system is paralysis. The results

M. Aulia (✉) · A. Arifin · D. Purwanto
Department of Electrical Engineering, Institut Teknologi Sepuluh Nopember, Surabaya, Indonesia
e-mail: masyitah.aulia1994@gmail.com

H. Triwiyanto et al. (eds.), *Proceedings of the 1st International Conference on Electronics, Biomedical Engineering, and Health Informatics*, Lecture Notes in Electrical Engineering 746, https://doi.org/10.1007/978-981-33-6926-9_36

obtained by the proportion of the population aged ten years and over who experience functional difficulties of 8.56% [2]. Patients with disabilities who cannot go up and down stairs need tools to help with daily mobility. In this case, a tool that is needed is a wheelchair, but for cases of paralysis in the upper and lower body parts that result in not being able to move conventional wheelchairs with the help of hands due to paralysis in both hands, then another solution is needed to run a wheelchair is to use electric wheelchairs that can be driven by utilizing bioelectric impedance signals.

The design of a wheelchair control command is based on changes in trapezoidal muscle impedance. Impedance measurement using bioelectric impedance instrumentation, there are three electrodes attached to the shoulder, namely on the right shoulder, left shoulder, and right in the middle of the spine. The change in impedance value occurs when the trapezius muscle moves, the greater the width of the muscle, the greater the impedance value, and vice versa the shorter the muscle widening the smaller the impedance value obtained. Any increase or decrease in the tilt angle will affect the speed of the wheelchair. The controller works when three inputs are entered, namely track slope, RPM speed, and rotary encoder sensor. These three inputs are processed in the fuzzification process. Fuzzy variables in the input value are processed by setting rules. The output of the rule will be a fuzzy variable and will undergo a defuzzification process. Then feed it back to the controller. Changes in the value of RPM in a wheelchair consisting of the slow, medium, and tight are influenced by the value of the slope of the track consisting of flat, slightly upward, and upward.

2 Materials

Impedance measurements use bioelectrical impedance with 3 electrodes, each attached to the right shoulder, left shoulder, and right in the middle of the spine [3]. The trapezius muscle impedance can change when the trapezius muscle moves. The impedance value will be greater when the muscle lengthens and will be smaller when the muscle shortens. Impedance changes in the trapezius muscle are used as a control command by providing a threshold for the bioelectrical impedance output. When the measured voltage value is greater than the specified threshold, the trapezius muscle movement is interpreted as a control command, where the detection uses edge detection, as shown in Fig. 1. The threshold is a way to translate the impedance change as a motion control command so that it can be read by the microcontroller. The block diagram of the whole system is shown in Fig. 2.

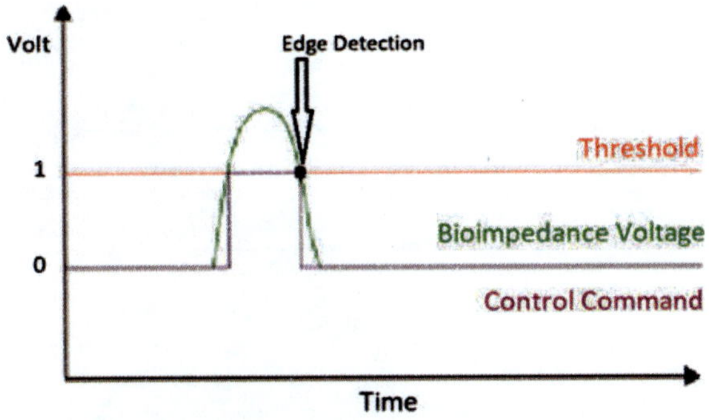

Fig. 1 Speed command giving process

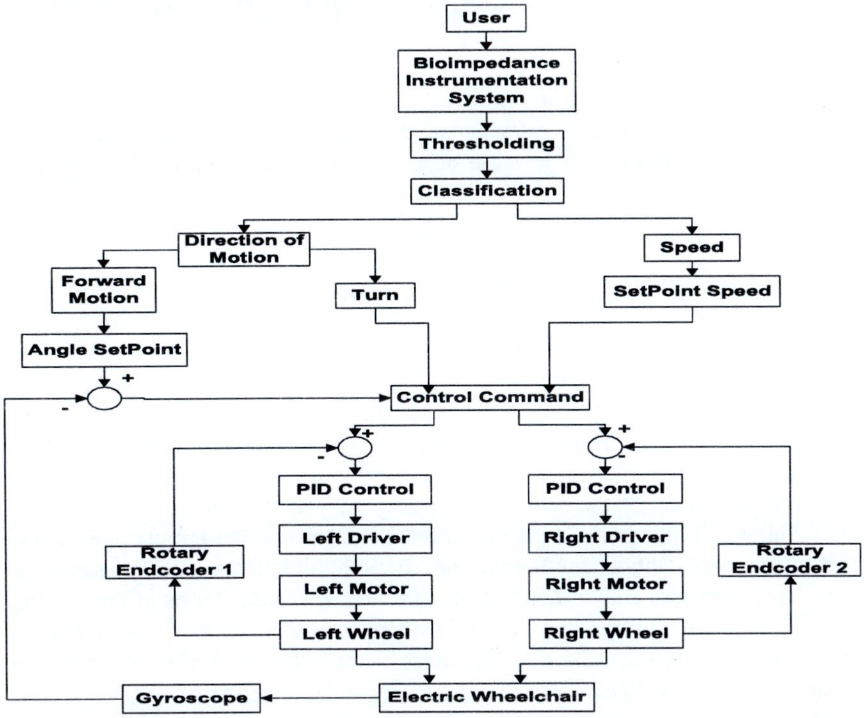

Fig. 2 Block diagram of the whole system

2.1 *Upper Trapezius Muscle*

The trapezius muscle is the muscle that makes up the structure of the human back. It's called a trapezius because its shape is similar to a trapezius shape. The upper trapezius muscle is part of the trapezius muscle located at the very top. Upper

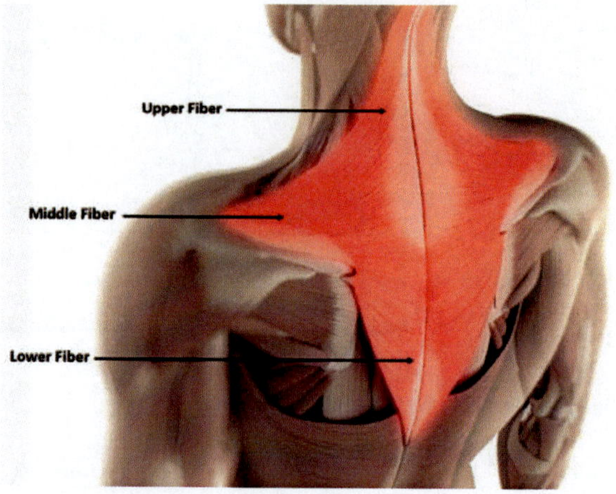

Fig. 3 Upper trapezius muscle

trapezius muscle fibers extending downward from the occipitalis up to the seventh cervical vertebrae and extend sideways to the acromion. This muscle often experiences tightness and stiffness because of its function as a stabilizer [4] (Fig. 3).

2.2 *Bioelectrical Impedance*

In the human body, there are many networks that are connected to each other; these networks contain electrical properties that can be utilized for human needs themselves. In research that has been done through these networks, bioimpedance can be used to help humans because bioimpedance is a resistance to the flow of current in the network [5]. The ability of current to pass through tissue in the body affects the frequency size model, if the network has a low frequency, then the current cannot pass through cell membrane capacitance but can flow through the cell area in the extracellular part. But when the network is with high frequency, resistivity in capacitance decreases and current can pass through the internal area of the cell [5].

To measure the bioimpedance signal in the body is done by using two methods, namely the two electrodes and four electrodes method. The method used this time is a method using three electrodes. The first electrode and the second electrode have the function to provide current, while the third electrode serves as a reference in measuring the output voltage from bioimpedance. The electrode placement will be explained in Fig. 5. The amount of bioimpedance can be determined by using Ohm's law calculation.

By using two integrated circuits, the first is a stimulation circuit that is enabled to generate alternating current sources with a frequency of 50 kHz and amplitude with a maximum value of 0.5 mA rms. The second is a series of instrumentations used to measure potential differences in a stimulated body. The magnitude of the voltage obtained from these measurements represents the magnitude of the value of the bioimpedance signal, so it can be said to be a system called the bioimpedance instrumentation system [5] (Figs. 4, 5, 6).

2.3 PID Controller

PID is an acronym for proportional, integral, and derivative. PID controller is a control that consists of three elements. This PID control was first used in 1939 and is used in almost every control. Investigations in Japan in 1989 showed that more than 90% of the controls used were PID controls and an advanced version of PID

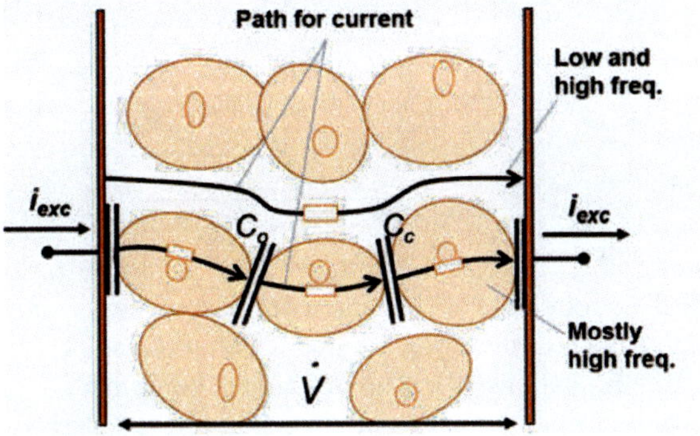

Fig. 4 Current flow on a network

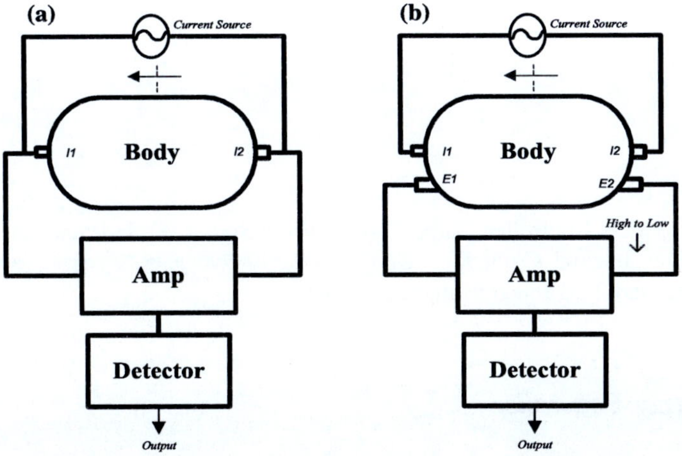

Fig. 5 Two methods for installing bioimpedance measurement electrodes, **a** two electrodes system, and **b** four electrodes system

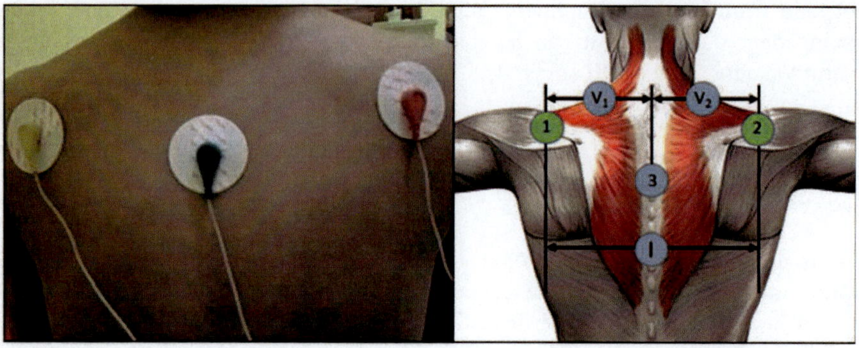

Fig. 6 Electrode placement in the body

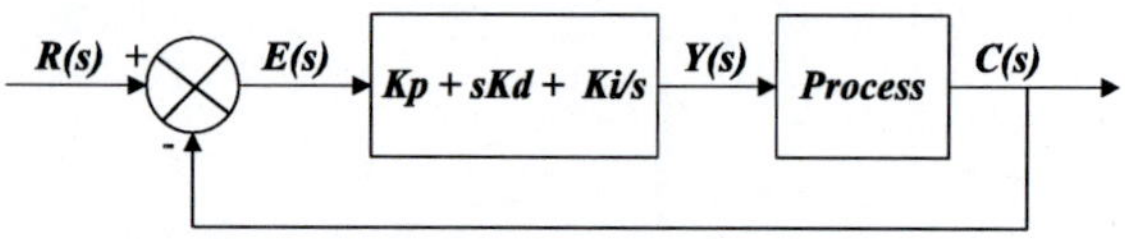

Fig. 7 PID controller

controls [6]. Tuning is an important parameter for the best performance of a PID controller. The PID controller can be tuned in various ways, including manual hand-tuning, Ziegler-Nichols tuning, tuning with Cohen-Coon parameters, and loop tuning, but this has limitations [7]. The additional combination of proportional, integral, and derivative actions is called proportional-integral-derivative action. The Control system block diagram with unitary feedback using PID control actions is shown in Fig. 7. Mathematically represented in Eqs. 1 and 2 below:

$$y(t) = K_p\left[e(t) + T_d\frac{d(e)}{d(t)} + \frac{1}{T_i}\int_0^t e(t)d(t)\right] \tag{1}$$

$$y(t) = \left[K_p e(t) + K_d\frac{d(e)}{d(t)} + K_i\int_0^t e(t)d(t)\right] \tag{2}$$

Where, $y(t)$ is Controller Output, $e(t)$ is Error Signal, K_p is Proportional Gain, $K_i = K_p/T_i$ is Integral Gain, $K_d = K_p$. T_d is Derivative gain, T_d is Constant time derivatives, and T_i is Integral time constant.

2.4 *Fuzzy Controller*

Fuzzy controllers are better than PID controllers because they can cover a wider range of operating conditions and operate with noise and interference from various

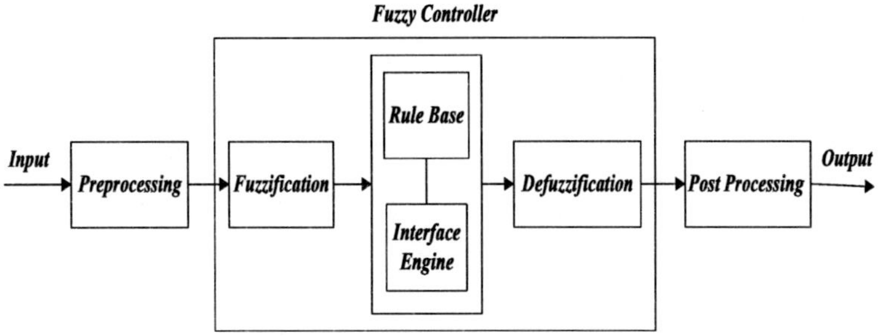

Fig. 8 Fuzzy logic controller

characteristics. Fuzzy control itself is widely used as an alternative to PID control due to the limitations possessed by PID control. Fuzzy Logic controller, as shown in Fig. 8, consists of four main parts of fuzzification, rule base, engine interface, and defuzzification.

3 Method

The design of the wheelchair control command is based on the change in impedance of the trapezius muscle. In measuring the value of impedance using bioelectrical impedance instrumentation, there are three electrodes attached to the right shoulder, left shoulder, and right in the middle of the spine. The change in the impedance value occurs when the trapezius muscle moves, the wider the muscle, the greater the impedance value obtained. Conversely, the shorter the muscle widening eats, the smaller the impedance value gets (Fig. 9).

In the stimulation and instrumentation circuit, bioimpedance is connected to STM32 as a control command. The stimulation circuit is a series of alternating current that has a maximum amplitude of 0.5 mA rms and a frequency of 50 kHz. The function of the circuit is to measure potential differences that exist in the body so that the source of current can be injected into the body through electrodes. The size of the measured voltage will affect the value of bioimpedance. Bioimpedance measurements will be changed in digital data so that STM32 can read it by utilizing the capabilities of the internal ADC of STM32 (Fig. 10).

3.1 Stimulation

The stimulation circuit consists of a square wave generator, low pass filter and Voltage controlled current source. Changes that occur in the bioimpedance signal will be measured using two electrodes attached to the body that will be amplified by

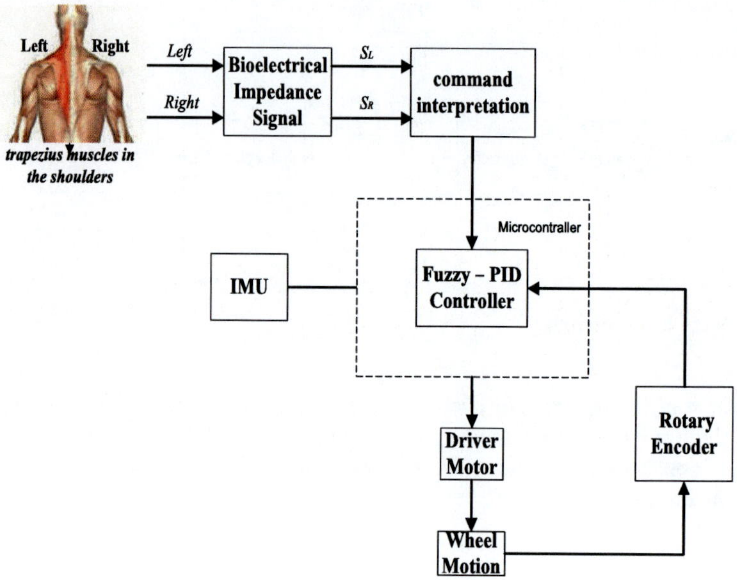

Fig. 9 Overall system diagram

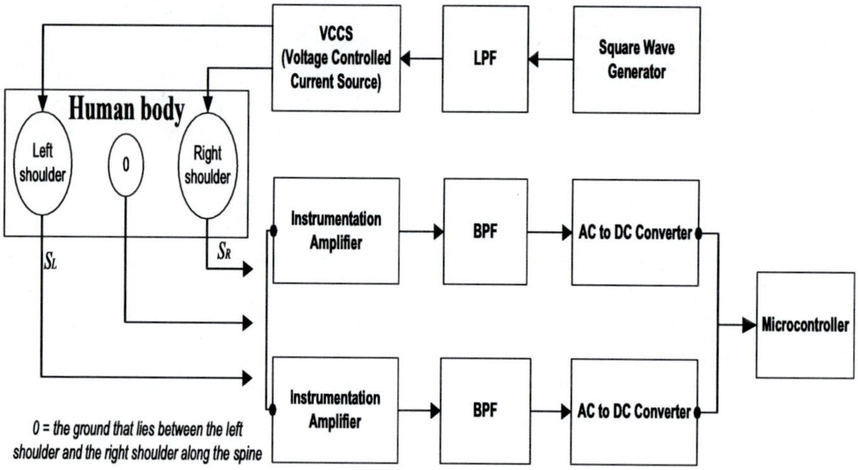

Fig. 10 Diagram of motor control with bioelectrical impedance signal

an instrumentation amplifier that is passed on the band pass filter so that it gets the desired frequency of 50 kHz.

3.2 Instrumentation

Using 3 op amps, LF412 and 2 unit LF353 which have a maximum voltage that can be passed by +12.7 V and −12.7 V.

3.3 Command Interpretation

The wheelchair can move forward when given motion commands, namely by raising the left and right shoulders simultaneously. When the shoulder is moved upwards, the bioimpedance signal will be read and send the command to the microcontroller to move the wheelchair. When the bioimpedance signal on the right shoulder is wider or the output signal is greater than the bioimpedance signal on the left shoulder, there will be a turning direction in the wheelchair, namely turning right. Vice versa, when the bioimpedance signal on the left shoulder is wider or the output signal is greater than the bioimpedance signal on the right shoulder, there will be a turning direction in the wheelchair, namely turning left. When the bioimpedance signal on the right shoulder and the left shoulder is greater than the threshold, then it is a command for the direction of forwarding motion for the wheelchair. This is shown in Fig. 11, namely the Command Interpretation Flow Chart.

3.4 Fuzzification

The controller works when three inputs are entered, namely the slope of the track, the speed of the RPM and the rotary encoder sensor. These three inputs are processed in the fuzzification process. Fuzzy variables at the input value will be processed by setting rules. The output of the rule will be a fuzzy variable and a defuzzification process will occur. The speed sensor measures the speed of the wheel to feed back to the controller. Changes in the RPM value in a wheelchair consisting of slow, medium, and fast are influenced by the slope value of the track consisting of flat, starting to tilt, and tilt (Figs. 12 and 13).

4 Result

4.1 Stimulation

The stimulation produces sinusoidal signals with a frequency of 50 kHz, and a constant current of 0.5 mA will then be injected into the body through electrodes. Stimulation consists of a square wave generator, low pass filter, and an inverting

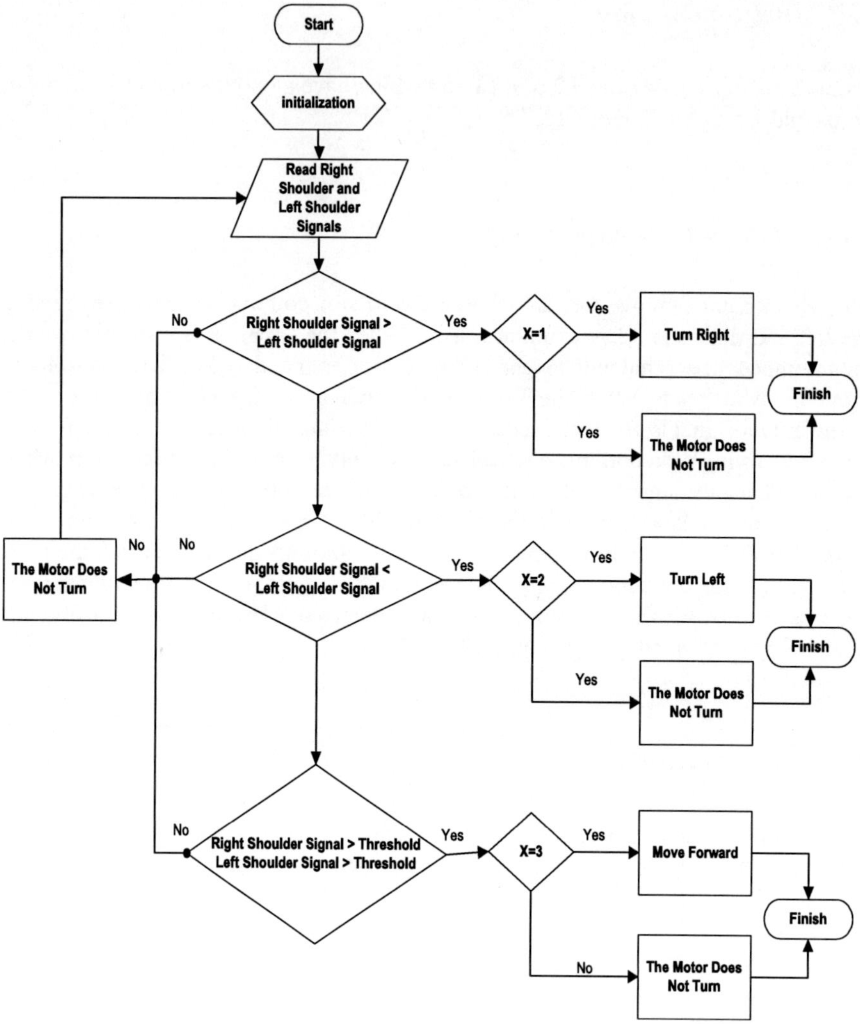

Fig. 11 Command interpretation flow chart

amplifier. Square wave generator functions to set the most optimal frequency in the measurement that is equal to 50 kHz. The signal generated by the square wave generator is then forwarded to the LPF to produce a perfect sinusoidal signal. A sinusoidal signal will be generated at a cut-off value of 50 kHz. The Inverting Amplifier circuit serves to regulate the amplification of sinusoidal signals generated by LPF so that we can easily adjust the signal amplitude at 2 V rms (Fig. 14).

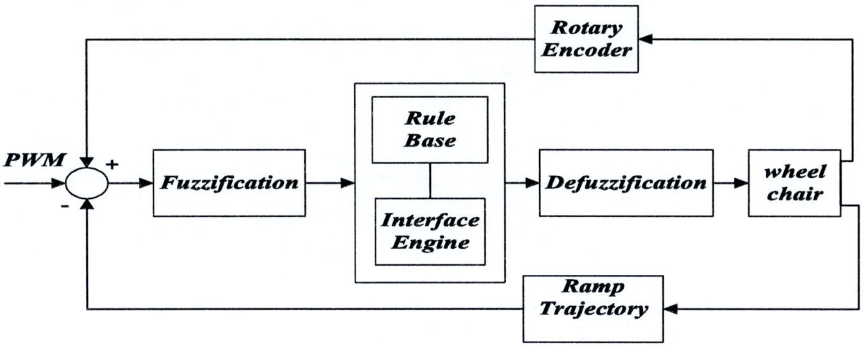

Fig. 12 Fuzzy logic block diagram

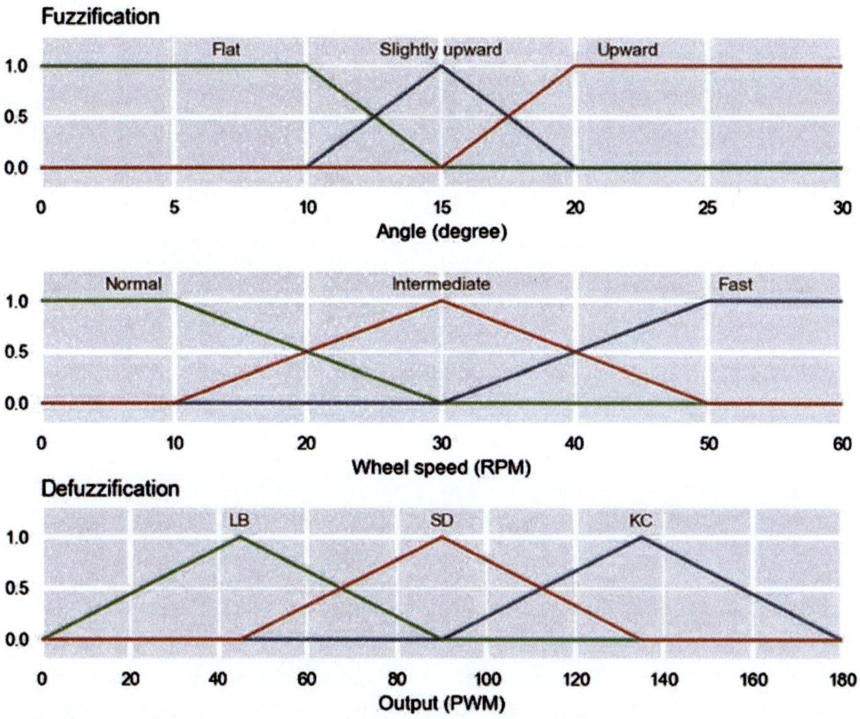

Fig. 13 Membership function of track slope, RPM and PWM speed

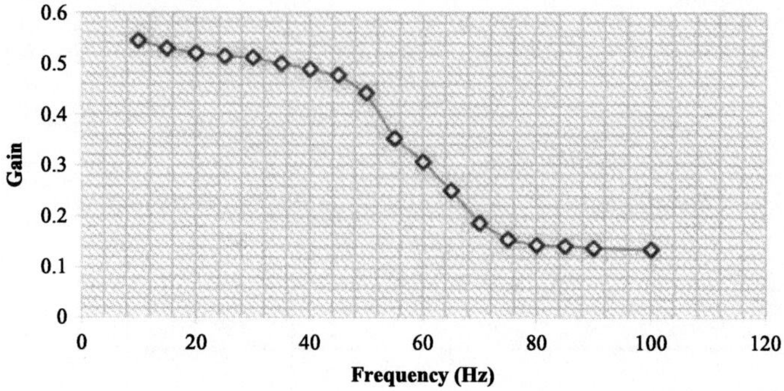

Fig. 14 LPF graph

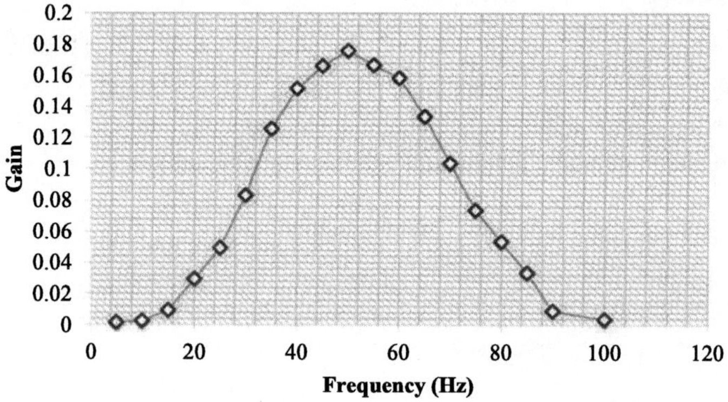

Fig. 15 BPF graph

4.2 Instrumentation

Instrumentation consists of the instrumentation amplifier, band pass filter, and AC to DC Converter. Strengthening of the instrumentation amplifier is produced by three op-amps, which show the results of a linear gain. The amount of Rgain obtained is ten times. BPF is done to get the cut off frequency between 48 and 55 kHz. From the test results, it was found that the center of frequency is located at 50 kHz. Look at Fig. 15. In AC to Dc Converter, the sinusoidal signal of 50 kHz as an input value of the function generator with varying amplitude values, the DC voltage will be measured.

4.3 Overall System Results

In 10 trials on 4 people whose weight was different. From the differences in the people produced differences in motor speed and differences in response from the bioimpedance signal. In the first person weighing 45 kg, the response to the reading of the bioimpedance signal is very slow, to move the wheelchair to move forward a number of movements of the shoulders, and the time lag between the forward motion command and the motorcycle is very long about 5 s. In the second person weighing 51 kg, the response from the bioimpedance signal is not so sensitive, when the left and right shoulders are moved upward, the wheelchair motor does not immediately respond to move forward, it takes a few seconds (approximately 3 s from the time of the motion command) until the wheelchair moves forward. In a third-person weighing 60 kg, the response from the bioimpedance signal produces a sensitive response, when the left and right shoulders are moved upward, the wheelchair motor moves forward immediately (approximately 1 s after the shoulder is moved up). In a fourth person weighing 75 kg, the response from the bioimpedance signal that is produced is so slow that it takes a long time and is carried out several times by motion commands by moving the left shoulder and right shoulder several times until the wheelchair can move forward.

4.3.1 Flat Trajectory

When moving forward on a flat trajectory with a slope of 0 and its RPM per-minute revolutions around the 40 s, it will provide a constant PWM rotation. In this experiment, 10 experiments were carried out with subjects with different body weights. In Fig. 16 shows that the inclination value is not constant on a flat trajectory and the RPM speed fluctuates so that the wheelchair speed also has an effect. In the figure, it can be seen that the success was obtained in subjects weighing 45 kg and 60 kg, where the angle reading and the RPM speed were constant. Whereas for subjects weighing 51 kg and 75 kg, the value of the slope angle of the track is negative, indicating it is a descending trajectory, but this does not affect the rotation at RPM so that the wheelchair is still running normally at a constant speed.

4.3.2 Upward Trajectory

When a wheelchair moves on an uphill track, it initially starts on a flat trajectory with a reading of the tilt angle of the track, which is 0°. When the wheelchair starts to rise on an upward trajectory, the IMU sensor will read the slope of the track and make the PWM speed change according to the increasing value of the slope angle of the track. This experiment was carried out on subjects with different body weights. The heavier the subject and the higher the angle of the trajectory, the faster the PWM speed (Fig. 17).

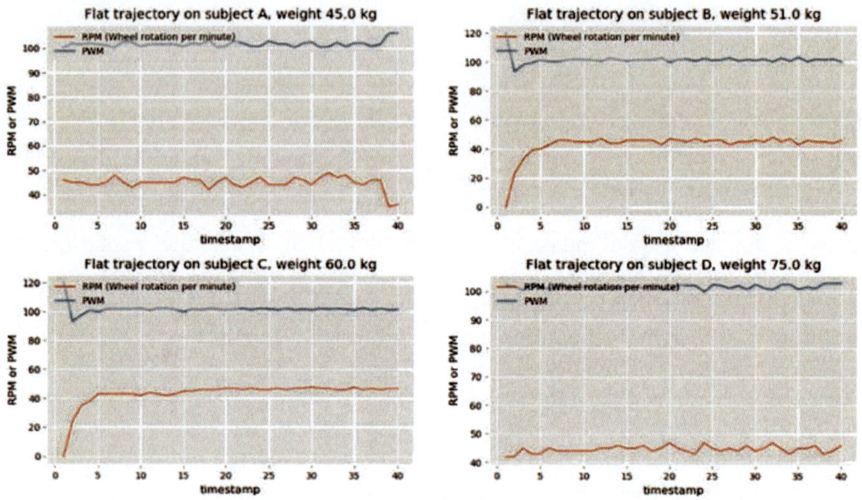

Fig. 16 PWM speed and RPM against flat trajectory with different subject weight

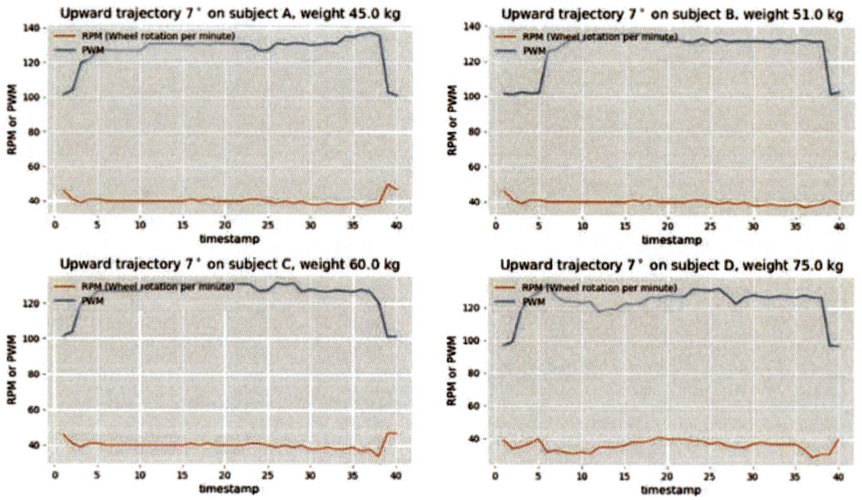

Fig. 17 PWM speed and RPM against an upward trajectory 7° with different subject weight

4.3.3 Downward Trajectory

When a wheelchair moves on a downward trajectory, it initially starts on a flat trajectory with a reading of the tilt angle of the track which is 0°. When the wheelchair starts to rise on the downward trajectory, the IMU sensor will read the

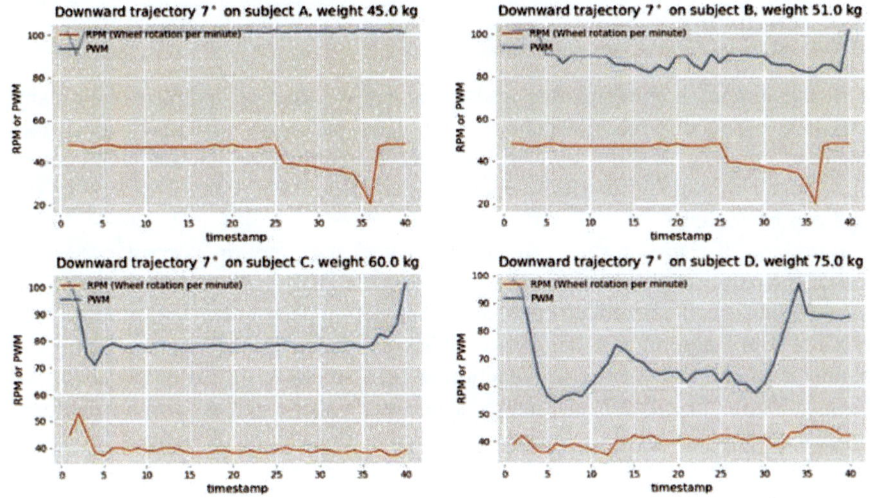

Fig. 18 PWM speed and RPM against an downward trajectory 7° with different weight of subjects A, B, C and D

slope of the track and make the PWM speed change according to the decreasing value of the slope angle of the track. This experiment was carried out on subjects with different body weights. The heavier the subject and the lower the tilt angle value, the slower the PWM rotation (Fig. 18).

5 Discussion

On a flat track, the PWM value of the motor is in the range of 100 for wheel RPM speeds of 40–50. Whereas in the upward trajectory, the PWM value is 120–140 for the same wheel speed, and in the downward trajectory, the PWM value is below 100. This difference shows that the Fuzzy-PID controller action is used to keep the wheel speed the same even though the slope of the track is different. This is necessary for the comfort of the wheelchair user so that there is no speed varies depending on the slope of the track. Then for different weights and the same speed, the required PWM value tends to be the same on a flat and upward path. However, it is different in the downward trajectory, where the PWM value will be smaller when the bodyweight is getting bigger. This result is very necessary to determine the effect of the angle of the track slope on the motor speed in a wheelchair.

The limitation in this study is the slope angle of the track not more than 10°. Research has been carried out in 2018 related to wheelchairs that can cross the upward trajectory, but in his research, the maximum limit of the slope of the track is 5.3° to get the stability of the motor rotation in a wheelchair [8].

6 Conclusion

With the aim of helping people with paralysis in order to mobilize their daily activities, especially for wheelchair users, it is necessary to know the correct electrode position on the user's back so that the application and development of knowledge about bioelectric impedance using the Fuzzy-PID control method on the road can be realized.

Based on the trial results, an electric wheelchair motion control system is designed by utilizing the bioelectrical impedance signal that is on the shoulders of the subject. The bioelectrical impedance signal produces a maximum voltage of 590 mV with a minimum voltage value of 50 mV. Electrodes were placed using the tetrapolar method, 2 electrodes functioned as a stimulus or current injection of 0.5 mA. While the other 3 functions as senders of voltage values from bioelectrical impedance signals from the subject's shoulders to the instrumentation system which is connected to the microcontroller which will instruct the electric wheelchair motion command. The electrode placement on the subject's back and the short width of the muscle on the subject as well as the subject's body weight affect the sensitivity of the reading of the bioelectrical impedance signal on the shoulder, this occurs because of a decrease in the value of the voltage resulting from the body's impedance results. The condition of fatigue or fatigue in the muscles also greatly affects the results of stress measurements from the body's impedance.

From the 10 experiments conducted, the success rate was 80%. The instability of the rotation of the left motor and right motor in a wheelchair when given a forward motion command occurs when the wheelchair is tested continuously without pause, the difference in rotation of the left motor and right motor on a wheelchair also occurs because the mechanical system of the wheelchair is not balanced between the two wheels front of the wheelchair, the front wheel to the left of the wheelchair is not the same position as the front wheel to the right of the wheelchair. The results of this trial also obtained a bioelectrical impedance signal which has a long response when given a motion command. The reading of the tilt angle of the track that changes according to the tilt of the wheelchair will affect the speed of the wheelchair motor. The greater the tilt angle of the track and the heavier the subject who uses a wheelchair when crossing the track up the speed of the wheelchair will increase, and the greater the tilt angle with a mild subject, the speed of the wheelchair will be relatively fast. And vice versa the smaller the slope angle of the track and the heavier the subject using a wheelchair, the speed of the wheelchair will slowly decrease. And the smaller the slope angle of the track with lighter subjects, the relative speed of the wheelchair increases.

For further research is to design an application to monitor the movement of wheelchairs used by persons with disabilities.

References

1. Fred S, Randy N (2015) Practical anatomy and physiology: the skeletal muscle system. Assoc Appl Psychophysiol Biofeedback 38:47–51
2. World Health Organization (2018) Disability and health
3. Gracia TJ (2009) Multichannel bioimpedance measurement master of science thesis tampere. University of Technology Biomedical Department Universitat Politecnica De Catalunya Enginyeria Electronica
4. Amit VN, Paul G, Aakanksha J, Gopichand R (2010) The efficacy of an integrated neuromuscular inhibition technique on upper trapezius trigger points in subjects with non-specific neck pain: a randomized controlled trial. J Manual Manupulative Therapy 18:37–43
5. Toivo P, Mart M, Dennis T (2011) Low-energy chirps for bioimpedance measurement. In: 34th International conference on telecommunications and signal processing (TSP), 18–20 Aug 2011
6. Araki M (2017) PID control control system, robotics and automation 2:694–696
7. Khan A, Rapal N (2006) Fuzzy PID controller: design, tuning and comparison with conventional PID controller. IEEE Int Conf Eng Intell Syst ICEIS 1:4244–0457
8. Maddalena S, Nicola G, Francesco DN, Nicola C (2020) Joint trajectory and fatigue analysis in wheelchair users. In: International conference on computer vision workshop, 27–28 Oct 2019
9. Huang Y (2010) Wheelchair control based on bioimpedance. Int J Appl Biomed Eng 3:13–15
10. Tsunami D (2005) Variable frequency bioimpedance instrumentation. In: Proceedings of the 26th annual international conference of the IEEE EMBS, San Francisco, CA, USA, 1–5 September
11. Philipe M, Christian F, Xavier D, Maurice D, Fabien D, Jean MN (2017) Morphological anatomy of the trapezius muscle, about 58 dissections: what to know before harvesting the muscular flap MOJ. Anat Physiol 4(4)
12. Taguchi H, Araki M (2000) Two degree of freedom PID controllers. In: Proceedings of the IFAC workshop on digital control: past, present and future of PID control, pp 91–96
13. IEEE, IEEE Citation Reference, [Online]. Available: www.ieee.org/documents/ieeecitationref.pdf
14. Kazuo T, Michio S (1992) Stability analysis and design of fuzzy control. Fuzzy Sets Syst 45:135–156
15. Hirokazu S, Atsushi K (2011) Disturbance road adaptive driving control of power-assisted wheelchair using fuzzy inference. In: Annual international conference of the IEEE engineering in medicine and biology society, 30 Aug to 3 Sept 2011
16. US Access Board (2004) Ramps and curb ramps Americans with Disabilities Act Standards. Washington DC
17. Huang Y, Pornchai P, Booncharoen W, Sawit T (2009) Development of a bioimpedance-based human machine interface for wheelchair control. In: 6th International conference on electrical engineering/electronics, computer, telecommunications and information technology, 6–9 May 2009
18. Barbara S, Zbigniew S, Dawid R, Aleksander S, Paweł K (2017) Bioimpedance spectroscopy monitoring—designing challenges and description of the acquired results. In: 24th International conference mixed design of integrated circuits and systems, 22–24 June 2017
19. Zhihong T, Wenhui X (2009) Electric wheelchair controller based on parameter self-adjusting fuzzy PID. In: International conference on computational intelligence and natural computing, 6–7 June 2009
20. Rudi H, Arista A, Yunafi'atul A, Farida HT (2017) The electric wheelchair control using electromyography sensor of arm muscle. In: International conference on information and communication technology and systems (ICTS), 12–12 Oct 2016

Unstable Walking Detection in Healthy Young Adults Using Postural Stability Index

Nurul Retno Nurwulan

Abstract Accelerometer is a common device being used in healthcare industry to recognize human daily activity as the early detection for the risk of fall. Past studies have been carried out in order to develop an effective human activity recognition using an accelerometer, either accelerometer in the form of dedicated motion sensors or the built-in triaxial accelerometer in smartphones. This study aimed to utilize the postural stability index (PSI) in discriminating the subtle changes in closely similar daily activities, such as walking on a flat surface, walking upstairs, and walking downstairs. The walking activities above were selected to see whether the PSI could detect the slight postural sway in the acceleration data. The dataset was collected from twenty-four subjects with a smartphone-based triaxial accelerometer inside the subjects' front pocket. The ensemble empirical mode decomposition (EEMD) was used to pre-processed the collected data. Then, the PSI values were obtained by calculating the complexity index of multiscale entropy (MSE) for each intrinsic mode function (IMF). The data calculation using paired t-test showed a significant difference between walking downstairs and walking on a flat surface ($p = 0.039$ and $p = 0.02$ for 2-tailed and 1-tailed t-test, respectively). The PSI value of walking downstairs was higher than walking on a flat surface. From this result, it is evident that walking downstairs is more challenging and less stable than normal walking. In conclusion, the PSI could be used for the early detection of unstable walking.

Keywords Accelerometer · Postural stability · PSI · EEMD · Multiscale entropy

N. R. Nurwulan (✉)
Sampoerna University, Jakarta 12780, Indonesia
e-mail: nurul.nurwulan@sampoernauniversity.ac.id

H. Triwiyanto et al. (eds.), *Proceedings of the 1st International Conference on Electronics, Biomedical Engineering, and Health Informatics*, Lecture Notes in Electrical Engineering 746, https://doi.org/10.1007/978-981-33-6926-9_37

1 Introduction

Unstable walking is an abnormality in walking that can be caused by disease related to the damage of the nervous system that controls the movement. It may appear as the after effect of illnesses, injury, and old age. Unstable walking is often difficult to notice, and it may develop to more serious problem if it is left untreated. The fall risk is greater in older adults' population, approximately 30% of older adults' population experience falls every year [1]. Falls may also happen to young adults as well [2, 3], especially if they have a history of injury or illnesses. Sleep deprivation increases the likelihood of falls because it may cause a lack of attentional control that lead falls [3, 4]. Attentional control is linked to walking performance, especially in older adults [4]. Active individuals, include young adults, tend to fall outdoors due to slip and trip [2, 5]. Whereas, older adults with illnesses tend to fall indoors [6]. Falls can cause further health issues physically and psychologically [7] both for young and older adults. Thus, early detection of unstable walking may help in preventing and minimizing fall risk.

In healthy subjects, the postural sway may not as significant as the fallers. Thus, it may be difficult to determine whether someone is having a risk of becoming a faller. The postural stability index (PSI) was proposed as a measure to distinguish the postural stability in healthy subjects [8]. This index was proposed as an early detection tool for the potential risk of falls. The performance of normal walking, walking with obstacles, and intentional falling in healthy young and older adults were evaluated and the PSI showed a promising result. Although the subjects in this past study were healthy, the tasks were very distinguishable. The PSI may not be as accurate if the tasks were only slightly different.

The current study aimed to utilize the PSI in discriminating the postural sway in healthy subjects while walking on a flat surface, walking upstairs, and walking downstairs. These walking tasks were chosen because of their slight differences, they are normal walking without any obstacles. With this evaluation, it can be seen whether the PSI can detect subtle changes in the postural stability of healthy subjects. Additionally, this study can also show which type of walking is less stable and need more attention in order to avoid falls.

The organization of this paper is as follows. The second section is the methodology which provides the information of data collection and theoretical background related to this study, namely ensemble empirical mode decomposition (EEMD), multiscale entropy (MSE), and postural stability index (PSI). Results and discussion are then presented in Sect. 3. Ultimately, the conclusion can be found in Sect. 4.

2 Materials and Method

The dataset used in this study was taken from the study by Malekzadeh et al. [9]. The data collection was done using the triaxial accelerometer built-in iPhone 6 s smartphone from twenty-four young adults with the age ranging from 18 to

46 years. The sampling frequency of data collection was 50 Hz. In this current study, walking on a flat surface, walking upstairs, and walking downstairs were selected due to the slight differences with one another. The dataset was pre-processed with 8-modes of ensemble empirical mode decomposition (EEMD) and the complexity index from the multiscale entropy (MSE) value was calculated for each intrinsic mode function (IMF). The postural stability index (PSI) value of each walking task was calculated by dividing the complexity index value of the dominant IMF with the total complexity index values for all IMFs [8].

2.1 Ensemble Empirical Mode Decomposition

Ensemble empirical mode decomposition (EEMD) is a powerful method for the non-stationary signals such as the human acceleration data [10]. The EEMD was introduced to overcome the drawbacks in empirical mode decomposition (EMD) by adding the white noise to the original signal. Then, the new signal with white noise is decomposed to obtain each layer of IMFs (IMF11, IMF12, …, $IMF1_n$). In the end, there will be $m \times n$ IMF components where m is the ensemble number and n is the layer of IMF. The results from the decomposition are then averaged.

$$\mathrm{IMF}_n = \frac{1}{m}\sum_{i=1}^{m}\mathrm{IMF}_n \tag{1}$$

2.2 Multiscale Entropy

Multiscale entropy (MSE) was proposed by Costa et al. [11] to calculate the complexity of human signal data. Since its introduction, it has shown promising results in various applications especially in the biomedical research field [11–13]. The MSE measures complexity of the time series data by building the consecutive coarse-grained data.

$$y_j^{\tau} = \frac{1}{\tau}\sum_{i=(j-1)\tau+1}^{j\tau} x_i, \quad 1 \le j \le \frac{N}{\tau} \tag{2}$$

where τ is the scale factor and N/τ is the length of the a coarse-grained.

The MSE uses sample entropy (SampEn) to calculate the entropy of each coarse-grained time series.

$$\mathrm{SampEn}(m, r, N) = -\ln\left(\frac{A}{B}\right) \tag{3}$$

where A is the total number of forward matches of length $m + 1$, and B is the total number of templates match of length m [11]. In order to obtain the complexity index (CI), the total value of the SampEn is accumulated.

$$\mathrm{CI} = \sum_{i=1}^{N} \mathrm{SampEn}(i) \tag{4}$$

2.3 *Postural Stability Index*

The postural stability index (PSI) was proposed in an attempt to distinguish the unbalance movement in healthy subjects. The postural difference between fallers and non-fallers is easy to recognize. However, when the subjects are all non-fallers with no history of neurological disorders or injuries, it is more challenging to discriminate against the non-fallers from fallers. The PSI uses the 8-modes EEMD as to pre-process the signal data before calculating the CI of each IMF and subsequently determine the stability index. The IMF3 is chosen as the dominant IMF because the frequency of IMF3 is closely related to the frequency of walking that ranging from 1.4 to 2.5 Hz [8, 14].

$$\mathrm{PSI} = \frac{\text{CI of IMF3}}{\text{CI of IMF1} + \text{CI of IMF2} + \ldots + \text{CI of IMF6}} \tag{5}$$

3 Results

The PSI is able to discriminate different balance states in healthy subjects. However, the tasks used in the evaluation of the PSI in the past study by Nurwulan et al. [8] were significantly different tasks, they were normal walking, walking with obstacles, and intentional falling. The question is, how good is the PSI in detecting the unbalance movement in healthy subjects if they are doing similar activity namely walking but in a slightly different situation. This current study aimed to see whether the PSI is still able to distinguish the slightly different activities in healthy subjects. Thus, the normal walking on a flat surface, walking upstairs, and walking downstairs, taken from the study by Malekzadeh et al. [9], were chosen for the evaluation. The PSI of all tasks done by each subject was calculated for comparison, as can be seen in Table 1.

The paired and independent t-tests were used to see whether the PSI of each task is different from one another (Table 2). From the paired t-test, it is evident that

Table 1 Calculated postural stability index

Subject	Upstairs	Flat	Downstairs	Subject	Upstairs	Flat	Downstairs
1	0.429	0.543	0.330	13	0.173	0.283	0.366
2	0.245	0.241	0.387	14	0.090	0.239	0.264
3	0.547	0.320	0.318	15	0.270	0.230	0.292
4	0.196	0.298	0.275	16	0.212	0.256	0.339
5	0.471	0.223	0.307	17	0.315	0.252	0.431
6	0.117	0.191	0.351	18	0.493	0.578	0.553
7	0.378	0.348	0.333	19	0.446	0.353	0.415
8	0.363	0.203	0.344	20	0.315	0.204	0.304
9	0.367	0.289	0.351	21	0.200	0.226	0.299
10	0.289	0.308	0.375	22	0.281	0.382	0.335
11	0.275	0.358	0.309	23	0.272	0.235	0.359
12	0.302	0.224	0.278	24	0.268	0.390	0.253

Table 2 Paired and independent t-test calculation

Paired t-test		
Activities	2-tailed	1-tailed
Upstairs–Flat	0.801	0.401
Upstairs–Downstairs	0.123	0.062
Downstairs–Flat	0.039	0.020
Independent t-test		
Upstairs–Weight	$p < 0.001$	$p < 0.001$
Upstairs–Height	$p < 0.001$	$p < 0.001$
Upstairs–Gender	0.014	0.007
Upstairs–Age	$p < 0.001$	$p < 0.001$
Downstairs–Weight	$p < 0.001$	$p < 0.001$
Downstairs–Height	$p < 0.001$	$p < 0.001$
Downstairs–Gender	0.028	0.014
Downstairs–Age	$p < 0.001$	$p < 0.001$
Flat–Weight	$p < 0.001$	$p < 0.001$
Flat–Height	$p < 0.001$	$p < 0.001$
Flat–Gender	0.012	0.006
Flat–Age	$P < 0.001$	$P < 0.001$

walking downstairs and walking on a flat surface are significantly different. Although the values of the PSI for both tasks seem different, the test showed that walking upstairs and downstairs are not different. The results of the independent t-test showed that the subjects' demographic characteristics such as weight, height, age, and gender affect the value of the PSI.

4 Discussion

Generally, the PSI values of walking upstairs (average of 0.305 ± 0.116) and walking downstairs (average of 0.340 ± 0.064) are greater than the PSI value of walking on a flat surface (average of 0.299 ± 0.1). However, the results in each subject are various. The U-shaped trend with the highest value in walking on a flat surface is shown by subjects 1, 4, and 24. Another U-shaped trend with the lowest value in walking on a flat surface can be seen in subjects 2, 15, 17, and 23. Increasing trend with walking upstairs as the highest value and walking downstairs as the lowest value is shown by subjects 6, 10, 11, 13, 14, 16, 18, 21, and 24. Whereas, the decreasing trend with walking upstairs as the lowest value is seen in subjects 3, 5, 7, 8, 9, 12, 18, and 29.

Considering there is no meaningful obstacle and difficulty, walking on a flat surface should be the most balanced movement. With regard to the calculated PSI values, it can be seen that the more balanced movement is the one with low PSI value. Therefore, walking downstairs should be the least balanced one. Both walking upstairs and downstairs are more challenging than walking on a flat surface [15]. Walking upstairs and downstairs require more balance skills. Walking upstairs requires more effort because we have to walk against the gravity. On the contrary, walking downstairs has more risk due to the acceleration added by gravity [15]. Therefore, walking downstairs is associated with a higher risk of falls. In addition, the psychological aspect of the subjects such as fear of falling down may increase the risk. To compensate with the challenges, the walking speed when people walking downstairs and upstairs is normally slower than walking on a flat surface [16, 17]. The subjects in this study are healthy young adults. Therefore, walking upstairs is not too different from walking on a flat surface.

The PSI is not able to discriminate walking upstairs and walking on a flat surface (p = 0.801). It also could not discriminate walking upstairs and walking downstairs. This inability to differentiate the walking tasks being evaluated may happen due to the sampling rate in data collection was 50 Hz, while the sampling rate in the past study was 30 Hz [8, 14, 18]. According to the previous researches, low sampling rate gave better accuracy in human daily activity recognition than the high sampling rate [18, 19]. Future researches evaluating the impact of the sampling rate might be able in explaining this phenomenon better. Another limitation in this current study is the subjects in this study were only the young adults' group, future studies involving older adults are important to see the performance of the PSI in distinguishing the slightly different tasks in older adults.

5 Conclusion and Future Work

This study evaluated the sensitivity of postural stability index (PSI) in evaluating activities with subtle differences such as walking on a flat surface, walking upstairs, and walking downstairs. By using activities with subtle differences, it can be seen how sensitive the PSI is in distinguishing human daily activities. The calculation using a paired-test showed that walking downstairs and walking on a flat surface are different. However, walking upstairs and downstairs were seen as no different. Similarly, walking upstairs and walking on a flat surface could not be distinguished. This phenomenon might happens because of the high sampling rate was used in data collection. As for the evaluation based on the PSI values, the least stable movement in this study was walking downstairs. This finding is in agreement with the past studies since walking downstairs is influenced by the additional acceleration from gravity. In addition, the psychological effect such as the fear of falling could make the subjects walk slower than usual. The current study has shown the ability of the PSI in detecting the unstable walking in healthy subjects although the differences are subtle. However, it was unable to detect the very subtle differences. Future studies evaluating the impact of sampling rate on the performance of the PSI may improve the sensitivity of the analysis.

References

1. Guirguis-Blake JM, Michael YL, Perdue LA, Coppola EL, Beil TL (2018) Interventions to prevent falls in community-dwelling older adults: a systematic review for the U.S. preventive service task force. J Am Med Assoc 319:1696–1704
2. Heijnen MJH, Rietdyk S (2015) Failure in adaptive locomotion: trial-and-error exploration to determine adequate foot elevation over obstacles. Hum Mov Sci 46:86–95
3. Kim SY, Kim SG, Sim S, Park B, Choi HG (2016) Excessive sleep and lack of sleep are associated with slips and falls in the adult Korean population: a population-based cross-sectional study. Medicine 95:e2397
4. Fernandez NB, Hars M, Trombetti A, Vuilleumier P (2019) Age-related changes in attention control and their relationship with gait performance in older adults with high risk of falls. Neuroimage 189:551–559
5. Selamaj G (2020) Impacts of mobile phone distractions on walking performance. Indonesian J Comput Eng Des 2(1):32–37
6. Nascimento CF, Duarte YAO, Lebrao ML, Filho ADPC (2017) Individual and contextual characteristics of indoor and outdoor falls in older residents of Sao Paolo, Brazil. Arch Gerontol Geriatr 68:119–125
7. McPee JS, French DP, Jackson D, Nazroo J, Pendleton N, Degens H (2016) Physical activity in older age: perspectives for healthy ageing and frailty. Biogerontology 17:567–580
8. Nurwulan NR, Jiang BC, Novak V (2019) Development of postural stability index to distinguish different stability scales. Entropy 21:314
9. Malekzadeh M, Clegg RG, Cavallaro A, Haddadi H (2019) Mobile sensor data anonymization. In: Proceedings of the international conference on internet of things design and implementation, Montreal, QC, Canada, pp 49–58
10. Wu Z, Huang NE (2009) Ensemble empirical mode decomposition: a noise-assisted data analysis method. Adv Adapt Data Anal 1:1–41
11. Costa M, Goldberger AL, Peng CK (2002) Multiscale entropy analysis of complex physiologic time series. Phys Rev Lett 89:068102
12. Nurwulan NR, Jiang BC (2016) Possibility of using entropy method to evaluate the distracting effect of mobile phones on pedestrian. Entropy 18:390
13. Faes L, Porta A, Javorka M, Nollo G (2017) Efficient computation of multiscale entropy over short biomedical time series based on linear state-space models. Complexity 2017:1768264

14. Nurwulan NR, Jiang BC, Novak V (2019) Estimation of balance-ability on healthy subjects using postural stability index. In: Proceedings of the 25th ISSAT international conference on reliability and quality in design, Las Vegas, NV, USA
15. Shieh WY, Ju YY, Yu YC, Lin CK, Lin YT, Cheng HYK (2016) Stair-walking performance in adolescents with intellectual disabilities. Sensors 16:1066
16. Tura A, Raggi M, Rocchi L, Cutti AG, Chiari L (2010) Gait symmetry and regularity in transfemoral amputees assessed by trunk accelerations. J Neuroengineering Rehabil 7:4
17. Koster G, Lehmberg D (2019) Walking on stairs: experiment and model. Phys Rev E 100:022310
18. Chang YP, Jiang BC, Nurwulan NR (2020) Revised stability scales of the postural stability index for human daily activities. Entropy 22:1188
19. Liang Y, Zhou X, Yu Z, Guo B (2013) Energy-efficient motion related activity recognition on mobile devices for pervasive healthcare. Mobile Networks Appl 19:303–317

Computational Study of Ventral Ankle-Foot Orthoses During Stance Phase for Post-surgery Spinal Tuberculosis Rehabilitation

Alfian Pramudita Putra, Akif Rahmatillah, Pujiyanto, Khusnul Ain, Nur Khafidotur Rodiyah, I. Putu Alit Pawana, Lolita Hapsari Dwi Syahananta, Mohammad Rizki Dwiatma, and Arief Sofian Hidayat

Abstract Spinal Tuberculosis could cause abnormalities in the lower extremity, even after the surgery and can be treated with Ankle-Foot Orthoses (AFO). The patient with that condition has to stabilize their body because it tends to fall forward. Thus, a ventral AFO is needed to support them. This study aims to evaluate AFO design by using Finite Element Method (FEM) with two different thickness (2 and 4 mm). The material used was a Polyethylene Terephthalate (PET). Three subphases in the stance phase were simulated, namely initial contact, midstance, and terminal stance. The external force in the simulation was based on the patient's weight (50 kg). The result showed that the highest stress was obtained from ventral AFO with a thickness of 2 mm at the terminal stance, 244.7 MPa. This value exceeded the Ultimate Tensile Strength (UTS) of PET which indicates the design would break. The ventral AFO with a thickness of 4 mm had lower stress than the UTS of PET. The strain of both designs was quite low with the maximum value of 0.019 from the ventral AFO with a thickness of 4 mm in the terminal stance. The deformation was also acceptable for both designs with the highest value of 39.67 mm from the ventral AFO with a thickness of 2 mm in the midstance. In

A. P. Putra (✉) · A. Rahmatillah · K. Ain · N. K. Rodiyah · L. H. D. Syahananta · M. R. Dwiatma · A. S. Hidayat
Biomedical Engineering Study Program, Department of Physics, Faculty of Science and Technology, Universitas Airlangga, Surabaya 60115, Indonesia
e-mail: alfian.pramudita@fst.unair.ac.id

A. P. Putra · A. Rahmatillah · K. Ain
Biomedical Signals and Systems Research Group, Faculty of Science and Technology, Universitas Airlangga, Surabaya 60115, Indonesia

Pujiyanto
Department of Physics, Faculty of Science and Technology, Universitas Airlangga, Surabaya 60115, Indonesia

I. P. A. Pawana
Department of Physical Medicine and Rehabilitation, Dr Soetomo General Academic Hospital, Surabaya 60286, Indonesia

H. Triwiyanto et al. (eds.), *Proceedings of the 1st International Conference on Electronics, Biomedical Engineering, and Health Informatics*, Lecture Notes in Electrical Engineering 746, https://doi.org/10.1007/978-981-33-6926-9_38

conclusion, the ventral AFO with a thickness of 4 mm could be used for post-surgery spinal tuberculosis patient's rehabilitation.

Keywords Ankle-Foot orthosis · Computational analysis · Rehabilitation · Spinal tuberculosis · Stance phase

1 Introduction

Spinal tuberculosis (Spinal TB) is a disease caused by tuberculosis bacteria that attack the spine. This type of TB is dangerous because it could defect the bone and cause paraplegia in the lower extremity. The motoric function of the spinal TB patient will drop and affect the daily activities [1, 2]. Some treatments that can help the spinal TB patients are restorative treatment by surgery and systemic treatment by consuming antibiotics [3]. After the surgery, the patients need to undergo rehabilitation to restore their motoric function, especially the lower extremity. By performing the rehabilitation, the patients could be more independent [2].

The rehabilitation of spinal TB could be done by wearing an orthosis for lower extremity, such as Ankle Foot Orthoses (AFO). This orthosis function as a stabilizer of its user in walking [4]. The spinal TB patients tend to fall forward due to their spine' weakness to stabilize the stature. Several types of AFO that could be used in treating the spinal TB patients, such as ventral AFO [5]. It is an AFO that has cuff in the front part to give more stability to its user and prevent it from falling forward. The user's ankle will be fixed, and the front part would be held by the cuff [6].

The manufacturing process of AFO usually takes some time due to its trial and error approach [7, 8]. The physician will give the prescription to the orthotist based on the condition of the patients, and the molded AFO will be worn by the patient and tested in the gait lab. However, if there is a problem in terms of design, size, comfort, or gait result, the manufacturing process should be repeated with a correction. This process will take a long time before the rehabilitation takes apart. Nowadays, Computer-Aided Design (CAD) is accessible due to its flexibility in terms of the design process, and also the designer could perform a simulation to observe the behavior of the design if the load is applied [9]. Finite Element Method (FEM) is one of the popular methods to simulate the design digitally. By applying a load that equals to the gait of the patients, an AFO design could be simulated initially before the manufacturing process is done [7–9]. The previous study mentioned that by using FEM, the concentrated stress could be avoided, and the design process could be optimized [9]. However, there is no study about the FEM of specific design, especially in the gait cycle. Thus, this study focuses on the computational study of ventral AFO for the post-surgery spinal TB patient to observe its behavior during the stance phase. By understanding the behavior of the AFO in the stance phase, the design process could be optimized by adapting the dimension to overcome the failure based on the simulation.

2 Materials and Methods

The design process of AFO started by collecting the secondary data of the spinal TB patient, especially the foot dimension and the weight. The anthropometry data for the AFO design was shown in Table 1. There were two designs of AFO with variation in the thickness; 2 and 4 mm. The design process used CAD software Solidworks 2016, as shown in Fig. 1.

The simulation of the AFO designs was started by discretization or meshing the design. The design was divided into small pieces called elements that will be simulated in the FEM. The material used in the simulation was polyethylene terephthalate with properties: density of 1420 kg/m^3, Young's modulus of 296 GPa, Poisson Ratio of 0.37, and Ultimate Tensile Strength of 57.3 MPa. The stance phase simulation's boundary condition is divided into two parts, which are the fixed constraint and loading. The fixed constraint is placed on the top of the design (in the cuff part). This condition indicates the unmovable part of the design. The loading in the stance phase is placed at the bottom of the footplate to represent the Ground Reaction Force (GRF) during the stance phase [10, 11]. The loading is divided into three subphases: initial contact, midstance, and terminal stance, as shown in Fig. 2. The loading was 500 N based on the patient's weight (50 kg) and applied vertically [12]. The result of the simulation was evaluated in terms of stress and deformation. Based on both parameters, the best design of AFO for post-surgery spinal TB patients was chosen. The limitation of this method is that the result depends on the design of AFO. The anthropometry information of the proposed user is the main parameter that affects the complete result and analysis.

3 Results and Discussions

The design of ventral AFO was successful based on the anthropometry data of post-surgery spinal TB patients. The result of the simulation was shown in Figs. 3, 4, 5, 6, 7 and 8. Figures 3, 4 and 5 showed the design's stress during the initial contact, midstance, and terminal stance, and Figs. 6, 7 and 8 showed the design's deformation during the initial contact, midstance, and terminal stance.

The AFO design's stress was placed in the curve connecting the rear part of the AFO and the cuff, as shown in Figs. 3, 4 and 5. The simulation result was tabulated

Table 1 The anthropometry data for AFO design

No.	Part of AFO	Size (cm)
1	Retromalleolar height	6.23
2	Cuff width	5
3	Cuff length	9
4	Foot length	24.3
5	Calf height	31.5

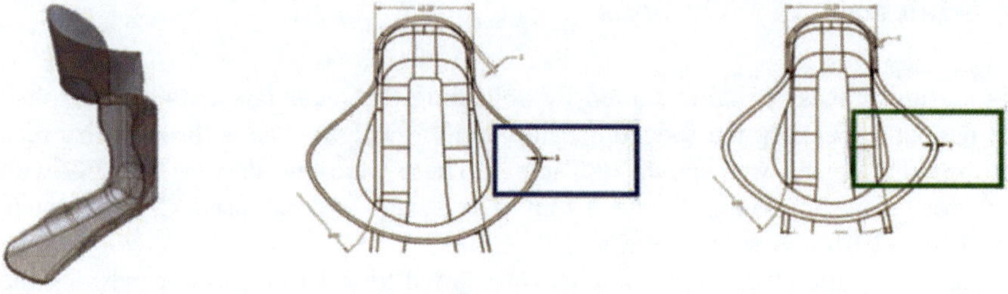

a b c

Fig. 1 The ventral AFO design for the post-surgery spinal TB rehabilitation, **a** full design, **b** design with thickness of 2 mm, and **c** design with thickness of 4 mm

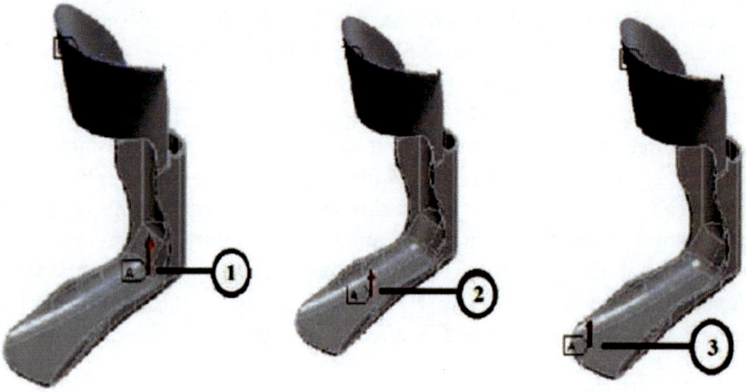

Fig. 2 The location of loading in three subphases; 1 terminal stance, 2 midstance, and 3 initial contact

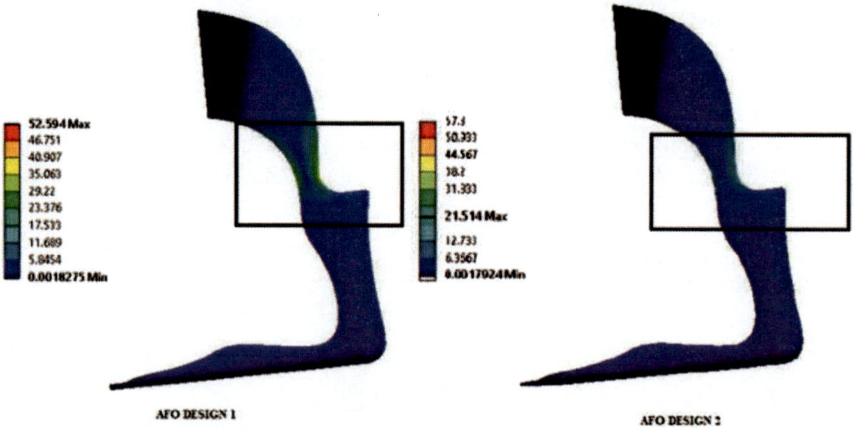

Fig. 3 The stress in AFO during initial contact

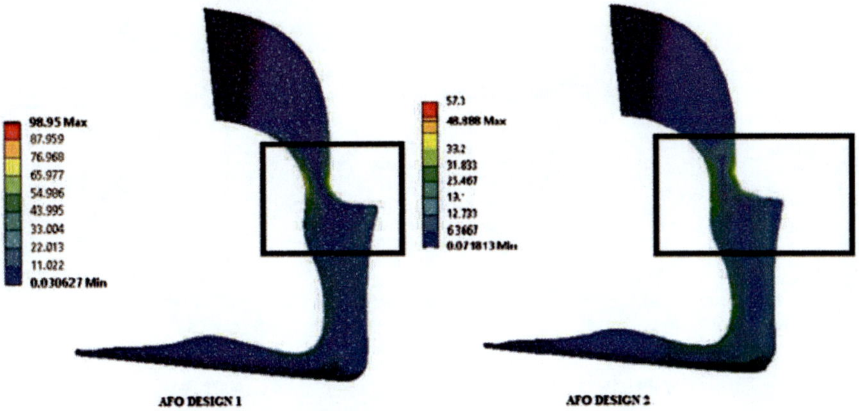

Fig. 4 The stress in AFO during midstance

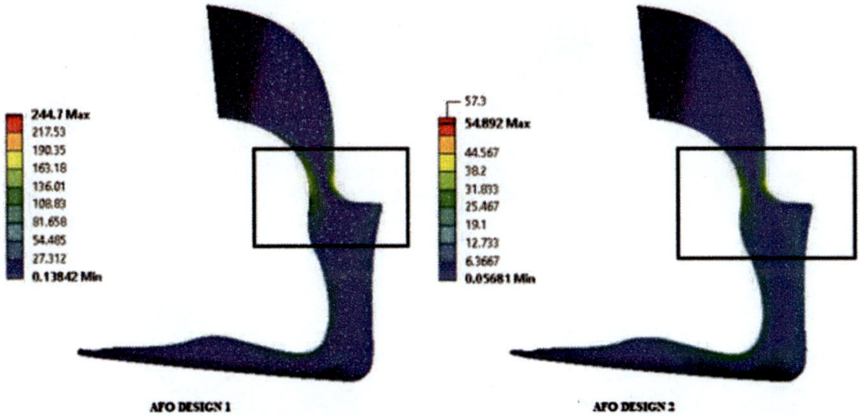

Fig. 5 The stress in AFO during terminal stance

in Table 2. This part was vital since it supports the cuff to stabilize the body of the user. The highest stress was found in AFO with a thickness of 2 mm. The thickness of the design determines its stiffness. The thicker the design, the stiffer the result. However, a high thickness design will give an uncomfortable feeling to the user due to its weight.

By using a thickness of 4 mm, the AFO design 2 would be sufficient in this case. The highest stress found in the simulation was 57.3 MPa (Fig. 3), which is lower or equal to the ultimate tensile strength of PET. PET is popular due to its toughness in a wide application. Moreover, it also has a high shock absorber and elasticity. This material could be a choice for AFO manufacturing besides common material such as polypropylene (PP) or DuraForm [8].

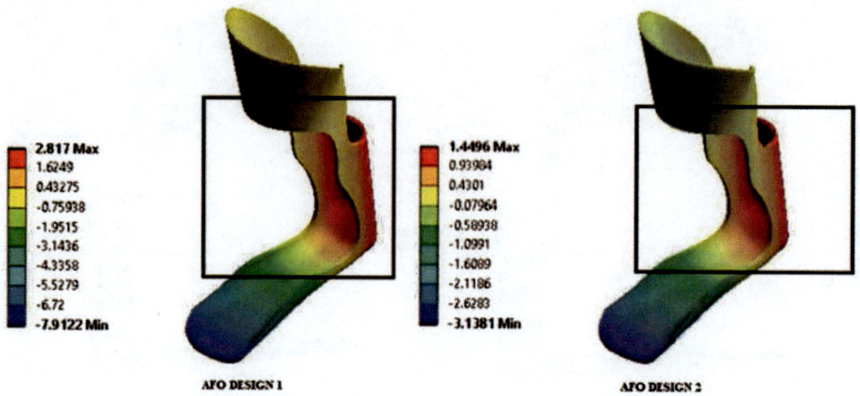

Fig. 6 The deformation in AFO during initial contact

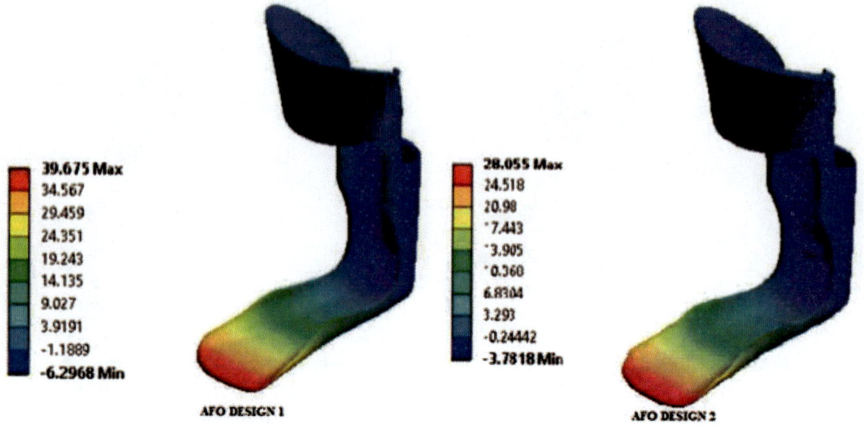

Fig. 7 The deformation in AFO during midstance

The AFO design with a thickness of 2 mm has maximum stress above the PET's ultimate tensile strength, which indicated that it would fail or break if a force of 500 N is applied to it. It occurred in the terminal stance. During this subphase, the user will give more force to the ground to lift the foot and enter the swing phase. The green area (Fig. 5) was concentrated in the curve between the front and rear parts of the AFO and several parts in the footplate. The stress in the footplate is undesired because it will affect the stability of the user. High concentrated stress will give low durability of the AFO due to the material's fatigue properties [13].

The deformation of AFO from the original position gives information about the stiffness of the design. The location of the applied force also determines the direction and the deformed part of the AFO. The simulation of initial contact (Fig. 6) that

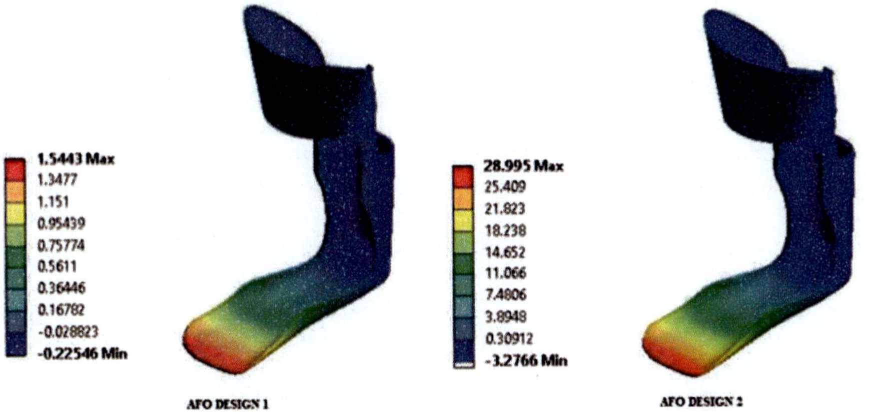

Fig. 8 The deformation in AFO during terminal stance

applied the load near the ankle gave a deformation in the rear part of the AFO below 3 mm, which is low. The front part of the footplate is barely moved. That behavior is caused by the fixed support location, which is in the upper part of the cuff. The fixed support has a role as a center of rotation when there is a load applied in the design. In the initial contact, the applied force has a short moment arm.

On the other hand, the moment arm of the applied force in the terminal stance is longer. The AFO design with a thickness of 4 mm is the best AFO in this study based on the result of stress and deformation. This AFO showed maximum stress in all the subphases in the stance phase that is lower than UTS of PET. However, the maximum stress in the terminal stance is just below the UTS of PET, which means that the AFO could be broken if the same load is applied several times [14–16]. Thus, it needs more improvement in the design or the material choice to have a better AFO result. The limitation of this is the use of the load, it is better to use dynamic loading of human walking to mimic the real condition. The load is not placed at a single position, but it is placed at the back of the AFO. It also moves along the way from the heel to the top of the foot, indicating the gait cycle.

Table 2 The stress and deformation of ventral AFO during stance phase

Subphase in stance phase	Minimum stress (MPa)	Maximum stress (MPa)	Minimum deformation (MPa)	Maximum deformation (MPa)
Initial contact AFO 1	0.002	52.594	−7.912	2.817
Initial contact AFO 2	0.002	21.514	−3.138	1.450
Midstance AFO 1	0.031	98.950	−6.300	39.675
Midstance AFO 2	0.007	48.890	−3.782	28.055
Terminal stance AFO 1	0.138	244.700	−0.220	1.544
Terminal stance AFO 2	0.057	54.890	−3.276	28.995

4 Conclusions

This study reported the computational analysis of ventral AFO for the post-surgery spinal TB patient to observe its behavior during the stance phase. The thickness of the AFO affects the stress and deformation of the design. The thicker the design, the higher the stress in the design, and the further the deformation from its original position. AFO design 2 with a thickness of 4 mm is sufficient to overcome the loading in the stance phase of post-surgery spinal TB patient with a weight of 50 kg. For future possibilities, the material of the AFO should be observed to obtain a better final design. The design should be improved in terms of the width of the cuff and the use of dynamic loading in the simulation to observe more real behavior.

Acknowledgements The author would like to thank Faculty of Science and Technology, Univeristas Airlangga for the funding of this study under the scheme of Faculty Excellent Research.

References

1. Rasouli MR, Mirkoohi M, Vaccaro AR, Yarandi KK, Rahimi-Movaghar V (2012) Spinal tuberculosis: diagnosis and management. Asian Spine J 6:294–308
2. Garg RK, Somvanshi DS (2011) Spinal tuberculosis: a review. J Spinal Cord Med 34: 440–454
3. Mehta JS, Bhojraj SY (2001) Tuberculosis of the thoracic spine. A classification based on the selection of surgical strategies. J Bone Joint Surg Br 83:859–63
4. Feng Y, Song Y (2017) The categories of afo and its effect on patients with foot impair: a systemic review. Phys Act Heal 1:8–16
5. Alam M, Choudhury IA, Mamat AB (2014) Mechanism and design analysis of articulated ankle foot orthoses for drop-foot. Sci World J 867869:1–15
6. Jamshidi N, Hanife H, Rostami M, Najarian S (2010) Innovation modelling the interaction of ankle-foot orthosis and foot by finite element methods to design an optimized sole in steppage gait. J Med Eng Technol 34:116–123
7. Cha YH, Lee KH, Ryu HJ, Joo IW, Seo A, Kim D, Kim SJ (2017) Ankle-foot orthosis made by 3D printing technique and automated design software. Appl Bionics Biomech 10468:1–6
8. Gomes G, Lourenço I, Oliveira J, Gomes M, Vale A, Freire L, Quental P, Policarpo H, Matos J (2017) Structural reinforcements on AFO's : a study using computer-aided design and finite element method. In: IEEE 5th Portuguese meeting on bioengineering (ENBENG), Portugal, pp 1–4
9. Marques MA, Mendes E, Ramos NV, Pinto VC, Vaz MA (2010) Finite element analysis of ankle foot orthosis to predict fracture conditions during gait finite-element analysis of ankle-foot orthosis to predict fracture conditions during gait. In: 1st ICH Gaia-Porto, Portugal
10. Williams SE, Gibbs S, Meadows CB, Abboud RJ (2011) Classification of the reduced vertical component of the ground reaction force in late stance in cerebral palsy gait. Gait Posture 34:370–373
11. Mulroy SJ, Eberly VJ, Gronely JK, Weiss W, Newsam CJ (2010) Effect of AFO design on walking after stroke: impact of ankle plantar flexion contracture. Prosthetics Orthot Int 34:277–292

12. Bas KWBS, Sjouke Z, Wiebren Z, Ida B (2012) Comparison of vertical ground reaction forces during overground and treadmill running. A validation study. BMC Musculoskelet Disord 13:235
13. Volpini M, Alves D, Horta A, Borges M, Reis P (2018) Orthosis and finite elements: a study for development of new designs through additive manufacturing. Int J Biomed Biol Eng 12:262–266
14. Abdelkader A (2018) Immediate effect of solid ankle foot orthosis versus gorund reaction ankle foot orthosis on balance in children with spastic diplegia. Biosci Res 15:1893–1898
15. Banga HK, Kalra P, Belokar RM (2018) Fabrication and customized design of kid's ankle foot orthosis by 3D printing. J Phys Conf Ser February 2019:1–10
16. Banga HK, Kalra P, Belokar RM, Kumar R (2020) Effect of 3D-printed ankle foot orthosis during walking of foot deformities patients. Lect Notes Mech Eng 275–88

The Implementation of EEG Transfer Learning Method Using Integrated Selection for Motor Imagery Signal

Aris Ramadhani, Hilman Fauzi, Inung Wijayanto, Achmad Rizal, and Mohd Ibrahim Shapiai

Abstract Brain-computer interface (BCI) is a system that can translate, manage, and recognize human brain activity. One of the devices used in the BCI system is Electroencephalogram (EEG). The brain signals produced by the EEG are diverse. One of them is the motor imagery signal. Motor imagery signal is used to translate the EEG signal into a specific movement. The performance of motor imagery signal classification is influenced by the number of training and testing data used. In most cases, the training data consists of a higher number of trials than the testing data. However, more trials cause higher subject variation. Previously study mentioned that this problem can be overcome by using transfer learning methods, which aimed at simplifying the training model. In this study, transfer learning in BCI is implemented using the integrated selection (IS) method, which simplifies the training model. Furthermore, IS is optimizing the data by removing the irrelevant channels of the EEG signals. Integrated selection uses the CUR matrix decomposition algorithm. The method split the data into two components, namely identity and historical data, represented by the C and UR matrix, respectively. The characteristic of the data from IS then calculated using three feature extraction methods. They are Fast Fourier Transform (FFT), Hjorth Descriptor, and Common Spatial Pattern (CSP). The features are then classified using the k-Nearest Neighbor (K-NN) method. The use of IS in the BCI system increases the accuracy of more than 6% and six-times faster processing time. In general, the integrated selection method is able to improve the performance of the BCI system.

Keywords BCI · EEG · Integrated selection · Motor imagery · Transfer learning

---

A. Ramadhani · H. Fauzi (✉) · I. Wijayanto · A. Rizal
School of Electrical Engineering, Telkom University, Bandung, Indonesia
e-mail: hilmanfauzitsp@telkomuniversity.ac.id

M. I. Shapiai
Malaysia Japan International Institute of Technology, Universiti Teknologi Malaysia, Kuala Lumpur, Malaysia

H. Triwiyanto et al. (eds.), *Proceedings of the 1st International Conference on Electronics, Biomedical Engineering, and Health Informatics*, Lecture Notes in Electrical Engineering 746, https://doi.org/10.1007/978-981-33-6926-9_39

1 Introduction

The Brain Computer Interface (BCI) is a system for translating, managing, and recognizing human brain activity. This method of recording follows an approach that does not require embedding of external objects into the brain. An example of measuring a brain signal is an electroencephalography (EEG) [1]. Electroencephalogram (EEG) is a tool that can be used to record the activity of electrons in the human brain placed on the scalp. EEG has shortcomings one of which is hindered by the time-consuming calibration repeatedly before use. This is a matter of two things, namely non-stationary noise and, high-dimensional brain signals and the components associated with the state of the brain are usually obstructed by noise, to accurately predict the state of the brain, a lot of data trains are needed to extract features and study the pattern of data classification appropriately [2]. Various methods to overcome the signal of EEG signals that are not desired or that are not intended, one of them is by transfer learning.

Transfer Learning uses the important structure or information of the selected data to define new data from the same class [3]. Some research on the transfer of learning in the brain wave signal is with the Feature method representation transfer which learns the overview of new features with spatial filtering using data collected and compiled in a matrix [2]. Other with Transfer Learning is implemented on EEG drowsiness detection to improve the performance of BCI-based EEG of sleepiness detection itself in previous studies [4]. Transfer Learning aims to simplify the training model. In this study, transfer learning in BCI will be implemented using the integrated selection method of the motor imagery EEG signal which in addition can simplify the training model of this method can also compress the dataset into a more optimal size. These results can be used as an alternative to the method of transfer learning in the future EEG which has improved performance and shortens processing time.

2 Methodology

2.1 *Brain Computer Interface*

BCI develops with its application system in the field of research. BCI can be used in the medical field as a preventive, detector and also nerve rehabilitation if it reaches a serious injury [1]. One of BCI modal is Electroencephalography (EEG). EEG is a device used to record electrical activity on the human brain by placing EEG on the scalp. EEG is one device that is done by non-invasive method. Some EEG channels are recorded simultaneously from multiple locations in the scalp section. The acquired signal is recorded using an electrode that detects the small charge generated by the brain cells [5]. The recorded signal waves are information about brain activity [6]. The information recorded by EEG is vibration, frequency, and brainwave or can be called Brain wave.

One of the applications of BCI is motor imagery (MI). MI's main objective is to aid the physically disabled people. Studies about MI are mostly focused on the movement of hands and feet. During the MI task, the participants need to imagine a specific movement of the body. This imagination then creates brain signals which recorded using EEG. By recognizing the brain wave pattern, researchers can create a system that can translate the signal into a prosthetic application using a robotic application [7]. In this study, EEG data set is obtained from University Medicine Berlin. The Data set contains the input of EEG signals of motion imagination, recorded from 5 healthy subjects. Subject is an adult age and in a healthy state. The information signal of motor imagery on this data recorded using 118 channel EEG.

2.2 *Integrated Selection*

Transfer Learning is a procedure to use processed data in a single task to improve the formation of another work [8]. Transfer learning captures the structure or important information of the selected data to find new data from the same class. Transfer Learning also provides a common structure for the same class data. The method of transfer learning is to find various structures in the variation of data between different set of data with common rules applied in different subjects [3]. One of the transfer learning method for BCI-EEG based is integrated selection. Integrated selection is the process of generating a smaller matrix of data sets. The smaller size of data will be optimized by defining the essential structure of the EEG signal. Thus, it will be executed at the time of the spatial selection and CUR transfer learning. Integrated selection will find and define the best time of the session and the signal channel in the selection of columns and rows using the method of energy calculation and optimized signal generated can improve the framework of the proposed decomposition of the CUR [3].

2.2.1 Spatial Selection

Spatial Selection is introduced as a channel selection technique. The spatial selection method is essentially the process of normalizing data in EEG signals and involving energy calculations. The Spatial Selection consists of two processes: energy extraction and energy selection. In energy extraction there are two methods of energy calculation: L2-norm and leverage score. In energy extraction, average energy channel is already calculated. This process is done by calculating the importance of each channel in the matrix on a dataset. Meanwhile, in the energy selection, there are two methods applied, i.e. manual and automatic selection [9]. In this research on energy extraction using the method L2-norm defined by Eq. (1).

$$p_j = \frac{\sum_{i=1}^{m} A(i,j)^2}{\sum_{i=1}^{m} \sum_{j=1}^{n} A(i,j)^2} \quad (1)$$

where p is the energy value, i is the row and j is the column. Further, A is the matrix of data, and m and n are the numbers of rows and columns, respectively. In this study, automatic mean method is used as an energy calculation method.

2.2.2 CUR Matrix Decomposition

CUR is the composition name of a matrix that can be configured to create an estimated matrix. C is a component of column in a matrix, R is the component of row in a matrix, and U is the form of component matrix that created by C, R, and the original matrix. The concept of transfer learning methods using the CUR matrix decomposition is to create the estimation of the original matrix compiled by the CUR matrix component. The UR matrix as the historical matrix for all subjects and some as the representative matrix of the subject. It is important to use table algorithms to create the appropriate UR matrix for best performance of transfer learning [3]. The UR matrix can be estimated by using two methods namely mean and selection. In mean method, matrix of the subject of the averaged experiment and combined to form a single matrix [3]. Then, single matrix is defined as the common UR matrix. Another case in the selection method, it performed based on the smallest value of the mean difference. Then, it is defined as the common UR matrix.

2.3 *Fast Fourier Transform (FFT)*

Fast Fourier Transform (FFT) is an efficient algorithm for calculating the coefficient of Discrete Fourier Transform (DFT) to a sequential finite of complex data [10]. DFT is used to convert discrete signal domain time into a frequency domain. But the conversion process takes a lot of time, so it uses the FFT method to reduce the complexity of the DFT computing by using the devide-and-conquer approach [11]. The formula of the DFT can be calculated by Eq. (2).

$$X(k) = \sum_{n=0}^{N-1} X(n).W_N^{nK} \quad (2)$$

where n, k is worth [0, N-1] and WNK = e-j2πk/N twiddle factor, $x(n)$ is the n sampling of discrete time signal and $x(k)$ is the sampling frequency on instant k.

2.4 Hjorth Descriptor

Hjorth Descriptor previously functioned to measure the health of people with an electroencephalogram (EEG) signal on a domain of time [12, 15]. Then Hjorth Descriptor is also used to measure Electromyogram (EMG) [13], and in the processing of lung sound [14]. This method includes three parameters i.e. activity, mobility, and complexity. These three parameters are used as a feature of each data [13].

Let σ_x become the standard deviation from $x(n)$, σ'_x is be the standard deviation from $x(n)'$ so σ''_x is the standard of the deviation $x(n)''$. Standard deviation $x(n)$ can be identified with the Eq. (3).

$$\sigma_{\bar{x}} = \sqrt{\frac{\sum_{n=0}^{N-1}(x(n)-\bar{x})^2}{N}} \quad (3)$$

With $\bar{x}$ can be identified with the Eq. (4).

$$\bar{x} = \frac{1}{N}\sum_{n=0}^{N-1} x(n) \quad (4)$$

Activities are defined as variations of the signal or standard squared deviations that can be defined by the Eq. (5).

$$\text{Activity} = \text{variance} = \sigma_x^2 \quad (5)$$

Mobility is defined in the Eq. (6) while complexity in Eq. (7).

$$\text{Mobility} = \text{M}_x = \frac{\sigma_{x'}}{\sigma_x} \quad (6)$$

$$\text{Complexity} = \text{FF} = \frac{\text{M}_{x'}}{\text{M}_x} = \frac{\sigma_{x''}/\sigma_{x'}}{\sigma_{x'}/\sigma_x} \quad (7)$$

2.5 Common Spatial Pattern (CSP)

The Common Spatial Pattern (CSP) is a method for determining the nature and characteristics of an EEG signal [16]. The CSP method is a very good method in terms of feature extraction. CSP can generate a spatial filter, which can define the multi-dimensional morphing data to be a component that is not correlated before [17]. To distinguish part of EEG data, CSP is a method that has good performance, by determining the maximum variant of one multi-channel signal and simultaneously CSP can minimize other variants. CSP is perfect method to distinguish the various mental conditions caused by human motor movements, as CSP focuses on the synchronization occurring in the location section of the motor sensor cortex [18]. In this method it uses eight extraction features which are the most excellent feature results among the values of other extraction features.

2.6 K-Nearest Neighbor (K-NN)

k-NN Classification calculates the distance between test data and the training data. The keyword in this classification is distance, by determining the value of K in the calculation process [19]. The following classification stages, by collecting the training data which is a combination of variables. Then the second, comparing the input data to an existing reference. Further, take consideration at the closest point. The last step is to capture the most points for each sample [20]. The k Parameter used on this research is $k = 1$, $k = 3$, $k = 5$.

3 Result and Discussion

3.1 Channel Selection Mapping

Attempts to filter the dataset to optimal size by removing the irrelevant. The selected channel is defined based on the highest energy from 118 channels to 23 channels. Based on the result of channel selection mapping, the 23 selected channels is represented in motor cortex, and occipital lobe area. It confirmed that the channel selection method can define the best representative channel where it mapped in appropriate location for motor imagery stimulation in motor cortex and occipital for visual stimulation. The mapping of selected channel in a subject can be seen in Table 1.

3.2 Classification Accuracy

The conducted test in this study aim to calculate the performance of the classification accuracy and computational time process of BCI System. The accuracy is calculated by the schemes on the BCI system using the Integrated Selection (IS) mean and Integrated Selection (IS) selection methods compare with the BCI system without these methods. The tests conducted consist of three different feature extraction methods in the BCI system; those are Fast Fourier Transform (FFT), Hjorth Descriptor, and Common Spatial Pattern (CSP) as the extraction feature and k-Nearest Neighbor (K-NN) as the classification.

Table 1 Channel mapping

No	Subject	Normal (118 channel)	Selected Channel (23 channel)
1	aa	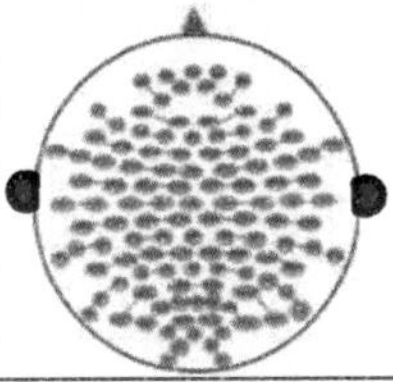	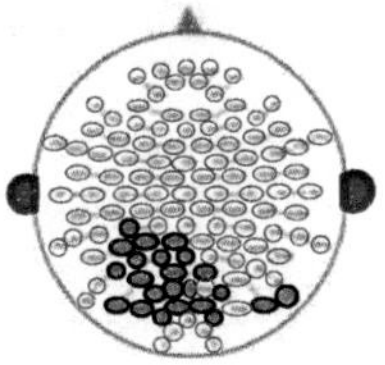
2	al	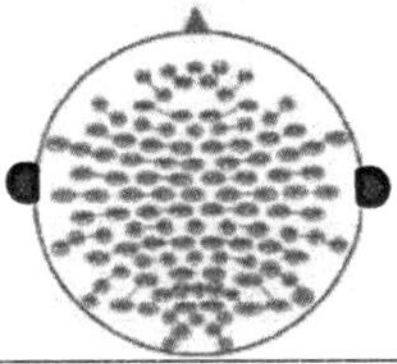	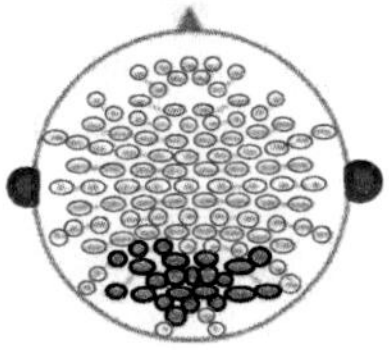
3	av	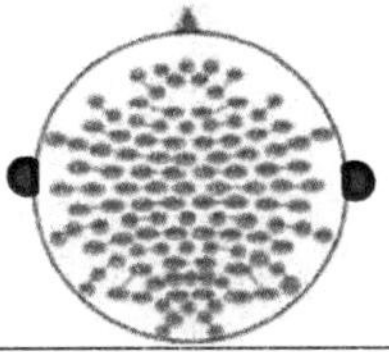	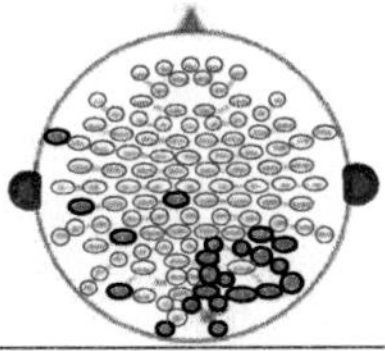
4	aw	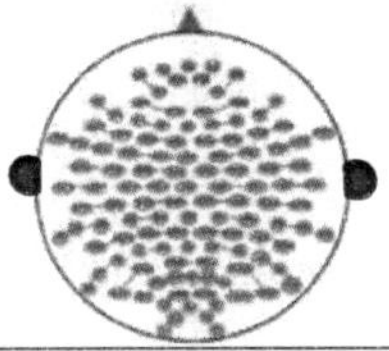	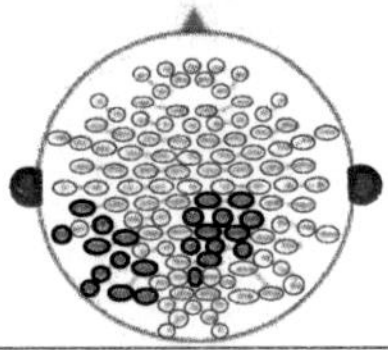
5	ay	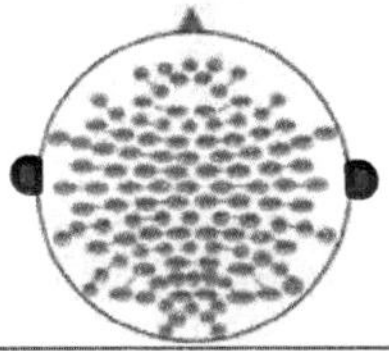	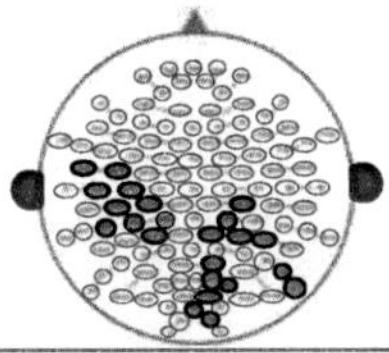

In the results of the test, IS mean method always increased in the average accuracy on each K = 1 parameter which becomes the best parameter of k-NN as classifier from each scenario that was tested. Generally, accuracy of the BCI system using IS selection was increased 6.3% for feature extraction FFT and CSP methods in all k value of k-NN. More than 50% of IS Mean and IS Selection methods in BCI system give better results. However, in general, this system can increase the highest average accuracy up to 0.06. That means, there is one optimal matrix in the experiment as a representative UR matrix that can represent all matrix experiments for all subjects. Referring to the result of subject channel mapping, the composition of the selected channel by spatial selection method differs for each subject. It because of the non-stationary and non-linear brain signal. However, the stimulated area on the scalp are similar for each subject.

According to a research [21], the working area of the brain for the motor imagery lies on the cortex and visual areas. Besides that, based on the classification accuracy test result, CSP is the best feature extraction method for two classes motor imagery signal compare to FFT and Hjorth descriptor methods. It reinforces the previous study statement that CSP method very suitable to proceed motor imagery signal for BCI-EEG based. In computational time calculation, Integrated selection method (mean and selection) was proven can reduce the time process more than 68%. Thus it gives the opportunity to the BCI-EEG to be implemented in the real world application. This could happen because the BCI system with IS method proceed fewer number of channels. The detail information of classification accuracy and computational time in second (in the bracket) can be seen in Tables 2, 3, and 4.

Table 2 Comparison of k-NN classification accuracy using FFT

Subject	K = 1			K = 3			K = 5		
	Normal	IS mean	IS	Normal	IS mean	IS	Normal	IS mean	IS
aa	0.52 (49.9)	0.45 (7.3)	0.52 (10.1)	0.54 (23.9)	0.54 (4.4)	0.54 (4.7)	0.52 (22.5)	0.52 (4.7)	0.53 (5)
al	0.46 (72.4)	0.45 (14.1)	0.46 (14.4)	0.51 (68.8)	0.45 (14.2)	0.47 (14.8)	0.50 (73.5)	0.53 (13.9)	0.43 (14.3)
av	0.52 (10.7)	0.54 (2)	0.61 (2.1)	0.57 (23.2)	0.50 (1.8)	0.57 (2)	0.57 (23.4)	0.54 (1.8)	0.54 (1.9)
aw	0.36 (14.4)	0.60 (1.3)	0.60 (1.3)	0.50 (7.8)	0.46 (1.3)	0.53 (1.2)	0.60 (7.5)	0.43 (1.1)	0.70 (1.3)
ay	0.66 (3.6)	0.61 (0.7)	0.55 (0.7)	0.44 (4.6)	0.55 (0.6)	0.50 (0.6)	0.38 (4.6)	0.50 (0.5)	0.44 (0.6)
Avg.	0.50 (30.2)	0.53 (5.1)	0.55 (5.7)	0.51 (25.7)	0.50 (4.4)	0.52 (4.7)	0.51 (26.3)	0.50 (4.4)	0.53 (4.6)

Table 3 Comparison of k-NN classification accuracy using Hjorth descriptor

Subject	K = 1			K = 3			K = 5		
	Normal	IS mean	IS	Normal	IS mean	IS	Normal	IS mean	IS
aa	0.56 (0.91)	0.59 (0.26)	0.55 (0.3)	0.61 (0.86)	0.56 (0.28)	0.44 (0.31)	0.54 (0.89)	0.57 (0.32)	0.50 (0.33)
al	0.50 (1.09)	0.52 (0.34)	0.52 (0.37)	0.50 (1.11)	0.53 (0.38)	0.50 (0.34)	0.56 (1.1)	0.47 (0.35)	0.47 (0.41)
av	0.59 (0.57)	0.57 (0.18)	0.42 (0.2)	0.61 (0.51)	0.66 (0.21)	0.54 (0.21)	0.59 (0.53)	0.57 (0.21)	0.52 (0.21)
aw	0.53 (0.38)	0.56 (0.15)	0.53 (0.13)	0.46 (0.36)	0.46 (0.16)	0.50 (0.17)	0.53 (0.39)	0.56 (0.14)	0.60 (0.16)
ay	0.44 (0.26)	0.61 (0.1)	0.55 (0.12)	0.44 (0.28)	0.44 (0.12)	0.44 (0.13)	0.44 (0.26)	0.44 (0.13)	0.50 (0.12)
Avg.	0.52 (0.64)	**0.57 (0.2)**	0.51 (0.22)	0.53 (0.62)	**0.53 (0.23)**	0.48 (0.23)	0.53 (0.63)	**0.52 (0.23)**	0.52 (0.24)

Table 4 Comparison of k-NN classification accuracy using CSP

Subject	K = 1			K = 3			K = 5		
	Normal	IS mean	IS	Normal	IS mean	IS	Normal	IS mean	IS
aa	0.51 (0.28)	0.54 (0.14)	0.48 (0.12)	0.52 (0.3)	0.55 (0.11)	0.50 (0.12)	0.52 (0.24)	0.60 (0.19)	0.57 (0.13)
al	0.84 (0.25)	0.61 (0.12)	0.62 (0.13)	0.86 (0.26)	0.60 (0.13)	0.60 (0.13)	0.85 (0.27)	0.61 (0.13)	0.61 (0.13)
av	0.54 (0.15)	0.57 (0.1)	0.61 (0.09)	0.59 (0.18)	0.57 (0.1)	0.64 (0.1)	0.59 (0.2)	0.59 (0.11)	0.61 (0.1)
aw	0.60 (0.15)	0.66 (0.09)	0.60 (0.1)	0.60 (0.14)	0.60 (0.1)	0.60 (0.09)	0.60 (0.13)	0.53 (0.09)	0.60 (0.09)
ay	0.44 (0.11)	0.88 (0.07)	0.94 (0.09)	0.61 (0,12)	0.88 (0.09)	0.94 (0.09)	0.66 (0.12)	0.88 (0.11)	0.94 (0.1)
Avg.	0.59 (0.18)	**0.65 (0.1)**	**0.65 (0.1)**	0.63 (0.2)	0.64 (0.1)	**0.65 (0.1)**	0.64 (0.19)	0.64 (0.12)	**0.67 (0.11)**

4 Conclusion

Based on the research that has been done on this test, we can conclude that the IS method in the imagination of motion EEG signal dataset could be implemented and increase the BCI system accuracy. The feature extraction from all the experiments in this research obtained the highest accuracy results using CSP; this reinforces the previous research statement which concluded that CSP is the most accurate feature extraction method for the imagination of motion EEG signals. The accuracy performance of the BCI system using the K-NN classification method with a parameter value of K = 1 and CSP feature extraction increased to more than 6%. The BCI system using the IS method can increase computational time six times faster than the original BCI.

References

1. Abdulkader SN, Atia A, Mostafa M-SM (2015) Brain computer interfacing: applications and challenges. Egypt Inf J 16:213–230. https://doi.org/10.1016/j.eij.2015.06.002
2. Wang P, Lu J, Zhang B, Tang Z (2015) A review on transfer learning for brain-computer interface classification. In: 2015 5th International conference on information science and technology, ICIST 2015. https://doi.org/10.1109/ICIST.2015.7288989
3. Fauzi H, Shapiai MI, Khairuddin U (2020) Transfer learning of BCI using CUR algorithm. J Signal Process Syst 92:109–121. https://doi.org/10.1007/s11265-019-1440-9
4. Wei CS, Lin YP, Wang YT, Jung TP, Bigdely-Shamlo N, Lin CT (2016) Selective transfer learning for EEG-based drowsiness detection. In: Proceedings—2015 IEEE international conference on systems, man, and cybernetics, SMC 2015, pp 3229–3232. https://doi.org/10.1109/SMC.2015.560
5. Bi L, Fan XA, Liu Y (2013) EEG-based brain-controlled mobile robots: a survey. IEEE Trans Hum Mach Syst. https://doi.org/10.1109/TSMCC.2012.2219046

6. Kannathal N, Choo ML, Acharya UR, Sadasivan PK (2005) Entropies for detection of epilepsy in EEG. Comput Methods Programs Biomed 80:187–194. https://doi.org/10.1016/j.cmpb.2005.06.012
7. Sun L, Feng ZR (2016) Classification of imagery motor EEG data with wavelet denoising and features selection. In: 2016 International conference on wavelet analysis and pattern recognition (ICWAPR), pp 184–188. IEEE. https://doi.org/10.1109/ICWAPR.2016.7731641
8. Jayaram V, Alamgir M, Altun Y, Scholkopf B, Grosse-Wentrup M (2016) Transfer learning in brain-computer interfaces. IEEE Comput Intell Mag 11:20–31. https://doi.org/10.1109/MCI.2015.2501545
9. Fauzi H, Shapiai MI, Setiawan NA, Jaafar J, Mustafa M (2017) Channel selection for common spatial pattern based on energy calculation of motor imagery EEG signal. In: 2017 International conference on control, electronics, renewable energy and communications (ICCREC), pp 33–39. IEEE. https://doi.org/10.1109/ICCEREC.2017.8226692
10. Sipasulta RY, Lumenta ASM, Sompie SRUA (2014) Simulasi Sistem Pengacak Sinyal Dengan Metode FFT (Fast Fourier Transform). E-JOURNAL Tek. ELEKTRO DAN Komput. https://doi.org/10.35793/jtek.3.2.2014.4448
11. Farihah SN, Lee KY, Mansor W, Mohamad NB, Mahmoodin Z, Saidi SA (2016) EEG average FFT index for dyslexic children with writing disorder. In: ISSBES 2015—IEEE student symposium in biomedical engineering and sciences: by the student for the student. https://doi.org/10.1109/ISSBES.2015.7435880
12. Hjorth B (1973) The physical significance of time domain descriptors in EEG analysis. Electroencephalogr Clin Neurophysiol 34:321–325. https://doi.org/10.1016/0013-4694(73)90260-5
13. Mouzé-Amady M, Horwat F (1996) Evaluation of Hjorth parameters in forearm surface EMG analysis during an occupational repetitive task. Electroencephalogr Clin Neurophysiol Electromyogr Mot Control. https://doi.org/10.1016/0924-980X(96)00316-5
14. Rizal A, Hidayat R, Nugroho HA (2015) Determining lung sound characterization using Hjorth descriptor. In: 2015 International conference on control, electronics, renewable energy and communications (ICCEREC), pp 54–57. IEEE. https://doi.org/10.1109/ICCEREC.2015.7337053
15. Rizal A, Hadiyoso S (2015) ECG signal classification using Hjorth Descriptor. In: 2015 International conference on automation, cognitive science, optics, micro electro-mechanical system, and information technology (ICACOMIT), pp 87–90. IEEE. https://doi.org/10.1109/ICACOMIT.2015.7440181
16. Tao R, Ren H, Peng X (2017) Modeling, design and simulation of systems. Asian Simul Conf 752:249–260. https://doi.org/10.1007/978-981-10-6463-0
17. Arvaneh M, Guan C, Ang KK, Quek C (2011) Optimizing the channel selection and classification accuracy in EEG-based BCI. IEEE Trans Biomed Eng 58:1865–1873. https://doi.org/10.1109/TBME.2011.2131142
18. Samek W, Kawanabe M, Muller KR (2014) Divergence-based framework for common spatial patterns algorithms. IEEE Rev Biomed Eng 7:50–72. https://doi.org/10.1109/RBME.2013.2290621
19. Hlaing KNN, Gopalakrishnan AK (2016) Myanmar paper currency recognition using GLCM and k-NN. In: 2016 2nd Asian conference on defence technology ACDT 2016, pp 67–72. https://doi.org/10.1109/ACDT.2016.7437645
20. Kaundanya VL, Patil A, Panat A (2015) Performance of k-NN classifier for emotion detection using EEG signals. In: 2015 International conference on communication and signal processing ICCSP 2015, pp 1160–1164. https://doi.org/10.1109/ICCSP.2015.7322687
21. Fauzi H, Shapiai MI, Shah Abdullah S, Ibrahim Z (2018) Automatic energy extraction methods for EEG channel selection. In: 2018 International conference on control, electronics, renewable energy and communications (ICCEREC), pp 70–75. IEEE. https://doi.org/10.1109/ICCEREC.2018.8711995

Computer Aided Diagnosis for Early Detection of Glaucoma Using Convolutional Neural Network (CNN)

Yunendah Nur Fu'adah, Sofia Sa'idah, Inung Wijayanto, Nur Ibrahim, Syamsul Rizal, and Rita Magdalena

Abstract Glaucoma is an eye disease caused by an increase in eye pressure resulting in damage to the optic nerve and can cause blindness. An ophthalmologist makes the diagnosis of glaucoma by analyzing the fundus images that show the retinal structure. This manual diagnosis requires years of expertise and prone to error. Previous studies have designed a glaucoma CAD system based on Convolutional Neural Network (CNN) and showed promising results. This study proposes the CNN method consisting of three hidden layers that use 3 × 3 of the filter size with 16, 32, 64 output channels, fully connected layers, and sigmoid activation. The experiment is conducted using the RIMONE R2 fundus images dataset to classify normal and glaucoma conditions. From 455 fundus images, 75% are used as the training data, while the rest is used as the validation data. From the experiment, this study outperforms other previous studies by achieving 91.22% of accuracy. The glaucoma system detection that has been developed in this research, can be helpful for ophthalmologists to establish an initial diagnosis of glaucoma that can reduce the harmful effects of glaucoma.

Keywords Fundus · Glaucoma · CNN · RIMONE R2

1 Introduction

Glaucoma is a multifactorial neurodegenerative disease, which reduces human vision and may cause blindness. The main cause of glaucoma is the Intra Ocular Pressure (IOP). This condition can damage the optic nerve, which made the brain does not get image information from light receptors [1]. The retina and optic nerve changes often occur without symptoms and are not detected by diagnostic tests [2]. Early examination and medical treatment suggested by an ophthalmologist can help reduce the risk of glaucoma [1]. Based on data from the WHO, glaucoma is one of

Y. N. Fu'adah (✉) · S. Sa'idah · I. Wijayanto · N. Ibrahim · S. Rizal · R. Magdalena
School of Electrical Engineering, Telkom University, Bandung, Indonesia
e-mail: yunendah@telkomuniversity.ac.id

H. Triwiyanto et al. (eds.), *Proceedings of the 1st International Conference on Electronics, Biomedical Engineering, and Health Informatics*, Lecture Notes in Electrical Engineering 746, https://doi.org/10.1007/978-981-33-6926-9_40

the major causes of blindness globally after cataracts. More than 82% of all blind people are aged 50 years and over. In 2013, the number of people (40–80 years old) with glaucoma was 64.3 million and continued to increase until 2020 [3].

Ophthalmologists diagnose Glaucoma by analyzing the retinal structures. They are followed by analyzing ocular parameters such as Cup to Disk Ratio (CDR) and very high Rim to Disk Ratio (RDR). This requires expertise and accuracy. In diagnosing Glaucoma, ophthalmologists use several expensive devices such as the Heidelberg Retinal Tomography (HRT), Optical Coherence Tomography (OCT), Including Confocal Scanning Laser Ophthalmoscopy (CSLO) and relatively limited fundus imaging [4]. Several studies based on fundus image processing have developed for glaucoma detection. Previous studies mentioned that glaucoma disease is detected by localizing and segmenting fundus images to obtain the Optic Nerve Head (ONH) sections. The features are extracted using statistical measurement and classified using K-Nearest Neighbor (K-NN). The method achieves 95.24% accuracy, which tested in a private data set [5]. GeethaRamani et al. [6] did a segmentation process is performed to calculate the Cup to Disc Ratio (CDR) based on image processing. The study obtains an accuracy of 98.7% using a private dataset. In study [7], the feature extraction process is performed using the Empirical Wavelet Transform method, and the Support Vector Machine (SVM) classification method. The method is tested in a private dataset combined with the RIM-ONE dataset. They achieved 98.33% accuracy for the private data set and 81.32% for the RIM-ONE dataset.

In some previous studies, the researches carried out several important stages in designing a glaucoma detection system, such as the preprocessing and segmentation process that must be accurate, proper feature selection and optimization at the classification stage which greatly affect the system performance. Some studies are starting to use the Convolutional Neural Network (CNN) as the main method. CNN has the advantage that it can learn the deterministic features of raw data directly and provide a promising system performance in detecting Glaucoma. Studies by Memon et al. [8] and Bajwa et al. [9] are the examples of study which use CNN as the main method for detecting Glaucoma. They achieve an accuracy of 85% [8] and 87.4% [9], which tested in RIM-ONE [8] and ORIGA [9] dataset. In the previous studies, CNN model was designed using more than three hidden layers and used softmax activation. In this research, CNN model design will be done using three hidden layers and sigmoid activation, which is more effective for classifying two conditions such as normal and glaucoma.

2 Method

This study designed a detection system to classify glaucoma and normal condition based on image processing. The system used the CNN method with three hidden layers, which used 3×3 filter size of each layers and 16, 32, 64 output channels

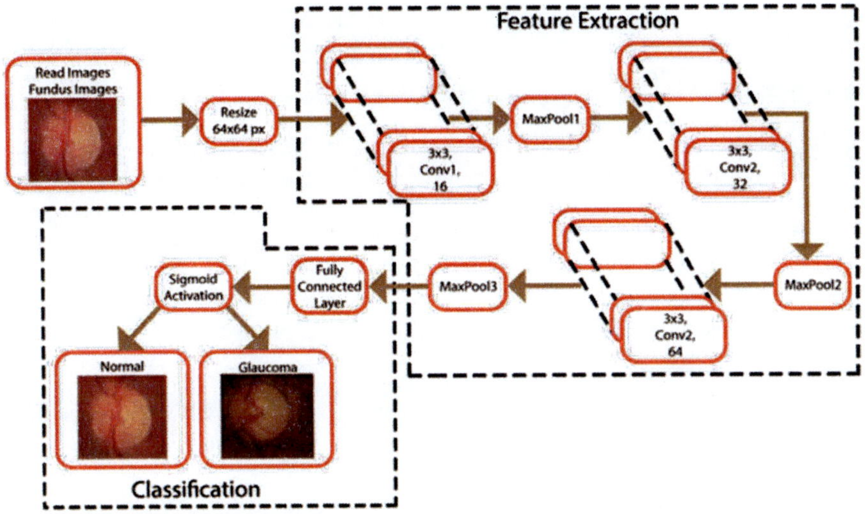

Fig. 1 The proposed system model of CNN for glaucoma detection

respectively. Furthermore, fully connected layers and sigmoid activation used to classify normal and glaucoma conditions. In general, the CNN model proposed in this study is shown in Fig. 1.

2.1 Dataset

This study uses RIM-ONE R2 dataset. The dataset has 455 fundus images, consist of 255 fundus images in normal condition and 200 fundus images in glaucoma condition. The distribution of training data and validation data in this study are 75% and 25%, respectively. Thus, the training data used are 341 fundus images, while the validation data are 114 fundus images. The data is then resized with a size of 64 × 64 to be processed at the next stage.

2.2 Convolutional Neural Network

Convolutional Neural Network (CNN) is one of the Deep Neural Networks, which implemented for image recognition [10]. CNN is a development of the Multilayer Perceptron (MLP). MLP accepts one-dimensional input data and propagates the data on the network to produce output. The CNN data propagated on the network are two-dimensional [11]. Thus, it can only be used on data that has a

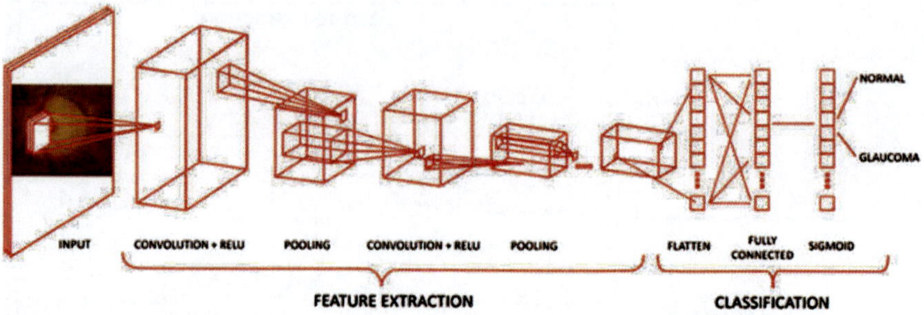

Fig. 2 The architecture of CNN

two-dimensional structure such as image data. In general, CNN consists of a Feature Extraction Layer and Classification Layer, which shown by the CNN architecture in Fig. 2.

The feature extraction layer consists of convolutional layers and pooling layers. Convolutional layers convert images with convolution processes to produce feature maps that show the original image's unique characteristics. Convolutional layers operate differently from other neural network layers that use connection weights. The convolutional layers use convolutional filters to produce a feature map [10].

Furthermore, the convolutional layer's activation process uses Rectified Linear Units (ReLU) activation to increase the training stage on the neural network so it can minimize errors and saturation. In this study, the ReLU activation function is used at each hidden layer of the neural network. The ReLU activation function is shown in (1) [12].

$$f(x) = \begin{cases} x, \cdots x > 0 \\ 0, \cdots x \leq 0 \end{cases} \tag{1}$$

The ReLu activation function changes the negative pixel value on the image to 0 on the feature map. The pooling layer on the feature extraction layer serves to reduce the size of the layer. There are two types of pooling methods, namely maximum pooling, which sees the maximum value and mean pooling that looks for the average value. An illustration of the pooling process can be seen in Fig. 3 [10].

Based on Fig. 3, it can be seen that the Pooling Layer reduces the size of the image, the image which was originally sized 4 × 4 to 2 × 2 without losing significant information. To avoid overfitting and help generalize at the training stage, this study used a dropout at the last hidden layer. The dropout consists of setting to zero the output of each hidden neuron according to the probability value used. Hence when the neurons in CNN are dropped out, the neurons do not contribute to the forward pass stage and do not participate in the back propagation stage [13].

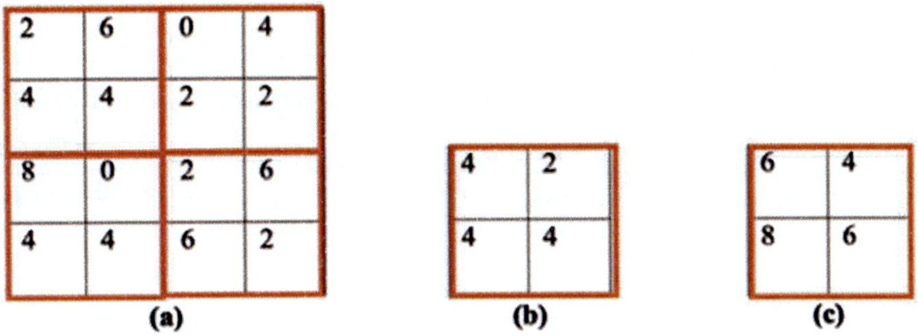

Fig. 3 Illustrate of pooling layer, **a** the 4 × 4 pixel input image, **b** mean pooling, **c** maximum pooling

2.3 Classification Layer

The classification stage consists of flattening stages to change feature maps, which are multidimensional arrays into one-dimensional arrays [14]. The fully connected layers emit vectors K, where K is the number of classes that can be predicted by the network. This study used two classes, namely normal and glaucoma. In the last stage, the sigmoid activation function is used following equation, which showed in (2) [15]. It can be seen that the sigmoid activation function transform the input value x into the range of 0–1.

$$S(x) = \frac{1}{1 + e^{-x}} \quad (2)$$

Table 1 shows the summary of the proposed CNN model as well as the output of each layer that affects the image size.

Table 1 Details of CNN model proposed

Layer type	Output shape	Parameter	Layer type	Output shape	Parameter
Input image	64,64,3	0	Convolution	16,16,64	18,496
Convolution	64,64,16	448	ReLU	16,16,64	0
ReLU	64,64,16	0	Max pooling	8,8,64	0
Max pooling	32,32,16	0	Dropout	8,8,64	0
Convolution	32,32,32	4640	Flatten	4096	0
ReLU	32,32,32	0	Dense	2	8194
Max pooling	16,16,32	0	Sigmoid	2	0

3 System Performance

This study uses accuracy, recall, precision, and f1 scores to measure the performance. The calculation is shown in (3), (4), (5) and (6) [9]. True Positive (TP) shows the exact glaucoma data detected as glaucoma, True Negative (TN) shows normal detected as normal data, False Positive (FP) shows glaucoma detected normal data while False Negative (FN) shows normal detected glaucoma data.

$$\text{Accuracy} = \frac{TP + TN}{TP + FP + TN + FN} \tag{3}$$

$$\text{Recall} = \frac{TP}{TP + FN} \tag{4}$$

$$\text{Precision} = \frac{TP}{TP + FP} \tag{5}$$

$$F1 \cdots \text{Score} = 2 \times \frac{\text{recall} \times \text{precision}}{\text{recall} + \text{precision}} \tag{6}$$

4 Result and Discussion

The RIM-ONE R2 dataset used in this study consist of 455 fundus images for glaucoma and normal conditions. The number of training data used is 341 fundus images. On the other hand, the amount of test data used is 114 fundus images for 67 normal condition images and 47 glaucoma conditions. For glaucoma and normal conditions, fundus images are trained using the CNN model with Adam optimizer learning rate 0.001, and loss binary cross-entropy. Performance parameters measured in this study are accuracy, recall, precision, F1 score, and loss. The model of accuracy and the loss of the proposed model is shown in Fig. 4.

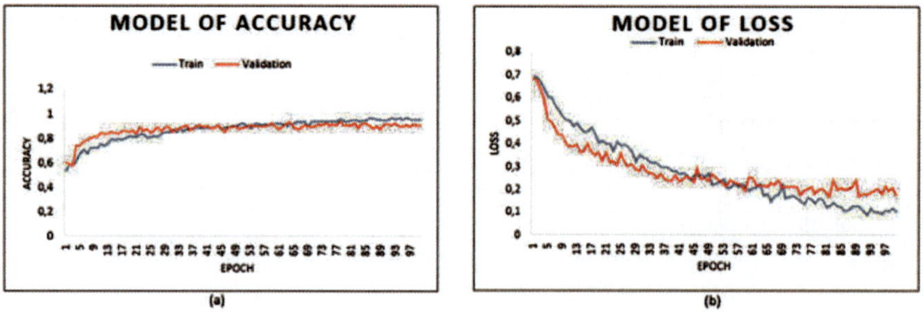

Fig. 4 **a** Accuracy of the proposed model, **b** loss of the proposed model

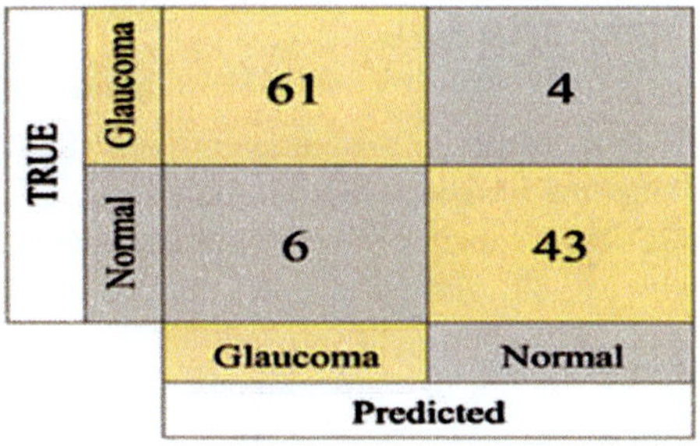

Fig. 5 Confusion matrix of validation data

Based on the experiment conducted in this study, the accuracy increases for each iteration (epoch), and the difference in accuracy between the training data and the validation data accuracy is not much different, as shown in Fig. 4a. Based on these results, it can be concluded that there is no overfitting of the system designed using the proposed model. Figure 4b shows a decrease in the value of the loss at each iteration (epoch) with a value that is not much difference between the value of loss training and loss validation. It can be concluded that learning errors that occur both for training data and test data achieved are minimum so that the model can recognize normal conditions and glaucoma conditions with the best accuracy performance of 91.22%, and loss of 0.1758.

Based on the Confusion Matrix shown in Fig. 5, it can be seen that from 114 validation data used, 104 data are successfully classified according to their class. Other parameters used to evaluate system performance are precision, recall, and F1-score, which have a range of values from 0 to 1 (a value of 1 indicates no error). Based on the data shown in Table 2, the value of system performance parameters is closed to 1. This condition shows that the CNN model can classify glaucoma and normal conditions with high accuracy and minimal missclassification.

Compared to some previous studies, which used RIM ONE data set and Convolution Neural Network with softmax activation as the main method to classify normal and glaucoma conditions, the proposed CNN method with sigmoid activation outperforms the previous studies. The sigmoid activation that used in the classification layer has proven to be more precise in classifying two conditions.

Table 2 Performance of CNN model proposed

Class	Precision	Recall	F1-Score	No of images
Glaucoma	0.91	0.94	0.92	65
Normal	0.91	0.88	0.90	49
Total	0.91	0.91	0.91	114

5 Conclusion

In this research, a computer-aided diagnose system for the early detection of glaucoma based on digital image processing is designed. The CNN model used in this study consists of three hidden layers. Each of them is using 3 × 3 filter sizes with 16, 32, and 64 channel outputs, a fully connected layer, and sigmoid activation. The experiment showed that the proposed CNN model is able to classify raw fundus image datasets directly into glaucoma conditions and normal conditions with an accuracy of 91.22%, loss of 0.1758, and the value of precision, recall, an f1-score average of each amounted to 0.91. In further research, a system for the classification of glaucoma conditions can be developed based on its severity.

References

1. Ahmad H, Yamin A, Shakeel A, Gillani SO, Ansari U (2014) Detection of glaucoma using retinal fundus images. In: 2014 International conference on robotics and emerging allied technologies in engineering (iCREATE), pp 321–324. IEEE. https://doi.org/10.1109/iCREATE.2014.6828388
2. Carrillo J, Bautista L, Villamizar J, Rueda J, Sanchez M, Rueda D (2019) Glaucoma detection using fundus images of the eye. In: 22nd Symposium image signal processing artificial vision STSIVA 2019—conference proceedings, pp 1–4. https://doi.org/10.1109/STSIVA.2019.8730250
3. Nucci C, Osbornec NN, Bagetta G, Cerulli L (2008) Glaucoma: an open-window to neurodegeneration and neuroprotection. Preface Prog Brain Res 173:173. https://doi.org/10.1016/S0079-6123(08)01145-X
4. Kim M, Han JC, Hyun SH, Janssens O, Van Hoecke S, Kee C, De Neve W (2019) Medinoid: computer-aided diagnosis and localization of glaucoma using deep learning. Appl Sci 9:2357–2362. https://doi.org/10.3390/app9153064
5. Septiarini A, Khairina DM, Kridalaksana AH, Hamdani H (2018) Automatic glaucoma detection method applying a statistical approach to fundus images. Healthc Inform Res 24:53–60. https://doi.org/10.4258/hir.2018.24.1.53
6. GeethaRamani R, Dhanapackiam C (2014) Automatic localization and segmentation of optic disc in retinal fundus images through image processing techniques. In: International conference on recent trends in information technology automatic
7. Maheshwari S, Pachori RB, Acharya UR (2017) Automated diagnosis of glaucoma using empirical wavelet transform and correntropy features extracted from fundus images. IEEE J Biomed Heal Inf 21:803–813. https://doi.org/10.1109/JBHI.2016.2544961
8. Memon I, Ursani AA, Bohyo MA, Chandio R ()2019 Automated diagnosis of glaucoma using deep learning architecture. Eng Sci Technol Int Res J 3. https://doi.org/10.2174/1574362414666190906112910
9. Bajwa MN, Malik MI, Siddiqui SA, Dengel A, Shafait F, Neumeier W, Ahmed S (2019) Correction to: two-stage framework for optic disc localization and glaucoma classification in retinal fundus images using deep learning. BMC Med Inf Decis Mak 19(136). https://doi.org/10.1186/s12911-019-0842-8. BMC Med Inform Decis Mak 19:1–16. https://doi.org/10.1186/s12911-019-0876-y
10. Kim P (2017) MATLAB deep learning. Apress, Berkeley, CA. https://doi.org/10.1007/978-1-4842-2845-6

11. Noeman A, Handayani D (2020) Detection of Mad Lazim Harfi Musyba images uses convolutional neural network. IOP Conf Ser Mater Sci Eng 771. https://doi.org/10.1088/1757-899X/771/1/012030
12. Kim P (2017) MATLAB deep learning: with machine learning, neural networks and artificial intelligence. Apress, Berkeley, CA
13. Wang L, Wen M, Wu Y (2019) Glaucoma detection based on deep convolutional neural network. Acta Microsc 28:331–338
14. Yamashita R, Nishio M, Do RKG, Togashi K (2018) Convolutional neural networks: an overview and application in radiology. Insights Imaging 9:611–629. https://doi.org/10.1007/s13244-018-0639-9
15. Feng J, Lu S (2011) Performance analysis of various activation functions in artificial neural networks. Int J Artif Intell Expert Syst 1. https://doi.org/10.1088/1742-6596/1237/2/022030

Invasive Ductal Carcinoma (IDC) Classification Based on Breast Histopathology Images Using Convolutional Neural Network

Nor Kumalasari Caecar Pratiwi, Yunendah Nur Fu'adah, Nur Ibrahim, Syamsul Rizal, and Sofia Saidah

Abstract Invasive Ductal Carcinoma (IDC) is the most common sub-type of all breast cancers that affected adult women worldwide. IDC can spread to other areas of the body such as liver, lungs and even bones. The process of identifying and categorizing breast cancer sub-types accurately is a very important clinical task. IDC Diagnosis requires extremely serious measures, such as surgery and radiation therapy. Diagnosis based on pathological imagery is no less difficult, requiring a microscope and manual learning to classify it as positive or negative cancer. This process is very time consuming and conveys many errors due to human cognitive limitations. The existence of a system which can automatically perform such work, is expected to save time and reduce the error rate diagnose. This study proposed IDC and Non IDC classification by analyzing the Breast Histopathology Images using Convolutional Neural Network (CNN) method. The dataset consisted of 1020 IDC images, the same number is also used for Non-IDC. The model was composed of CNN with three hidden layers plus one fully connected layer with sigmoid activation. An evaluation is carried out to see the performance of the proposed method by using a matrix of precision, recall, F1, and accuracy. The experimental results show that the proposed method provides precision, recall, F1-score of 0.93 and 93% accuracy. This study is expected to be validated for later use in assisting medical authorities for conducting clinical diagnoses.

Keywords Invasive ductal carcinoma (IDC) · Breast cancer identification · Convolutional neural network (CNN)

N. K. C. Pratiwi (✉) · Y. N. Fu'adah · N. Ibrahim · S. Rizal · S. Saidah
School of Electrical Engineering, Telkom University, Bandung, Indonesia
e-mail: caecarnkcp@telkomuniversity.ac.id

H. Triwiyanto et al. (eds.), *Proceedings of the 1st International Conference on Electronics, Biomedical Engineering, and Health Informatics*, Lecture Notes in Electrical Engineering 746, https://doi.org/10.1007/978-981-33-6926-9_41

1 Introduction

Breast cancer affects 2.1 million women every year, and also causes the highest death rates in women caused by cancer. According to WHO, in 2018, there were at least 627,000 women died of breast cancer [1]. Invasive Ductal Carcinoma (IDC) or usually referred to Infiltrating Ductal Carcinoma, is the most common subtype/pathological type of all breast cancers [2]. Invasive shows that the cancer has invaded or spread to the surrounding breast tissue. Ductal means that cancer starts in the milk glands/lobules, while carcinoma refers to cancer whose growth begins in the skin or other tissues that cover internal organs. Over time, invasive ductal carcinoma can spread to other areas of the body such as liver, lungs and even bones. The development of breast cancer begins with the initiation and expansion of deep tumor cells in the breast, characterized as Atypical Ductal Hyperplasia (ADH). These cells then develop into Duct Carcinoma In Situ (DCIS). When tumor cells spread outside the mammary, hence the condition of the cancer has been classified in stages as an Invasive Ductal Carcinoma (IDC) [3] (Fig. 1).

Early diagnosis of breast cancer is very important, to support a good prognosis process and so that survival rates can be even higher. Several studies related to the classification of breast cancer have been done by several previous researchers. In 2017, Hamsagayathri and friends conducted a breast cancer classification study using decision tree classifier with Wisconsin Breast cancer dataset [4]. The aim of the research conducted by Hamsagayathri is to make a comparative study of various decision tree classification algorithms and determine the best algorithm for breast cancer classification, especially for the Wisconsin Original dataset. The dataset is divided into three classes; original, prognostic, and diagnostic. First of all, the input image will be preprocessed by the system, namely data cleaning and data reduction. Data cleaning process will replaces the missing attribute values with the mean values. Meanwhile, data reduction is removing irrelevant and redundant attributes from the dataset that are less significant in classification. The analysis process is done by comparing the performance of the J48 algorithm, RepTree, Random Tree and Priority based decision tree. The results showed that Priority-based decision tree algorithm has the best performance with an accuracy of 93.63%. Overall, the

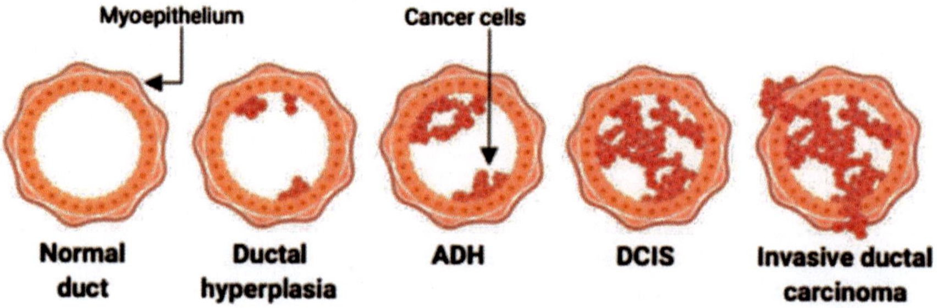

Fig. 1 The development of breast cancer [3]

system performs fairly well, but keep in mind that a serious disadvantage of the decision tree algorithm is high complexity, making it more prone to over-fitting, and it is also possible that the small trees may be under-fitted [5]. Both cases triggered the system to lose its accuracy. In addition, it also requires larger memory and longer computation time.

Karthik and friends have conducted research related to the classification of malignant and benign breast cancer using the Deep Neural Network (DNN) [6]. This study was experimented using Wisconsin Breast Cancer Dataset (WBCD) from UCI repository, divided into two classes, called benign (patient without cancer) and malignant (patients with cancer). This data will then be carried out by using Recursive Feature Elimination (RFE) feature selection. The feature selection serves to eliminate ambiguity and reduce data complexity. The research result states that the limitation of this system is that it takes a long time for the training process.

Yun Jiang and friends also done the study related to breast cancer classification using Convolutional Neural Networks (CNN) with SE-ResNet model [7]. This study used Breast Cancer Histopathological Image (BreaKHis) dataset, contains 7909 images, divided into 2480 benign images and 5429 malignant images. The flow of this research starts from the image augmentation process. Each image is given the same augmentation technique, consisting of a shifting process in height and width with a factor of 0.125, horizontal flip, and constant fill mode. This dataset then resized to 224×224 and normalized with Zero-mean normalization. The entire network will be trained end-to-end through a back propagation scheme using SGD optimizer. At the end, the softmax function algorithm is used as a classifier. For binary classification, the system achieved a performance of between 98.87 and 99.34%. Whereas for multi-classification, the system achieved performance between 90.66 and 93.81%. The results of this study suggest the use of the Gauss error scheduler. This scheme is used for a new learning rate scheduler which frees the user from adjusting the learning rate parameters for the SGD algorithm. SGD removes redundancy by performing one update at a time. So, SGD is usually faster and can also be used to study online. SGD often performs weight updates causing the objective function to fluctuate greatly [8].

In 2019, Ray and friends write the results of research related to the classification of benign and malignant breast cancer with supervised machine learning [9]. In his research, at least four classifiers were used, they are Gaussian Naive Bayes, Decision Tree, K-Nearest Neighbors and Random Forest. This study used the Coimbra Breast Cancer dataset for predictive analysis of the numerical dataset, in the form of cancer biomarkers. While for image analysis, the Kaggle dataset was used in the form of breast histopathology images. The image is divided into two classes, namely benign and malignant. The entire dataset is divided into training data and testing data, with a composition of 75 and 25%, respectively. Numerical data is used to analyze breast cancer based on different biomarkers such as Age, Body Mass Index (BMI), Glucose, Insulin, Homeostatic Model Assessment (HOMA), Lectins, Adiponectin, Resistin, and MCP. The test results for numerical data show that the Decision Tree and Random Forest classifiers provide promising results with an accuracy score of 70%. From this classification algorithms, it was found that the most relevant biomarker with the presence of breast cancer is a BMI (Body Mass Index) and Resistin. Meanwhile, the test results for breast histopathology image showed that the Random Forest classifier gave the best performance, with F1-score of 92%.

From several previous studies discussed above, mostly settled on the use of algorithms with a high level of complexity. In addition, most studies divide the class into benign and malignant. Thus, in this study we propose a simple CNN-based model that can classify breast cancer conditions into IDC and Non-IDC conditions. Although the system was built with a simple CNN modeling, it is expected that the system will be able to work with a high level of performance.

2 Material and Method

Convolutional Neural Network (CNN) is a deep network that imitates how visual cortex of human's brain process and recognizes the images [10] (Fig. 2).

CNN architecture consists of neural layers that play a role in the process of feature extraction and another neural layers that function as classifiers. The CNN model consists of at least four components; convolution layer, pooling layer, activation function, and fully connected layer [11]. Convolutional and pooling layer included into feature extraction layer. Convolutional layer generates an output images called feature map [10]. The feature map will describe the unique features of the original images. Convolutional layer contains filters, that assigned to convert the image. For example, suppose an images with 4 × 4 sized is convoluted with a 2 × 2 filter, the feature maps result becomes (Fig. 3).

The Rectified Linear Unit (hence the name ReLU) can be used to increase the non-linearity of the CNN [12]. The ReLU activation function works with the operating principle of a threshold for each input element whose value is less than zero [13]. This RELU activation will convert input values that are less than zero (negative pixel value) and are forced to zero.

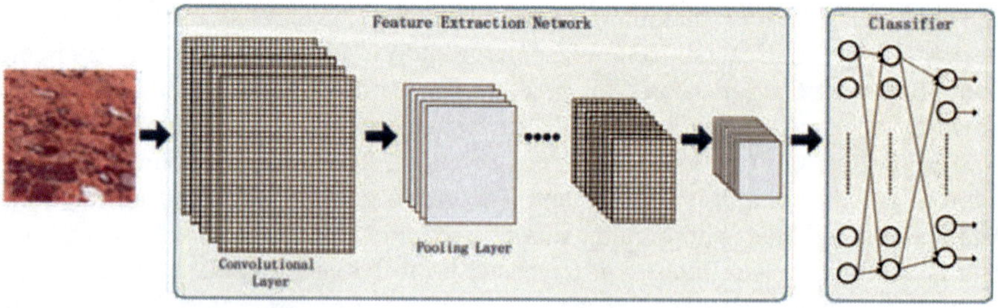

Fig. 2 Typical architecture of CNN

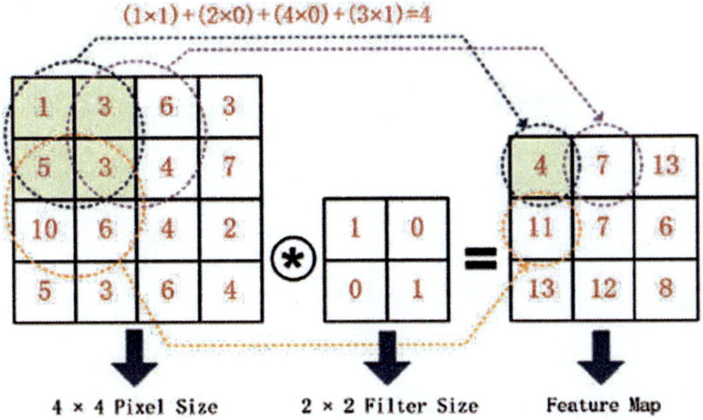

Fig. 3 The convolution process

$$f(x) = \max(0, x) = \begin{cases} x_i; \, if x_i \geq 0 \\ 0; \, if \, x_i < 0 \end{cases} \quad (1)$$

The main idea of pooling layer is to down-sampling or reduce the complexity of the process at the next layer [14]. Complexity reduction is accomplished by reducing the size of the image, by combining neighboring pixels into one value. The neighboring pixels are usually selected from square matrix, and the representative value set as the mean or maximum value of selected pixels (Fig. 4).

There are many algorithms that can be used as classifiers in neural networks. Sigmoid classifier returns the output value which falls in the range of 0 or 1, mainly used for binary data classification [15]. The equation for sigmoid classifier produces the curve in *S* shape.

$$f(x) = \frac{1}{1 + e^{-x}} \quad (2)$$

Fig. 4 The resultant cases of pooling using two different method

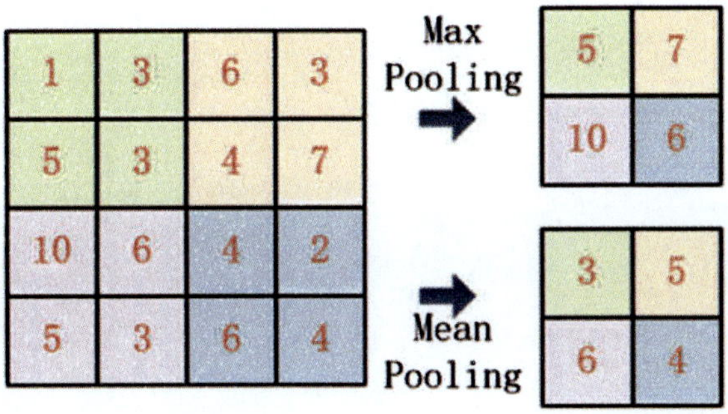

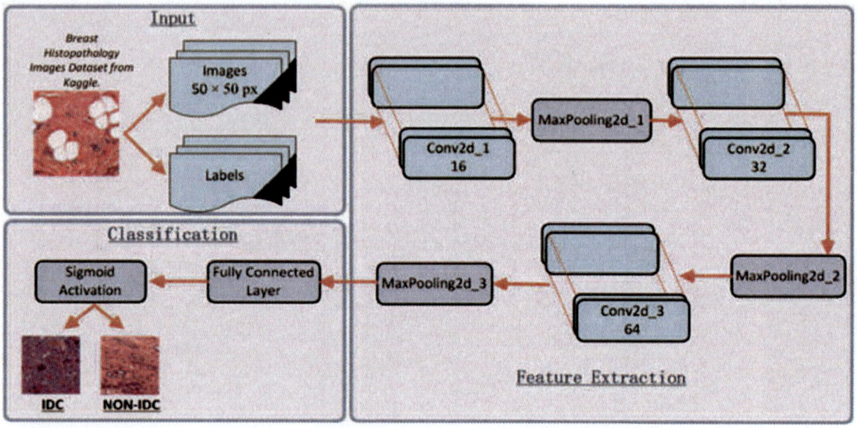

Fig. 5 The proposed model for invasive ductal carcinoma (IDC) detection

CNN offers a better level of image identification when using deeper extraction neural networks (using more layers). But with more layers, it makes the training process more difficult and CNN to be impractical, even over-fitting. Over-fitting is basically a state when a network cannot learn effectively for a number of reasons, one of which is the complexity of the model used [16]. The proposed CNN model consists of three convolutional layers, with max pooling layer, RelU activation and sigmoid classifier. The learning rate of 0.001 using in Adam, SGD and RMSProp Optimizer with Binary-Crossentropy for loss (Fig. 5).

3 Result and Discussion

An evaluation is carried out to see the performance of the proposed method by using a matrix of precision, recall, F1, and accuracy. Equations 3–6 show how precision, recall, F1-Score, and accuracy are derived, respectively. These four value are the most frequently used as performance indicators for Convolutional Neural Network modeling.

$$Precision = \frac{TP}{TP + FP} \tag{3}$$

$$Recall = \frac{TP}{TP + FN} \tag{4}$$

$$F1 - Score = 2 \times \frac{Precision \times Recall}{Precision + Recall} \tag{5}$$

$$Accuracy = \frac{TP + TN}{TP + TN + FP + FN} \quad (6)$$

From the equations above, it can be explained that precision talks about how accurately the model we designed can predict positive, compared to the amount of data that is truly positive. In the case of IDC breast cancer detection, False Positive (FP) means that the image that is Non-IDC (actual negative) breast cancer has been identified as IDC breast cancer. The Recall parameter is used in calculating how many Actual Positives are captured by the model and labeled as True Positive (TP). F1 Score parameters are very necessary to know the balance between Precision and Recall.

The dataset consists of 2040 breast histopathology images, 1020 each for IDC and Non-IDC. The dataset is taken from Kaggle breast histopathology images dataset [17, 18]. Total data will be divided into 75% (1530 images) as training data and 25% (510 images) as validation data. This dataset will serve as input for the designed CNN model. In this study, an evaluation is carried out to see the performance of the proposed model by using a matrix of precision, recall, F1, and accuracy. Total iteration for training data is 100 times (100 epoch).

Based on the results of system testing shown in Fig. 6, data related to system performance comparisons based on the optimizer algorithm are provided. At least four optimizers were studied, namely Adam, SGD, RMSProp and Nadam. Adam provides the best validation accuracy performance when compared to other optimizer algorithms. The accuracy of model validation when using the Adam optimizer is 93%. Nadam gave the second best performance for performing IDC and Non-IDC classification for the breast histopathology dataset. The accuracy of model validation when using the Nadam optimizer is 90%. Then followed by the RMSProp optimizer, with a validation accuracy of 87%. However, although Nadam and RMSProp provide fairly good performance, the value of this accuracy is very fluctuating. It can be seen from the graph, there are many spikes or derivatives in the accuracy value. Meanwhile, the Adam optimizer tends to be stable by continuing to show an increase in accuracy at each iteration (epoch). After Adam, Nadam

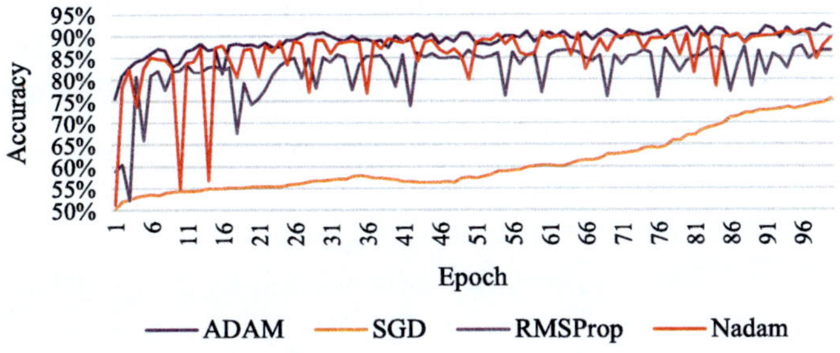

Fig. 6 The accuracy of proposes model

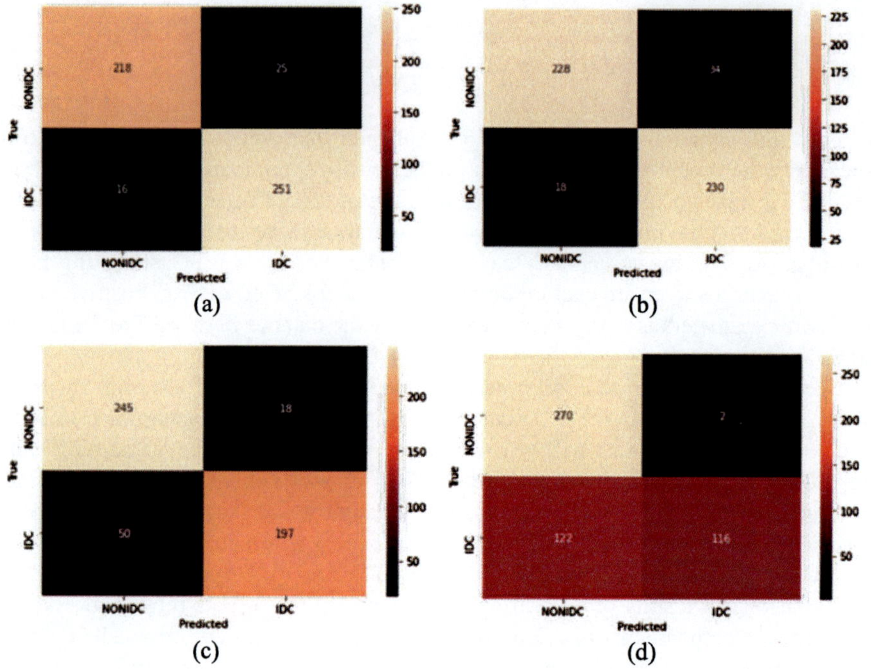

Fig. 7 Confusion matrix of proposes model, **a** Adam, **b** Nadam, **c** RMSProp and **d** SGD

and RMSProp, the SGD optimizer provided the worst performance for the system. The system validation accuracy when using the SGD optimizer is only 76%. The proposed model is also not over-fitting and can be used to recognize IDC and Non-IDC conditions with the best accuracy performance of 93%.

From the confusion matrix listed in Fig. 7, we can find the value of precision, recall and F1-score for each optimizer.

As seen from the graph, the SGD optimizer provides the worst precision values for Non-IDC datasets. This means that the SGD optimizer has minimal ability to recognize IDC images, there are about 122 IDC images predicted to be Non-IDC. Vice versa, the worst recall occurs for the SGD optimizer for the IDC dataset. This means that the system made many prediction errors on the Non-IDC image, which actually turned out to be IDC.

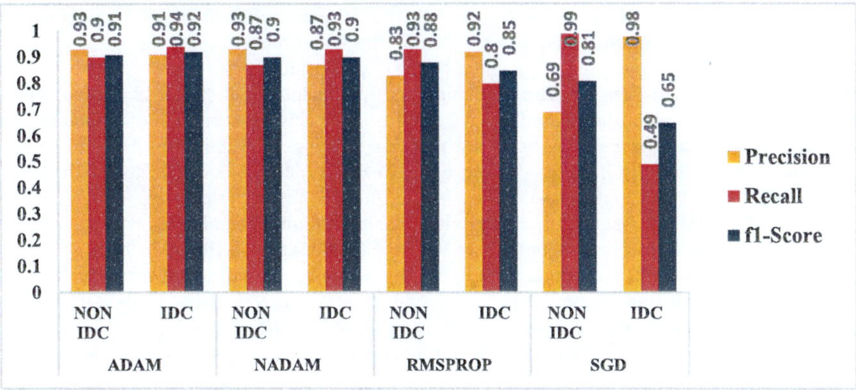

Fig. 8 The precision, recall and f1-score of proposed model

4 Conclusion

System for early detection of IDC and Non-IDC breast cancer conditions based on histopathology images using Convolutional Neural Network is carry out by using 3 hidden layers, RelU activation, max pooling layer and fully connected layers with sigmoid classifier. At least four optimizers were studied; Adam, SGD, RMSProp and Nadam. Adam provides the best accuracy performance when compared to other optimizer algorithms. Based on testing that has been done, the proposed CNN model is able to classify into IDC and Non-IDC conditions with the best accuracy of 93%, and the value of precision, recall, F1-score are 0.93. This study is expected to be validated for later use in assisting medical authorities for conducting clinical diagnoses.

References

1. Organization WH. Breast cancer. https://www.who.int/cancer/prevention/%0Adiagnosis-screening/breast-cancer/en/. Last accessed 04 Sept 2020
2. Saadallah F et al (2019) Case report coexistence of invasive ductal breast carcinoma and fibroadenoma. Pan African Med J 8688, 1–4. https://doi.org/10.11604/pamj.2019.33.139.17140
3. Tower H et al (2019) The immune microenvironment of breast cancer progression. Cancers MDPI 11, 1–15. https://doi.org/10.3390/cancers11091375
4. Hamsagayathri P, Sampath P (2017) Performance analysis of breast cancer classification using decision tree classifiers. Int J Curr Pharm Res 9(2):19–25
5. Polaka I, Tom IE (2010) Decision tree classifiers in bioinformatics. Sci J Riga Tech Univ 44:119–124. https://doi.org/10.2478/v10143-010-0052-4
6. Sekaran K et al (2018) Breast cancer classification using deep neural networks. Knowl Comput Its Appl 227–241. https://doi.org/10.1007/978-981-10-6680-1

7. Jiang Y et al (2019) Breast cancer histopathological image classification using convolutional neural networks with small SE-ResNet module. Plos One (Pone) J 1–21
8. Ruder S (2016) An overview of gradient descent optimization
9. Ray R et al (2019) Classification of Benign and Malignant breast cancer using supervised machine learning algorithms based on image and numeric datasets classification of benign and malignant breast cancer using supervised machine learning algorithms based on image and nume. J Phys Conf Ser Int Conf Biomed Eng (ICoBE) 1372(1):1–6. https://doi.org/10.1088/1742-6596/1372/1/012062
10. Kim P (2014) MATLAB deep learning: with machine learning, neural networks and artificial intelligence, 1st ed. Apress, Seoul, South Korea. https://doi.org/10.1007/978-1-4842-2845-6
11. Indolia S et al (2018) Conceptual understanding of convolutional neural network—a deep learning approach. Proc Comput Sci 132:679–688. https://doi.org/10.1016/j.procs.2018.05.069
12. Wu J (2017) Introduction to convolutional neural networks. Nanjing, China
13. Nwankpa CE et al (2018) Activation functions : comparison of trends in practice and research for deep learning, pp 1–20
14. Albawi S, Mohammed TA (2017) Understanding of a convolutional neural network. In: International conference on engineering and technology (ICET). IEEE, Antalya, Turkey, pp 1–6. https://doi.org/10.1109/ICEngTechnol.2017.8308186
15. Chauhan K, Ram S (2018) Image classification with deep learning and comparison between different convolutional neural network structures using tensorflow and keras. Int J Adv Eng Res Dev 5(2):533–538
16. Shea KO, Nash R (2015) An introduction to convolutional neural networks, pp 1–11
17. Janowczyk A, Madabhushi A (2016) Deep learning for digital pathology image analysis : a comprehensive tutorial with selected use cases. J Pathol Inf 7(29) (2016). https://doi.org/10.4103/2153-3539.186902
18. Cruz-roa A et al (2014) Automatic detection of invasive ductal carcinoma in whole slide images with Convolutional Neural Networks. Med Imaging 2014 Digit Pathol 9041, 216, 1–15. https://doi.org/10.1117/12.2043872

Drowsiness Detection Based on EEG Signal Using Discrete Wavelet Transform (DWT) and K-Nearest Neighbors (K-NN) Methods

Cahyantari Ekaputri, Yunendah Nur Fu'adah, Nor Kumalasari Caecar Pratiwi, Achmad Rizal, and Alva Nurvina Sularso

Abstract Drowsiness generally occurs due to lack of sleep. Drowsiness can trigger various problems, such as decreasing productivity, damaging emotions, even to the point of causing serious accidents, both on the highway or in the workplace environment. One possible way to detect drowsiness is by using an Electroencephalographic (EEG) signal. EEG is a test used to evaluate the electrical activity in the brain. This research proposed a system that can detect drowsiness based on EEG signal using Discrete Wavelet Transform (DWT) as feature extraction and K-Nearest Neighbor (K-NN) as classification method of drowsy and normal conditions. At a preliminary stage, the system would perform a pre-processing to minimize noise signals using normalization and grounding magnitude. Feature extraction of these EEG signals was then decomposed using DWT function whereas the K-NN method is used to classify the EEG signals either in normal or drowsy conditions. The K-NN is done by Euclidean Distance Method. The private dataset consists of 60 signals, divided into 30 signals to normal and drowsy each. This research used DWT with eight-level decomposition of Alpha and Beta signals, and 3 wavelet family types (Coiflet, Symlet and Biorthogonal). Based on the results of tests conducted, EEG signals was decomposed using 3 different types of wavelet family generally provides accuracy values that are not much of a difference while selecting different K values for K-NN classification affects the accuracy. In conclusion, the value of k = 5 is the optimum value to classify normal dan drowsy condition. This condition is in accordance with the K-NN theory in which a greater k value can reduce noise in the classification process so it can improve accuracy of the system. This condition provides system performance with the highest accuracy around 90–100% for any type of wavelet family.

C. Ekaputri (✉) · Y. N. Fu'adah · N. K. C. Pratiwi · A. Rizal
Telkom University, Bandung, Indonesia
e-mail: cahyantarie@telkomuniversity.ac.id

A. N. Sularso
Akademi Teknik Telekomunikasi Sandhy Putra, Jakarta, Indonesia

H. Triwiyanto et al. (eds.), *Proceedings of the 1st International Conference on Electronics, Biomedical Engineering, and Health Informatics*, Lecture Notes in Electrical Engineering 746, https://doi.org/10.1007/978-981-33-6926-9_42

Keywords Drowsiness detection · Discrete wavelet transform (DWT) · K-Nearest network (K-NN) · EEG signal

1 Introduction

Drowsiness is defined as the need to fall asleep as the result of both the circadian rhythm process and the need to sleep [1]. Drowsiness can trigger various problems, such as decreasing productivity, damaging emotions, even to the point of causing serious accidents, both on the highway or in the workplace environment. Drowsiness causes disturbances in concentration. If this occurs at the wrong time, it can be a major cause of making mistakes in work or activities

In more serious cases, drowsiness is one of the main causes of traffic accidents and has significant implications for life safety [2, 3]. Driving within a long duration is very potential to cause fatigue [4]. Manifestations of fatigue that often occur usually arise drowsiness. When planning to travel within long duration, it must be ensured that the driver is in his best condition, accustomed to being awake longer and having no or little drowsiness in the process. Several ways can be done to detect drowsiness, for example through facial expressions (the frequency of blinking and yawning) [5], or other methods using photoplethysmography signal [6] and EEG signal.

EEG signal measurements are carried out to record activities brain in the form of electrical signals [1–18]. In drowsy conditions, the measured EEG signal is able to display a unique signal shape and provide important information [7]. High-quality EEG signals are obtained from a measurement system consisting of several elements needed, from electrodes with conductive media, amplifiers with filters, analog-to-digital (A/D) converters to recording devices. The micro-volt signal recorded by the electrodes on the scalp will be processed by the amplifier into a signal within a certain voltage range. The amplifier output signal will then be converted from analog to digital format by A/D converter, and finally stored through a recording device [8] (Fig. 1).

Several studies related to the detection of drowsiness based on EEG signals have been carried out by previous researchers. Research on hybrid model for EEG-based drowsiness detection was completed by Budak et al. [10]. This research built a detection system using Alex-Net and VGG-Net feature extraction. After the feature extraction process was complete, Tunable Q-factor Wavelet Transform (TQWT) was used to decompose EEG signals into related sub-bands. This research provided results an average accuracy of 94.3%.

The study related to classification of micro-sleep (MS) from baseline utilizing linear and non-linear features derived from electroencephalography (EEG) had been done by Bijay et al. [11]. The EEG signal was recorded from five brain regions, such as frontal, central, parietal, occipital, and temporal. This study used 55 features extracted from EEG signals. Furthermore, these features would be processed using a wrapper-based method. The selected feature then was put into the Linear

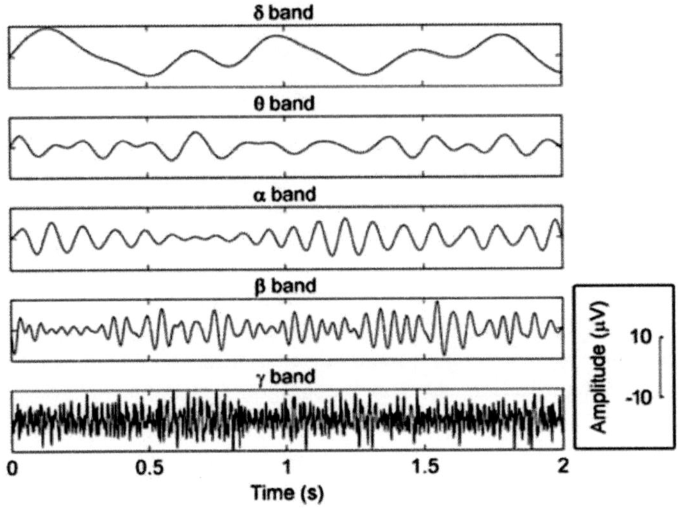

Fig. 1 Rhythmic EEG activity patterns, divided into five frequency bands: delta (δ, <4 Hz), theta (θ, 4–8 Hz), alpha (α, 8–13 Hz), beta (β, 13–30 Hz), and gamma (γ, >30 Hz) [3]

Discriminant Analysis (LDA) or Quadratic Discriminant Analysis (QDA), which could then automatically distinguish the baseline from the MS state. The best classification performance of the proposed algorithm is an F1 value of 87.11%.

Yurui Ming and colleagues have completed the research related to EEG-Based Drowsiness Estimation for Driving Safety Using Deep Q-Learning [12]. The results of this study indicated that the deep Q-network (DQN) model could properly track variations in the state of mind from testing EEG data. These results confirmed that the model is feasible and practical to be used as a new computing paradigm.

Non-invasive devices involved in the detection of drowsiness by using Electroencephalography (EEG) based on machine learning models had been done by Sanurak Natnithikarat et al. [13]. The results demonstrated a correlation between the predicted Karolinska sleepiness Scale (KSS) from the biometrics to the actual KSS from the user input. The conclusion of this research was that the proposed approach could be developed to be applied to monitor mental fatigue in other more realistic scenarios.

EEG based drowsiness detection using K-Nearest neighbor was done by Purnamasari et al. [14]. The EEG signal was processed using Fast Fourier Transform (FFT) to extract its features. These features were classified using K-Nearest Neighbor (KNN). The proposed system produced the highest accuracy of 95.24% using the value of k = 3 and four brain waves as features, namely Delta, Theta, Alpha, and Beta waves. Chunwu Wang and colleagues completed the research related spectral analysis of EEG during micro-sleep events via driver monitoring system to characterize drowsiness [15].

Findings from these studies focused on the ability of EEG signals in the Delta and Alpha spectrum bands to characterize micro-sleep events. From some of the research results above, it is recommended to conduct further studies related to the drowsiness detection by using other methods. The private dataset that was used for this study consists of 60 signals, each divided into 30 signals to normal and drowsy. This study using DWT with eight-level decomposition, devoted to the alpha and beta signals, and 3 wavelet family types (Coiflet, Symlet and Biorthogonal) where drowsiness detection in the previous research studies used Delta, Theta, Alpha and Beta signal.

This research conducted a drowsiness detection study using the Discrete Wavelet transform (DWT) and K-Nearest Neighbor (K-NN) methods. Wavelet is a common method which is used for image processing and computer vision. Several applications of wavelet utilization, such as recognition, detection, image capture and compression. Wavelet transformations have become very popular because of their complete theoretical nature, great flexibility for selecting bases and using computational processes that tend to be simpler [16]. While the KNN as a classification algorithm has several advantages, including being non-deterministic, effective for small numbers of datasets and producing high accuracy [17].

2 Materials and Methods

2.1 EEG Datasets

This research used a MindWave mobile headset by NeuroSky equipped with a single EEG sensor to record the electrical activity of the brain for classifying which EEG signal occurring during normal and drowsy condition. It has EEG electrode sensor which is put on the forehead, the reference and ground electrode which are tucked behind the ear, on/off feature with Bluetooth pairing switch, indicator lamp and powered by battery.

Data collection was conducted by putting NeuroSky MindWave mobile headset to a participant's head to record EEG signals (under participant's consent) for a minute. The first data collection intended for training data was conducted to 30 participants with two conditions setting of normal and drowsy for 1 minute each. For recording EEG signals under normal conditions, participants were asked to remain in normal conditions by focusing their mind, regulating breathing and adjusting their body position as comfortable as possible. When recording EEG signals for normal and concentrated conditions, participants were also invited to chat and performed various activities such as moving the limbs, flickering and playing games on smartphone. Whereas for recording EEGs for drowsy condition, data collection was carried out at night while all participants slept. The next data collection for the test data was conducted to 30 different participants for normal and

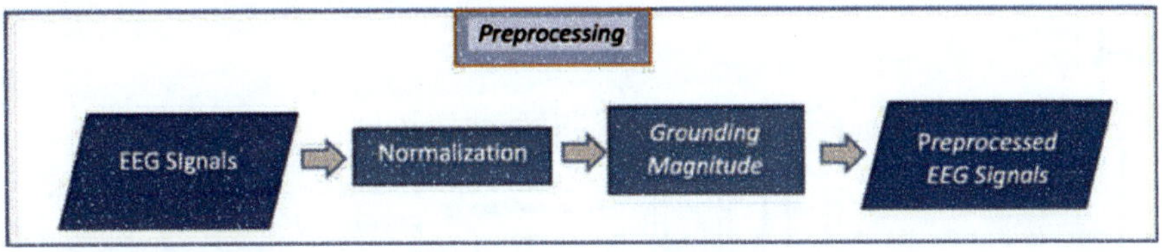

Fig. 2 Steps of pre-processing as follows

drowsy conditions under the same treatment. In addition, participants were also asked to state their feelings during the data collection process in both conditions.

2.2 *Pre-processing*

Pre-processing the EEG data needs to be conducted beforehand to minimize noise, which comes in the form of normalization and high amplitude grounding in the first second of recording, in order for the EEG signal can be analyzed and classified correctly. The flowchart of pre-processing steps is shown in Fig. 2.

Normalization is a process in which raw signal is reduced by its own average. Mathematically, normalization of EEG signal value is shown in Eq. (1).

$$\text{Normalised } X = X - \text{mean } X \tag{1}$$

where X is the EEG raw signal.

Grounding magnitude is the proses of removing noise that occurs when a device starts data retrieval process in the first 2 seconds. Amplitude value in the first 2 seconds which exceeds 200 or less than 200 will be grounded to 0.

2.3 *Discrete Wavelet Transform (DWT)*

Feature extraction was performed using wavelets. By utilizing the Discrete Wavelet Transform (DWT) function, the signal was broken down into two parts which shown in Fig. 3a. They were Approval Coefficients (AC) and Detailed Coefficients (DC). This process was done repeatedly to produce Approximation Coefficients and Detailed Coefficients into different levels of decomposition. That way, we got the feature value of frequency power band from that signal.

EEG signal could be decomposed based on their band frequencies, namely Alpha, Beta, Delta, Gamma and Theta on each channel which are shown in Fig. 3b. The wavelet family types used in this research were Symlet, Coiflet and

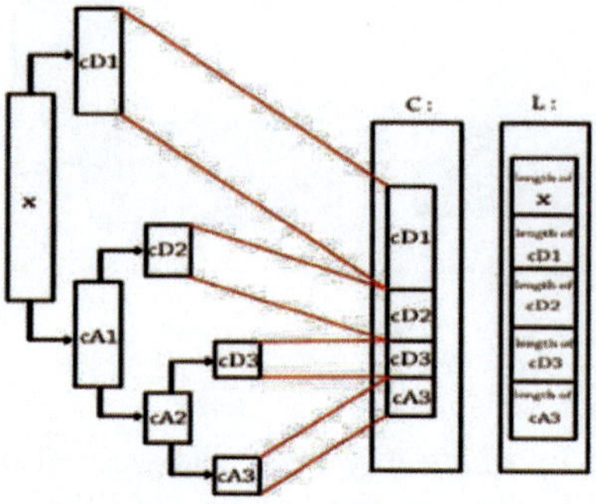

(a)

Frequency Range (Hz)	Frequency Band	*Frequency Bandwidth*
0-4	Delta	4
4-8	Theta	4
8-14	Alpha	6
14-32	Beta	18
32-64	Gamma	32
64-128	Noises	64

(b)

Fig. 3 **a** Decomposition using Discrete Wavelet Transform (DWT) and **b** frequency band

Biorthogonal to decompose EEG signals, so that Alpha and Beta signals were obtained which then be used in this study.

After decomposition of the signal to obtain Alpha and Beta signals using Discrete Wavelet Transform (DWT) was complete, statistical features in the form of means, variance, and standard deviation of the Alpha and Beta signals were then calculated to analyze which features could significantly distinguish normal and drowsy condition.

2.4 *K-Nearest Neighbors (K-NN)*

The K-Nearest Neighbors algorithm (K-NN) is a method for classifying objects, based on learning data that is in close proximity to the object. Distance is an approach used to determine identical aspect of two feature vectors, namely training features and test features. Measurement of distance in the K-NN method can be calculated using several methods, one of which is the Euclidean Distance. Mathematically, Euclidean Distance is shown in Eq. (2).

$$j(v_1, v_2) = \sqrt{\sum_{k=1}^{N} (v_1(k) - v_2(k))^2} \tag{2}$$

where:

j	The distance of test data to training data
$v_1(k)$	Test data of k with k = 1, 2, … N
$v_2(k)$	Training data of k, with k = 1, 2, …, N

The success parameter in this study is the accuracy of the system intended for classifying normal and drowsy conditions derived from the test results. System accuracy is a comparison between data giving the correct classification results to the amount of test data. Mathematically, the accuracy of the system is shown in Eq. (3).

$$\text{Accuracy} = \frac{\sum \text{success Data}}{\sum \text{Total Test Data}} \times 100\% \tag{3}$$

3 Result and Discussion

This research used dataset from 60 participants, which consist of 30 signals in normal condition and 30 signals in drowsy condition. At the feature extraction stage, we analyzed the effect of wavelet types (such as Coiflet, Symlet and Biorthogonal) on system performance while at the classification stage, an analysis were carried out regarding the effect of k values on system performance.

Figure 4 shows the raw EEG signal at normal state and at drowsy state in time domain. Based on the results shown in Fig. 1, it can be seen that there is an amplitude signal with the value exceeding up to 200. So, we had to remove the noise using grounded magnitude. Grounding magnitude is the process of removing noise that occurs when a device starts data retrieval in the first 2 seconds. Amplitude in the first 2 seconds that exceeds 200 or less than −200 will be grounded to 0. The single sided amplitude spectrum of raw EEG signal in frequency domain shown in Fig. 5. The figure also shows the comparison before and after pre-processing in the frequency domain. It can be seen that there was a very high amplitude value at 0 Hz before pre-processing and there was no amplitude value at 0 Hz after pre-processing.

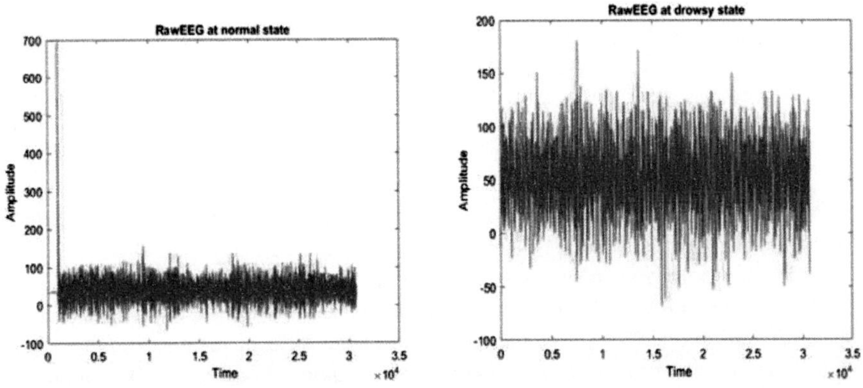

(a) (b)

Fig. 4 Raw EEG signal **a** normal state, **b** drowsy state

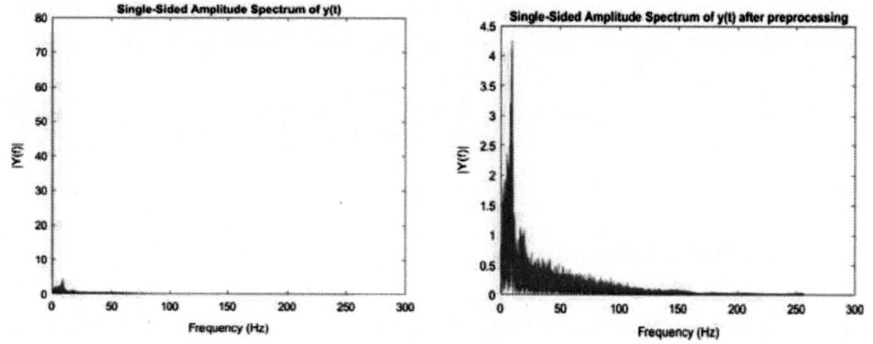

(a) (b)

Fig. 5 Pre-processing of raw EEG signal at normal state **a** before pre-processing and **b** after pre-processing

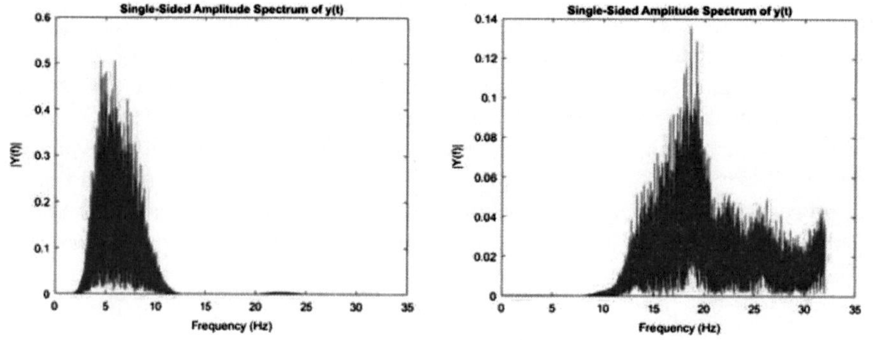

(a) (b)

Fig. 6 Drowsy state signal **a** Alpha signal and **b** Beta signal

EEG signals can be decomposed based on their band frequencies, namely Alpha, Beta, Delta, Gamma and Theta on each channel. In this research, the wavelet family of Coiflet, Symlet and Biorthogonal types were used to decompose EEG signals so that Alpha and Beta signals were obtained which later be used in the next stage.

Based on Fig. 6a, it can be seen that the Alpha frequency ranges around 5–12 Hz. Furthermore, Fig. 6b shows the range of Beta signal of around 10–32 Hz. After decomposition of the signal to obtain alpha and beta signals using Discrete Wavelet Transform (DWT), statistical features in the form of means, variance, and standard deviation of the alpha and beta signals would be calculated. The features value later be used in K-NN to classify normal and drowsy conditions.

Tests were carried out by analyzing the type of wavelet family used when decomposing the alpha signal and beta signal. The characteristic features used were

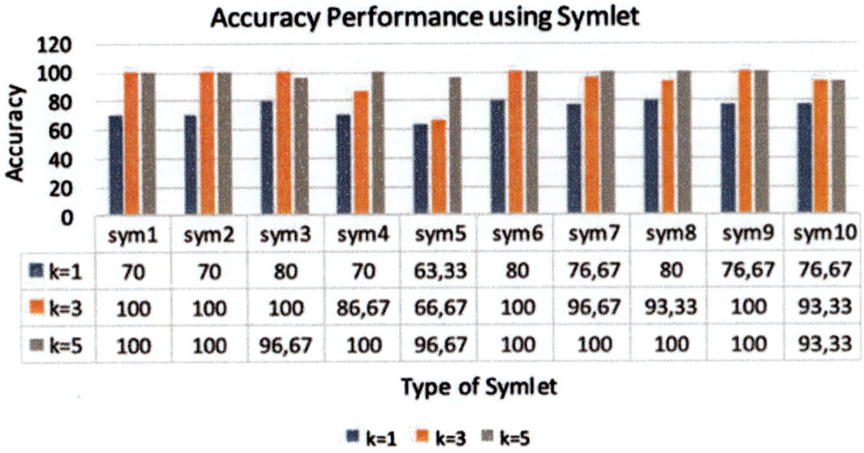

Fig. 7 Accuracy performance using Symlet

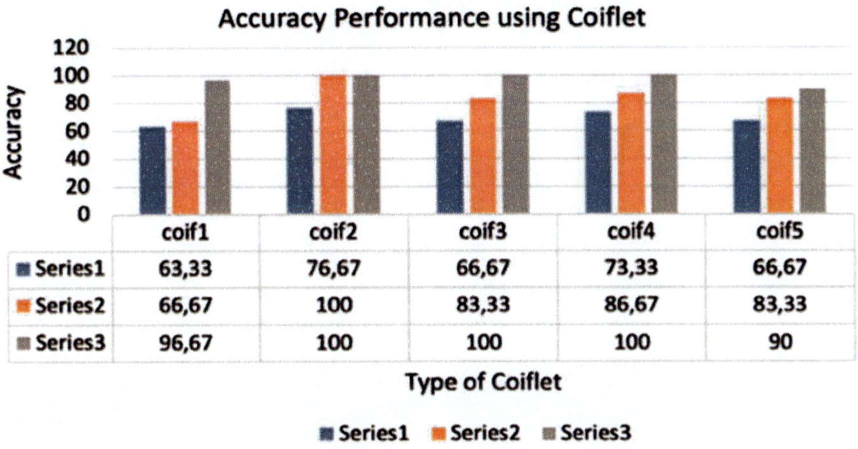

Fig. 8 Accuracy performance using Coiflet

mean, variance value and standard deviation of the alpha signal and the beta signal. At the stage of classification, the distance equation used was the Euclidean distance for the values k = 1.3 and 5. The results of the accuracy of the system for testing 30 test data (15 normal signal conditions and 15 drowsy signal conditions) are shown in Figs. 7, 8, and 9.

Based on the results of tests conducted, it can be concluded that the use of wavelet family types for alpha and beta signal decomposition generally gives a system accuracy value that is not much of a difference significantly for any wavelet family type. However, the accuracy of the normal and drowsy condition

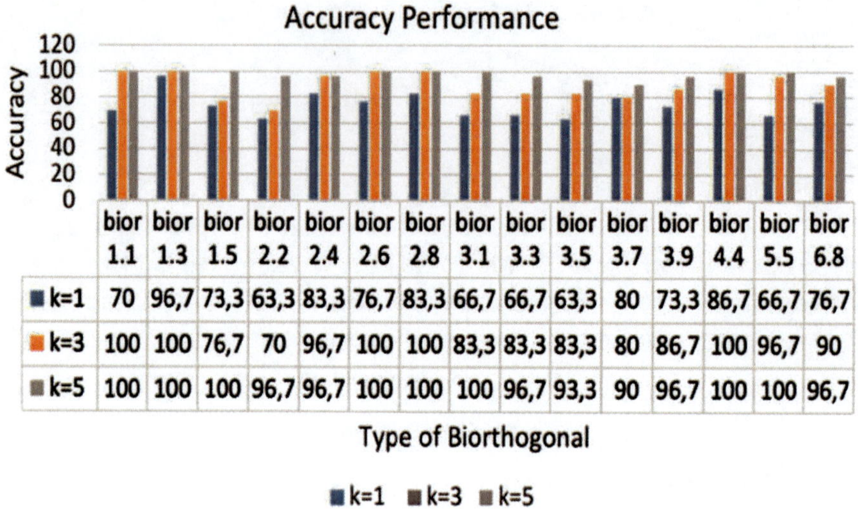

Fig. 9 Accuracy performance using Biorthogonal

Table 1 The performance comparison of the proposed drowsiness detection system with previous related studies

Authors	Method	Performance result
Budak et al. [4]	Tunable Q-factor Wavelet Transform (TQWT)	Accuracy of 94.3%
Bijay et al. [5]	Linear Discriminant Analysis (LDA) or Quadratic Discriminant Analysis (QDA)	F1 value of 87.11%
Purnamasari et al. [8]	Fast Fourier Transform (FFT) and K-Nearest Neighbor	Accuracy of 95.24%
Ekaputri et al. [18]	Discrete Wavelet Transform and K-Nearest Neighbor (**Proposed Method**)	Accuracy of 100%

classification system that has been designed is greatly influenced by the selection of k values at classification using k-NN. Based on the test results in this study, the value of k = 5 is the optimum value to classify normal dan drowsy condition. This condition provides system performance with the highest accuracy around 90–100 for any type of wavelet family. Table 1 shows the performance comparison of the drowsiness detection system developed in this study with previous related studies.

Based on Table 1, it can be seen that the drowsiness detection system using the proposed method, namely Discrete Wavelet Transform as a feature extraction method and K-Nearest Neighbor as a classification method gives the best performance with accuracy of 100%. Several factors did affect the performance of the drowsiness detection system that gives the best performance. This research used primary data in which the conditions of the data used were similar to the data acquisition process of the same stages which resulted in the pre-processing stage being less complex. Furthermore, the accuracy of the feature extraction using DWT to extract Alpha and Beta signal was valid, since these two signals were proven to provide significant information to distinguish normal conditions and drowsiness conditions. The calculation of statistical features of Alpha and Beta signals, such as mean, variance value and standard deviation, simplified the classification stage in recognizing each condition. The feature extraction results obtained in the previous stage and the proper k value at K-NN will affect the classification stage. Based on the result that is shown in Figs. 7–9, a greater k value gives the higher accuracy. This condition is in accordance with the K-NN theory in the notion that greater k value can reduce noise in the classification process, so it can really improve the accuracy of the system. To get the best performance, some experiments should be carried out to find the most optimal K value. Based on the results, it can be acknowledged that the drowsiness detection system developed in this study outperforms the previous studies.

4 Conclusion

The conclusion of this research is that the proposed approach can be developed and applied to monitor mental fatigue in other more realistic scenarios. Based on the results of tests conducted, it can be concluded that the use of wavelet family types for Alpha and Beta signal decomposition generally gives a system accuracy value that is not much of a difference significantly for any wavelet family type, but the accuracy of the normal and drowsy condition classification system that had been designed is greatly influenced by the selection of k values in classification using k-NN. Based on the test results in this study, the value of $k = 5$ is the optimum value to classify normal dan drowsy condition. This condition provides system performance with the highest accuracy around 90–100% for any type of wavelet family.

In the future, it is expected to continue designing a device such as a headset integrated with EEG electrodes. This device is expected to be able to detect drowsiness on drivers in the earliest stage and eventually be able to reduce the number of traffic accidents caused by drowsiness.

References

1. National Center on Sleep Disorders Research (2013) Drowsy driving and automobile crashes: report and recommendations
2. Omidyeganeh M, Javadtalab A, Shirmohammadi S (2011) Intelligent driver drowsiness detection through fusion of yawning and eye closure. In: 2011 IEEE international conference on virtual environments, human-computer interfaces and measurement systems proceedings. IEEE, pp 1–6

3. de Mello MT, Narciso FV, Tu KS, Paiva T, Spence DW, BaHammam AS, Verster JC, Pandi-Perumal SR (2013) Sleep disorders as a cause of motor vehicle collisions. Int J Prev Med 4(3):246
4. Liu D, Sun P, Xiao Y, Yin Y (2010) Drowsiness detection based on eyelid movement. In 2010 second international workshop on education technology and computer science, Vol 2. IEEE, pp 49–52
5. Deng W, Wu R (2019) Real-time driver-drowsiness detection system using facial features. In: IEEE Access, Vol 7. IEEE, pp 118727–118738
6. Kurian D, PL JJ, Radhakrishnan K, Balakrishnan AA (2014) Drowsiness detection using photoplethysmography signal. In: 2014 fourth international conference on advances in computing and communications. IEEE, pp 73–76
7. Oviyaa M, Renvitha P, Swathika R, Joe Louis Paul I, Sasirekha S (2020) Arduino based real time drowsiness and fatigue detection for bikers using helmet. In: 2020 2nd international conference on innovative mechanisms for industry applications (ICIMIA). IEEE, pp 573–577
8. Xia X, Li H (2019) EEG: neural basis and measurement. In: EEG signal processing and feature extraction. Springer, Singapore, pp 7–21
9. Lu X, Li H (2019) Electroencephalography, evoked potentials, and event-related potentials. In: EEG signal processing and feature extraction. Springer, Singapore, pp 23–42
10. Budak Umit, Bajaj Varun, Akbulut Yaman, Atila Orhan, Sengur Abdulkadir (2019) An effective hybrid model for EEG-based drowsiness detection. IEEE Sens J 19(17):7624–7631
11. Guragain B, Rad AB, Wang C, Verma AK, Archer L, Wilson N, Tavakolian K (2019) EEG-based classification of micro-sleep by means of feature selection: an application in aviation. In: 2019 41st annual international conference of the IEEE engineering in medicine and biology society (EMBC). IEEE, pp 4060–4063
12. Ming Y, Wu D, Wang Y-K, Shi Y, Lin C-T (2020) EEG-based drowsiness estimation for driving safety using deep Q-learning. arXiv preprint arXiv:2001.02399
13. Natnithikarat S, Lamyai S, Leelaarporn P, Kunaseth N, Autthasan P, Wisutthisen T, Wilaiprasitporn T (2019) Drowsiness detection for once-based workload with mouse and keyboard data. In: 2019 12th biomedical engineering international conference (BMEiCON). IEEE, pp 1–4 (2019)
14. Purnamasari PD, Yustiana P, Ratna AAP, Sudiana D (2019) Mobile EEG based drowsiness detection using K-nearest neighbor. In: 2019 IEEE 10th international conference on awareness science and technology (iCAST). IEEE, pp 1–5
15. Wang, Chunwu, Bijay Guragain, Ajay K. Verma, Lewis Archer, Shubha Majumder, Abdiaziz Mohamud, Emily Flaherty-Woods et al: Spectral Analysis of EEG During Micro-sleep Events Annotated via Driver Monitoring System to Characterize Drowsiness. In IEEE Transactions on Aerospace and Electronic Systems 56, no. 2, pp 1346–1356. (2019)
16. Jasim Wala'a N, Harfash Esra J (2018) Recognition Normal and Abnormal Human Activities by Implementation K-Nearest Neighbor and Decision Tree Models. Journal of Theoretical and Applied Information Technology 96(19):6423–6443
17. Jadhav SD, Channe HP (2016) Comparative study of K-NN, naive Bayes and decision tree classification techniques. International Journal of Science and Research (IJSR) 5(1):1842–1845
18. Ekaputri, C., Widadi, R. and Rizal A.: EEG Signal Classification for Alcoholic and Non-Alcoholic Person using Multilevel Wavelet Packet Entropy and Support Vector Machine. In 2020 8th International Conference on Information and Communication Technology (ICoICT). IEEE (2020)

Classification of White Blood Cell Abnormalities for Early Detection of Myeloproliferative Neoplasms Syndrome Using Backpropagation

Zilvanhisna Emka Fitri and Arizal Mujibtamala Nanda Imron

Abstract One of the diseases of white blood cells is myeloproliferative neoplasms syndrome where this disease is an abnormality in the bone marrow in excessive blood cell counts. Full Blood Count (FBC) is a type of examination that shows the patient's health status, blood cell abnormalities, and the presence of infection in the patient's body. However, the determination of cell abnormalities is still done manually based on the knowledge and experience of clinical pathology so that the determination of these abnormalities is subjective. Therefore we need a system that is able to classify white blood cell abnormalities automatically, objectively and accurately. This study uses digital image processing on peripheral blood smear images then feature extraction will be obtained which will be the input of the classification system. The features used are area, perimeter, metric and compactness, while the classification method used is the backpropagation method. The best backpropagation network architecture used is 4, 6, 8, 5, 2 with a variation of learning rates of 0.05 and 0.3 producing the best accuracy rate of 91.82% with the amount of training data that is 516 and testing data is 159.

Keywords Abnormalities · White blood cells · Myeloproliferative neoplasms syndrome · Backpropagation · Peripheral blood smear

Z. E. Fitri (✉)
Informatics Engineering, Department of Information Technology,
Politeknik Negeri Jember, Jember 68121, Indonesia
e-mail: zilvanhisnaef@polije.ac.id

A. M. N. Imron
Departement of Electrical Engineering, Electrical Engineering,
Universitas Jember, Jember 68121, Indonesia
e-mail: arizal.tamala@unej.ac.id

H. Triwiyanto et al. (eds.), *Proceedings of the 1st International Conference on Electronics, Biomedical Engineering, and Health Informatics*, Lecture Notes in Electrical Engineering 746, https://doi.org/10.1007/978-981-33-6926-9_43

1 Introduction

One of the human body's defense system that is able to protect the body from bacteria, viruses and pathogenic organisms is white blood cells or better known as leukocytes. There are 6 known types of leukocyte cells namely Polymorphonuclear (PMN), Neutrophil Bands, Lymphocytes, Monocytes, Eosinophils, and Basophils. The number of leukocytes can be used as a reference to identify the disease [1]. One of the diseases of white blood cells is myeloproliferative neoplasms syndrome, where the disease is an abnormality in the bone marrow in producing excessive blood cell counts. WHO classifies four diseases involving white blood cells in myeloproliferative syndrome, namely Chronic Myelogenous Leukemia (CML), Chronic Neutrophilic Leukemia (CNL), Chronic Eosinophilic Leukemia (CEL) and Primary myelofibrosis [2]. Full Blood Count (FBC) is a type of examination that shows the patient's health status, blood cell abnormality and the presence of infection in the patient's body [3]. In the FBC results, the patient's status will be categorized into two, namely the reduction in the number of leukocyte production (leucopenia) and the excess amount of leukocyte production (leucocytosis). A blood smear analysis takes into account flagged automated hematology results and enables the determination of whether a manual differential count should be performed. Therefore, peripheral blood smear examination along with manual differential leukocyte count (if necessary) and CBC provide the complete hematological picture of the patient [4]. But the problem that often occurs is the process of calculating leukocyte differences is still manually and subjectively dependent on the ability and experience of the analyst himself, so we need a system that is able to classify and calculate the difference in leukocytes automatically and objectively.

Some research references related to white blood cells. In 2010, research related to the introduction of leukocyte image patterns using image feature extraction methods. The features used are the image area, perimeter and euler number and the system is able to predict the five types of leukocytes with an error percentage of 30% [5]. Then in 2012, a system was developed to recognize the segmentation of the leukocyte nucleus in blood smear images by comparing two intelligent systems namely KNN and SVM [1]. The other research related to the identification of acute leukemia in microscopic blood images also used the KNN method with variations in K values resulting in an increase in accuracy of 94% at k = 5 [6]. Besides KNN, another method used for the introduction of white blood cells is the artificial neural network method. This method is used to recognize acute lymphoblastic leukemia (ALL) cells with an accuracy rate of 100%, but there is no mention of the type of artificial neural network algorithm used in the research [7]. The Learning Vector Quantization method or better known as LVQ is able to identify the ALL and AML blood images with the lowest accuracy rate of 70% with the variation of learning rate used [8]. Besides LVQ, Multilayer Perceptron method capable of classifying the white blood cells to the level of accuracy of 94.12% [9].

Based on the description above, the researchers developed a classification system for white blood cell abnormalities for early detection of myeloproliferative syndrome using an artificial neural network algorithm. This research is a development of our previous research. The first research, we compared two classification methods, namely LVQ and KNN to classify platelets on peripheral blood smear images. The accuracy rate using the KNN is 83.67%, while the accuracy rate using the LVQ is 74.75% [3]. The second research, we tried to use the backpropagation method to classify platelets. The results showed that both the KNN and Backpropagation methods were able to classify platelets in the AL color space. The accuracy rate of the KNN method is 83.26%, while the accuracy rate of the backpropagation method is 87.76% [10]. The third research, we tried to adopt the image processing techniques that we had done in previous research, but in this research we changed the object of our research from classifying platelets to classifying types of leukocytes as early detection of myeloproliferative syndromes. In that research, we varied the value of k to get the best accuracy results from the KNN method. The level of accuracy of the KNN method for classifying leukocytes is 94.3% with a K value of 23 [11]. Based on the exposure of our previous research results, we tested the backpropagation method to classify the types of leukocytes and compared the results with the classification method that we had done in our previous research.

2 Materials and Methods

In this research, the data used are peripheral blood smear images in Essential Thrombocythemia (ET) patients on our previous research. There are 5 types of white blood cells consisting of Polymorphonuclear (PMN), Neutrophil Bands, Lymphocytes, Monocytes, and Eosinophils. Basophile cell image data does not exist, because based on the results of examination of peripheral blood smear patients these cells were not found [11]. These data are in accordance with laboratory results based on ET patients, where the examination of the peripheral blood smear shows that the white blood cell count is usually normal or slightly increased and no basophil cells are found [12]. The data used is an image measuring 301 × 301 pixels with a variation of white blood data as shown in Fig. 1. The method used in this study also adopted our previous research [3, 10], but the difference was the feature parameters used. The feature used is not using the Gray Level Co-Occurrence Matrix feature but morphological features such as area, perimeter, metric and compactness of the variation of white blood cells [11]. Several research stages are shown in Fig. 2.

2.1 Color Conversion

The first stage is the variation of white blood cells carried out the process of color conversion from the RGB color space to another color space. Because RGB

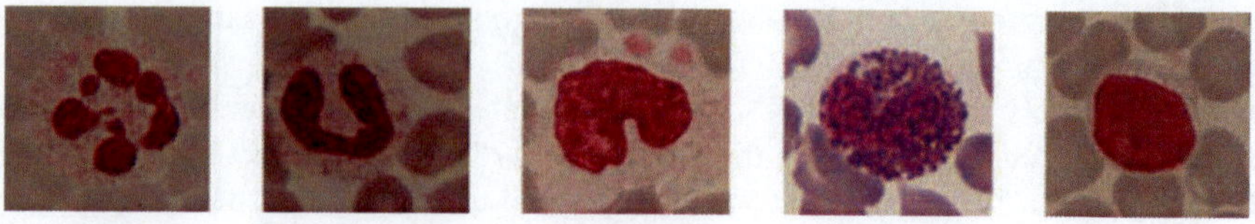

Fig. 1 Variations in abnormalities of white blood cells

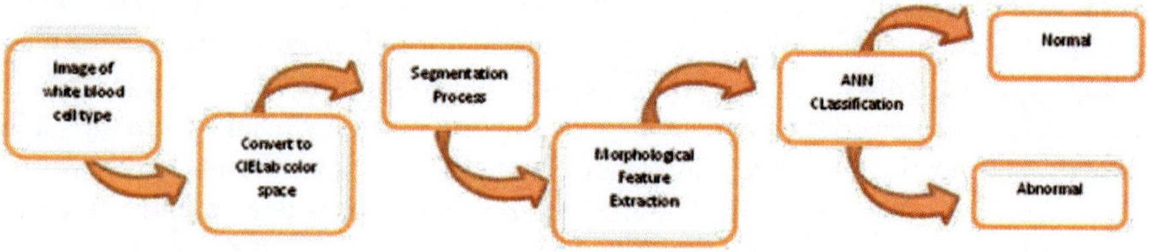

Fig. 2 System block diagram

colorspace is difficult to segment, so the image must be converted to another color space such as HSV color space or CIELab color space [3]. RGB color space cannot be directly converted to CIELab color space, so it must be converted to XYZ color space then converted to CIELab color space. After successfully converting to the CIELab color space, do the separation between the components in the color space. Then do the process of reducing between components so that a new color space is formed, namely the AL color space as shown in Fig. 3. AL color space is obtained from the process of subtracting color components A from color components L [3, 10, 11].

2.2 *Segmentation Process*

The second stage is the process of segmentation in the image of white blood cells. This segmentation process serves to separate objects from the background. The separation process uses the thresholding process with Eq. (1), thus forming a binary image.

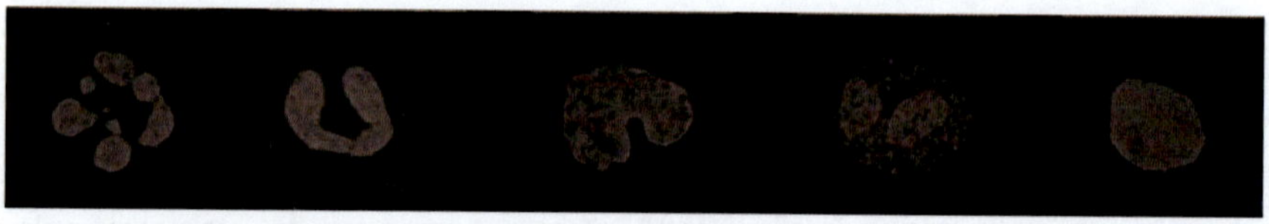

Fig. 3 Image of white blood cells in the AL color space

$$a(x, y) = \begin{cases} 1, & a(x, y) \geq T \\ 0, & a(x, y) < T \end{cases} \tag{1}$$

2.3 *Feature Extraction*

The function of the feature extraction process is taking on the characteristics of the object that we examine. In this experiment, morphological feature extraction which consists of area, perimeter, metric and compactness of a variety of white blood cells. The equation used to find the metric value in Eq. (2) and compactness value in Eq. (3).

$$a(x, y) = \begin{cases} 1, & a(x, y) \geq T \\ 0, & a(x, y) < T \end{cases} \tag{2}$$

$$\text{Compactness} = \frac{P^2}{A} \tag{3}$$

2.4 *ANN Classification*

Artificial Neural Network (ANN) is an information processing technique whose principle is similar to the workings of the nervous system in humans. Neural Networks consist of a large number of information processing elements (neurons) that are interconnected and work together to solve a particular problem, so in general to solve classification or prediction problems. The relationship between neurons is called weight and to get certain functions can be done by conducting training that adjusts the weight value of each neuron. Generally ANN is trained so that the input leads to a specific target output, therefore the training process is called supervised learning [13]. In this research the ANN algorithm used is a backpropagation algorithm. Backpropagation is also known as the Multi Layer Perceptron (MLP) where there are many hidden layers that are used to update the weighting value [10]. The input parameters of the backpropagation method are area, perimeter, metric and compactness.

3 Experiment and Result

In this research used data that consists of a variety of white blood cells of normal and abnormal white blood cells obtained in Fig. 4. There is a difference between normal white blood cells and abnormal white blood cells that can be seen from the

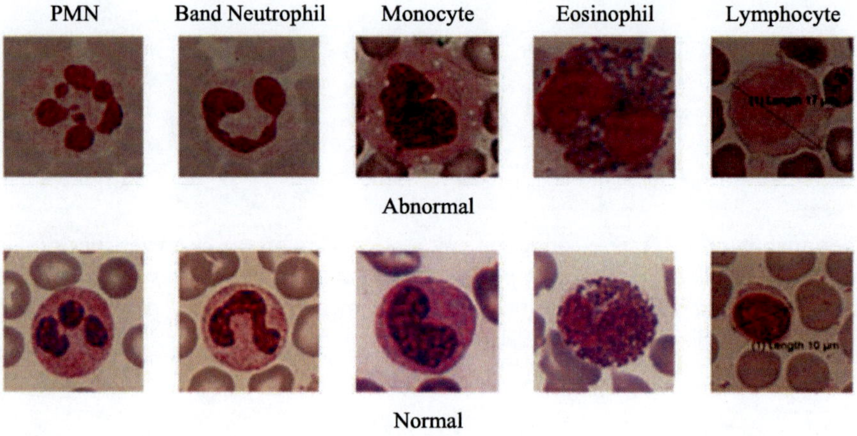

Fig. 4 Variations in normal and abnormal white blood cells

Fig. 5 The difference in size between normal and abnormal lymphocyte cells

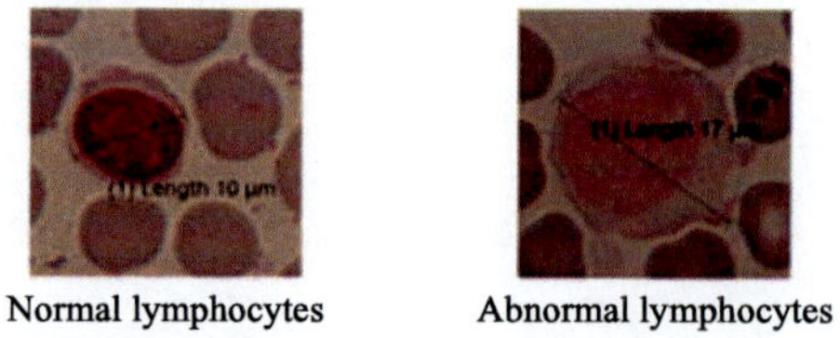

cell size and the number of lobe nuclei as in Fig. 5, so to distinguish the two can be seen in the size and shape of the lobes or commonly called morphological features.

Figure 5 shows that the size of abnormal lymphocyte cells is greater than normal lymphocyte cells. The diameter of abnormal lymphocyte cells is 17 μm while the diameter of normal lymphocyte cells is 10 μm. But before extracting the morphological features of white blood cells, we must do the segmentation process. In the explanation above, the segmentation process functions to separate the object of research with the background using the thresholding process with Eq. (1). In this research several times the threshold value was tested, 50, 90 and 100 so the results are shown in Table 1.

Table 1 shows that the best threshold value is 90. This is because images with a threshold value of 90 are able to represent the best objects and separating objects from the background are better when compared to the threshold values of 50 and 100. After the segmentation process, do the morphological feature extraction process. The features used are area, perimeter, metric and compactness so values are obtained as shown in Table 2.

Table 2 shows that there are differences in the value of feature extraction from normal white blood cells and abnormal white blood cells. This can be seen from the four values of morphological features in each image. The area, perimeter and compactness values of the abnormal white blood cell images are greater than

Table 1 Binary imagery with variations in threshold value (T)

PMNA88	Threshold value (T)		
	50	90	100
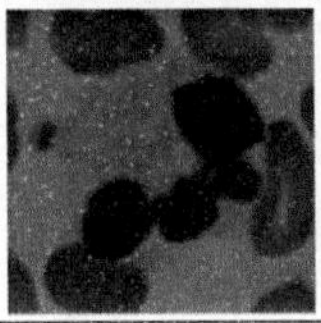	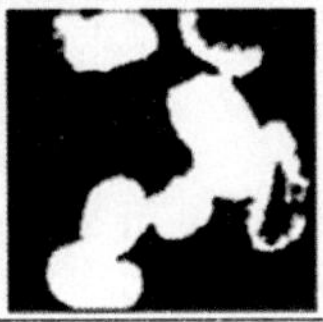	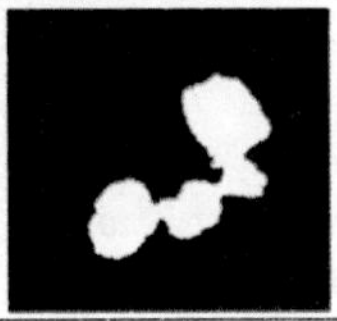	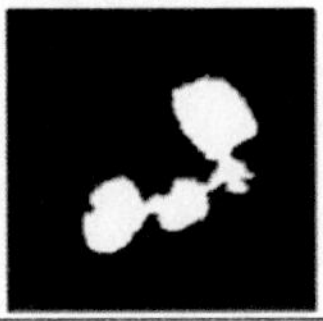

Table 2 The difference between normal and abnormal wbc is based on feature values

Type of white blood cells	The features			
	Area	Perimeter	Metric	Compactness
Normal	8087	626	0.26	48.46
Abnormal	9905	832	0.18	69.89

normal white blood cells, but the abnormal white blood cell metric values are smaller than normal white blood cells. This morphological feature value will be input to the classification method so that the system can distinguish normal white blood cells from abnormal white blood cells. The classification method used is the backpropagation method, which consists of two processes, namely training and testing. The amount of data in the training is 516 while the amount of testing data is 159 data. In determining the network architecture, several experiments were carried out, namely using five different network architectures, as in Table 3, while Table 4 shows the accuracy of the system in the testing process with a variation in learning rate. In this training process using a momentum value of 0.2 and an epoch value of 10,000.

Table 3 shows that the five architectures can be grouped into three based on the number of hidden layers. In some experiments, the accuracy of the test system stability is obtained when using the three hidden layer with variations in the

Table 3 The percentage of system accuracy in training with a variety of network architecture models and learning rates

Network architecture					Learning rate			
Input layer	Hidden layer			Output layer	0.05	0.1	0.3	0.5
4	3	–	–	2	92.82	93.41	89.53	89.34
4	6	–	–	2	89.92	89.92	91.08	92.63
4	6	3	–	2	93.21	93.60	80.23	89.34
4	4	2	–	2	83.14	83.53	83.14	82.95
4	6	8	5	2	93.22	93.99	92.25	91.67

Table 4 The percentage of system accuracy in testing with variety of learning rates

Network architecture					Learning rate			
Input layer	Hidden layer			Output layer	0.05	0.1	0.3	0.5
4	6	8	5	2	91.82	91.20	91.82	89.94

learning rate. The percentage of system training accuracy of at least 91.67% and a maximum of 93.99% with a learning rate of 0.1, so that the architecture used in this research is a network architecture with three hidden layers. Each hidden layer has a number of nodes or neurons: 6 nodes in the first hidden layer, 8 nodes in the second hidden layer, and 5 nodes in the third hidden layer with a root mean square error parameter of 0.2. The relationship between the number of hidden layers with input and output must be proportional, so the system gets the best accuracy. The number of nodes in each hidden layer must be adjusted to the number of inputs and outputs. The number of hidden layers serves to increase system accuracy when the values between classes have a high level of similarity to their input parameters. Based on the results of the training, then do the testing process systemnya accuracy percentage shown in Table 4. Table 4 shows that the number of hidden layer used is 3 with a variation of learning rate to obtain the best system accuracy percentage is 91.82% with a learning rate variation of 0.05 and 0.3.

4 Discussion

This research is a development of our previous research. In research [3, 10], it was aimed to classify platelets and compare them with leukocytes. This is because on the microscopic examination of ET patients, it was found that giant platelets based on size and appearance had similarities with the shape of young lymphocytes. The three classification methods have been compared: LVQ, KNN and Backpropagation, so that it is found that Backpropagation is the best method of classifying platelets as early detection of myeloproliferative syndromes. Based on the results of these two studies, we adapted the image processing technique, especially the color conversion technique, so that the AL color space was best represented in representing the shape and size of leukocyte cells. Then we changed the feature extraction, from texture feature extraction to morphological feature extraction. The results of the morphological feature extraction obtained four parameters, namely area, perimeter, metric and compactness. This feature becomes the input of the classification method. In research [11], the classification system we use is the KNN which has an accuracy rate of 94.3% with a variation of the K value of 23, but in this research, we used the backpropagation classification method. Our results show that the best network architecture is 4, 6, 8, 5, 2 with a training accuracy of 93.22% and testing accuracy of 91.82%. The difference in accuracy between the KNN and Backpropagation methods is not far away. This is due to the grouping of only two classes, so that KNN can classify better according to a simple classification concept. However, the KNN and backpropagation methods will be further tested for class grouping in greater numbers.

5 Conclusions

The backpropagation method is able to classify the abnormality of white blood cells with the best accuracy rate of 91.82% with 516 training data and 159 testing data. These results are due to variations in the types of white blood which are made into two classes: normal class and abnormal class. In addition, there is a closeness to the morphological feature values between the abnormal class and the normal class so that it also affects the classification process. To improve and develop further research, several steps must be done, it is necessary to add additional parameters such as texture, add the class used, and compare with other methods to find an accurate method of classifying abnormalities white blood cells.

References

1. Huang D-C, Hung K-D, Chan Y-K (2012) A computer assisted method for leukocyte nucleus segmentation and recognition in blood smear images. J Syst Softw 85(9):2104–2118
2. Bain BJ (2015) Blood cells—a practical guide, Fifth edn. Wiley, United KIngdom
3. Fitri ZE, Purnama IKE, Pramunanto E, Purnomo MH (2017) A comparison of platelets classification from digitalization microscopic peripheral blood smear. In: 2017 international seminar on intelligent technology and its applications (ISITIA). IEEE, Surabaya, pp 356–361
4. Wahed A, DasGupta A (2015) Hematology and coagulation: a comprehensive review for board preparation, certification and clinical practice
5. Fifin DR (2010) Pengenalan pola citra leukosit dengan metode ekstraksi fitur citra, p 5
6. Susilawati I (2016) Identifikasi penyakit leukimia akut pada citra darah mikroskopis, vol 12, no 1, p 6
7. Saputra GD, Syidada S (2017) Pengenalan Sel Acute Lymphoblastic Leukemia (ALL) dengan Menggunakan Metode Jaringan Syaraf Tiruan, p 4
8. Putra FM (2017) Penerapan Learning Vector Quantization 3 (LVQ3) untuk Mengidentifikasi Citra Darah Acute Lymphoblastic Leukemia (ALL) dan Acute Myeloid Leukemia (AML). Universitas Islam Negeri Sultan Syarif Kasim Riau, Riau
9. Fauzi H (2018) Klasifikasi citra sel darah putih berdasarkan nilai ekstraksi fitur citra menggunakan multilayer perceptron. Universitas Gadjah Mada, Yogyakarta
10. Nanda Imron AM, Fitri ZE (2019) A classification of platelets in peripheral blood smear image as an early detection of myeloproliferative syndrome using gray level co-occurence matrix. J Phys Conf Ser 1201:012049

11. Fitri ZE, Syahputri LNY, Imron AMN (2020) Classification of white blood cell abnormalities for early detection of myeloproliferative neoplasms syndrome based on k-nearest neighbor. Sci J Inf 7(1):7
12. Anderson S (2013) Anderson's atlas of hematology, p 607
13. Praida AR (2008) Pengenalan penyakit darah menggunakan teknik pengolahan citra dan jaringan syaraf tiruan, p 9

Non-Complex CNN Models for Colorectal Cancer (CRC) Classification Based on Histological Images

Nur Ibrahim, Nor Kumalasari Caecar Pratiwi, Muhammad Adnan Pramudito, and Fauzi Frahma Taliningsih

Abstract Colorectal cancer become a significant public health issue and is the world's second leading cause of death from cancer. Cancer becomes a very dangerous disease, because it gives no visible signs at an early stage. Signs of cancer will usually only be seen if it is in the third stadium or the last stadium, where the cancer has spread to surrounding organs. Early diagnosis of colorectal cancer is highly needed because treatment choices are decided and the period of survival is heavily affected. This paper proposes the Convolutional Neural Network (CNN) for detecting four classes of colon cancer. The data-set consists of 2500 images, divided into Tumor, Complex, Lymphoma and Stroma. This data set represents a selection from the Institute of Pathology, University of Heidelberg, Germany, consist of 150 × 150 px textures in histological pictures. The proposed system consist of two hidden convolutional layers, a fully connected layer and use Adam Optimizer with learning 0.001, and trained 10 times (epochs = 10). The result of the proposed system is 83% accuracy.

Keywords Non-compex CNN · Colorectal cancer · Early diagnosis

1 Introduction

Colorectal cancer found in the large intestine (colon) organ, whereas rectal cancer is cancer that occurs in the rectum. If the cancerous tissue is found from the large intestine (colon) to the rectum, it is called by colorectal cancer [1]. The third most common cancer diagnosed in men and women in the United States is colorectal cancer (CRC) [2]. In 2020, the number of colorectal cancer cases in the United States reached 104,610 new cases of colon cancer and 43,340 new cases of rectal cancer, according to figures published by the American Cancer Society [2]. Although there is almost the same risk of diagnosing colorectal cancer in men and

N. Ibrahim (✉) · N. K. C. Pratiwi · M. A. Pramudito · F. F. Taliningsih
Telkom University, Bandung, West Java, Indonesia
e-mail: nuribrahim@telkomuniversity.ac.id

H. Triwiyanto et al. (eds.), *Proceedings of the 1st International Conference on Electronics, Biomedical Engineering, and Health Informatics*, Lecture Notes in Electrical Engineering 746, https://doi.org/10.1007/978-981-33-6926-9_44

women, there is a higher risk of developing colorectal cancer: around 1 in 23 (4.4%) in men and 1 in 25 (4.1%) in women [2]. Early detection, improved and advanced treatment techniques, and lifestyle changes such as diet modification and increased exercise awareness have contributed to changes in the number of colon cancer cases in the world [3]. The important highlight is to do early detection, where by detecting cancer as early as possible can increase the chances of patient's recovery. In addition, the cost of an early detection test is far cheaper when compared to the cost of treatment, if the cancer has entered an advanced stage and spread to other body organs. Therefore, it is very important for everyone to do an early detection of cancer, especially if you have been known to have a family history of cancer. Some things that can be done in the early detection of colon cancer are through vague blood tests and Fecal Immunochemical Test (FIT) which are done at least once a year. If the results of this test are positive, then a colonoscopy should be continued.

Early diagnosis of colon cancer is very important, to support a good prognosis process and so that survival rates can be even higher. Many studies have been performed by several previous researchers linked to the identification of colon cancer. Tina and colleagues performed colon cancer prediction research on various magnified colon biopsy images [4]. The first process in the system designed was that a colon biopsy image would be converted to HSV color. Then proceed with feature extraction using Dual-Tree and double-density 2-D wavelet transform. Random Forest is used for the classification algorithm. The results of this study indicate an accuracy of 85.4%. Biswas and his friends have conducted research regarding the classification of colon diseases in the colonoscopy film [5]. This study proposes a method based on colonoscopy videos to identify colon diseases using Cross-Wavelet Transform (XWT), classified using Multi-class Support Vector Machine (MSVM). The results showed that XWT-MSVM produced recognition rate of 98.46%, much better compared to other well-known benchmark procedures. Automatic detection of polyps on CT colonography image for colon cancer diagnosis is a research that has been completed by Akshay M. Godkhindi and Rajaram M. Gowda [6]. In his study, the Convolution Neural Network (CNN) used image processing techniques by applying a deep learning algorithm and the results will be contrasted with classical algorithms for machine learning. As classifiers using Local Binary Patterns (LBP) and Histogram Driven Gradient (HOG), the classic machine learning algorithms used in the feature extraction are Random Forest (RF) and k-Nearest Neighbors (KNN). The results showed the accuracy of the proposed method for intestinal segmentation using CNN was 87%, superior to Random Forest (85%) and KNN (83%). Yuan Hong and colleagues have also completed research on colon cancer diagnostic based on the Empirical Mode Decomposition (EMD) and Least-Support Vector Machines (LS-SVM) [7]. The test results show that the EMD and LS-SVM have better results for classification, which can accomplish the objective of classification in the case of fewer samples. The colon cancer detection analysis using local image descriptors was carried out by Suvidha Tripathi et al. [8]. In this research, several image descriptors are explored for the identification of computer-assisted colon cancer. Five recent local descriptors have been established, namely LCOD, RSHD, LWP, LDEP and LBDP. Proposals using LCOD and RSHD descriptors have been provided based on the assessment of parameter comparisons. Nor Kumalasari and colleagues also completed the research with the title K-Nearest Neighbor for colon cancer identification [9]. The system built in this study is able to detect and classify the condition of the colon into normal (healthy), carcinoma, and lymphoma with a maximum accuracy of 68.52%.

The research studies that have been mentioned above, tend to use complex computational processes, the CNN architecture used has a deeper layer, requires a computer with high specifications and often takes relatively longer computation time for training process. This has led the authors to conduct research related to colon cancer detection using a simpler model, but produces a reliable system performance.

2 Material and Method

Colorectal cancer is a malignancy that originates in the colon tissue, consisting of the colon (the longest part of the large intestine) and/or rectum (the last small part of the large intestine before the anus) [10]. In Indonesia, colorectal cancer is the third largest type of cancer. In 2008, Indonesia ranked fourth in ASEAN countries, with an incidence rate of 17.2 per 100,000 population and it is predicted to increase continuously from year to year [11]. Previous epidemiological studies have shown that the age of colorectal cancer patients in Indonesia is younger than colorectal cancer patients in developed countries. More than 30% of cases are acquired in patients aged 40 years or younger, whereas in developed countries, patients aged less than 50 years are only 2–8% [12]. Early detection and classification of colorectal cancer is needed so that the right curative therapy can be done while the cancer still at the early stage. Therefore, this research aims to design a system that can classify kinds of colorectal cancer based on histological images.

Convolutional Neural Network (CNN) is one of machine learning algorithm that recently used for image processing. Some previous research in biomedical image processing also use CNN method to identify and classify kinds of disease, like in [13, 14].

CNN architecture can usually be divided into 2 blocks; the extraction block of features and the classification block. The extraction function block is composed of a convolution layer and a pooling layer. A set of convolution layer and pooling layer is called hidden layer. Convolution layer will generate an output images called featured map [15], and pooling layer reduce the featured map size. These featured map will be proceed in classification block that consist of fully connected layer, and this block will generate the result of classification process.

In this paper, the proposed CNN architecture consist of 2 hidden layers, and 1 fully connected to classify CRC histological images into 4 classes (see Fig. 1). Each convolution layer is added with Rectified Linear Unit (RelU) activation function to

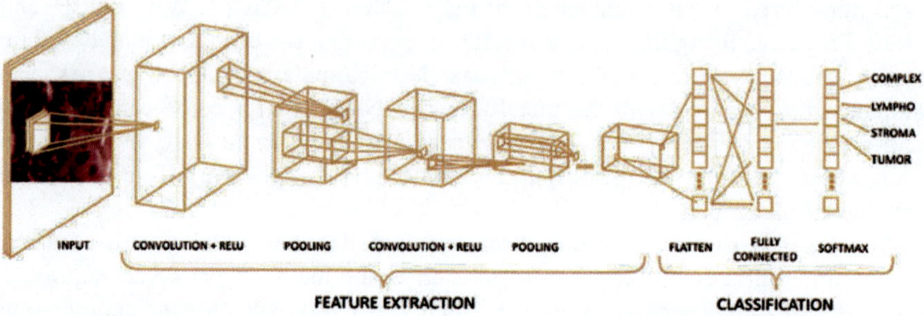

Fig. 1 Proposed CNN Architecture for CRC classification into four classes

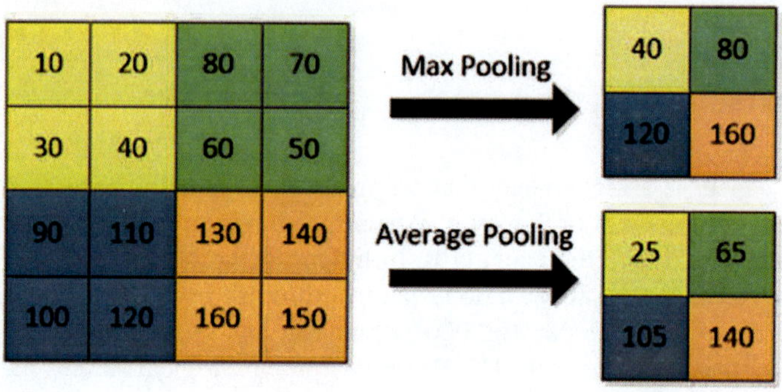

Fig. 2 The output of pooling layer using two different methods

increase the complexity and give the non-linearity in the CNN [16], so that the neurons will be deactivated only if the input value is less than zero. To put it simply, RelU will convert the negative pixel value to zero.

Pooling layer is used to reduce data size, by combining neighbor pixels into one pixel value, and the methods can be set as the maximum or average value. For example, suppose a feature map with 4 × 4 size is pooled with 2 × 2 pool size and 2 × 2 stride, so the feature map size will be 2 × 2 (see Fig. 2).

Performance of proposed CNN model will be evaluated through confusion matrix, accuracy and loss value. The amount of dataset used in this research is 2500 CRC histological images, which consist of 625 images for each class (COMPLEX class, LYMPHO class, STROMA class, and TUMOR class), and divided into training data (1875 images) and validation data (625 images). The source of dataset is from Kaggle [17].

3 Result and Discussion

Figure 3 show the output of each layers in feature extraction block, and Table 1 show the layer configuration and parameters in proposed CNN model.

Based on Table 1, the size of CRC historical images is resized to 64 × 64 pixel and inserted into CNN model. In both convolution layers, a filter with size 3 × 3 and channel output 8 is configured, along with RelU activation function. Max Pooling is done at feature maps that generated from both convolution layers. Classification is done with Softmax activation in fully connected layer. Categorical Crossentropy for loss evaluation and Adam optimizer with learning rate 0.001 for are used. Thus, the proposed CNN model was trained with 10 iterations (see Figs. 4 and 5).

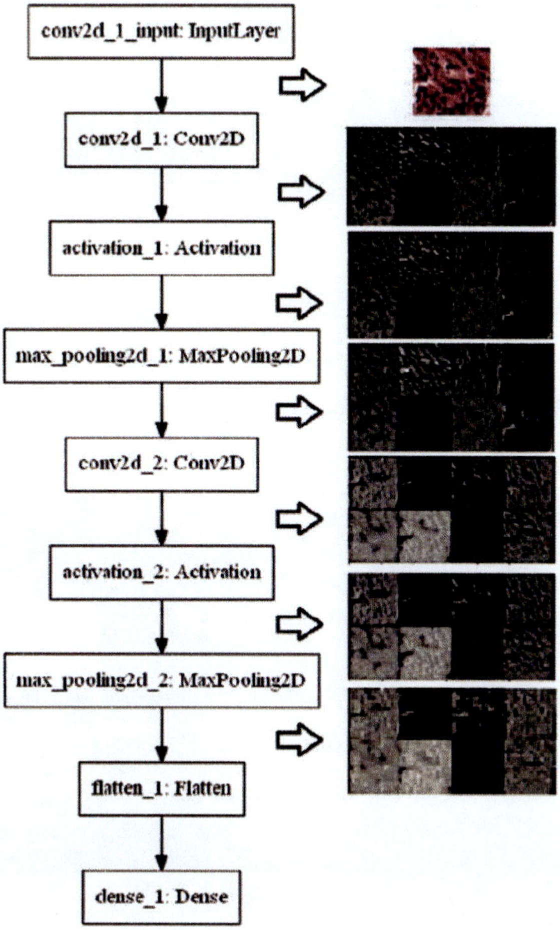

Fig. 3 Output of each layers in feature extraction block

Table 1 Summary of proposed CNN model

Layer (type)	Output shape	Parameter
Conv2d_1 (Conv2D)	(None, 64,64,8)	224
Activation_1 (Activation)	(None, 64,64,8)	0
MaxPooling2d_1 (Max pooling)	(None, 32,32,8)	0
Conv2d_2 (Conv2D)	(None, 32,32,8)	584
Activation_2 (Activation)	(None, 32,32,8)	0
MaxPooling2d_2 (Max pooling)	(None, 16,16,8)	0
Flatten_1 (Flatten)	(None, 2048)	0
Dense_1 (Dense)	(None, 4)	8196

Total Parameters: 9004
Trainable Parameters: 9004
Non-trainable parameters: 0

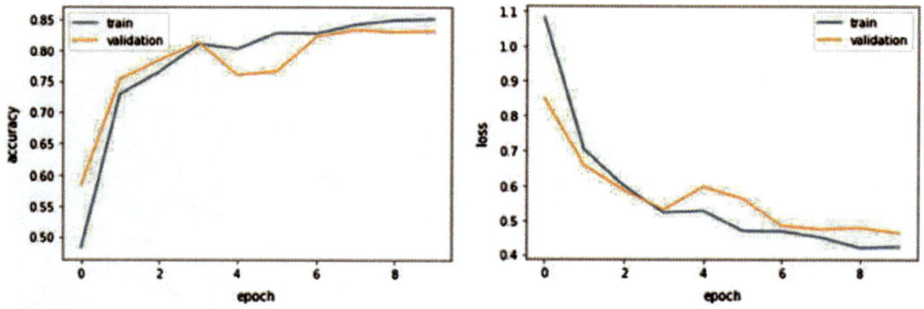

Fig. 4 The accuracy and loss value of CNN Model

Fig. 5 Confusion matrix of CNN model

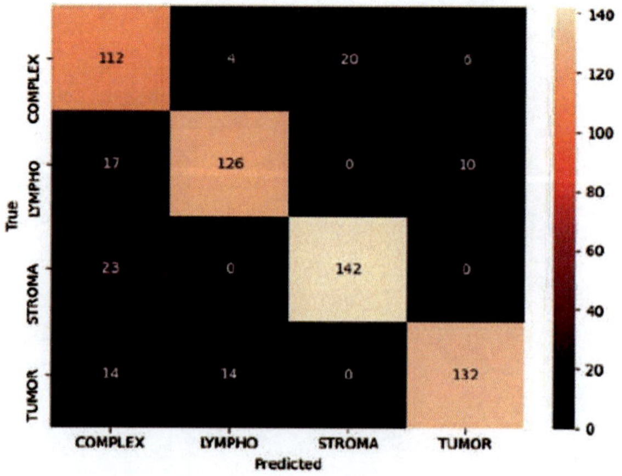

Figure 4 shows that the increase of accuracy and the decrease of loss between training accuracy and validation accuracy for epoch 10 times is not too far, so it can be concluded that the proposed CNN model is not over-fitting. Even the accuracy value of validation data is 83%, the loss value is 0.48. To figure out more, the proposed model is tested to classify using validation data images. 5 Figure shows that each class can be classified correctly more than 80% (89% for LYMPHO class, 87% for TUMOR class, and 83% for STROMA class), except for COMPLEX class that 72% correctly classified. These results show that COMPLEX class images has more identical value when compared with the other classes.

4 Conclusion

A system to Classify Colorectal Cancer (CRC) based on histological images has been built using CNN model that consist of two hidden layers with RelU activation and one fully connected layer with softmax activation for classifier. From the testing result, the proposed CNN model is able to classify CRC histological images into four classes (COMPLEX class, LYMPHO class, STROMA class, and TUMOR class) with the accuracy 83% and loss 0.48. For future work, the system can be improved by using another model and add pre-processing before training step to get higher accuracy and loss.

References

1. Get the facts about colon cancer. https://coloncancercoalition.org/get-educated/what-you-need-to-know/colon-cancer-facts/. Last accessed 23 July 2020
2. Siegel RL (2020) Colorectal cancer statistics. CA Cancer J Clin 70(3):145–164
3. Hislop G (2020) Trends and risk factors for colorectal cancer. BCMJ Clin Artic 42(3): 131–135
4. Babu T, Gupta D, Singh T, Hameed S (2018) Colon cancer prediction on different magnified colon biopsy images. In: Tenth international conference on advanced computing (ICoAC), pp 277–280
5. Biswas M, Bhattacharya A, Dey D (2016) Classification of various colon diseases in Colonoscopy video using Cross-Wavelet features. In: International conference on wireless communications, signal processing and networking (WiSPNET), pp 2141–2145
6. Godkhindi AM, Gowda RM (2017) Automated detection of polyps in CT colonography images using deep learning algorithms in colon cancer diagnosis. In: International conference on energy, communication, data analytics and soft computing (ICECDS), pp 1722–1728
7. Hong Y, Wei H, Zeng-Li L (2011) Research for the colon cancer based on the EMD and LS-SVM. In: Fourth international conference on intelligent computation technology and automation, pp 888–891
8. Tripathi S, Mishra S, Singh SK (2016) Routine colon cancer detection using local image descriptors. In: IEEE region 10 conference (TENCON), pp 2062–2065
9. Pratiwi NKC, Magdalena R, Fuadah YN, Saidah S (2019) K-Nearest Neighbor for colon cancer identification. J Phys Conf Ser 1367:1–10

10. American Cancer Society (2014) Colorectal cancer facts & figures 2014–2016. Atlanta
11. Kimman M, Norman R, Jan S, Kingston D, Woodward M (2012) The burden of cancer in member countries of the association of southeast asian nations (ASEAN). Asian Pac J Cancer Prev 13(2):411–420
12. Abdullah M, Sudoyo AW, Utomo AR, Fauzi A, Rani AA (2012) Molecular profile of colorectal cancer in Indonesia: Is there another pathway? Gastroenterol Hepatol Bed Bench 5 (2):71–78
13. Nasr-Esfahani E (2016) Melanoma detection by analysis of clinical images using convolutional neural network. In: 38th annual international conference of the IEEE engineering in medicine and biology society (EMBC), pp 1373–1376
14. Shin Y, Balasingham I (2017) Comparison of hand-craft feature based SVM and CNN based deep learning framework for automatic polyp classification. In: 39th annual international conference of the IEEE engineering in medicine and biology society (EMBC), pp 3277–3280
15. Kim P (2017) MATLAB deep learning: with machine learning, neural networks and artificial intelligence, 1st edn. Apress, Seoul, South Korea
16. Wu J (2017) Introduction to convolutional neural networks. Nanjing, China
17. Colorectal histology MNIST, Collection of textures in colorectal cancer histology. https://www.kaggle.com/kmader/colorectal-histology-mnist. Last accessed 23 July 2020

Performance Comparison of Classification Algorithms for Locating the Dominant Heel Pain Using Electromyography Signal

Ghifari Indra Gunawan, Desri Kristina Silalahi, Husneni Mukhtar, Dandi Trianta Barus, and Dien Rahmawati

Abstract The prevalence of heel pain is commonly associated with injuries, infections, nervous system problem or a non-neutral type of the foot posture. The diagnosis of heel pain can be done by a physical examination, medical records, imaging (X-Ray), Magnetic Resonance Imaging (MRI), and analysis of electromyography (EMG). An accurate diagnosis must be made to specify the appropriate treatment but it is often very difficult due to the complex anatomy of heel. The aim of this study, therefore, is to predict and compare the location of heel pain using several classification algorithms and feature extractions. In this work, the EMG signal recording is performed on three locations of human heel, namely plantar, midfoot, and posterior heel. For feature extraction step, the EMG signal is processed in the frequency domain after its frequency has been sampled (625 Hz) and filtered (butterworth filter order of 4, 10, and 300 Hz). The used extraction features are MNF, MDF, Spectral Movement, and Power Spectrum Deformation while the used classification algorithms are Support Vector Machine (SVM), adaboost, and xgboost. The results in this research are that the comparisons of prediction accuracy on heel pain location using adaboost and xgboost methods are 91 and 82%, respectively and using the linear Kernel SVM, RBF, polynomial, and sigmoid methods are 64, 73, 73, and 55%, repectively. Adaboost is the best classification algorithm among the others for predicting the location of heel pain. The developed model provides an alternative identifying tool because knowing the specific anatomic location of heel pain may help the medical practitioners in guiding the diagnosis and determining the initial or specific treatment.

Keywords Heel pain · Electromyography · Support vector machine · Adaboost · Xgboost

G. I. Gunawan · D. K. Silalahi · H. Mukhtar (✉) · D. Rahmawati
Faculty of Electrical Engineering, Telkom University, Bandung, Indonesia
e-mail: husnenimukhtar@telkomuniversity.ac.id

G. I. Gunawan · D. T. Barus
Biospin Laboratory, Telkom University, Bandung, Indonesia

D. T. Barus
Faculty of Informatics Engineering, Telkom University, Bandung, Indonesia

H. Triwiyanto et al. (eds.), *Proceedings of the 1st International Conference on Electronics, Biomedical Engineering, and Health Informatics*, Lecture Notes in Electrical Engineering 746, https://doi.org/10.1007/978-981-33-6926-9_45

1 Introduction

The diversity of human daily activities can be undertaken by the controlled cooperation among the organ systems. During the activity, sometimes there is pain or discomfort in certain body parts such as shoulder, arms, legs and heels. Heel pain is a general term for symptoms of pain that occurs in the heel. In general, most adults over the age of 40 years feel the initial heel pain, but children and adolescents at the age of 8–13 years are also subjected to this pain, commonly in the lateral area (back heel) [1]. Some factors causing the emergence of the heel pain are associated with injuries, infections, nervous system problems [1] and the abnormal posture [2]. Heel pain is classified into several types based on the location of the appearance of pain. They are types of symptoms, patient age and the undertaken activity [3]. Several methods are performed by the medical staffs to diagnose the heel pain such as the physical examination, medical records, analysis of X-Ray images, Magnetic Resonance Imaging (MRI), and Electromyography (EMG) [1, 4].

Wynne et al. [5] in his research measured the electrically and mechanically reflex activities in muscles of the plantar fascitis. O'Brien and Byrden [6] offered the parameters for electrodiagnostics of patients with tarsal tunnel syndrome. In this research, there were 12 parameters offered, one of which was performed by the electromyography (EMG) analysis on the adductor halucis and the digital quinti adductor muscles. The results of the research conducted by O'Brien reported that the abnormality of 68% subjects suspected to the tarsal tunnel syndrome. Moussa et al. [7] in his research explained that there are the abnormalities in the adductor digiti quinti and adductor hallucis brevis muscles. The diagnose of the research is that the subject was suspected to tarsal tunnel syndrome, or no motor unit response to the muscle. However, none of the research used the machine learning technology to detect the location of heel pain.

The purpose of this research is to predict the location of heel pain using several classification algorithms and feature extractions in order to compare several developped machine learning models in locating the EMG signal-based heel pain. Each two electrodes are attached on the plantar and the posterior of heel with the intention of recording the EMG signals. These signals then are processed in the frequency domain in order to obtain the feature extraction as the input for the developed machine learning.

2 Material and Method

2.1 *Data Set of EMG Signal*

This research used a MyoWare™ muscle sensor (AT-04-001) module and two channels of Ag/AgCl electrodes (25.4 mm × 25.4 mm in size). These two-EMG electrode channels were placed on two locations namely the posterior and plantar

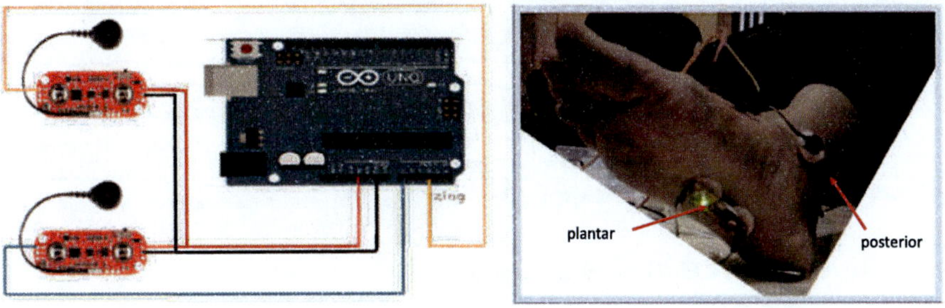

Fig. 1 The electrical schematic for EMG signal measurement (left) and the placement position of the electrodes (right)

areas, exactly on Calcaneus Tendon (TC) and Flexor Digitorum Brevis (FDB). Figure 1 shows the electrical schematic for EMG signal measurement and the position of the electrodes. For experiment purpose, the subjects used in this study consisted of five men and two women adults with age (45 ± 4) years and BMI (23.78 ± 2.26) kg/m^2.

This EMG signal recording was carried out in time-series for the subjects who were in the relaxed condition after running on a reflection carpet for 5 min. The running activity was performed to stimulate pain in the heel. This recording was taken for 3 min by 625 Hz of frequency sampling and repeated until 10 times after each participant has rested for 5 min.

2.2 *Signal Processing*

The EMG signal processing was carried out using a personal computer (intel CORE i3-6006 on a 2.00 GHz CPU, 4 GB RAM, Windows 10). After the EMG signals from plantar and posterior heel were sensed and sampled in microcontroller, as shown in Fig. 2, a 4th order butterworth was used to filter the EMG signals with a cut-off frequency 10 and 300 Hz on PC before further processing. The use of kind of this filter was based on some references of papers, such as in [8–10], which performed EMG researches in lower body, namely legs. Figures 3 and 4 show the comparison both unfiltered and filtered EMG signals, respectively.

A Fast Fourier Transform (FFT) was used to convert the filtered signal from time domain into the frequency domain. This conversion produced the spectral density of the EMG signals, where the calculation of the spectral density is shown in Eq. (1). For the term of the feature extraction, the Power Spectrum Density (PSD) calculations were performed using Eq. (2). This PSD calculation was needed for several feature extraction methods used in this research.

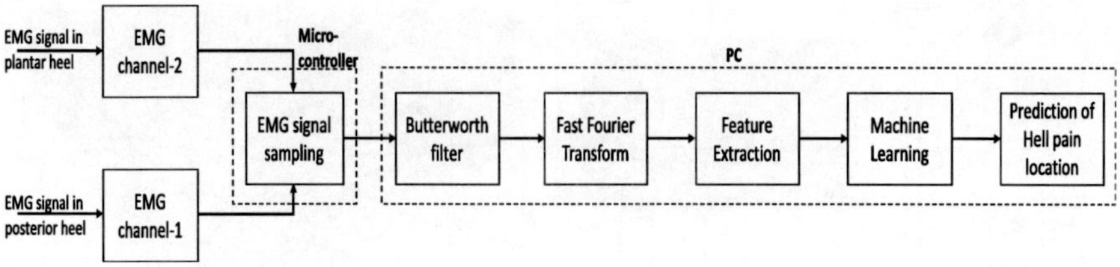

Fig. 2 Diagram block of EMG signal processing

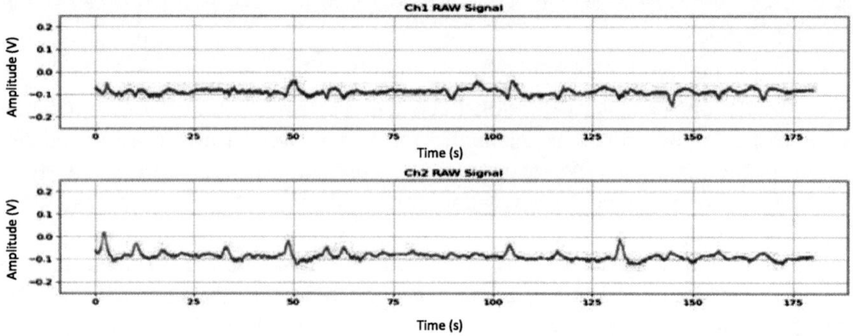

Fig. 3 Raw EMG signal

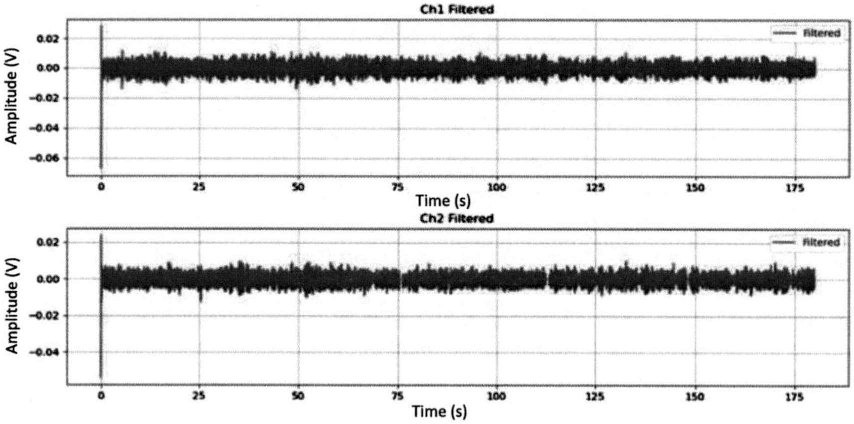

Fig. 4 Filtered EMG signal

$$y[k] = \sum_{n=0}^{N-1} e^{-2\pi j \frac{kn}{N}} x[n] \quad (1)$$

$$PSD = (y[k])^2 \quad (2)$$

For the machine learning process, a set of EMG sampling signal was processed to obtain the unique values from the spectral information using several feature extraction set methods. These feature extraction data were labeled with 3-training classes, namely plantar-burning, plantar-achy, and posterior and were trained with the developed machine learning model.

2.3 Feature Extraction

Feature extraction is a feature vector form of a signal used as a signal pattern identifier. Parameters of Modified Median Frequency (MMDF), Modified Mean Frequency (MMNF), and Spectral Moments (SM) were chosen because they are commonly used to recognize the EMG signal characters and capable to track the changes in muscle fatigue over time [11]. The used feature extractions in this research study are shown in Table 1.

2.4 Classifier

Three classifiers used in this study are Adaboost, Xgboost, and Support-Vector Machine (SVM). The comparison of the accuracy results for the three classifiers

Table 1 Set of the feature extraction

Set of feature extraction	Mathematical model
Modified Median Frequency (MMDF) [12]	$\sum_{j=1}^{MMDF} A_J = \sum_{J=MMDF}^{M} A_J = \frac{1}{2}\sum_{j=1}^{M} A_j$
Modified Mean Frequency (MMNF) [12]	$\sum_{j=1}^{M} f_j A_j \Big/ \sum_{j=1}^{M} A_j$
Spectral Moments (SM) [13]	$SM_1 = \sum_{l=1}^{M} P_l f_l$ $SM_2 = \sum_{l=1}^{M} P_l f_l^2$ $SM_3 = \sum_{l=1}^{M} P_l f_l^3$
Power spectral deformation (Ω) [14]	$\Omega = \frac{\sqrt{SM_2/SM_0}}{SM_1/SM_0}$

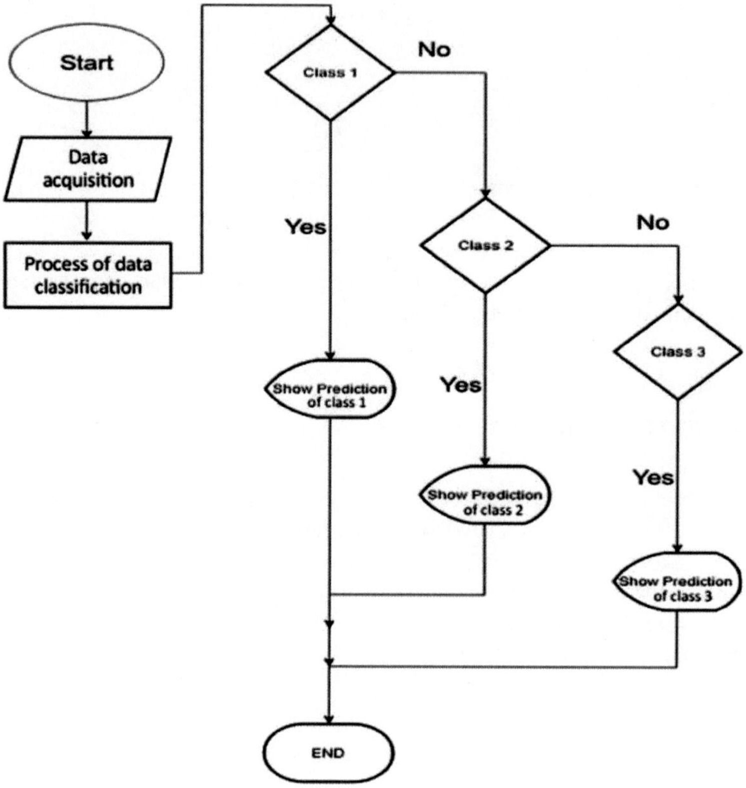

Fig. 5 Flowchart of the classification process

was conducted to find the best machine learning model for this study. There are 3 classes tested in the development of the three models, namely class 1 (a burning pain sensation in the plantar foot), class 2 (a sharp or piercing pain in the plantar foot), and class 3 (the emergence of pain in the posterior foot). The classification process of the developed model was shown in the flowchart of Fig. 5.

Adaboost

A boosting algorithm, such as AdaBoost (Adaptive Boosting) proposed by Freund and Schapire [15], can be used in the classification and the regression problems. Boosting is one of the ensamble methods used to improve the performance of a model by reducing the occurrence of bias and variance [16]. Initially in the classification problem, the boosting method only can be used for binary classification. But over time, the boosting method was developed and used for multiclass classification problems with no exception [17–19]. In general, this method is a collection of several weak classifiers that will be converted into strong classifiers.

In other words, this algorithm reduces the errors from the weak classifiers so that it creates a strong classifier that has a better performance. The formula of AdaBoost model is described in Eq. (3),

$$H(x) = sign\left(\sum_{t=1}^{T} a_t h_t(x)\right) \tag{3}$$

where h_t is the output of the t classifier (value -1 or $+1$), T is the used weak classifier, a_t is the used weight in the t classifier determined by AdaBoost. Hence, the final result is only a linear combination of all weak classifiers.

Classifiers are trained one by one, then the probability of each training example will be updated and used as the training set for the next classifier. The first classifier (t = 1) is trained with the same probability for all training examples. Then the output weight α for the classifier will be calculated using Eq. (4) after the training process.

$$\alpha_t = \frac{1}{2}\ln\left(\frac{1-\in_t}{\in_t}\right) \tag{4}$$

The output weight (α_t) is affected by the classifier's error rate ($\in_t$), where $\in_t$ is the number of misclassifications in the training set divided by the size of the training set. Then α_t is as the first classifier after the training process, while the weight training example is updated by using Eq. (5).

$$D_{t+1}(i) = \frac{D_t(i)\exp(-\alpha_t y_i h_t(x_i))}{z_t} \tag{5}$$

where D_t is a weight vector for each training sample in a set of the training, and i is the example of the training number. The formula above is used in updating the weight for the i training example. The value of D_t is a distribution calculated by adding all probabilities to 1 [20], hence a weight normalization has to be done by dividing each weight by the sum of all weights (z_t). The correct output for the example of training (i) is called y_i, and the predicted output from the classifier t is $h_t(x_i)$.

Xgboost

A scalable machine learning system, XGBoost (Xtreme Gradient Boosting), is an implementation of the Gradient Boosting algorithm [22, 23] for tree boosting [23]. It is often used in machine learning and data mining competitions, such as Kaggle due to its excellent performance and high computing speed. XGBoost is able to solve problems such as regression, classification, and ranking.

Support Vector Machine (SVM)

SVM is a type of a supervised learning system for both classification and regression. SVM is defined as a system that uses linear hypothesis functions with high

Table 2 The SVM kernel used in developed model

Kernel type	General description	Mathematical modeling
Linear kernel	It is the simplest kernel used to separate linear data	$k(x, x') = x^T x' + c$
Polynomial kernel	It is a model commonly used for non-linear data	$k(x, x') = (x, x')^d$ $k(x, x') = ((x, x') + 1)^d$
Radial Basis Function (RBF)	It is a model that produces a linear solution if there is a discontinuity	$k(x, x') = exp\left(-\frac{x-x'}{2\sigma^2}\right)$
Sigmoid (MLP / hyperbolic tangent)	The kernel is adapted from the field of neural networks	$k(x, x') = \tanh(\rho(x, x') + e)$

dimensional features and is trained using optimization learning algorithm with statistical learning bias [24]. The SVM algorithm looks for the hyper planes with a maximum degree of the separation and the data grouping with the help of the support vectors. Support vector becomes the maximum margin reference modeled in Eq. (6) and serves to separate and classify data using the hyperplanes [24].

$$\arg max\left\{\frac{1}{w} min\left[t_n\left(w^T k(x, x') + b\right)\right]\right\} \tag{6}$$

where, w is weight, $t_n = 1, 2, 3, \ldots, N$ is target value, $k(x, x')$ is kernel function and b is bias parameter. There are several types of kernels that can be used in developing the SVM machine learning models. Kernels help to separate the non-linier and difficult data. The description of the kernel types used in this study are presented in Table 2.

2.5 *Performance Evaluation*

The performance of machine learning model is evaluated by the accuracy value. Several additional parameters are precision and recall. Equations (7–9) explain the calculation of accuracy (acc), precision, and recall [25]. Accuracy is a ratio of the true prediction consisting of a true positive (t_p) and a true negative (t_n) to the overall data. The overall data includes the summation of the true positive (t_p), the false positive (f_p), the true negative (t_n) and the false negative. Precision is a ratio of the positive true prediction compared to the overall positive predicted outcome. While, recall is a ratio of the true positive predictions to overall true positive data [25].

$$acc = \frac{tp + tn}{tp + fp + tn + fn} \tag{7}$$

$$precision = \frac{tp}{tp + fp} \tag{8}$$

$$recall = \frac{tp}{tp + tn} \tag{9}$$

3 Result

The class classification of the heel pain location from the acquired EMG signals of plantar and posterior of heel were processed in three developed models. These models were used in aiming to compare their performance and find the most suitable classifier for this study. One of the processing results (process steps shown in Fig. 2) of the EMG signals of heel are shown in Fig. 6. Three types of the developed machine learning models used in this classification of heel pain are SVM model, SVM-Adaboost model, and SVM-Xgboost model with three data classifications for each model. The data standardization is carried out using Eq. (10) before doing the training process,

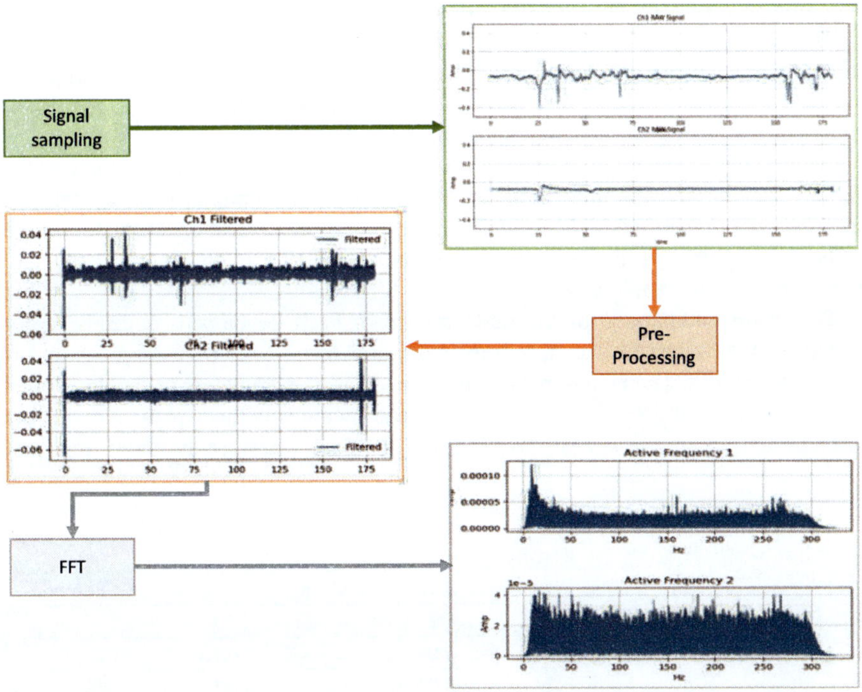

Fig. 6 Signal Processing of the EMG signals of heel

Table 3 Mean and standard deviation of feature extractions for each channel

Fitur-Channel	Mean	Standard deviation
MMDF-Ch1	2.27969124e+00	3.13631470e+01
MMDF-Ch2	3.78407374e−01	2.47874037e−01
MMNF-Ch1	1.32903957e+02	6.11728349e+02
MMNF-Ch2	1.41688642e+02	3.21585683e+02
SM1-Ch1	3.26032871e−01	1.62940924e+00
SM1-Ch2	3.32030017e−03	1.23379133e−04
SM2-Ch1	3.85257171e+01	2.39581759e+04
SM2-Ch2	3.17349730e−01	3.65839668e−01
SM3-Ch1	6.61836231e+03	7.09953139e+08
SM1-Ch2	5.76826607e+01	5.33538634e+03
PSD-Ch1	1.27239614e+00	1.76379481e−02
PSD-Ch2	1.22767675e+00	1.32390778e−02

$$z = \frac{(x - u)}{s} \tag{10}$$

where x is the sample data, u is the training data sample mean, and s is the standard deviation of the training data sample. Table 3 shows the mean and standard deviation data of each channel's features.

The scaling process of each feature data per channel obtained using the mean and standard deviation values, shown in Table 3, describes the value distribution for each feature set. The higher the standard deviation value, the wider the distribution of feature values for each data sample.

Some parameters of each kernel (shown in Table 4) are adjusted to get the highest accuracy during the testing process. Those parameters of each kernels are used into the developed SVM model. The results of classification of heel pain are influenced by the parameters of each kernels in SVM models, Adaboost, and Xgboost.

The result comparison of the performance of each developed model is represented by the values of accuracy, precision, and recall of each testing model, as shown in Table 5. The testing results of the evaluation parameters of the developed SVM model are the class classification of the location of heel pain. Among the classifiers used in the SVM model, the Adaboost classifier provides the best

Table 4 Adjustment of the SVM parameter

Kernels	Parameters			
	C	Coeff	Gamma	Degree
Linear	1	0.1	0.1	3
RBF	0.1	0.1	0.1	1
Poly	0.1	0.1	0.1	3
Sigmoid	0.1	0.1	0.1	1

Table 5 Comparison of the performance of SVM models, Adaboost, and Xgboost

Classifier	Accuracy (%)	Precision (%)	Recall (%)
SVM Linear	64	75	68
SVM Polynomial	73	83	70
SVM RBF	73	61	89
SVM Sigmoid	55	18	33
Adaboost	91	91	84
Xgboost	82	82	74

performance results in the classification testing. The values of accuracy, precision, and recall of this clasiifier are 91, 91, and 84%, respectively. While the Sigmoid SVM is the poorest classifier in providing the performance results, where the accuracy, precision and recall values of the classification are below 60%.

4 Discussion

In this research, there are 3 classes, namely plantar-achy, plantar burning and pain in posterior leg. When there is pain, appear fluctuation in EMG signal and increasing in the peak value of EMG signal amplitude compared to the EMG signal without pain. A healthy EMG signal appears more flattened with less signal fluctuation and less amplitude peaks.

The signal sampling process done by using microcontroller. Microcontroller is able to provide an average sampling rate of 625 Hz per second, and is considered sufficient to avoid frequency shift because the high cut-off frequency value of the Butterworth 4 order filter is 300 Hz. The use of a higher sampling rate is expected to be able to increase the sampling rate value and clarify the shape of the recorded signal to be closer to the original signal shape.

Increasing the sampling rate will giving the option to determine the characteristics of the filter being developed. One of the reasons for choosing the cut-off frequency at 10–300 Hz in this research was to adjust the sampling rate specification of 625 Hz. By increasing the sampling rate for both plantar and posterior signal recording, it will provide more options for using filters such as filters with cut-off frequency values at 20 and 450 Hz [8] and the use of bandpass filters with bandwidths of 10–500 Hz [9]. The different filter designs used will provide different spectral information. Different spectral information will give different feature values. The comparison of each filter design used as input for feature extraction can provide opportunities for improving the performance of the machine learning system being developed.

AdaBoost model has the best performance with an accuracy of up to 91%. This means that the model successfully predicts each test data according to the actual class. The SVM model developed has an accuracy level of under 75%. The model being developed will provide an alternative tool for medical personnel in diagnosing the location and type of heel pain. Of course, other diagnostic methods are needed for better diagnostic accuracy. The performance of machine learning models that use EMG can be hampered by noise in the signal that can appear at any time.

The main concern in this research is the development of alternative tools for medical personnel who can help predict the type and location of heel pain. The more easy the operation of this prediction system, will increasingly provide convenience for medical personnel. In addition, the development of the model must continue to be done so that the performance of the model remains better.

5 Conclusion

This research was carried out to compare several classification algorithms and feature extractions for finding the best machine learning model from the three tested model to classify the heel pain location. The use of the selected features also resulted in a fairly good level of accuracy for each tested model. AdaBoost's model is the best machine learning model with an accuracy of 91% in this study. We expect that this developed model may help the medical practitioners especially in department of medical rehabilitation to diagnose and analyse the location of heel pain of the patients. Future research should be more focus on expanding the class classifications and increasing the amount of the training data and tests to improve the performance of the developed machine learning model.

References

1. Agyekum EK, Ma K (2015) Heel pain: A systematic review. Chinese J Traumatol Eng Ed 18:164–169
2. Irving DB, Cook JL, Young MA, Menz HB (2007) Obesity and pronated foot type may increase the risk of chronic plantar heel pain: a matched case-control study. BMC Musculoskelet Disord 8:1471–2474
3. Tu P, Bytomski JR (2011) Diagnosis of heel pain. Am Fam Physician 84:909–916
4. Sawyer GA, Wang JH, Digiovanni CW (2014) Plantar and medial heel pain: diagnosis and management. J Am Acad Orthop Surg 22:372–380
5. Wynne MM, Burns JM, Eland DC, Conatser RR, Howell JN (2006) Effect of counterstrain on stretch reflexes, hoffmann reflexes, and clinical outcomes in subjects with plantar fasciitis. J Am Osteopath Assoc 106:547–556
6. O'Brien C, Byrden R (2017) Tarsal tunnel syndrome—a new way to diagnose an old problem. World J. Neurosci 7:172–180
7. Moussa A, Chakhachiro Z, Sawaya RA (2018) Posterior tibial nerve lymphoma presenting as tarsal tunnel syndrome: a case report. J Foot Ankle Surg 57:167–169
8. Henriksen M, Aaboe J, Bliddal H, Langberg H (2009) Biomechanical characteristics of the eccentric Achilles tendon exercise. J Biomech 42:2702–2707

9. Moyne-Bressand S, Dhieux C, Dousset E, Decherchi P (2018) Effectiveness of foot biomechanical orthoses to relieve patients suffering from plantar fasciitis: is the reduction of pain related to change in neural strategy? Biomed Res Int 2018:1–17
10. Rozanski GM, Huntley AH, Crosby LD, Schinkel-Ivy A, Mansfield A, Patterson KK (2020) Lower limb muscle activity underlying temporal gait asymmetry post-stroke. Clin Neurophysiol 131:1848–1858
11. Nazmi N, Rahman MAA, Yamamoto SI, Ahmad SA, Zamzuri H, Mazlan SA (2016) A review of classification techniques of EMG signals during isotonic and isometric contractions
12. Phinyomark A, Limsakul C, Phukpattaranont P (2009) A novel feature extraction for robust emg pattern recognition. J. Comput 1:71–80
13. Toledo-pérez DC, Rodríguez-reséndiz J, Gómez-loenzo RA (2019) Support vector machine-based emg signal classification techniques: a review. Appl Sci 9:4402–4430
14. Kendell C, Lemaire ED, Losier Y, Wilson A, Chan A, Hudgins B (2012) A novel approach to surface electromyography: An exploratory study of electrode-pair selection based on signal characteristics. J Neuroeng Rehabil 9:24–32
15. Freund Y, Schapire RE (1997) A decision-theoretic generalization of on-line learning and an application to boosting. J Comput Syst Sci 55:119–139
16. Breiman L(2000) Bias, variance, and arcing classifiers. Tech Rep 460, Stat Dep Univ Calif pp 1–17
17. Freund Y, Schapire RE (1996) Experiments with a new boosting algorithm. In: Proceedings of 13th International Conference Mach. Learn, pp 148–156
18. Schapire RE, Singer Y (1999) Improved boosting algorithms using confidence-rated predictions. Mach Learn 37:297–336
19. Friedman J, Hastie T, Tibshirani R (2000) Additive logistic regression: a statistical view of boosting (With discussion and a rejoinder by the authors). Ann Stat 28:337–407
20. Schapire RE (2013) Explaining adaboost. Empir Inference 37–52
21. Friedman JH (2001) Greedy function approximation: a gradient boosting machine. Ann Stat 29:1189–1232
22. Friedman JH (2002) Stochastic gradient boosting. Comput Stat Data Anal 38:367–378
23. Chen, T, Guestrin, C (2016) XGBoost: a scalable tree boosting system. In: KDD '16 Proceedings of 22nd ACM SIGKDD international conference knowledge discovery and data mining Medication, pp 785–794
24. Jakkula V (2011) Tutorial on support vector machine (SVM). School EECS, Washington State University, 1–13 (2011)
25. Hossin M, Sulaiman MN (2015) A review on evaluation metrics for data classification evaluations. Int J Data Min Knowl Manag Process 5, 01–11

The Optimal Scan Delay of Contrast Media Injection for Diagnosing Abdominal Tumors (Image Quality and Radiation Dose Aspects of Abdominal CT Scan)

Siti Masrochah, Ardi Soesilo Wibowo, Jeffri Ardiyanto, Fatimah, and Agung Nugroho Setiawan

Abstract Abdominal tumors due to malignancy in the liver often occurred in Abdomen CT Scan patients. To obtain a good and accurate image quality can be done by setting the scan delay and improper timing of contrast media injection. It will have an impact on the image of the tumor and also the patient dose. The purpose of this study is to determine the values of scan delay that also fulfilled the radiation protection aspects. The research was done by using 40 image samples resulted from 5 scan delay (60, 65, 70, 75, 80 s). Assessment was determined by calculated the Region of Interest (ROI) of object and dose which analyzed by Friedman tests. There was a difference in image quality. The results of dose calculations showed an increase in dose for each additional scan delay. Suggest for getting the optimal image quality with 70 s scan delay and the maximum scan delay with 75 s is still accepted for patients. The radiation dose is 24.54 mGy with maximum scan delay, which under the regulation of Bapeten and safe for the patients. The results of this study can give the recommendation for scan delay setting in abdominal CT scan to diagnose the abdominal tumor.

Keywords Scan delay · Contrast media · Abdominal CT scan · Image quality · Radiation dose

1 Introduction

Today many abdominal abnormalities that need to be enforced by CT scan diagnostic support include the presence of abdominal tumors due to malignancy in the liver, which can lead to death. Malignancy is a term for diseases in which abnormal

S. Masrochah (✉) · A. S. Wibowo · J. Ardiyanto · Fatimah · A. N. Setiawan
Department of Radiodiagnostic and Radiotherapy Technic,
Poltekkes Kemenkes Semarang, Semarang, Indonesia
e-mail: masrochah@poltekkes-smg.ac.id

H. Triwiyanto et al. (eds.), *Proceedings of the 1st International Conference on Electronics, Biomedical Engineering, and Health Informatics*, Lecture Notes in Electrical Engineering 746, https://doi.org/10.1007/978-981-33-6926-9_46

cells divide without control and can invade nearby tissues. Malignant cells can also spread to other parts of the body through the blood and lymph systems. There are several main types of malignancy. Carcinoma is a malignancy that begins in the skin or in tissues that line or cover internal organs. Malignancy also called cancer [1].

In the enforcement of clinical diagnoses of cancer, a precise and accurate radiological examination is required. Hepatocellular carcinoma (HCC) is the most common primary liver malignancy and is a leading cause of cancer-related death worldwide. In the United States, HCC is the ninth leading cause of cancer deaths [2]. A total of 30,640 new liver and intrahepatic bile duct cancers were estimated to occur in 2013 in addition to 21,670 deaths [3]. HCC occurred more often in males than females (2.4:1), with a higher incidence in Eastern and Southern Asia, Middle and Western Africa, Melanesia, and Micronesia/Polynesia [4].

In order to obtain the right and accurate image quality, CT parameters are needed to adjust properly. The two main output aspects are image quality of the abdominal pathologies and the patient dose is safe (radiation safety). For this reason, studies are needed in the selection of CT scan parameters. Scan delay is a scanning parameter on a CT scan that is set when the examination was done using contrast media. After the computer completes image processing through the reconstruction of the matrix and algorithm, the results will be converted into a numerical scale, which are called as Hounsfield unit (HU). The purpose of windowing itself is the method used to be able to display images according to what they want to display, by changing the contrast of the image into Window width and Window level [5].

Change windowing incorrectly will have an impact on the edge enhancement of the CT scan image produced. Likewise, the result of selecting parameters can cause the radiation dose received by the patient to change. On the other hand, in accordance with the principle of radiation protection in conducting radiological examinations, an optimization principle is needed, to get obtaining optimal image results with sufficient radiation and limitation principle, that is limiting the safe dose for each radiation examination, so that in-depth studies on edge enhancement and dosage are needed radiation produced due to changes in window width and radiation dose on Abdomen CT Scan [6, 7].

The previous research, scan delay on Multi Slice CT (MSCT) scan was valuable for detection pathologies in abdominal CT, such as focal liver lesion [8], abdominal trauma [9] and routine abdominopelvic studies [10]. In this study, subjective image quality evaluation of liver, stomach, intestine, kidney and spleen images were evaluated, and radiation dose measurements were performed on the different scan delay. So, it is necessary to do further studies on edge enhancement.

2 Method

The population in this study was a CT scan of the patients with abdomen mass/tumor, with sample size using the formula [11]:

$$n = \frac{N}{1 + N(e)^2} \tag{1}$$

With:

n Sample size required
N Population
E The desired level of trust (precision) (95% confidence level, e value = 0.05)

Then the minimum sample size is 29,573 (rounded up 30 people).

The study was conducted on 40 patients. Patients consisted of 25 men and 15 women. Detailed description of sample characteristics by sex as shown on Table 1. Seventeen patients with age 51–60 years old, fourteen patients are 40–50 years old and nine patients are 61–70 years old, as shown on Table 2.

The process of making axial slice in cases of abdominal tumor with variations in scan delay changes 60, 65, 70, 75, 80 s.

Research location in Radiology Installation of SMC Hospital Semarang. The research steps are:

1. Research preparation

   a. Patient Preparation

      (1) The patient is given an explanation of the procedure to be examined.
      (2) There is no special preparation. The patient is only asked to remove objects that can interfere with images such as hairpins, earrings, necklaces, and dentures.

   b. CT Scan procedure

      (1) Position of the patient: supine on the examination table, both hands raised above the head, so that the abdomen is free of hand artifacts.
      (2) Position of the object: the upper limit is as high as the xyphoideus process and the lower limit is as high as the symphysis pubis, the midline of the body is in the middle of the table.
      (3) Scan routine Abdomen parameters:

Rotation Time	0.5 s
Detector Configuration	64 × 0.6 mm
Detector Configuration	64 × 0.6 mm
Pitch	0.6
KVP	120 kV

Table 1 Sample description by sex

Sex	Count	Percentage (%)
Male	25	62.5
Female	15	37.5
Total	40	100

Table 2 Sample description by age

Age (yr)	Count	Percentage (%)
40–50	14	35
51–60	17	42.5
61–70	9	22.5
Total	40	100

Quality Ref.mAs	210
Image thickness	5.0 mm.
Kernel	B30f
Iterative Reconstruction	Salfire (Power 3.0)
Contrast medium	Iopamiro 370
Flow rate	3 ml/s
Pressure	325 psi

(4) Scanning stages:

Stage I	AP projection scanogram
Stage II	Scanning without contrast/plain media
Stage III	Scanning the post phase of insertion of contrast media is carried out with the same scanning parameters for the patient to be examined. That is:

(a) Location of tracker/ROI at the same location for each variation of the study that is in descending aorta as high as a carina.
(b) The value of HU is recorded in a predetermined table.
(c) Record Dosage by looking at CT dose index (CTDI) calculations.

2. Data Processing and Analysis

a. Quality Analysis of Abdomen Image Enhancement
Based on the results of the ROI calculation for each determined object and delay scan changes from all samples, tabulation was conducted and then the data normality test was carried out. If the data distribution was normal, then a T-test was conducted to see the difference in the quality of Image Enhancement CT scans due to scan delay changes.
b. Radiation Dose Analysis
To see the difference in radiation dose based on data measured by CT dose index (CTDI) on CT Scan monitor. Linear Regression test is carried out. The statistical test can be used to see the effect of delay scan changes on the radiation dose obtained.

3 Result and Discussion

There is example of ROI in images resulted from this acquisition process. The Fig. 1 shows the value of HU in liver (a) and kidney (b).

After the ROI results are collected, the data normality test was done to see the data distribution. Because the number of samples is only 40, the significance value seen is Kolmogorov so that the results show that the normality test (p-value < 0.05) obtained abnormal data, therefore it is continued with the Friedman Statistics Test to determine the difference in delay variation. The following are the results of the Friedman Test for the whole organ.

Based on the Table 3, for the whole organ in each delay variation that is the significance of 0.002 ($p < 0.05$) which means there is a difference between each delay variety for the entire organ. Based on the results of the highest mean rank in 70-s delay with mean rank 3.75 and the lowest is 60 s with mean rank 2.50 Then after the Friedman test on the whole organ Friedman test was carried out for each organ to determine the difference in delay variation in each area.

The Friedman Test found that intestinal organs, liver and stomach were found to be different in the variation of delay, but in spleen and kidneys, there were no difference, as shown in Table 4. The highest mean rank of the liver organ is a 70-s delay with 4.38 and the lowest mean rank is a 60-s delay with a value of 2.25. In the mean rank intestinal organ, the highest was 70 s delay with 4.25 and the lowest mean was 80 s delay with a value of 1.75. The highest mean rank in the spleen organ is a 70-s delay with 3.31 and the lowest mean rank is 75 s delay with a value of 2.75. The highest mean rank gastric organ was a 70-s delay with 4.50 and the lowest mean rank was a 60-s delay with 1.94. In the mean rank kidney, the highest was delay 65 s with 4.00 and the lowest mean was 60 s delay with a value of 3.13. The difference in HU value on delay scan changes in each organ can be seen in Fig. 2.

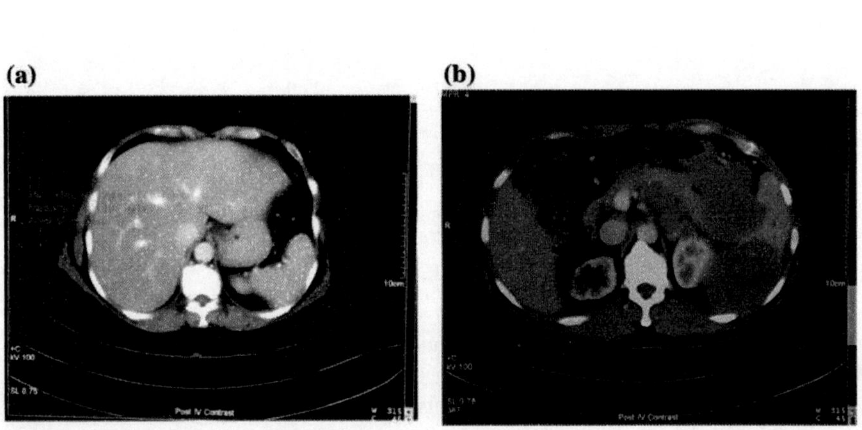

Fig. 1 Example of taking ROI in certain organs (a) Liver, (b) Kidney

Table 3 Test results of different Friedman tests

No	Delay (s)	Mean rank	Significance	Meaning
1	60	2.50	0.002	Difference
2	65	3.08	0.002	Difference
3	70	3.75	0.002	Difference
4	75	2.97	0.002	Difference
5	80	2.67	0.002	Difference

Table 4 Results of different tests on delay and HU of each organ

Organ	Scan delay (s)	Mean rank	*P* value	Meaning
Liver	60	2.25	0.050	Difference
	65	2.38		
	70	4.38		
	75	2.88		
	80	3.13		
Intestine	60	2.13	0.008	Difference
	65	3.25		
	70	4.25		
	75	3.63		
	80	1.75		
Spleen	60	2.88	0.965	No difference
	65	3.00		
	70	3.31		
	75	2.75		
	80	3.06		
Stomach	60	1.94	0.024	Difference
	65	3.00		
	70	4.50		
	75	2.88		
	80	2.69		
Kidney	60	3.13	0.319	No difference
	65	4.00		
	70	2.50		
	75	2.75		
	80	2.63		

The result of radiation dose in abdominal CT examination due to changes in scan delay, as displayed on Fig. 3.

Based on the results of measurements of radiation doses obtained from all samples obtained in the scan delay calculation using 90 ml contrast media with a flow rate of 3 ml/s, the lowest dose obtained on 60 s scan delay was 20.23 mGy

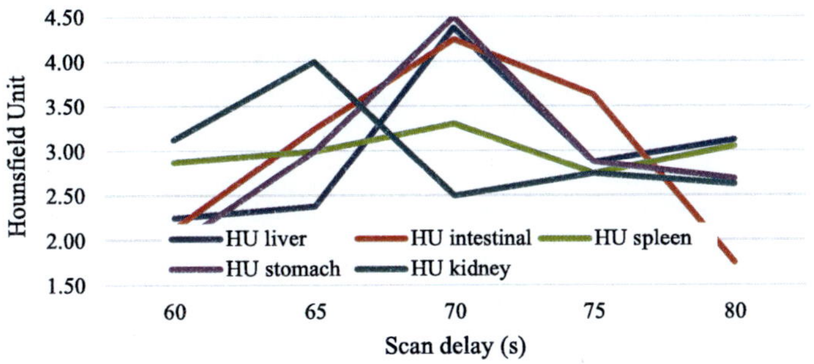

Fig. 2 HU value of the five organs in abdominal CT

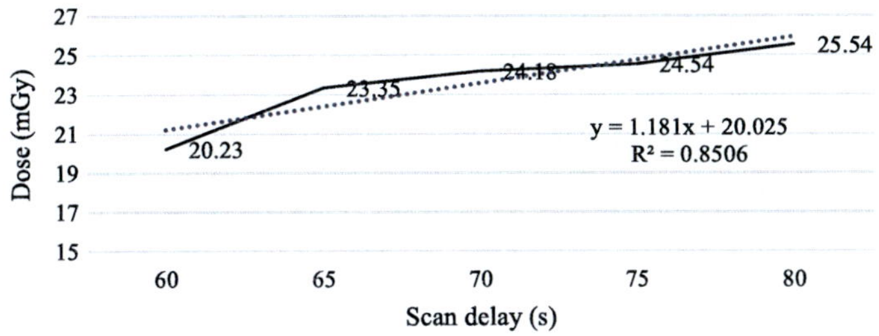

Fig. 3 Graph of time delay versus radiation doses

and the highest dose on 80 s scan delay was 25.54 mGy. According to the regulation as outlined in the Badan Pengawas Tenaga Nuklir (Bapeten) regulation, it was set that the dose guide level for the examination of adult Abdomen MSCT was 25 mGy for each scan [12]. Seeing the results of this measurement, the 60 s delay scan up to 75 s is declared safe because it is still below 25 mGy, while the 80 s delay scan has exceeded 25.54 mGy, so for patient safety it is not recommended to use an 80 s scan delay because it exceeds the dosage guide determined by Bapeten.

3.1 The Image Quality of Liver in CT Scan Abdominal Examination Due to Changes in Scan Delay

The image quality of the abdominal scan results in a general difference in the value of HU, which states that the level of enhancement increases up to the edge enhancement at a certain time. For each organ, the level of abdominal enhancement has a certain time difference. The quality of the liver image and surroundings with changes of scan delay shows that the longer the delay time is set, the HU value of the liver and surrounding images increases, this is due to a long time, the contrast media that will reach the organ increases the HU value high. Based on the highest edge enhancement image on the 70-s delay scan with a value of HU 4.38. This is the right time to describe the portal vein, so that the HU value is highest, after that it will decrease [13].

3.2 Differences in the Quality of Liver Image Examination of Abdominal MSCT Due to Changes in Scan Delay

In general, based on the results of statistical tests, there are differences in the quality of abdominal images with a *p*-value of 0.02 < 0.05, which means that there are differences between scan delay 60, 65, 70, 75 and 80 s.

Getting peak enhancement requires a longer delay than the arterial, venous and port phases. Based on the results of this study, if you are going to look at the liver organs in the parenchyma phase certain delay times are needed according to each organ by looking at the graph above at the peak of the enhancement. This result is also shown on previous study [14, 15].

In accordance with the statistical results, there is a difference in delay scan of the image of the organ, that is in the liver, intestine and stomach. Liver peak enhancement appears at a value of 70 s with a mean rank value of 4.8. while the peak enhancement of the intestine is evident at 70 s with a mean rank value of 4.25, and the peak enhancement of the stomach is evident in the scan delay of 70 s, the mean rank value is 4.5 for stately spleen organs. for the liver, organs are very clear on a 70-s delay scan [16].

Based on the results of statistics for Kidney and Spleen organs there were no significant differences with p value > 0.05. This is because the results of the calculation of HU do not show significant differences in the combustion with the surrounding organs.

3.3 Differences in Radiation Dose on Abdominal CT Scan Examination Due to Changes in Scan Delay

The results of the dose calculation with CTDI showed an increase in the dose for each additional scan delay time. This is indicated by the lowest dose value on the 60-s scan delay of 20.23 mGy, and the highest on the 80-s scan delay at a dose of 25.54 mGy. These results are appropriate with previous study. The longer delay scan, then the length of time per gap between one x-ray beam to another x-ray beam rotation. Pitch smaller than 1.0 indicates overlap between one X-ray beam and the other resulting in double irradiation of the tissue, so the measured radiation dose in CTDI is also greater. This is in accordance with the results of statistical tests with the regression equation as follows: $y = 1{,}181x + 20{,}025$ with $R^2 = 0.8506$, which means that the dose increase is caused by delay scan time 1,181 with chi-square 0.8506 which means the delay scan is strong enough to cause an increase in radiation dose. Looking at the results of this study, in order to obtain a good level of edification, it is also necessary to pay attention to the radiation dose produced and measured in CTDI [17].

3.4 Radiation Dose on Abdominal MSCT Examination Due to Changes in Scan Delay According to Bapeten's Regulation

The results of this study indicate the selection of scan delay on the Abdomen CT dose value obtained was lowest on a 60-s delay scan with a dose of 20.23 mGy. And the highest was 80 s scan delay with a dose of 25.54 mGy. Based on the regulation, the diagnostic guide for the allowable dosage for an abdominal CT scan is 25 mGy [7]. Thus, for the selection of delay scans that produce doses below 25 mGy is a delay scan 60–75 s.

4 Conclusion

Scan delay changes produce different image quality in liver, stomach, intestine, kidney and spleen organs with peak enhancement and highest HU value on 70 s and decrease in 80 s. There are differences in the image quality and dose radiation of the overall abdominal image. The value of $R^2 = 0.806$, which means there is an increase in radiation dose with an increase in scan delay. The optimum scan delay is 70–75 s with maximum dose of 24.54 mGy, as the best image of edge enhancement in tumors (HU = 4.38), which confirm safety dose to reference dose medical radiographic as low with dose as the Bapeten's regulation.

References

1. National Cancer Institute, NCI Dictionary of Cancer Terms. https://www.cancer.gov/publications/dictionaries/cancer-terms/def/malignancy
2. Centers for Disease Control and Prevention (CDC) (2010) Hepatocellular carcinoma - United States, 2001–2006. MMWR. Morb. Mortal. Wkly. Rep. 59, 517–20.
3. Crissien AM, Frenette C (2014) Current management of hepatocellular carcinoma. Gastroenterol Hepatol (N. Y)10:153–161
4. Ferlay J, Shin HR, Bray F, Forman D, Mathers C, Parkin DM (2010) Estimates of worldwide burden of cancer in 2008: GLOBOCAN 2008. Int J cancer 127:2893–2917. https://doi.org/10.1002/ijc.25516

5. Seeram E (2016) Computed tomography : physical principles, clinical applications, and quality conol
6. Seeram E, Sil J (2013) Computed tomography: physical principles, instrumentation, and quality control. https://doi.org/10.1007/978-1-4471-4703-9_5.
7. Grover S, Kumar J, Gupta A, Khanna L (2002) Protection against radiation hazards: regulatory bodies, safety norms, does limits and protection devices. Indian J Radiol Imaging 12:157–167
8. Anderson SW, Varghese JC, Lucey BC, Burke PA, Hirsch EF, Soto JA (2007) Blunt splenic trauma: delayed-phase CT for differentiation of active hemorrhage from contained vascular injury in patients. Radiology. https://doi.org/10.1148/radiol.2431060376
9. Anderson SW, Varghese JC, Lucey BC, Burke PA, Hirsch EF, Soto JA (2007) Blunt splenic trauma: delayed-phase CT for differentiation of active hemorrhage from contained vascular injury in patients. Radiology. https://doi.org/10.1148/radiol.2431060376
10. Chan MG, Cassidy FH, Andre MP, Chu P, Aganovic L (2014) Delayed imaging in routine CT examinations of the abdomen and pelvis: is it worth the additional cost of radiation and time?. Am. J. Roentgenol. https://doi.org/10.2214/AJR.12.10468
11. Israel GD (1992) Determining sample size 1 the level of precision. Lev Precis 1–5
12. Bapeten (2011) Perka Bapeten Nomor 8 Tahun 2011 tentang Keselamatan Radiasi dalam Penggunaan Pesawat Sinar-X Radiologi Diagnostik dan Intervensional. Jakarta
13. Neseth R (2000) Procedures and documentation for CT and MRI. http://books.google.com/books?id=dYJrAAAAMAAJ
14. Abimanyu B, Rusyadi L, Taufiq T (2017) Analisis Informasi Citra Anatomi Fase Late Artery dengan Variasi Time Scan Delay pada Pemeriksaan MSCT Abdomen. J Imejing Diagnostik 3:213–219. https://doi.org/10.31983/jimed.v3i1.3187
15. Choi SY, Lee I, Seo JW, Park HY, Choi HJ, Lee YW (2016) Optimal scan delay depending on contrast material injection duration in abdominal multi-phase computed tomography of pancreas and liver in normal Beagle dogs. J Vet Sci 17:555–561. https://doi.org/10.4142/jvs.2016.17.4.555
16. Knollmann F, Coakley F (2006) Multislice CT: principles and protocols. Elsevier Saunders, Philadelphia
17. LW G (2008) Principles of CT: multislice. CT J Nucl Med Technol 36:57–68

Effect of mAs on the Radiation Doses Received by Eyes Organ at Cranium Examination

Ayu Wita Sari and Stanislaus Yudianus Sam

Abstract The study aims to see the effect of mAs to radiation doses on eye organs with the phantom cranium and to know the right mAs at cranium examination with phantom objects. So that the radiation dose received is the smallest organ. This type of research is quantitative with an experimental approach. The object was exposed using mAs; 8, 12, 16, 32, 63. Radiation dose measurements were carried out using a radiation device. The results of the first measurement that the radiation dose received by the eye organ in the phantom cranium is 0.05 mSv, the second measurement the radiation dose received by the eye organ is 0.11 mSv, the third is 0.17 mSv, the fourth measurement is 0.41 mSv, the fifth measurement is 0.77 mSv. This is influenced by mAs showing a small quantity of X-ray mAs, which will cause the number of electron clouds produced small so that when making images on the results of the radiograph, determine the amount of X-ray quantity that affects the radiation dose received by the object. A good density value is at mAs 32, producing a usable density in the normal range of 1, 23 with the radiation dose received on eyes organ are 0.41 mSv.

Keywords mAs · Radiology · Eyes organ · Radiation doses · Density

1 Introduction

Conventional x-ray is the device used to establish the diagnosis with the source of the x-ray tube with the benefit to assess the anatomical results of an object. X-rays have biological effects that can cause biological changes in tissues in organs in radiation. X-rays (Roentgen) have the same ability as gamma rays in ionizing the objects in its path, so that both are also known as ionizing rays. If this ionization process occurs in the soft tissues of organs and fluids in the human body, it can cause cell damage, gene mutations, free radical formation, and cancer cells.

A. W. Sari (✉) · S. Y. Sam
School of Health Guna Bangsa, Yogyakarta, Indonesia
e-mail: ayu.0221@gmail.com

H. Triwiyanto et al. (eds.), *Proceedings of the 1st International Conference on Electronics, Biomedical Engineering, and Health Informatics*, Lecture Notes in Electrical Engineering 746, https://doi.org/10.1007/978-981-33-6926-9_47

The standard Exposition Factor is used on cranium inspection the AP projection is 85 kV with output a dose of 1781 mGy with mAs of 12. Viewed from the side anatomy, one of the organs exposed to radiation during cranium examination are eyes [1].

One of the factors of radiation dose is mAs. It's one component in the formation of radiographs where mAs effect on radiation intensity. High mAs settings can reduce the density and increase the dose of radiation received by the patient. One of the effects of radiation that need to be considered is the effect of radiation received by radiation workers on the eye organs [2]. The standard exposure factor used on cranium examination the anterior posterior projection is 85 kV with output a dose of 1,781 mGy, mAs of 12. Viewed from the side anatomy, one of the organs exposed to radiation during cranium examination are eye lens [3]. The eyes lens is one organs or body tissues that have sensitivity to radiation large enough. In publication 103, ICRP (International Commission for Radiation Protection) states that the threshold dose for cataracts is on the eye lens is 5 Gy for acute exposure and >8 Gy for exposure divided or prolonged. To prevent these cataracts, The ICRP then sets a dose limit value for the eyepiece of 150 mSv per year for radiation workers and 15 mSv per year for the general public [4]. Recommends a reduction in the Dose Limit Value of the eye lens for radiation workers from 150 to 20 mSv in one year and in one particular year not beyond 50 mSv [5, 6].

Based on this latest study, it was found that there are several effects deterministic, especially effects with very slow manifestations, in which the threshold dose is lower than previously estimated. For lenses eye, the threshold dose value is now estimated at 0.5 Gy, or about 10 times lower than previous estimates. Therefore, ICRP then revised the dose limit value for the eye lens to 20 mSv per years, averaged over five years, and not in one particular year may exceed 50 mSv. If dose more than doses limit value has been determined to cause cataracts in the eyes [7]. In the Anterior Posterior cranium examination one of the organs affected by exposure radiation is the eye. From some of the above it states that the dosage high radiation can cause eye organ damage such as cataract [8]. Cataract, or opacification of the lens, is one of the largest causes of visual impairment and blindness worldwide and may be classified into three main forms: nuclear, cortical and posterior subcapsular (psc), according to its anatomic location [9]. However, in the field it is not yet known how many doses are received by the patient's eye organ during cranium examination with the mAs commonly used in the field. Because in the field variations of mAs are on use so varied that the number of doses is not yet known Cranium examination especially specifically eye organs. For that, I am interested to research on effect of mAs on eye radiation doses on cranium examination.

2 Method

This research is a quantitative research with take radiation dose measurements with an experimental approach. The location of this research is in the Laboratory Departement of D3 Radiodiagnostic Technique STIKES Guna Bangsa Yogyakarta. The independent variable in this experimental study is the exposure factor. The dependent variable in this experimental study was the radiation dose received by the eye organ. The variables that must always be controlled in this study are X-ray tube, focus film distance, kV, radiation field area, and processing film. The object we use phantom cranium.

2.1 Instrumentation

As for the tools used in research are:

- X-Ray conventional that name diagnostic x-ray unit, model number SF 100 BY, serial number 150,014 kV max 80, mA max is 100 and time max is 3.2 s.
- Dosimeter to measurement of radiation dose.
- Densitometer to measurement of optical density.

2.2 Procedure

Cranium examination with phantom is performed instead organ. The dose of radiation exposure was measured using detector radiation dosimeter. The method is as follows:

- Cranium is positioned on the examination table
- Exposure factors are adjusted with different variations of mAs from 40, 32, 24, 16, 8 and kV stand by 70 kV
- Radiation dose placed measuring devices around the eyes
- Exposed and measured the radiation dose produced at the detector and record the results.

2.3 Data Analysis

Data from measurements with survey meters are included in the table and graphed using Microsoft Office Excel 2013. Results measurements with dosimeter entered in tabular form and averaged so that you can know the radiation dose received at organs around the eye at different variations of mAs. Processing results and data analysis is then concluded and adjusted for NBD radiation in eye organs determined by IRCP and the best advice about receiving doses and can be determined the smallest dose varies mAs without reducing the optimal density.

3 Result and Discussion

A dose of radiation has been measured by the eye organ using Antero Posterior (AP) projection with phantom cranium in the laboratory Radiology. That measurement using mAs variation exposure with x-ray conventional. The results of measurements of radiation doses received by the eye organ are presented in form of a table as in Table 1.

Researchers focus on measuring radiation dose received by the eye organ using a phantom cranium by using a radiation gauge that is the dosemeter placed between the eyes. Based from the results of Table 1 results of the first measurement the radiation dose received by the eye organ in phantom cranium is 0.05 mSv using mAs 8 and kV 70, in the second measurement of radiation dose received by the eye organ is 0.17 mSv using 16 mAs and kV 70, in the third exchange with the exposure factor mAs 24 and kV 70 are obtained radiation dose received by the eye organ in these measurements is 0.29 mSv, the fourth measurement was carried out using the exposure factor mAs 32 and kV 70 obtained the dose of radiation received by the eye on the measurement that is 0.41 mSv, the fifth measurement was carried out using the exposure factor mAs 40 and kV 70 showed the radiation dose received by the organ the eye is 0.57 mSv.

Based on the results of changes in mAs will be effect on the radiation deposition received by the cranium phantom object where the higher the mAs we use, the radiation dose received the object will increase. This will be seen in (Fig. 1).

Based on graph one can be seen an increase in the radiation dose received by eye organ objects in phantom cranium from the use of low mAs eight and the highest is 40. Changes in the value of the radiation dose in each change mAs. Milliampere second (mAs) is the multiplication of amperes with the exposure time (s). The mAs value is identical to the number of radiation doses that are given at the time of making the picture. Reduction in radiation dose is proportional by reducing the value of mAs. mAs shows a small quantity of X-ray mAs will cause the number of

Table 1 The results of measurements of radiation doses

mAs	Measured dose (mSv)			Total (mSv)	Dose average (mSv)
	I	II	III		
8	0.05	0.05	0.05	0.15	0.05
16	0.17	0.17	0.17	0.51	0.17
24	0.29	0.28	0.30	0.87	0.29
32	0.40	0.41	0.41	1.22	0.41
40	0.56	0.56	0.58	1.70	0.57

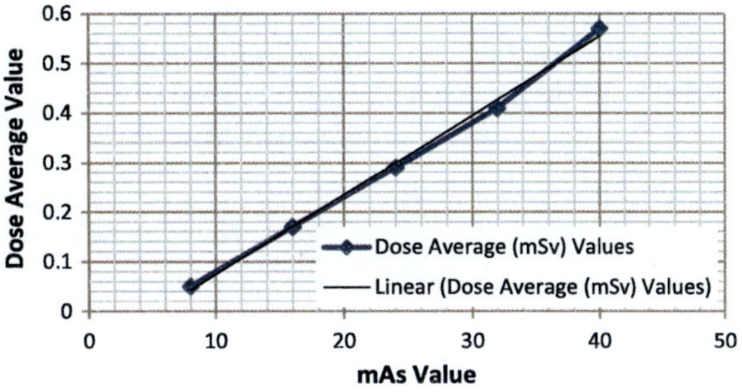

Fig. 1 Graph of radiation dose values based on changes in mAs

electron clouds produced to be small so at the moment making images on the radiograph determine the amount of X-ray quantity thus affecting the radiation dose received by the object. In this study, changes in mAs affect changes in film density radiographs. Changes in mAs affect the quantity of radiation. A linear regression method was used to curve-fit the measured dose versus mAs [10]. So that when mAs is increased the film density is higher as in Table 2 where changes in mAs affect density on the radiograph.

Density measurements were made at three points namely point 1 (soft tissue), point II (bone), point III (density outside the object). Three points to determine the density whole radiograph. After the measurement is done then it is calculated manually using the density formula and using a densitometer. Density on film will be described in (Fig. 2).

Figure 2 illustrates the value of mAs that changes determine high and low density values on the radiograph. This because mAs will increase the quantity of x-rays received by the film thus affecting the degree of blackness in the film. Vulnerable value of density or use density is 0.25–2.0 [11]. A performance phantom was used to evaluate the effect of the different mAs settings on resolution. There was some loss in low contrast resolution at 6 and 20 mAs; however, the resolution was identical at 40 and 100 mAs [12]. Based on the results above can be connected between optical density with the radiation dose value received like Table 3.

From Table 3 it can be seen that the higher the mAs given, the higher the radiation dose received as well as the optical density is directly proportional.

Table 2 Result of optical density measurement on phantom radiograph cranium with variation mAs

mAs	Optical density			Optical density average
	Point I	Point II	Point III	
8	0.05	0.03	1.43	0.48
16	0.67	0.63	1.56	0.95
24	0.67	0.66	1.60	0.98
32	1.20	0.73	1.77	1.23
40	1.66	1.29	2.26	1.74

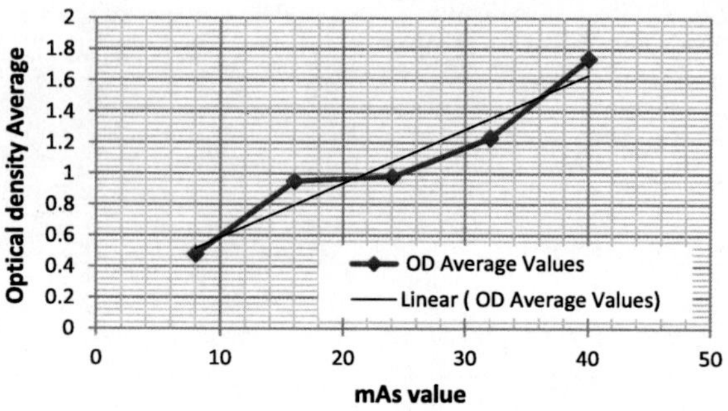

Fig. 2 Graph value of density with respect to variations in mAs

Table 3 Value of change in density with respect to radiation dose

mAs	Optical density	Radiation doses (mSv)
8	0.48	0.05
16	0.95	0.17
24	0.98	0.29
32	1.23	0.41
40	1.74	0.57

However, in mAs 16 there is an abnormal optical density value of 0.95. This is probably caused by the lack of attention on the processing time of the film. Although the results are directly proportional to the radiation dose received by the eye in the mAs variation, it is still safe, which is less than 20 mSv per year while the optimal optical density values are at mAs 32 and 40. If a radiation worker with a workload of 50–100 actions per year, the value of the radiation dose received is 260–700 mSv per year. This radiation doses has exceeded the recommended dose limit value [13].

4 Conclusion

Changes in mAs affect the radiation received by the eye on cranium examination. The greater the mAs, the greater the radiation received will be vice versa. The greater the radiation is given, the optical density is increasingly optimal. Based on the results of radiographs produced on these measurements, the good value density is at mAs 32, which results in a density of use within the normal range of 1.23 with the radiation dose received by the organ the eye on the cranium object is 0.41 mSv.

References

1. Bruce Rollins (2016) Smith: Merril's atlas of radiographic positioning and radiologic procedures 2, Thirteen edn. Elsevier. St. Louis, Missouri
2. Arifin Z, Setiawati E, Putri AA, Hidayanto E, Reskianto AD (2020) Measurement of eye lens doses estimation in interventional radiology. J Phys Conf Ser 1524(1):012018. IOP Publishing
3. Nikupaavo U, Kaasalainen T, Reijonen V, Ahonen SM, Kortesniemi M (2015) Lens dose in routine head CT: comparison of different optimization methods with anthropomorphic phantoms. Am J Roentgenol 204(1):117–123
4. German Commission on Radiological Protection: Radiation-induced cataracts. German (2009)
5. McNair A (1980) Radiation quantities and units. International commission on radiation units and measurements (ICRU). Washington Report, p 33
6. Stewart FA, Akleyev AV, Hauer-Jensen M, Hendry JH, Kleiman NJ, MacVittie TJ, Aleman BM, Edgar AB, Mabuchi K, Muirhead CR, Shore RE, Wallace WH (2012) ICRP 41(1–2)
7. Shore RE, Neriishi K, Nakashima E (2010) Epidemiological studies of cataract risk at low to moder-ate radiation doses (not) seeing is believing. Radiat Res 174:889–894
8. Kleiman NJ (2010) Radiation cataract. In: Radiation protection new insights in radiation risk and basic safety standards. European Commission Proceedings of the working party on research implications on health and safety standards of the article. 31 Group of Experts 145, pp 81–95
9. Reid J, Gamberoni J, Dong F, Davros W (2010) Optimization of kVp and mAs for pediatric low-dose simulated abdominal CT. Am J Roentgenol 195(4):1015–1020
10. Bushong SC (2017) Radiologic Science for Technologists: physics, biology, and protection, Eleventh edn. Elsevier, Houston Texas
11. Haaga JR, Miraldi F, Macintyre W, LiPuma JP, Bryan PJ, Wiesen E (1981) The effect of mAs variation upon computed tomography image quality as evaluated by in vivo and in vitro studies. Radiology 138(2):449–454
12. Matsubara KV, Lertsuwunseri, Srimahachota, Krisanachinda S, Tulvatana A, Khambhiphant W, Sudchai B, Rehani W (2017) Phys Med Eur J Med Phys, 1–4
13. Wrixon AD, Barraclough I, Clark MJ, Ford J, Diesner-Kuepfer A, Blann B (2004) Safety report series no. 13. International Atomic Energy Agency (IAEA)

Development of Phantom Radiology Using Eggshells Powder as Bone Genu Material

Ayu Wita Sari, Putri Winda Loja Bimantari, and Nadela Putri Sakhia

Abstract Eggshells have never been used to create phantoms as bone substitutes so far. Eggshells are easy to find and commonly thrown into the waste bin. The phantom is very important in the field of radiological engineering, especially for practicums on campus to avoid X-ray radiation. The price of a phantom sold in the market is hundreds of millions. This study aims to make a Phantom using eggshell powder as a basic material for bones, especially genu, and to calculate the optical density values in bones made from eggshell powder. The main advantage of this research is that it uses a simple method and easy to find the basic materials so that the manufacturing costs are lower. By using eggshell powder, it is expected to produce Phantom products that are comparable in structure to those made in factories. The method used in this research is an experiment. Provide a comparison between the main material and the companion material; they are 1:1, 1:2, and 1:3. After the experiment is carried out, it is printed based on the appropriate comparison. The result obtained was the 1:1 ratio of the ingredients to be stronger and dry faster than the ratio of 1:2 and 1:3. The optical density value of the radiograph obtained was 0.2. Based on the references value, 0.2 on the bone radiograph included in the bright or radiopaque interval. The radiographs obtained did not show the trabecular structure. So that for the further research it is necessary to add additional materials to replace trabecular.

Keywords Phantom · Radiology · Eggshells · Bone · Genu

1 Introduction

Radiology is a medical science that interprets the body's organs using the emission of radiation wave, both electromagnetic wave and mechanical waves to diagnose diseases. It makes the human body an important object in the imaging process using

A. W. Sari (✉) · P. W. L. Bimantari · N. P. Sakhia
School of Health Guna Bangsa, Yogyakarta, Indonesia
e-mail: ayu.0221@gmail.com

H. Triwiyanto et al. (eds.), *Proceedings of the 1st International Conference on Electronics, Biomedical Engineering, and Health Informatics*, Lecture Notes in Electrical Engineering 746, https://doi.org/10.1007/978-981-33-6926-9_48

X-rays, CT-Scan, MRI, USG, and nuclear medicine [1]. In the radiology learning process, students are required to master radiology examination techniques with various examination positions and patient conditions. Therefore, during the practicum in the radiology laboratory, students will repeatedly practice using X-ray to be skilled in taking radiology images appropriately. In this case, the use of human objects dangerous due to X-ray exposure to the object. The level of exposure to electromagnetic waves of various frequencies significantly changes in line with technological developments which raises concern that exposure to the electromagnetic wave can adversely affect physical health.

The radiological examination uses radiation as a key component, including in practicum in the laboratory. Radiation exposure can be harmful to the body. Thus, it is crucial to minimize the effects of radiation, especially for students and lecturers. One of the efforts to minimize the effect is through using radiological phantoms so that there is no exposure to humans. On the other hand, the use of radiological phantoms also creates a new issue due to its expensive price. Hence, not all radiology education institutes can afford it.

Phantom is a prop for knowledge of body anatomy used by education in patient house and equipment testing equipment. Function phantom is a prop that is learning media that contains the characteristics of concepts and competencies that are studied. While phantom functions as a special test tool, radiology as a tool in measuring eligibility of certain radiological tools. Our discussion on applications will be limited to the phantoms used with photons and electrons since most medical applications utilize those particles. The last section is devoted to speculative discussion on what types of phantom and material will be developed in the near future [2]. Based on the benefits of using phantoms then some research related to manufacture phantom has done a lot of one of them namely the manufacture of Indian female pelvic phantom aims to design and develop similar to the original organs especially imitating pelvic dimensions of Indian women with use the available network substitutes locally and cost-effective properties according to need [3]. A technique is presented for the production of polymer-based phantom materials from solid polymer powders and various compounds added to adjust x-ray attenuation [4].

Using available data for photon attenuation and tissue composition, a computer code was developed for the optimization of the composition of phantom materials for diagnostic radiology [5] and phantoms containing iodine details with clinically relevant iodine concentrations are required to systematically study dose requirements, for quality assurance and optimizing exposure parameters and protocols for contrast enhanced dual energy mammography (CEDEM) applications [6]. Physical and visual measures suggest our low-cost phantom has suitable anatomical characteristics for X-ray imaging. Our phantom could have utility in dose and image quality optimisation studies [7] and the phantom has physical characteristics (in terms of spinal deformity) and radiological characteristics [8]. The price of a phantom sold in the market is hundreds of millions. It is expected that the discovery of this organic phantom (made from eggshells) has almost the same quality as a bone at a more economical price. After successfully conducting this research, the phantom product can be patented and marketed to various agencies. Moreover, radiological engineering students no longer face radiation exposure during practicum. It has been widely known that repeated exposure to X-ray radiation can cause somatic and/or genetic effects.

To investigate whether the phantom shape was suitable for dose evaluation, organ doses in the same scan protocol were compared between the 3-yr-old head and commercially available anthropomorphic phantoms having approximately the same head size. The doses of organs in both phantoms were equivalent. The authors' designed paediatric head phantom will be useful for dose evaluation in paediatric head CT examinations [9]. The knee joint or genu is one of the most complex joints in the human body. The femur, tibia, fibula, and patella are held together into a complex group by ligaments [10]. Movement of bending and straightening as well help every human movement, for example, walking, running, up, and down the stairs. Most of the bodyweight and movement is supported by knee joint [11].

Eggshells have never been used to create phantoms as bone substitutes so far. Eggshells are easy to find and commonly thrown into the waste bin. The eggshells are composed of a three layered structure, namely, the cuticle, sponge (foam) and lamellar layers. The cuticle layer is a transparent protein that coats the surface of the eggshells. This layer coats the pores on the eggshells, but steam and CO_2 gas can still pass through it [12]. The sponge (foam) and lamellar layers form a matrix composed of protein fibbers bound to calcium carbonate ($CaCO_3$) crystals or commonly called calcite, with a ratio of 1:50. This foam layer is the largest part of the eggshells layer. It consists of protein and a limestone layer of calcium carbonate, calcium phosphate, magnesium carbonate, and magnesium phosphate [13].

Typically, the bone composition consists of 60% organic material, 30% organic material and 10% water. Organic material is a bone mineral that contains sufficient calcium, particularly calcium phosphate carbonate or called apatite carbonate and other minerals. An organic bone material such as calcium (Ca) and phosphorus (P) are abundant. However, some other minerals are limited, such as bicarbonate (HCO_{3-}), magnesium (Mg), sodium (Na), Potassium (K), copper (Cu), zinc (Zn), manganese (Mn), and others [14]. Based on the explanation above, the composition of eggshells and human bones is almost similar and it encourages the researcher to conduct this study.

2 Method

This experimental study created genu phantom using eggshells as bone substitutes. The research was carried out in the laboratory of School of Health Guna Bangsa Yogyakarta and workshop anatomy of Gadjah Mada University for five months and then tested. The tools and the materials used in this study were eggshells flour as the main ingredient for genu phantom, gypsum flour, water, silicon rubber, catalyst, blender, pestle, scales, basins, glue, stirrer, fan, cutter, X-ray beam, radiology cassettes, film and markers.

The process of creating eggshells flour was started with collecting unused eggshells from sellers who use egg as cooking ingredients. Then the eggshells were cleaned of the white skin layer, washed with water and then dried under the sun. After drying, it was continued with the refining process by grinding the eggshells into smaller pieces, and it was processed using a blender to get fine flour texture.

Then the material concentration for bones was tasted to get the desired result with three trials, namely 1:1 ratio with the composition of 150 g of eggshell flour, 150 g of gypsum flour, and 25 ml of water. Second, 1:2 ratio was used with the composition of 150 g of gypsum flour, 300 g of eggshell flour, and 50 ml of water. The third ratio is 1:3 used the composition of 150 g of gypsum flour, 450 g of eggshells flour, and 100 ml of water.

After the material concentration test, it was continued with creating phantom using silicon rubber and catalyst with a ratio of 350 ml of silicon rubber and 10 ml of catalyst each then mixed and stirred until evenly distributed. Then the silicon material was poured into a container to create a phantom. To ensure that the result is almost similar to the original bone, then it was tasted by taking radiograph images after being exposed using an X-ray beam. Then the optical density was measured using a densitometer.

3 Result and Discussion

In this study, the experimental results of the concentration of materials were obtained, as shown in Fig. 1. Based on these three ratios, a good result to use for making phantom is a ratio of 1:1 because it is not brittle, dries quickly, and is denser than the other ratio.

After experimenting with 3 different ratios, the exposure was made to see the density of the material, as shown in Fig. 2. Then the material with a 1:1 ratio was printed using a genu bone mold.

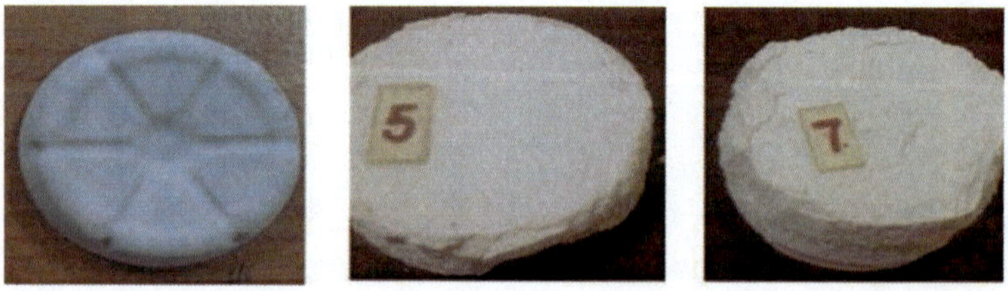

a b c

Fig. 1 The result of the material concentration test from eggshells flour with **a** 1:1 ratio, **b** 1:2 ratio and **c** 1:3 ratios

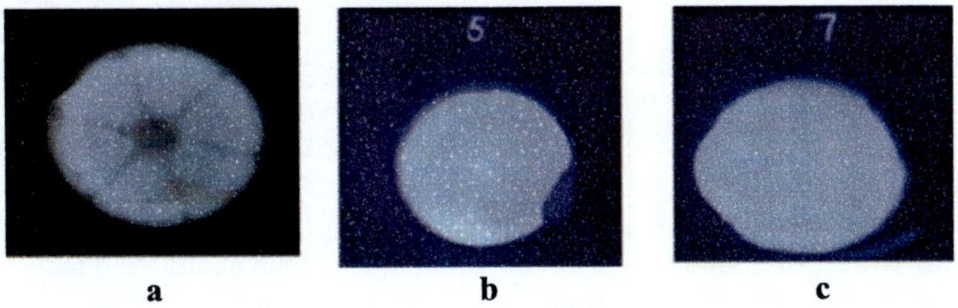

Fig. 2 The result after exposure using X-ray with a 1:1 ratio, b 1:2 ratio and c 1:3 ratios

An experiment using eggshells managed to produce genu phantoms, which consist of the femur, fibula, tibia, and patella. The ingredients were eggshell powder, gypsum powder, and water as a solvent.

Figure 3 presents genu phantoms made from eggshells which consist of powder parts, namely the femur, fibula, tibia, and patella. The genu phantom was successfully printed using a meld made of silicon rubber. The genu phantoms obtained still have many holes because the ingredients are not perfectly mixed. The composition of the ingredients was 1: 1 consisting of eggshell powder, gypsum powder, and a few ml of water as the solvent. This composition was selected so that the product will not easily brittle, breaks, and dry when it is put into the meld.

The genu phantoms that have been designed with genu anatomical structure were tested using a conventional X-ray beam from Shanghai Guanzheng type SF 100 BY brand with a serial number of 150014. The image receptor used was $18 \times 24\ cm^2$ with an exposure factor of 10 mAs, a voltage of 60 kV, and a focus film distance of 100 cm.

The radiograph result presented in Fig. 4 already looks almost similar to the real bone when exposed. Bones are white or have radiopaque characteristics when exposed to X-rays. Meanwhile, non-bone will be radiolucent or black because X-rays hit the free air without any absorption from certain materials. The result of this study was still in the form of bones, and it would be better if in the form of soft

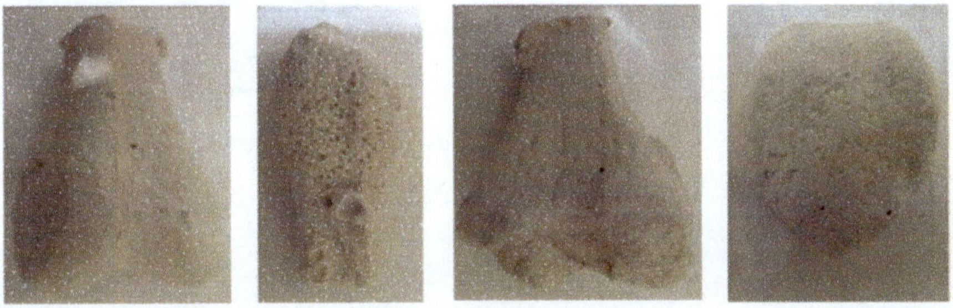

Fig. 3 The result of genu phantom made from eggshells powder with 1:1 ratio from left to right femur, fibula, tibia and patella

tissue using acrylic material. Thus, it shows the greyish color and the boundaries between the soft tissue and the bones, even the fishy smell of the bones will also be covered with the soft tissue. In this case, if the phantom is completely composed of bones and soft tissue, it will be suitable for teaching material or practicum in the radio-diagnostic study program. Therefore, there is no need to use humans as samples or experiment objects. Further, the material is easy to find and to be formed according to human bones. For further research, it is crucial to test the quality of the radiographs produced. The processed radiograph is analysed in the densitometer, a device that has a light source focused through a pinhole. A light-sensing device is positioned on the opposite side of the radiograph. The radiographic film is positioned between the pinhole and the light sensor, and the amount of light transmitted through each step of the radiographic image is measured. The result of radiograph density measurement using a densitometer is presented in Table 1.

Optical density is the degree of blackening of the finished radiograph. Optical density has a numeric value and can be present in varying degrees, from completely black, in which no light is transmitted through the radiograph, to almost clear. Whereas black or radiolucent is numerically equivalent to an Optical density of 3 or greater clear or radiopaque is less than 0.2 [15]. Based on Table 1, the value of optical density from the densitometer the average optical density value for 5 measurements was 0.20. Based on reference, the percentage of radiopaque in bone was too high. Thus, the bones appear very light or bright, and no visible trabecular on the bones. For the component structure, there are some shortcomings, including greyish trabecular lines. The bones are not strong enough because the meld and the

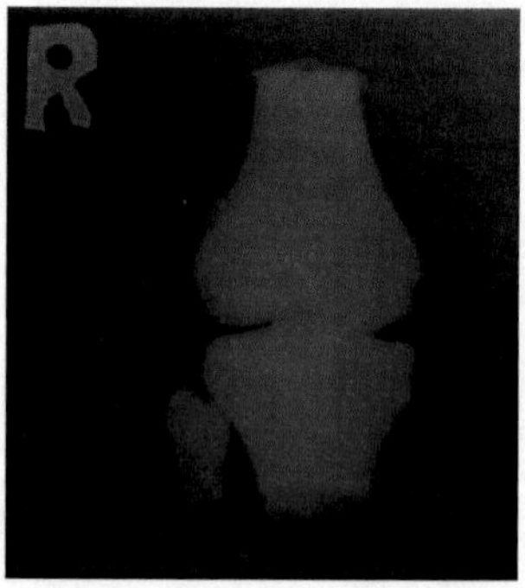

Fig. 4 Radiograph of genu phantoms from eggshells

Table 1 The optical density value of genu phantom radiographs made of egg shells

Measure	Optical density	Average of optical density
1	0.24	0.20
2	0.35	
3	0.16	
4	0.16	
5	0.11	

tools for producing eggshell flour are still very simple. For further research, it is still necessary to add ingredients to complement the bone structure.

4 Conclusion

The phantom has been successfully created using a ratio of 1:1 with 150 g of eggshell powder, 150 g of gypsum, and 25 ml water. The optical density value on the radiograph is an average of 0.20 more radiopaque (light). The radiographs obtained did not show the trabecular structure. So that for further research, it is necessary to add additional materials to replace trabecular.

References

1. Bontrager KL, Lampignano JP (2010) Textbook of positioning and related anatomi, 4th edn. The CV Mosby, St. Louis
2. Watanabe Y, Constantinou C (2006) Phantom materials in radiology. Encycl Med Dev Instrum
3. Shrotriya D, Yadav RS, Srivastava RN, Verma TR (2018) Design and development of an Indigenous in house tissue-equivalent female pelvic phantom for radiological dosimetric applications. Ir J Med Phys 15(3):200–205
4. Homolka P, Nowotny R (2002) Production of phantom materials using polymer powder sintering under vacuum. Phys Med Biol 47(3):47. IOP Publishing
5. Homolka P, Gahleitner A, Prokop M, Nowotny R (2002) Optimization of the composition of phantom materials for computed tomography. Phys Med Biol 47(16):2907
6. Leithner R, Knogler T, Homolka P (2013) Development and production of a prototype iodine contrast phantom for CEDEM. Phys Med Biol 58(3):N25
7. Ali AM, Hogg P, Johansen S, England A (2018) Construction and validation of a low cost paediatric pelvis phantom. Eur J Radiol 108, 84–91
8. Alrehily F, Hogg P, Twiste M, Johansen S, Tootell A (2020) Development and validation of a bespoke phantom to test accuracy of Cobb angle measurements. Radiography 26(2):78–87
9. Yamauchi-Kawaura C, Fujii K, Akahane K, Yamauchi M, Narai K, Aoyama T, ... Ikeda M (2015) Development of age-specific Japanese head phantoms for dose evaluation in paediatric head CT examinations. Radiat Prot Dosim 163(2):188-201
10. Ballinger PW, Frank ED (2003) Merill's atlas of radiograpic positions and radiologic procedures, vol 3, 10th ed. Mosby Ohio
11. Arya RK, Jain V (2013) Osteoarthritis of the knee joint An overview. J Indian Acad Clin Med 14(2):154–162
12. King'ori AM (2011) Review of the factors that influence egg fertility and hatchability in poultry. Int J Poult Sci 10:483–492
13. Gowsika D, Kokila S, Sargunan K (2014) Experimental investigation of egg shell powder as partial replacement with cement in concrete. Int J Eng Trends Tech
14. Constantini N, Leburn C (2014) Bone health. handbook of sports medicine and science the female athlete
15. Bushong SC (2013) Radiologic science for technologists. E-book: physics, biology, and protection. Elsevier Health Sciences. Elsevier, Texas

Comparison of Radiation Dose and Image Noise in Head Computed Tomography with Sequence and Spiral Techniques

Yeti Kartikasari, Darmini, Siti Masrochah, and Dwi Rochmayanti

Abstract Head CT Scan techniques in clinical can use sequence and spiral technique, but the problems is dose not been routinely recorded and noise have not been assessed. This study was to determine the profile value of radiation doses and image noise in sequence and spiral technique, and also relationship between SAFIRE-Head MSCT. Quasi-experimental research design with one group pretest-posttest method to determine the effect of reducing tube voltage (kVp) 130, 110, 80 to radiation doses and image noise within and without SAFIRE. Measurements of CTDIvol, TLD and image noise. Data was analysis by Anova test followed by post hoc test. The result, there is a difference dose and noise of the spiral and sequence techniques on all variations of tube voltage. Radiation dose increases according to tube voltage and the sequence technique gives a higher dose by CTDIvol. On TLD's measurements, doses in the eyes and thyroid are lower when using spiral techniques. High value of tube voltage produced smaller image noise. The higher level of strange (S5) SAFIRE produced lower image noise. Examination with low tube voltage in spiral technique would be reduce radiation dose (CTDIvol). However, sequence technique reduce radiation dose at the eyes and thyroid gland.

Keywords CT head · Sequence · Spiral · Dose · Image noise

1 Introduction

Head CT Scan examination has two techniques, namely the sequence and spiral technique. The spiral technique is more widely used because it is faster in the scanning process. Selection of tube voltage (kVp) used to produce a image with good detail and also the resulting less noise but dose will be high. Therefore it is

Y. Kartikasari (✉) · Darmini · S. Masrochah · D. Rochmayanti
Radiodiagnostic and Radiotherapy Health Polytechnic, Health Ministry of Semarang, Semarang, Indonesia
e-mail: yeti.kartikasari@gmail.com

H. Triwiyanto et al. (eds.), *Proceedings of the 1st International Conference on Electronics, Biomedical Engineering, and Health Informatics*, Lecture Notes in Electrical Engineering 746, https://doi.org/10.1007/978-981-33-6926-9_49

very necessary to setting tube voltage as a scanning parameter to reduce radiation radiation to the patient, but will be able to produce optimal image quality. To improve image quality, especially reducing noise on MSCT examination of the head with low doses can be done using the reconstruction technique of Iterative Reconstruction (IR) algorithm. IR technique is an aiming algorithm reconstruction to reduce noise and maintain clarity in imaging within anatomical structures [1]. Some CT scan manufacturers such as Siemens have provided IR techniques, namely Sinogram Affirmed Reconstruction (SAFIRE) [2]. There are two reconstructions in Head CT, namely Filter Back Projection and SAFIRE with level 1–5. The doses resulting from both spiral and sequence techniques are not routinely recorded and observed. The radiation dose on a CT scan is very high because it get a primary dose and a secondary dose at the same time per scanning. CT dose guide rate for adult patients the average dose of multiple scans on a CT scan of the head is 50 mGy [3]. CT scan have also been displayed on the monitor for estimated dose values in the form of CTDIvol (CT Doses Index, measured in mGy) and Dose Length Product (DLP).

2 Materials and Methods

This type of research is quantitative descriptive with a quasi experimental approach. The research design used was a one group pretest-posttest design to determine the effect of tube voltage reduction at 130, 110, 80 kVp and the use of SAFIRE on radiation dose and image noise. After knowing the results of the measurements of CTDIvol, TLD and image noise then the data was tested with the Anova test followed by a post hoc test. Data was collected at Tugurejo Hospital Semarang with the object of the study was Phantom. Data collection is done by scanning CT head of Phantom with sequence and spiral techniques at 130, 110, and 80 kVp. Others parameter tube current 240 mAs, slice thickness 5 mm, pitch 0.95, FOV 206 mm was under controlled. Measurement of eye and thyroid radiation doses with TLD, seen in Fig. 2. After scanning, dose of CTDIvol will appear on the consul's monitor screen. The results of the CT head image are then in the ROI (Region of Interest) to measure the value of the noise image. The results of measurements of radiation doses and image noise are recorded in a table for data analysis. The research concept is as follows (Fig. 1).

3 Results

This research was carried out measurements of radiation doses and image noise. For radiation dose measurements obtained from CTDIvol values. To determine the dose affected in the eye and thyroid TLD chips are used that are mounted on the right eye, left eye and thyroid (Table 1).

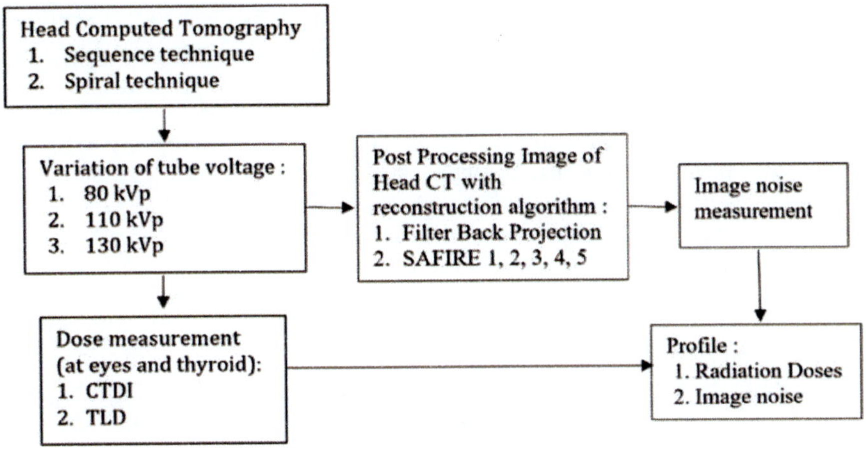

Fig. 1 Diagram block of research concept

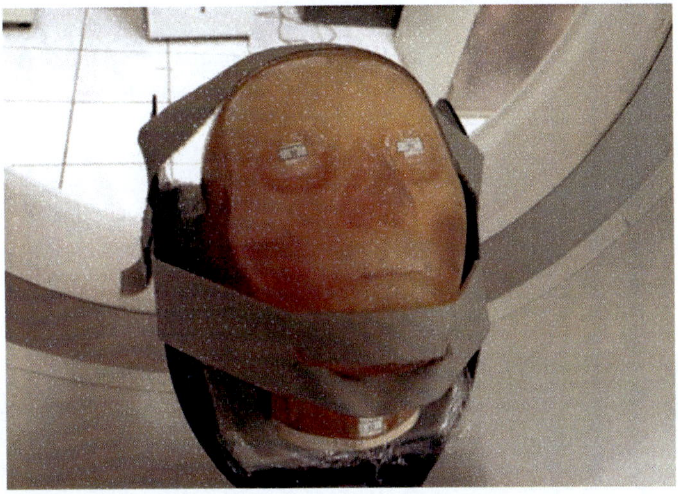

Fig. 2 Placement of TLDs in the right and left eyes and on the thyroid

Table 1 Radiation dose between spiral and sequence techniques (CTDIvol)

No	kVp	Radiation dose on spiral technique (mGy)	Radiation dose on sequence technique (mGy)
1.	130	55.30	65.15
2.	110	38.46	45.28
3.	80	15.64	18.42

Radiation doses was increases linier to tube voltage, and sequence techniques provide a higher dose than spiral. Both techniques show the same dose reduction, i.e. when the tube voltage is pass down from 130 to 110, CTDIvol reduce 30%, while the decrease at 110 to 80 is 59%.

According Table 2, Masurement using TLD, dose in the eye and thyroid gives results that spiral technique has a higher dose than the sequence technique, the increase in the dose is also proportional to the increase in the given tube voltage. To Find the diferrences of radiation dose in each tube voltage use an annova test.

Table 3 showed that Annova statistical test results ρ value <0.05, which means, there is a significant difference in the CTDIvol radiation dose between the use of the spiral technique and the sequence of MSCT Head examinations on the tube voltage adjustment of 130, 110, and 80 kVp.

The graph on Fig. 3 shows that the radiation dose (measure on CTDIvol) has decreased with the decrease in tube voltage. In the spiral technique with 130 kVp radiation dose is 55.3 mGy; in the 110 kVp setting a dose of 38.46 mGy; at 80 kVp a dose of 15.64 mGy was obtained. For the use of sequence techniques it produces higher doses than the spiral, at 130 kVp the dose is 65.15 mGy; at 110 kVp the dose obtained was 45.28 mGy; whereas at 80 kVp the dose obtained was 18.42 mGy.

Radiation dose at eyes and thyroid, which is measured with TLD, has decreased with the decrease in tube voltages. Dose at sequence techniques is lower than the spiral technique. The dose received by the eye is still below the cataract threshold value which is below 0.5 Gy. Whereas in the thyroid, sequence techniques also provide a dose that is still below the thyroid threshold dose which is below 1.1 mGy, see in Figs. 4, 5 and 6. The ALARA principle states that the radiation dose given to patients must be as low as possible without loss of diagnostic information and maintaining optimal image quality [4, 3] (Figs. 7 and 8).

Table 2 Radiation dose in eyes and thyroid (TLD)

Tube voltage	Right eye (mGy)		Left Eye (mGy)		Thyroid (mGy)	
	Spiral	Sequence	Spiral	Sequence	Spiral	Sequence
130	59.79	53.64	60.57	53.95	2.08	1.79
110	42.29	37.14	45.46	33.26	1.35	1.34
80	18.44	13.79	16.55	15.17	0.50	0.39

Table 3 Result of Annova test tube voltage adjustment to CTDIvol radiation doses

	Technique	Tube voltage	ρ value
Radiation dose	Spiral Sequence	130	0.000 (<0.05)
		100	
		80	

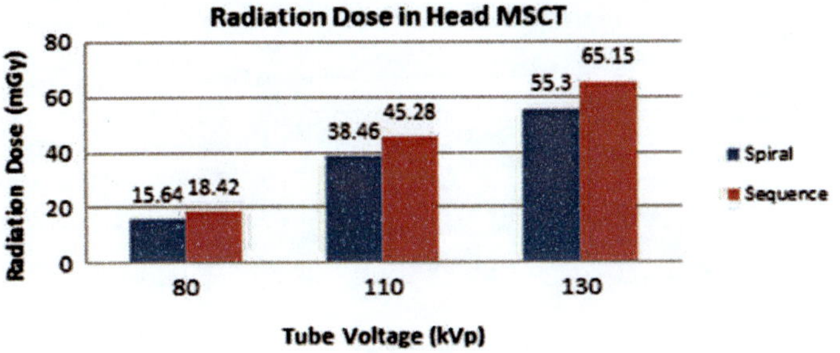

Fig. 3 Graph of comparison of tube voltage to radiation dose (CTDIvol) of Head MSCT between sequence and spiral technique

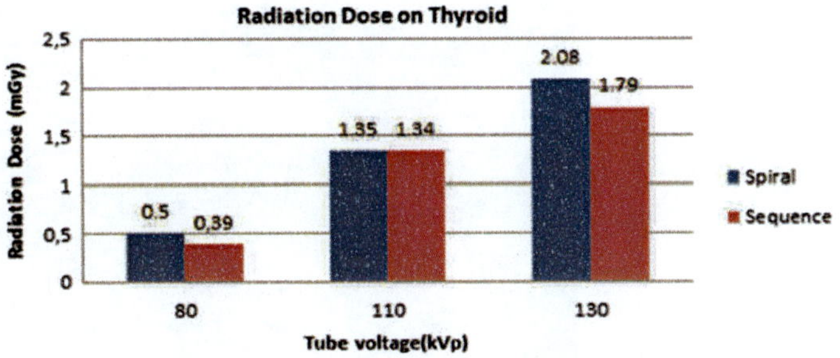

Fig. 4 Comparison radiation dose on thyroid with TLD measurement between sequence and spiral technique

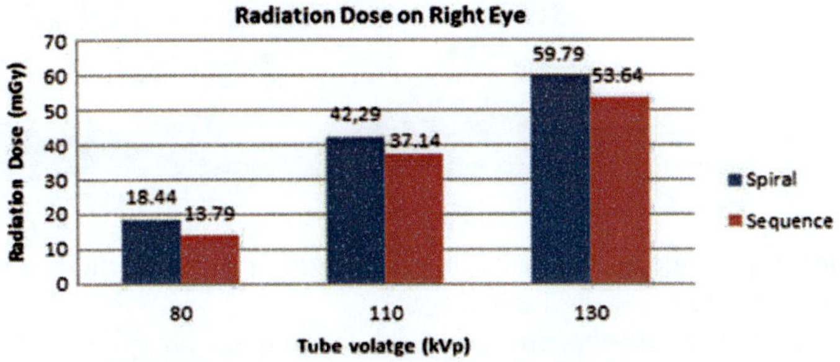

Fig. 5 Comparison radiation dose on right eye with TLD measurement between sequence and spiral technique

Image noise on CT Scan Head examination the highest value is in the 80 kVp with spiral technique and strange level 1. Whereas in the sequence technique the highest image noise value is on the use of 80 kVp. The lowest image noise generated by the 130 kVp spiral technique with strange level 5. When compared, the

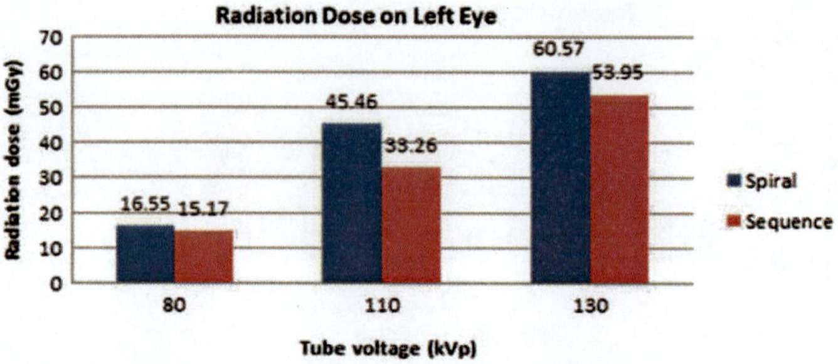

Fig. 6 Comparison radiation dose on left eye with TLD measurement between sequence and spiral technique

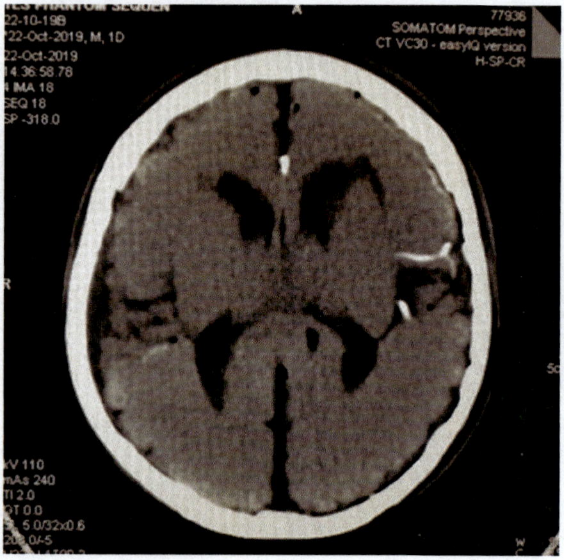

Fig. 7 Image of axial Head CT

value of the spiral image noise noise is lower than the sequence technique in the use of 130, 110 or 80 kVp, see in Table 4.

According Table 5, Anova test results of image noise on spiral and sequence techniques produce ρ value 0.000 < 0.05, showing that there are differences in image noise in both techniques. In addition, according to the results of the study, the higher the tube voltage (kVp), less image noise. The higher the level of strange used (S5) in the spiral technique, the image noise was less.

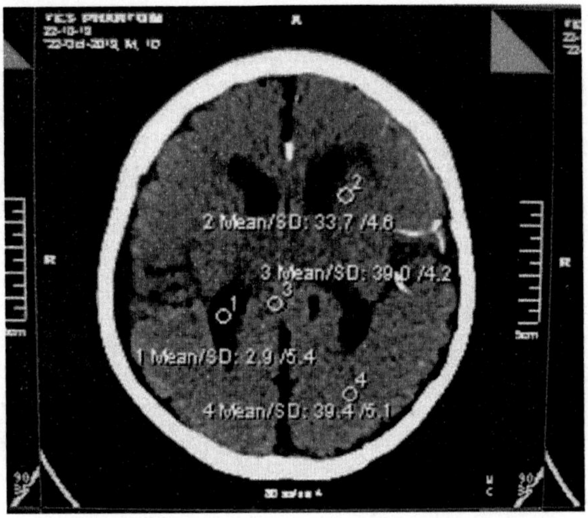

Fig. 8 Image of axial head CT with SAFIRE reconstruction

Table 4 Result of image noise measurement between Spiral and sequence Technique

Image noise (SD)	Tube voltage (kVp)		
	130	110	80
Spiral			
Filter back projection	1.3	1.7	2.4
SAFIRE 1	1.6	2.4	3.6
SAFIRE 2	1.5	1.5	1.5
SAFIRE 3	1.4	1.6	3.0
SAFIRE 4	1.2	1.3	2.5
SAFIRE 5	1.0	1.1	2.1
Sequence	1.6	2.1	3.3

Table 5 Results the difference in the value of image noise in spiral and sequence techniques on the MSCT Head with Anova test

Technique	Tube voltage	ρ value
Spiral Sequence	130	0.000
	110	
	80	

4 Discussion

Result shows that radiation dose (measure on CTDIvol) has decreased with the decrease in tube voltage and masurement using TLD, dose in the eye and thyroid gives results that spiral technique has a higher dose than the sequence technique, the increase in the dose is also proportional to the increase. Radiation dose influenced by technique was used. On CT Scan with the sequence technique, the patient table moves forward first and then the x-ray tube exposed while rotating around the patient. By using this sequence technique, the time needed for one shooting is longer because one round of gantry only produces one piece of image, so the radiation dose released is also greater. Whereas the CT Spiral (continuous) technique that is the patient's table moves forward and simultaneously the x-ray tube exposes while surrounding the patient. The duration of this process is determined by the extent of the object to be examined, the type of organ or tissue. This type already uses multi-slice so that the time needed for one image taken is shorter because one round of gantry can produce two or more pieces of image and the resulting more detailed than a single slice. In addition, the radiation dose is directly proportional to the square with the tube voltage (kVp2). So that the selection of high tube settings, will provide a higher radiation dose.

Tube voltage is the intensity of x-ray photons and the ability of x-rays to penetrate organ tissue. The tube voltage will determine the energy and intensity of the x-ray photon and is directly related to the radiation dose. Mathematically the tube voltage is directly proportional to the radiation dose. Exponentially changes in radiation dose between 2.5 and 3.1 times. So the higher the tube voltage used, the higher the radiation dose produced [5]. In other literature also mentioned if the radiation dose is influenced by several factors, one of which is the setting of the tube voltage (kVp). Reduction of tube voltage from 120 to 100 kVp can reduce radiation dose by 30% due to linear radiation dose with tube voltage [6]. Reduction in tube voltage was very effective in reducing the radiation dose [7].

Noise is influenced by variations in the attenuation coefficient of each organ and the number of x-ray photons captured by the detector. The attenuation coefficient is defined as the standard deviation (SD) of the Hounsfield Unit (HU). The attenuation coefficient and the number of x-ray photons captured by the detector are influenced by the energy and intensity of the x-ray photons that penetrate an organ, which in low tube voltage regulation will cause the photon to attenuate to the organ or be absorbed by the object rather than passed on to the detector. Whereas the high tube voltage will cause more x-ray photons to penetrate the organ or object and be captured by the detector. This difference is indicated by the CT number (HU value). The higher the tube voltage regulation, the standard deviation CT number obtained is lower, and the noise obtained is also low. Noise is directly related to the number of x-ray photons that contribute to image formation or determine fluctuations in CT number values in homogeneous tissue or material [8]. Noise is inversely proportional to the tube voltage. A decrease in tube voltage will result in increased noise [5]. In this study, the tube voltage adjustment that provides low noise values is the 130 kVp tube voltage. However, the radiation dose given is too high. At 80 kVp tube voltage will provide a low radiation dose. However, the noise given is too high. Thus, based on the results of this study the tube voltage adjustment that is able to provide optimal image quality (less noise) and radiation doses is 110 kVp.

There is an increase in the value of image noise between scanning without SAFIRE and after the use of SAFIRE level strange 1, the highest increase in image noise at 80 kVp tube voltage with an image noise value of 3.6. The strange level 1 produces a more image noise. However, the graph also shows that at the use of strange levels 2–5, image noise will decrease. The lowest noise image value that is equal to 1.0 is generated by strange level 2 at 110 kVp tube voltage and strange level 5 at 130 kVp.

This noise reduction is in accordance with the level of SAFIRE strength level, i.e. the higher the use of SAFIRE strength level, the noise obtained will be lower. Noise reduction occurs due to the use of reconstruction with SAFIRE. SAFIRE is a reconstruction algorithm that works on raw data and image space data. The Head of MSCT image reconstruction process using SAFIRE is done in two ways, namely reconstruction of raw data and reconstruction of image data space. Reconstruction of the image space data is carried out by means of Filter Back Projection (FBP), namely statistical optimization, where there is a stratified sum of several data projections. Reconstruction on the results of this procedure are measured back projection. This process will occur repeatedly according to the chosen strength level.

The results of the reconstruction that occurred on the raw data and image space data then made a comparison, so that the comparison is obtained to a minimum. The above process will be repeated continuously in accordance with the selection of strength levels. This repetition is called iteration (iterative). The results obtained are images with low noise and sharpness. Setting a low SAFIRE strength level, fewer iterations will occur, so that the image will appear more noise. Whereas in setting a high SAFIRE strength level, iterations will occur more frequently, so that the image results obtained will appear smoother. The use of SAFIRE is able to reduce noise and still maintain the sharpness of the image (sharpness) [9]. SAFIRE is an iterative reconstruction advance technique that uses two projections, namely space (raw) data and image data space, where iterations occur in each space arranged according to scanning needs [10]. In images with low exposure factors, the noise will increase. After reconstruction with SAFIRE, the image obtained was smoother [11]. SAFIRE can reduce noise by 50–60% compared to using FBP [9, 12]. In other literature also mentions the results of images with a strength level of SAFIRE 1 i.e. the image will appear more noise. While on the strength level setting of SAFIRE 5 (S5) the image will appear smooth [10]. Increase SAFIRE reducing noise [13]. However, in the use of SAFIRE it is also necessary to pay attention to the patient's pathology, especially in the regulation of SAFIRE strength levels. Because setting the highest SAFIRE strength level does not always produce an optimal image [2].

5 Conclusion

There is a difference in the dose value on the MSCT Head of the spiral and sequence techniques in the variation of the tube voltage values of 130, 110 and 80 kVp. The radiation dose increases according to the increase in tube voltage and the sequence technique gives a higher dose than the spiral technique using CTDIvol. Based on dose measurements by the TLD badge, receiving doses in the eye and thyroid are lower by using the sequence technique.

MSCT image noise of spiral and sequence techniques on the variation of tube voltage values of 130, 110, and 80 kVp show the higher the tube voltage the image noise was less.

The relationship between the increase in strange level SAFIRE (1–5) with image noise is the higher the level of strange used (S5) the image noise is less and the image will be smoother.

Although the dose measured by TLD on all objects was still below the range, the use of increased tube voltage would cause the dose to increase as well. It is recommended to use optimal tube voltage. Using high SAFIRE, noise is reduced, but object detail is reduced. Further research is needed to determine the optimal tube voltage and the use of reconstruction algorithms that can produce better image quality

Based on TLD measurements. head CT scan using the sequence technique gives a lower dose than spiral. Because of using algorithm reconstruction SAFIRE (S-5) in spiral technique, it is possible setting lower tube voltage, so it can be decreasing doses and noise less.

References

1. Paper S, Ardley N, Buchan K, Lau K (2013) Efficacy of a liver detection algorithm for noise reduction in abdominal CT, pp 1–11
2. Exhibit S, Inoue T, Yamaguchi M, Bessho Y (2013) Assessment of a sinogram-affirmed iterative reconstruction (SAFIRE) on visual detection performance in chest phantom containing nodule ground-glass opacity, pp 1–10
3. Badan K, Tenaga P (2011) Available: chrome-extension://ohfgljdgelakfkefopgklcohadegdpjf/https://jdih.bapeten.go.id/unggah/dokumen/peraturan/81-full.pdf
4. Dalehaug I (2013) Optimization in CT, no. June, pp 1–77
5. Mcdermott S, Otrakji A, Kalra M (2017) Radiation dose optimization in CT, pp 557–561
6. Kubo T (2019) Vendor free basics of radiation dose reduction techniques for CT. Eur J Radiol 110:14–21
7. Kalra MK et al (2013) Sinogram-affirmed iterative reconstruction of low-dose chest CT: effect on image quality and radiation dose. Am J Roentgenol 201(2)
8. Busberg JT (2002) The essential physics of medical imaging
9. Ghetti C, Palleri F, Serreli G, Ortenzia O, Ruffini L (2013) Physical characterization of a new ct iterative reconstruction method operating in sinogram space. J Appl Clin Med Phys 14(4): 263–271
10. Grant K, Raupach R (2012) SAFIRE: Sinogram Affirmed Iterative Reconstruction (2012). Available: http://www.medical.siemens.com/siemens/en_US/%0Agg_ct_FBAs/files/Definition_AS/Safire.pdf
11. Singh S et al (2014) Radiation dose optimization and thoracic computed tomography. Radiol Clin North Am 52(1):1–15
12. Bodelle B et al (2014) Acute intracranial hemorrhage in CT: Benefits of sinogram-affirmed iterative reconstruction techniques. Am J Neuroradiol 35(3):445–449
13. Greffier J, Fernandez A, Macri F, Freitag C, Metge L, Beregi JP (2013) Which dose for what image? Iterative reconstruction for CT scan. Diagn Interv Imaging 94(11):1117–1121

Wrapper Subset Feature Selection for Optimal Feature Selection in Epileptic Seizure Signal Classification

Inung Wijayanto, Rudy Hartanto, and Hanung Adi Nugroho

Abstract Epilepsy is diagnosed by assessing the brain signal using an electroencephalograph (EEG). The assessment relies on manual visual inspection, which required experience and years of training. A computer-aided diagnose system can help neurologists assess the EEG signal. This study explores the epileptic condition by decomposing EEG signals using three levels of wavelet packet decomposition (WPD). Three orders of Daubechies mother wavelets are used. Since EEG is a non-stationary biological signal, an entropy measurement using the Shannon entropy is used to extract the signals' information. The next process is combining the features from all levels of the decomposed signals producing 14 number of features. This study reduces the number of features using the wrapper feature subset selection (WFSS) method. The searching algorithm used is the sequential backward (SBS) and forward (SFS) selection method. The multilayer perceptron neural network (MLPNN) is used for the classification method. The system achieves the highest accuracy of 91% by using seven number of features obtained from WPD (db2) + WFSS(SBS) + MLPNN. The minimum number of features is obtained using WPD(db16) + WFSS(SFS) + MLPNN, which produces six features. While the use of WFSS(SFS) in db16 produces six features with the highest increase of accuracy by 22%. This indicates that the use of WFSS can obtain an optimal number of features set and can improve the system's performance.

Keywords Epilepsy · EEG · Seizure · WPD · WFSS

I. Wijayanto (✉) · R. Hartanto · H. A. Nugroho
Department of Electrical and Information Engineering, Universitas Gadjah Mada, Yogyakarta, Indonesia
e-mail: inung.wijayanto@mail.ugm.ac.id

I. Wijayanto
School of Electrical Engineering, Telkom University, Bandung, Indonesia

H. Triwiyanto et al. (eds.), *Proceedings of the 1st International Conference on Electronics, Biomedical Engineering, and Health Informatics*, Lecture Notes in Electrical Engineering 746, https://doi.org/10.1007/978-981-33-6926-9_50

1 Introduction

Epilepsy is a brain disease, which characterized by short electrical spikes in the brain waves that leads to muscle spasm, convulsions, and loss of consciousness. This disease is spread all over the world, affecting more than 50 million people [1]. Lehnertz defined the conceptual definition of epilepsy as "a disorder of the brain characterized by an enduring predisposition to generate epileptic seizures and by neurobiological, cognitive, psychological, and social consequences of this condition" [2]. This conceptual definition requires at least one occurrence of seizure. However, epidemiologic researchers need an operational definition. Therefore, Thurman et al. define a person with epilepsy is when there are two unprovoked seizure occurs at least 24 h [3]. This operational definition is in line with the definition from the International League Against Epilepsy (ILAE) [4].

Neurologist mostly used EEG for diagnosing epilepsy. The diagnosis is conducted manually using visual inspection in the EEG recording, which requires experiences and a lot of time. The tedious, tiresome, and subjective process may lead to misinterpretation of the EEG signals [5]. Therefore, the continuous development of a computer-aided diagnose system is highly needed. Many studies have been conducted to detect the seizure and non-seizure conditions by locating the ictal period in the EEG recording [6–10]. From the machine learning (ML) point of view, the seizure detection process is challenging. It requires adequate data for training the classifier to reduce miss detection, low accuracy, and false alarms. Moreover, since the morphology of seizure among patients is inconsistent [11], a suitable feature extraction method plays an important role in detecting seizures in EEG recording.

The EEG signal's interpretation must follow the nature of EEG, which are non-stationary, non-linear, complex, and tends to be random. Therefore, a complexity-based analysis using entropy is suitable to analyze the EEG signal [12]. The use of complexity-based measurement has been conducted in studies that analyzing the EEG signal. Studies about Alzheimer's dementia detection system in EEG signals show lower complexity is found in patients with dementia [13, 14]. Similar studies about complexity measurement also performed in the epileptic EEG signals. Li et al. [15] measure the distribution entropy (DistEn) in EEG recording to classify the normal, interictal, and ictal condition of EEG. They measure the DistEn in full recording, one, and five-second non-overlapped window. The study is able to show significant differences between the normal, interictal, and ictal conditions ($p < 0.001$). Further research conducted using a combination of DistEn and Fuzzy entropy (FuzzyEn) obtained 93% as the highest accuracy in classifying normal and epileptic group (ictal and preictal) [16]. Moreover, the entropy calculation can be conducted in a multilevel scenario, which produces 94.3% of accuracy to classify normal, interictal, and ictal conditions [8]. Other multiscale calculation using entropy shows a significant result, producing 97.7% of accuracy [17].

The aforementioned studies were conducted using short term EEG recordings. The feature set produced by the proposed methods is fed directly to the classifiers.

A complete seizure detection system in the EEG signal should have a feature selection process [18]. Therefore, this study develops a seizure detection system that applies the wrapper feature subset selection as feature selection method to obtain the optimal number of features and improves the seizure detection system's performance.

2 Materials and Methods

The general process of epileptic seizure classification in this study is started by decomposing the signal using three levels of wavelet packet decomposition (WPD). This study investigates the use of Daubechies (db) wavelet functions in three different orders (db2, db8, and db16) to fit for the system. Each level of the decomposed signal then extracted using Shannon entropy (ShEN) to find the signal information, which produces 14 features for each order (regular feature set). The wrapper feature subset selection (WFSS) method then performed to select the best features (selected feature set). The multilayer perceptron neural network (MLPNN) is used to classify the regular and the selected feature set into three conditions: normal, interictal, and ictal. Finally, we analyze the system's performance by comparing the result. The general process of this study is shown in Fig. 1.

2.1 Bonn University Dataset

The EEG dataset used in this study is taken from Bonn University, which reported by Andrzejak et al. [19]. The dataset has five classes (Set A—Set E) representing three different conditions. The normal (Set A and Set B), interictal (set C and set D), and ictal classes (set E). The signal is recorded using 173.6 Hz of sampling frequency for 23.6 s. This study uses 100 data from each set B, set C, and set E with a total of 300 data. These sets are representing the three epileptically conditions. Figure 2 shows example of each class of EEG signals used in this study. Figure 2 shows the example of each class of EEG signals used in this study.

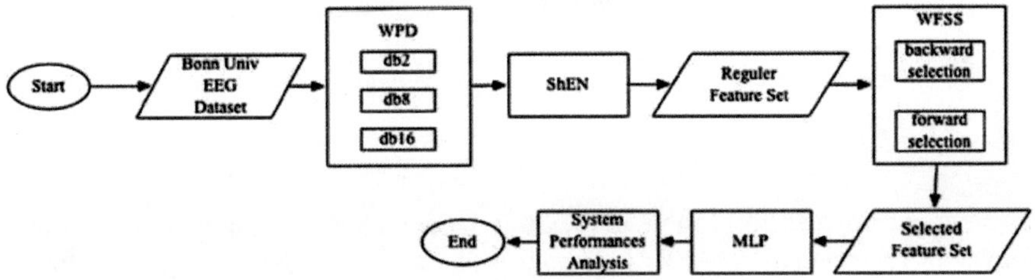

Fig. 1 General process of epileptic EEG signal classification

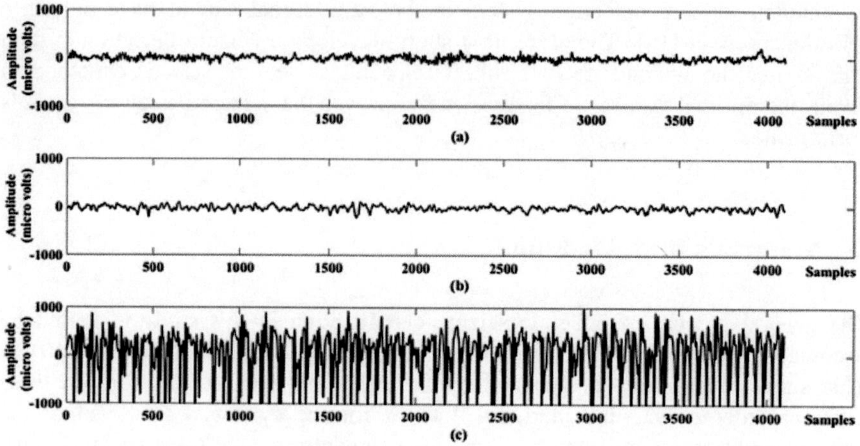

Fig. 2 The EEG signal representing three conditions; **a** normal, **b** interictal, **c** ictal

2.2 *Wavelet Packet Decomposition*

Wavelet packet decomposition (WPD) is a decomposition method that can be used to analyze a non-stationary signal such as EEG. A discrete signal $x[n]$ is decomposed into wavelet coefficients using DWT by shifting the wavelet functions (mother wavelets) [20]. Mother wavelet is a function that has certain periods and various amplitudes which localized in time and frequency. This study uses Daubechies as the mother wavelet since it has the ability to eliminate the noise in the EEG signal [21]. Three wavelet orders are used in this study to find out the correlation of the mother wavelet's order with the accuracy of the system. The DWT process is started by deciding the decomposition levels (N_k). In the first level, the signal $x[n]$ passed to a set of low and high-pass filters generating two signals called the detail (D_k) and approximation (A_k). For the next level ($N = 2$), the (A_k) is processed as the next input $x[n]$. This process is repeated until it reached the maximum decomposition levels (N_k). Since WPD is the extension of DWT, the decomposition process is executed for the (D_k) and the (A_k). Based on the decomposition process, the DWT produces $N + 1$ wavelet coefficients, while WPD produces 2^N. This study uses three levels of WPD, where the topology is illustrated in Fig. 3.

2.3 *Shannon Entropy*

Shannon entropy (ShEN) is able to measure the complexity of signal through time-frequency representation (TFR) [22], and it has a fast computation [23]. ShEN is expressed using (1).

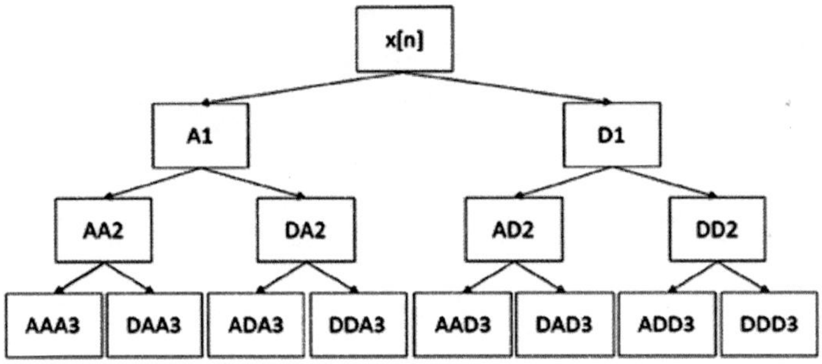

Fig. 3 The WPD process

$$ShEN = \sum_{i=1}^{n} P(x_i)\log_b \frac{1}{P(x_i)} \quad (1)$$

Here, $P(x_i)$ is the probability of occurrence of x_i and $b > 1$ [24].

2.4 *Wrapper Feature Subset Selection*

Determining the best subset feature from a feature set by observing the contribution for separating classes is the main objective of a feature subset selection (FSS). There are two methods for FSS, the filter, and the wrapper approach. The filter approach is conducted by calculating the feature's quality based on the data's intrinsic information, which gives faster computation and low complexity. On the other hand, the wrapper approach used the classifier accuracy to calculate the performance. It takes longer processing time but gives better performance [25]. This study uses two types of WFSS, the sequential forward selection (SFS), and sequential backward selection (SBS).

The SFS added the feature set to an empty candidate sequentially. Each feature is tested using the classifier algorithm. Then the best feature is combined with the next feature, which fed again to the classifier. This process is repeated until the system found the highest accuracy. The SBS works in the opposite way from the SFS. It removes features from the feature set sequentially. First, a feature set is used to find the best accuracy, and then one feature is removed in the next process. If the accuracy is not showing a significant decrease, then the feature is permanently deleted. The process is repeated until the removal brings a significant decrease to accuracy [26].

Figure 4 shows the searching process, which started by initiating the state space and initial space. The state space is a Boolean vector consisting of one bit per

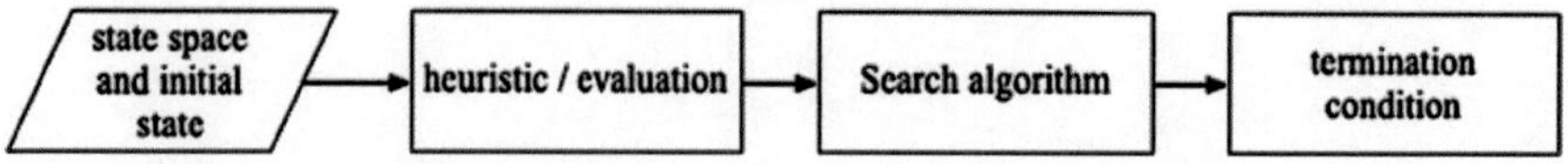

Fig. 4 The searching process of WFSS

Table 1 The best-first algorithm [25]

1	Put the initial state on the OPEN list,
2	Get the state from OPEN with max $f(w)$, $v = \arg\max_{w \in OPEN} f(w)$
3	Remove v from OPEN, add v to CLOSED
4	If $f(v) - \varepsilon > f(BEST)$, then BEST $\leftarrow v$
5	Expand v; apply all operator to v
6	For each child not in the CLOSED or OPEN list, evaluate and add to the OPEN list
7	If BEST changed in the last k expansions, go to 2
8	Return BEST

feature, while the initial state is an empty set. Five-fold cross-validation is used as the evaluation process, which is repeated multiple times. A small penalty is set to 0.1% for each feature. The search algorithm used in this study is the best-first search method, followed by a termination condition. The best first searching algorithm is shown in Table 1.

2.5 *Multi-layer Perceptron Neural Network*

The multilayer perceptron neural network (MLPNN) is a feed-forward artificial neural network, which operates fast and requires a smaller training set. It consists of three layers, the input, output, and hidden layers [27]. The hidden layer has an important role in transferring the information from the input to the output layer. The number of hidden layers is obtained by trial and error since it has no analytical method in determining the number of hidden layers [28]. Each of the hidden layer's neuron (j) is multiplied with the respective connection weights (w_{ij}) then sum the input signal x_i impinging onto it. The output is described as (2).

$$y_j = f \sum w_{ij} x_i \tag{2}$$

where f is the activation function such as thresholding, hyperbolic tangent, and the sigmoid function.

3 Result

This study is focused on observing the use of WFSS to select the features to increase system performance. Thus, this study compares the result before and after using the feature selection method. The experiment is conducted using three data classes, the normal, interictal, and ictal class (B-C-E). The typical signal of the normal, interictal, and ictal conditions is shown in Fig. 2. The interictal has a lower frequency and higher amplitude compared with the normal condition. Furthermore, the ictal condition has the lowest frequency and the highest amplitude compared to the two other conditions. The feature extraction process is done for each level (N) of WPD. There are 2^N features produced at each level. The first level produces two features. Four features are produced at the second level and eight features at the third level. Thus, the number of features produced for each signal is 14 features. To quantify the difference between the feature set in each class, one-way ANOVA is performed. The result showed in Table 2 indicate that each class has significant differences ($p < 0.05$). All the features are then classified using MLPNN with 10 cross-fold validation.

The first search method used in this study is the SBS, which refers to the searching sequence that begins with a full set of features. The process is started with the use of all features (14 features) then remove the insignificant features one by one using the best-first algorithm until there is no significant decrease in the system's performance. From the experiments, we obtained seven significant features in the WPD (db2) decomposed signals. On the other hand, the WPD (db8) and WPD (db16) obtained 9 and 11 significant features, respectively. The second method is the SFS method, which works in the opposite way of SBS. It started with an empty set, then added the features one by one to calculate the system performance. Next, when another feature is added, the system checks the performance. If there is a significant improvement, then the previously added feature is used as the selected feature. We obtained 9 and 10 number of selected features for WPD (db2) and WPD (db8), respectively. While the WPD (db16), we obtained six selected features. The detailed result is shown in Table 3.

Table 4 shows the complete classification result by using regular and the selected feature set. The system achieves the highest accuracy of 84.3% by using the 14 features and db2 as the mother wavelet. The accuracy is lower in the higher Daubechies order. Although the higher order of Daubechies mother wavelet can increase the smoothness of multiresolution analysis, it does not guarantee a better accuracy result [29].

Table 2 p-value using one-way ANOVA between feature sets for each mother wavelet used

Mother wavelet	p-value
db2	2.33×10^{-5}
db8	4.06×10^{-5}
db16	4.46×10^{-5}

Table 3 Selected features on SBS and SFS searching method

Mother wavelet	WFSS (SBS)	WFSS (SFS)
db2	1, 8, 9, 10, 12, 13, 14	2, 3, 4, 5, 8, 9, 10, 13, 14
db8	3, 4, 6, 8, 9, 10, 11, 12, 13	1, 2, 3, 4, 5, 6, 9, 10, 11, 13
db16	1, 3, 4, 5, 6, 8, 9, 10, 11, 12, 13	4, 7, 10, 11, 12, 13

4 Discussion

A significant result is achieved by applying the WFSS (SBS). The highest accuracy is obtained by selecting seven features (feature no.: 1, 8, 9, 10, 12, 13, and 14) from the three levels of WPD (db2). The accuracy is increased by 6.7% by using the selected features, from 84.3 to 90%. The highest increase of accuracy is 20.7%, which obtained by applying WPD (db16) + WFSS (SBS). Similar result also achieved by applying the WFSS (SFS). The system performance is increased from 5.7 to 22%. The least number of selected features is obtained by using a db16 wavelet filter. It produces 6 selected features (feature no.: 4, 7, 10, 11, 12, and 13) with 90.3% of accuracy. Shows that a higher order of Daubechies wavelet filter can produce the most significant increase in system performance. However, it does not guarantee the system to achieve the best accuracy. The highest accuracy in WFSS (SBS) is obtained in the lowest order of Daubechies mother wavelet. On the other hand, the highest accuracy of WFSS (SFS) is obtained in db8.

Based on the feature selection process using the wrapper technique, there are seven significant features out of 14 features that can be used to classify three conditions of the EEG signal. The WFSS(SFS) produce more features in the lower Daubechies' order, but it has higher accuracy in the higher-order compared to the WFSS(SBS). This happened because the best first algorithm in the WFSS(SBS) process is forcing the system to halt when the accuracy is decreased significantly. Furthermore, there is a possibility of performing an exhausted search to test all feature combinations, but it is not recommended due to the longer computation time.

Table 4 Comparison of system performances using all feature set and selected feature set

Mother wavelet	WPD + MLPNN		WPD + WFSS (SBS) + MLPNN		WPD + WFSS (SFS) + MLPNN	
	No. of features	Acc. (%)	No. of selected features	Acc. (%)	No. of selected features	Acc. (%)
db2	14	84.3	7	91	9	90
db8	14	74	9	90.3	10	90.7
db16	14	68.3	11	89	6	90.3

Table 5 Comparison with other studies

Author	Method	Feature reduction (%)	Performance improvement (%)
Assi et al. [30]	mRMR-Genetic Algorithm	98	4.71
Mursalin et al. [31]	Improved correlation-based feature selection	29	0.14
Sharmila et al. [32]	Best feature subsets based on estimation of mutual information	39	0
This study	WFSS (SBS)	50	6.7
	WFSS (SFS)	57	22

Assi et al. reduced the feature set up to 98% and increased the system performance up to 4.7% by using minimum redundancy maximum relevance (mRMR) combined with the genetic algorithm. Mursalin et al. used the improved correlation-based feature selection to obtain a 29% average feature reduction, increasing the system's performance by 0.14%. Sharmilla et al. can significantly reduce the feature set for 39%. The method in this study is outperformed the aforementioned study by producing the highest increase in system performance. The comparison is shown in Table 5.

5 Conclusion

This study performs a feature selection method to optimize the feature set of epileptic EEG signals. We decompose the signal using three levels of wavelet packet decomposition (WPD) with three orders of Daubechies mother wavelets. The decomposed signal is extracted using Shannon entropy measurement. This process produces 14 features for each order. The wrapper technique is done to select the most significant feature from each feature set. Two selection method is performed, the SBS and the SFS methods. The WFSS(SBS) method produces seven significant features and an accuracy of 91% as the best result. On the other hand, the WFSS(SFS) obtains ten significant features and 90.7% accuracy. By reducing the number of features, the classification process can be optimized and can be done faster. This study proves that the feature selection method is highly needed for analyzing the epileptic EEG signals. There is an opportunity to implement the feature selection method to the channel selection problem on multichannel EEG recordings.

Acknowledgements The Directorate General of Higher Education, Ministry of Research, Technology and Higher Education, Republic of Indonesia, funded this study through the Research Grant "Penelitian Disertasi Doktor" Universitas Gadjah Mada, No. 3125/UN1.DITLIT/DIT-LIT/PT/2020. This study also funded through the Research Grant "Program Rekoknisi Tugas Akhir" No.2488/UN1.P.III/DIT-LIT/PT/2020, from The Directorate of Research Universitas Gadjah Mada. The authors thank Telkom University that has provided a scholarship to study at Universitas Gadjah Mada and the Intelligent Systems research group in the Department of Electrical and Information Engineering Universitas Gadjah Mada for inspiring discussion and motivation.

References

1. World Health Organization (2019) WHO|Epilepsy: a public health imperative
2. Lehnertz K (2008) Epilepsy and Nonlinear Dynamics. J Biol Phys 34:253–266
3. Thurman DJ, Beghi E, Begley CE, Berg AT, Buchhalter JR, Ding D, Hesdorffer DC, Hauser WA, Kazis L, Kobau R, Kroner B, Labiner D, Liow K, Logroscino G, Medina MT, Newton CR, Parko K, Paschal A, Preux P-M, Sander JW, Selassie A, Theodore W, Tomson T, Wiebe S (2011) Standards for epidemiologic studies and surveillance of epilepsy. Epilepsia 52:2–26
4. International League Against Epilepsy (1993) Guidelines for epidemiologic studies on epilepsy. Commission on epidemiology and prognosis, International league against epilepsy. Epilepsia 34:592–596
5. Iasemidis LD (2003) Epileptic seizure prediction and control. IEEE Trans Biomed Eng 50:549–558
6. Rajendra Acharya U, Vinitha Sree S, Alvin APC, Suri JS (2012) Use of principal component analysis for automatic classification of epileptic EEG activities in wavelet framework. Expert Syst Appl 39:9072–9078
7. Wang L, Xue W, Li Y, Luo M, Huang J, Cui W, Huang C (2017) Automatic epileptic seizure detection in EEG signals using multi-domain feature extraction and nonlinear analysis. Entropy 19:222
8. Wijayanto I, Rizal A, Hadiyoso S (2018) Multilevel wavelet packet entropy and support vector machine for epileptic EEG classification. In: Proceedings—2018 4th international conference on science and technology, ICST 2018
9. Shaikh MHN, Farooq O, Chandel G (2019) EMD analysis of EEG signals for seizure detection. In: Lecture notes in electrical engineering. pp 189–196
10. Siuly S, Alcin OF, Bajaj V, Sengur A, Zhang Y (2019) Exploring Hermite transformation in brain signal analysis for the detection of epileptic seizure. IET Sci Meas Technol 13:35–41
11. Panayiotopoulos CP (2010) A clinical guide to epileptic syndromes and their treatment. Springer, London
12. Sanei S, Chambers JA (2007) EEG signal processing. Wiley, Ltd
13. Simons S, Espino P, Abásolo D (2018) Fuzzy entropy analysis of the electroencephalogram in patients with Alzheimer's disease: is the method superior to sample entropy? Entropy 20:21
14. Hadiyoso S, Mengko TLER, Zakaria H (2019) Complexity analysis of EEG signal in patients with cognitive impairment using the Hjorth descriptor. Proceedings—2019 2nd international conference bioinformatics, biotechnology Biomedical Engineering—Bioinformatics and Biomedical Engineering BioMIC 2019, pp 0–4
15. Li P, Yan C, Karmakar C, Liu C (2015) Distribution entropy analysis of epileptic EEG signals. In: 2015 37th annual international conference of the ieee engineering in medicine and biology society (EMBC). IEEE, pp. 4170–4173
16. Li P, Karmakar C, Yearwood J, Venkatesh S, Palaniswami M, Liu C (2018) Detection of epileptic seizure based on entropy analysis of short-term EEG. PLoS ONE 13:e0193691

17. Rizal A, Hadiyoso S (2018) Sample entropy on multidistance signal level difference for epileptic eeg classification. Sci World J 2018:1–6
18. Wijayanto I, Hartanto R, Nugroho HA, Setiawan NA (2019) A study on signal complexity measurement for epileptic seizure detection. In: 2019 IEEE 9th international conference on system engineering and technology (ICSET). IEEE, pp 320–325
19. Andrzejak RG, Lehnertz K, Mormann F, Rieke C, David P, Elger CE (2001) Indications of nonlinear deterministic and finite-dimensional structures in time series of brain electrical activity: Dependence on recording region and brain state. Phys Rev E 64:061907
20. Kevric J, Subasi A (2017) Comparison of signal decomposition methods in classification of EEG signals for motor-imagery BCI system. Biomed Signal Process Control 31:398–406
21. Mamun M, Al-Kadi M, Marufuzzaman M (2013) Effectiveness of wavelet denoising on electroencephalogram signals. J Appl Res Technol 11:156–160
22. Moukadem A, Dieterlen A, Brandt C (2013) Shannon entropy based on the S-transform spectrogram applied on the classification of heart sounds. In: ICASSP, IEEE international conference on acoustics, speech and signal processing—proceedings. IEEE, pp 704–708
23. Naidu MSR, Rajesh Kumar P, Chiranjeevi K (2018) Shannon and Fuzzy entropy based evolutionary image thresholding for image segmentation. Alexandria Eng J 57:1643–1655
24. Borowska M (2015) Entropy-based algorithms in the analysis of biomedical signals. Stud Logic Gramm Rhetor 43:21–32
25. Kohavi R, John GH (1997) Wrappers for feature subset selection. Artif Intell 97:273–324
26. Marill T, Green DM (1963) On the effectiveness of receptors in recognition systems. IEEE Trans Inf Theory 9:11–17
27. Orhan U, Hekim M, Ozer M (2011) EEG signals classification using the K-means clustering and a multilayer perceptron neural network model. Expert Syst Appl 38:13475–13481
28. Hazarika N, Chen JZ, Tsoi AC, Sergejew A (1997) Classification of EEG signals using the wavelet transform. In: Proceedings of 13th international conference on digital signal processing. IEEE, pp 89–92
29. Daubechies I (1990) The wavelet transform, time-frequency localization and signal analysis. IEEE Trans Inf Theory 36:961–1005
30. Assi EB, Sawan M, Nguyen DK, Rihana S (2015) A hybrid mRMR-genetic based selection method for the prediction of epileptic seizures. In: 2015 IEEE biomedical circuits and systems conference (BioCAS). IEEE (2015)
31. Mursalin M, Zhang Y, Chen Y, Chawla NV (2017) Automated epileptic seizure detection using improved correlation-based feature selection with random forest classifier. Neurocomputing 241:204–214
32. Sharmila A, Geethanjali P (2018) Epileptic seizure detection from EEG signals using best feature subsets based on estimation of mutual information for support vector machines and naïve bayes classifiers. In: Lecture notes in electrical engineering, pp 585–593

Preliminary Study of EEG Characterization Using Power Spectral Analysis in Post-stroke Patients with Cognitive Impairment

Sugondo Hadiyoso, Hasballah Zakaria, Tati Latifah E. R. Mengko, and Paulus Anam Ong

Abstract Post-stroke dementia (PSD) or post-stroke cognitive impairment can occur in one-third of stroke sufferers. Therefore, we need a detection protocol so that patients get treatment early. Electroencephalogram (EEG) analysis is one of the methods to study deteriorating brain function where visual observation is commonly used. However, this method requires expert experience and time-consuming. Therefore, in this study, a method for characterizing EEG waves in post-stroke patients with cognitive impairment is proposed by calculating and analyzing quantitative EEG (QEEG) parameters. This study proposes a linear QEEG method through the power spectral analysis approach to characterize post-stroke patients with cognitive impairments and normal subjects. This study used a resting-awake EEG dataset collected from nineteen participants consisting of ten normal subjects, five post-stroke patients with mild cognitive impairment, and four post-stroke patients with dementia. The experiment results showed significant differences in the relative power between the three groups. These include (1) increase in delta activity and simultaneously a decrease in alpha, beta and gamma activity in dementia patients, (2) Significant differences (p-value < 0.05) on these bands are most commonly found on the frontal area electrodes and (3) there is linearity between power spectral density and the severity of dementia. This preliminary study showed that relative power analysis could be a discriminant feature among normal, post-stroke patients with mild cognitive impairment and post-stroke patients with dementia. It is hoped that the proposed method can be used to assist doctors in the early detection of post-stroke dementia and monitor the progress of dementia.

Keywords Post-stroke dementia · QEEG · Power spectral · Early detection

---

S. Hadiyoso (✉) · H. Zakaria · T. L. E. R. Mengko
School of Electrical Engineering and Informatics, Bandung Institute of Technology, Bandung, Indonesia
e-mail: sugondo@telkomuniversity.ac.id

P. A. Ong
Departement of Neurology, Faculty of Medicine, Padjadjaran University/
Dr. Hasan Sadikin General Hospital, Bandung, Indonesia

H. Triwiyanto et al. (eds.), *Proceedings of the 1st International Conference on Electronics, Biomedical Engineering, and Health Informatics*, Lecture Notes in Electrical Engineering 746, https://doi.org/10.1007/978-981-33-6926-9_51

1 Introduction

Stroke is a leading cause of physical disability and cognitive impairment. Even minor strokes can affect executive and cognitive function, consequently affecting the quality of life and ability to work. However, the fact that physical disability receives more attention than cognitive impairment [1]. Whereas cognitive deterioration also contributes to the deterioration of the patient's health condition [2, 3]. Stroke patients will develop 30% of dementia post six months after stroke onset [4]. About 20–25% of subjects will experience delayed dementia [5].

Risk factors will increase with age, where the risk of vascular dementia doubles every five years. Based on Riskesdas data in 2013, the stroke prevalence rate was 7% and increased to 10.9% in 2018 [6]. The proportion of strokes increases at the age of more than 55 years by more than 30%, this is proportional to increasing age. With a vast number of older adults with stroke risk factors, Indonesia will encounter a large number of vascular dementia. Vascular dementia is a form of cognitive impairment associated with blood vessel disease in the brain. Vascular dementia (VaD), contributes around 20% of dementia cases worldwide [7].

Various instruments are available to assess cognitive status, with some specific instruments for post-stroke dementia. Cognitive can be assessed using the Mini-Mental State Examination (MMSE) or Montreal Cognitive Assessment (MoCA) test [8]. Diagnosis through biomarkers has also been proposed, including genetic polymorphisms, cerebrospinal fluid, and microRNA profiles profiles [9, 10]. Furthermore, imaging techniques are an essential diagnostic tool for post-stroke dementia. For example, MRI, CT, or PET imaging is a crucial neuroimaging modality and has high sensitivity and specificity for detecting pathological changes, including small vessel disease that causes cognitive impairment [11–13]. However, this modality requires specific equipment that is relatively expensive, takes a long time, and risks that can be caused when carried out periodically in a short time [14].

Over the past several decades, electroencephalogram (EEG) has the potential to observe brain cortical abnormalities associated with cognitive impairment and dementia [15]. EEG waves correlate with function, dysfunction, and diseases of the central nervous system due to neuronal cell death in areas of the brain. Thus the EEG can be thought to complement diagnostic criteria related to cognitive impairment. Quantitative EEG or (QEEG) techniques can provide numerical information about EEG wave characteristics related to brain disorders. Several studies have focused on using QEEG to study characteristics, evaluate the severity or differentiate types of dementia, as reported in [14–20]. The final goal of processing the EEG signals related to dementia is to obtain specific distinguishing characteristics and obtain the highest accuracy.

Although the studies that have been proposed cannot be compared directly because of differences in data sources, EEG recording techniques, or EEG devices, which are used, the studies that have been reported are generally useful to support the hypotheses of other related studies. Thus the EEG will be able to be a tool in diagnosing cognitive dysfunction.

In this paper, a preliminary study was conducted to characterize EEG signals in post-stroke patients with cognitive impairment. The aim is to compare EEG wave patterns in patients with cognitive impairment and normal subjects so that this analysis can be used for detection in the future. Quantitative analysis on EEG waves, which is proposed, is the power spectral on conventional EEG bands, including delta (δ), theta (θ), alpha (α), beta (β), and gamma (γ). We use wavelet transforms for segmenting the traditional EEG band. Then the power spectral is calculated for each band. Measurement of spectral power from EEG waves is expected to provide a specific point of view if there is impaired cognitive function. Thus, this can be a tool for the detection of abnormalities.

As a reminder, the paper is organized as follows: Sect. 2 is a material and method that describes the EEG recording and the method used in EEG characterization. The results of the calculation of relative power parameters followed by statistical analysis is explained in Sect. 3. The last section is the conclusion and future work of the research.

2 Material and Method

The stages of EEG signal characterization in this study are shown in Fig. 1. These stages include the signal pre-processing stage for noise removal, then the segmentation of the EEG band (delta, theta, alpha, beta, and gamma) using wavelet transform. The next stage, power spectral measurement, uses Welch's periodogram and then performs the relative power calculations on each EEG band. The last stage is the significance of the difference test and analysis. The details of these methods are presented in the following sub-sections.

2.1 EEG Recording

In this preliminary study, we involved 19 subjects with 10 normal control subjects, five post-stroke patients with mild cognitive impairment, and four post-stroke patients with dementia. Post-stroke patients are validated based on brain CT scans

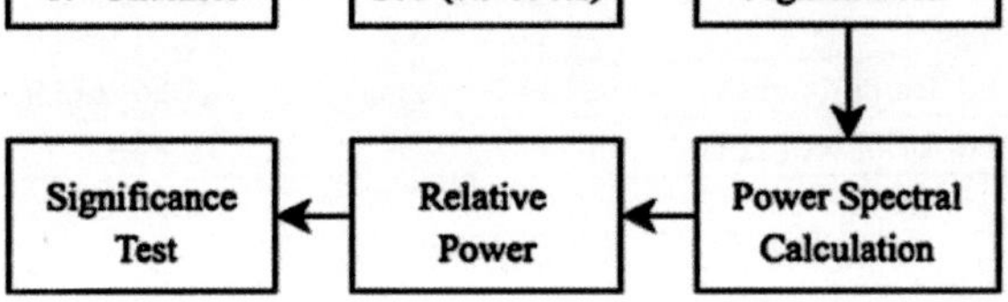

Fig. 1 The proposed characterization method

by neurologists. The subjects' cognitive status was determined by psychologists and neurologists, who were confirmed based on the MoCA-Ina test and interviews. All groups consisted of men and women with a ratio of almost 50%. Control subjects were selected with the following criteria: healthy, not indicated neurological disorders and physiological disorders and had never suffered a brain injury. Subjects were considered normal, post-stroke cognitive impairment, and post-stroke dementia if they have a score of more than 23, 19–23, and 0–18, respectively. All volunteers agreed to participate in this study by filling in informed consent. Clinical data from the patient and control groups are presented in Table 1.

The EEG recording was done with the Cadwell Easy III Amplification System. The electrodes are placed on the skin according to the standard 10–20 system with 19 electrodes (Fp1, Fp2, F7, F3, Fz, F4, F8, T3, C3, Cz, C4, T4, T5, P3, Pz, P4, T6, O1, and O2) and two reference electrodes including A1 and A2. All EEG signals have a sampling frequency of 250 Hz. Power noise was filtered with a 50 Hz notch filter. These settings are performed in a recording software application. The recording was done in a comfortable and quiet room with dim lighting. EEG recording was done in a conscious, relaxed, eyes closed, lying on a bed for five minutes. Digital data of raw EEG signals are stored in European Data Format (*. EDF). The cognitive test and EEG recording were carried out at Hasan Sadikin Hospital, under the supervision of a neurologist. The ethics committee approved the protocol in this study of the Hasan Sadikin Hospital, Bandung, Indonesia.

2.2 *Quantitative EEG/QEEG*

Quantitative EEG (QEEG) is a computer-based analysis of a continuous EEG signal. Raw digital EEG data recorded results are then analyzed and compared with the reference database of normal subjects. QEEG parameters include absolute power, relative power, symmetry, coherence, the correlation across the phase spectrum, and peak frequency [20]. The results of the QEEG analysis are displayed

Table 1 Clinical data from the control group and patient group

	Normal control	Patients	
		Cognitive impairment no dementia	Dementia
Number of samples	10	5	4
Gender (M/F)	6/4	3/2	2/2
Age	57.9 ± 3.6	59.2 ± 4.08	59 ± 5.59
Education (years)	14.2 ± 2.53	10.6 ± 3.91	11.75 ± 4.5
Stroke onset (month)	–	9.8 ± 6	15.25 ± 2.87
MoCA-Ina	26 ± 1	20 ± 1	9.75 ± 4.4

in the form of statistical tables and topographic maps. Thus, differences in the normative set can be observed to support the diagnosis.

In this study, one of the QEEG parameters which are analyzed is the power spectral. Power spectral describes the energy distribution of a series of signals in the frequency domain. The magnitude of the power spectral can be expressed in Power Spectral Density (PSD), which is the power of a signal as a function of frequency. In this study, spectral information from EEG signals was obtained through mathematical transformations, namely Wavelet Transform and Welch Periodogram method. The methods used in this study are explained in the following sub-sections.

2.3 Wavelet Transform

Wavelet Transform (WT) is a signal analysis method that is commonly used in biological signals with non-stationary properties such as EEG. Wavelet can characterize signals locally and in detail according to scale. Therefore, WT is suitable for analyzing non-stationary signals or has transient components within a short time. Wavelet transform is an analysis tool in the time-frequency domain which produces a series of orthonormal signals and matches those generated by the wavelet function.

The wavelet will divide data into several different frequency components using a resolution that is appropriate to the scale. Thus, there is a process of translation and dilation of the wavelet basis function to the analyzed signal. Mathematically the wavelet function is expressed as follows:

$$W_x^{\psi}(\tau, s) = \frac{1}{\sqrt{|s|}} \int x(t)\psi * \left(\frac{t-\tau}{s}\right) \mathrm{d}t \quad (1)$$

In this study, WT was used as a filter bank for segmenting signals into conventional EEG bands, including delta (δ), theta (θ), alpha (α), beta (β), and gamma (γ) with Daubechies-2 (DB2) as mother wavelet. The signal was decomposed to 5 levels according to the sampling frequency used to generate these bands. The frequency of wavelet decomposition in EEG segmentation is shown in Table 2.

Table 2 Wavelet decomposition (Sub-band) and correspondence with EEG frequency bands

Sub-band	Frequency band (Hz)	EEG frequency
D2	31.25–62.5	Gamma (γ)
D3	15–31.25	Beta (β)
D4	7.5–15	Alpha (α)
D5	3.75–7.5	Theta (θ)
A5	0–3.75	Delta (δ)

2.4 Relative Power Analysis

Relative power is measured as spectral power on the band, which is observed to the total power of all EEG bands. The absolute power of the five EEG bands is then estimated using the Welch Periodogram, and then the relative power can be measured. The following equation is the estimated spectral power using Welch [21], which is calculated on each EEG band.

$$\breve{P}_{xx}^{W} = \frac{1}{U}\sum_{i=0}^{U-1}\breve{P}_{xx}^{i}(f) \tag{2}$$

where

$\breve{P}_{xx}^{i}(f)$ Spectral estimation $X_i(n)$
$\breve{P}_{xx}^{W}$ Spectral estimation Welch
U Window normalization function.

The signal power was segmented with a duration of 2 s and a 50% overlap to get representative power estimation results and EEG records. The number of n-segments then averaged the measured power. Furthermore, relative power can be calculated using Equation below.

$$P_{\text{relative}} = \frac{P_{\text{abs}(i)}}{\sum_{fL}^{fH} P_{\text{abs}}} \tag{3}$$

where $P_{\text{abs}(i)}$ is the power of the selected frequency and [fL, fH] are the frequency bands of delta, theta, alpha, beta and gamma.

2.5 Statistical Analysis

Statistical analysis is intended to measure the significant difference in the relative power parameters between the patient group and the normal control group. As the primary analysis, we investigated whether there was a statistically significant difference in EEG's relative power between the patient group and the normal group. We apply a one-way analysis of variance (ANOVA) to test the significance of the relative power for each EEG electrode. The difference in relative power between groups is considered to have significance if the p-value < 0.05. This statistical calculation is performed in Excel.

3 Results and Discussion

This section presents the results of power spectral measurements including relative power and statistical analysis. This is followed by an explanation and discussion related to these results.

3.1 Power Spectral Analysis

The Welch measurement results on 19 electrodes with a frequency range of 1–60 Hz in normal subjects are shown in Fig. 2. From the results of these measurements, it can be seen that the EEG wave power spectrum tends to be dominant in the alpha (7.5–15 Hz) frequency band.

Meanwhile, the results of Welch measurements from post-stroke no dementia patients are shown in Fig. 3. From these measurements, it can be seen that the EEG wave power spectra in some electrodes tend to be dominant in low frequencies that are the delta band, whereas the power spectra of post-stroke dementia patients show that the signal power is dominant in the delta band in all electrodes. The Welch estimation results for dementia patients are shown in Fig. 4.

Figures 2 and 4 show examples of spectra Welch estimation results for dementia patients and normal subjects. Figure 2 shows that the power spectral of EEG in normal subjects has a higher power at the frequency of 7.5–15 Hz or dominant on

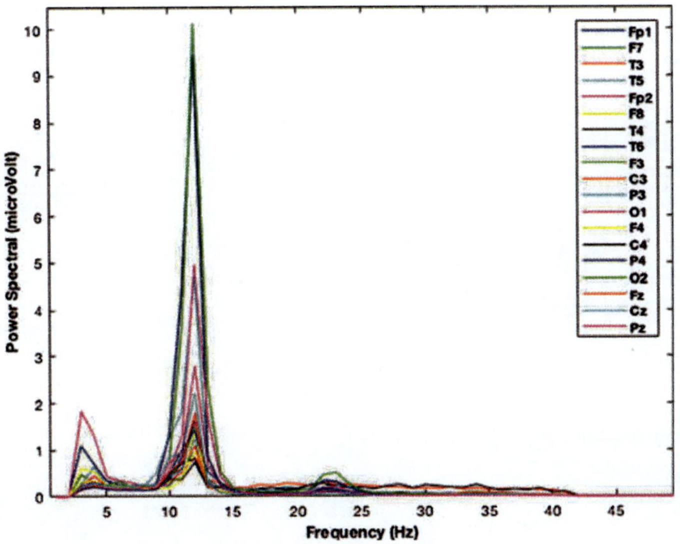

Fig. 2 Power spectrum on 19 electrodes EEG from Subject normal-1

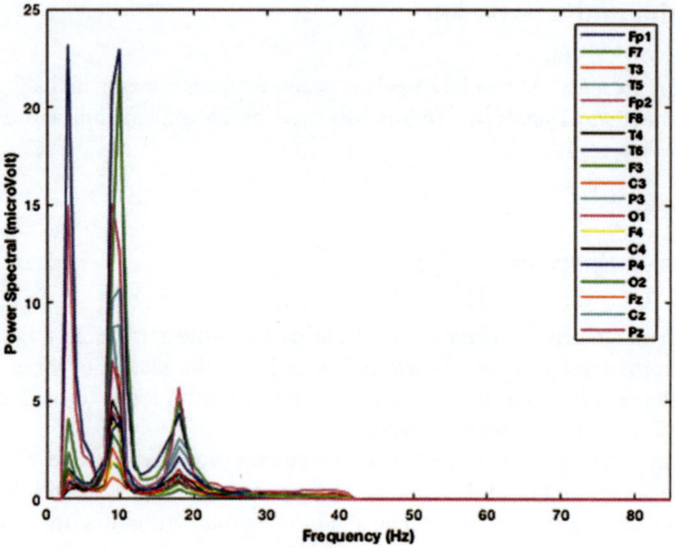

Fig. 3 Power spectrum on 19 electrodes EEG from post-stroke no dementia patient-1

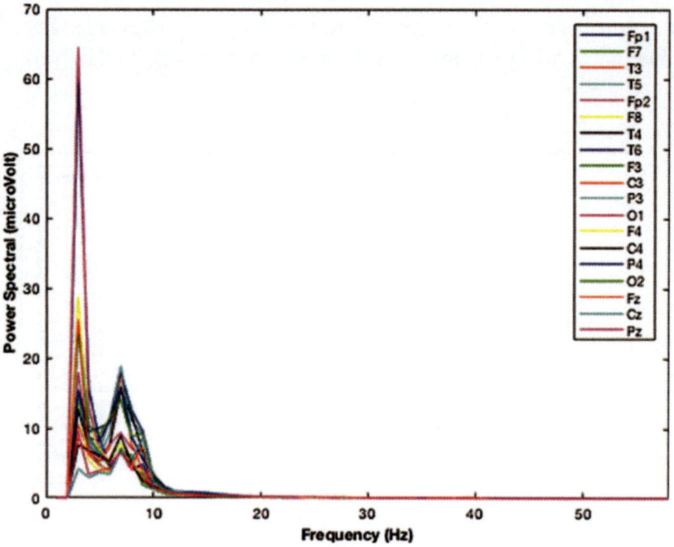

Fig. 4 Power spectrum on 19 electrodes EEG from post-stroke with dementia patient-1

the alpha band. On the contrary, in Fig. 4, it can be seen that the spectral power of EEG in patients with dementia has a higher power at a lower frequency of 1–4 Hz or dominant on the delta band. This represented that the EEG wave of dementia patients increased in power in the delta frequency and was followed by a decrease in the alpha frequency. In other terms, there is a slowing of the EEG wave.

3.2 *Relative Power and Statistical Analysis*

The relative power spectrum of each EEG band is measured using Eq. 3. Relative power can mean a normalization process because the magnitude of EEG varies between person. Thus, the relative power can eliminate bias that causes misinterpretation. The results of the average relative power for each group are presented in Table 3. The alpha ratio decreased in the dementia group showing that in dementia there was a decrease in alpha power and an increase in delta power compared to the normal group. These results show a more detailed depiction of the shift of power spectral on the 19-EEG electrodes. EEG signals in post-stroke with dementia subjects become slower, meaning that the power in the EEG spectrum is

Table 3 The ratio of relative power of each group

Channel	Normal		Post-stroke no dementia		Post-stroke dementia	
	α/δ	α/θ	α/δ	α/θ	α/δ	α/θ
Fp1	1.931	1.604	0.416	1.335	0.244	0.798
Fp2	1.631	1.459	0.430	1.346	0.277	0.908
F7	1.370	1.533	0.837	1.516	0.287	0.624
F3	2.825	1.757	1.299	1.911	1.250	1.085
Fz	2.857	1.553	1.976	2.040	1.178	1.194
F4	2.395	1.670	1.491	2.057	1.192	1.316
F8	1.197	1.256	0.907	1.650	0.430	0.994
T3	2.846	1.682	1.870	1.792	0.508	0.798
C3	2.383	1.776	2.130	2.038	1.382	1.133
Cz	2.354	1.381	3.168	1.927	1.366	1.300
C4	2.531	1.560	3.181	2.548	1.214	1.262
T4	2.297	2.185	1.998	2.066	1.138	1.238
T5	6.257	2.059	4.031	2.677	1.291	1.234
P3	3.258	1.973	4.880	3.849	1.068	1.076
Pz	2.625	1.668	2.407	2.630	0.841	1.153
P4	3.401	2.223	5.439	3.543	1.355	1.424
T6	7.724	2.832	5.602	2.684	4.443	2.809
O1	5.335	2.359	4.433	3.892	1.263	2.018
O2	6.679	2.760	4.204	3.527	2.758	3.514

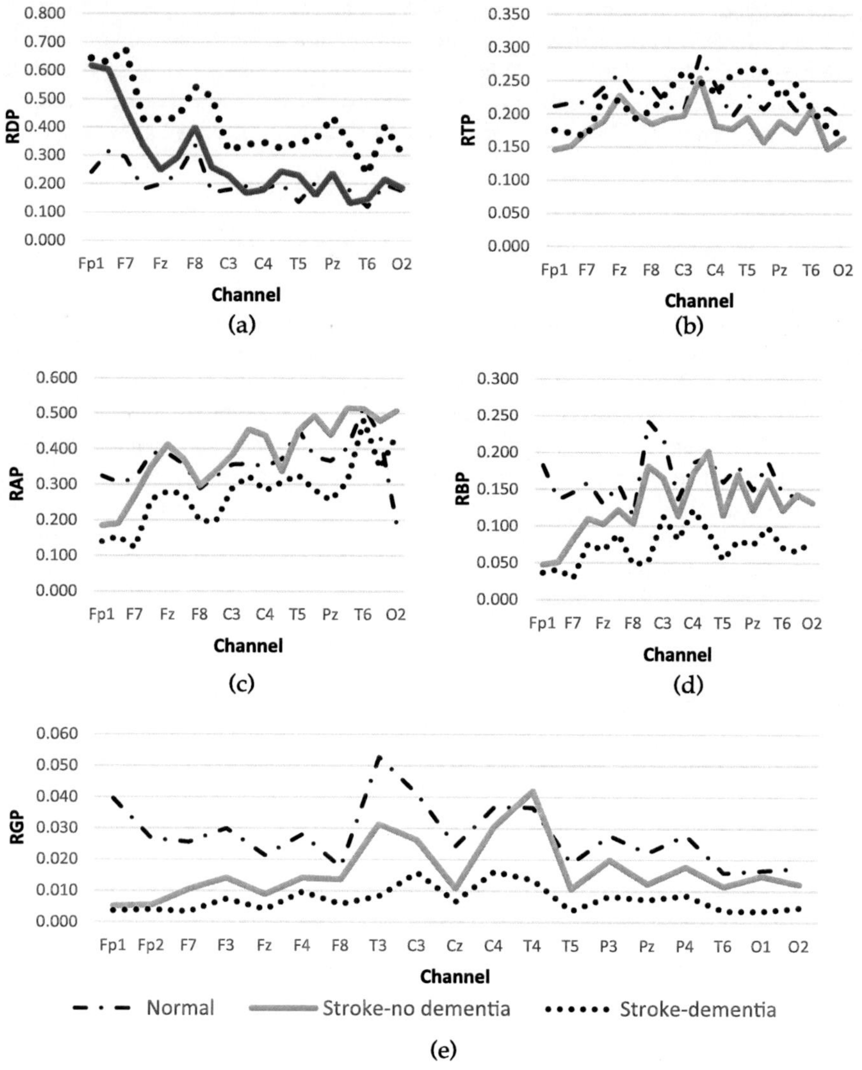

Fig. 5 The relative power in the **a** delta, **b** theta, **c** alpha, **d** beta and **e** gamma bands of each group

concentrated at lower frequencies. For clarify, Fig. 5 shows the relative power in the delta, theta, alpha, beta and gamma bands of each group.

In post-stroke dementia patients showed a higher trend of delta band power than the normal group. However, slow EEG waves do not occur in all electrodes. We also highlighted the average relative power of delta, beta, and gamma in no dementia patients having a trend to be between normal and dementia groups. There is linearity between the power of the EEG signal and the severity of dementia, as reported in the study [22–26].

The ANOVA test among groups was then carried out to confirm the significance of the difference in the relative power characteristics of each band. The ANOVA test results are presented in Table 4. Based on statistical measurements, the three groups show differences in relative power. Most significant differences (p-value < 0.05) are found on the delta, alpha, beta, and gamma bands. The relative delta power in the dementia group was higher than the normal group, as explained in the study [27], in cases of vascular dementia. Then simultaneously decrease in power in alpha, beta, and gamma bands [27, 28]. Significant differences in the delta, alpha, and gamma waves were mostly found in electrode at the frontal area (p-value < 0.05). In the case of cerebrovascular disease, the density of the delta rhythm in the frontal area will increase as a result of dementia [29].

The different characteristics between normal and cognitive impairment conditions can be caused by different brain conditions due to the degradation of some neurons. Delta waves occur when a deep sleep condition or conscious condition in person who has brain disorders [25, 30]. Whereas in normal subjects, the existence of alpha waves occurs when in a conscious condition, relax, and eyes closed [25].

The results of this preliminary study showed a correlation between power spectral and the severity of dementia. This study can be used as a marker of

Table 4 The test results of significance differences in the relative power of each EEG band

Channel	Delta	Theta	Alpha	Beta	Gamma
Fp1	0.000*	0.121	0.021*	0.004*	0.008*
Fp2	0.012*	0.107	0.021*	0.002*	0.002*
F7	0.015*	0.300	0.045*	0.052	0.142
F3	0.033*	0.507	0.198	0.02*	0.001*
Fz	0.041*	0.628	0.212	0.005*	0.000*
F4	0.135	0.719	0.474	0.049*	0.016*
F8	0.214	0.199	0.391	0.025*	0.043*
T3	0.001*	0.761	0.086	0.001*	0.024*
C3	0.139	0.170	0.503	0.073	0.158
Cz	0.027*	0.631	0.208	0.031*	0.016*
C4	0.061	0.163	0.174	0.207	0.415
T4	0.201	0.113	0.481	0.099	0.150
T5	0.053	0.221	0.264	0.000*	0.007*
P3	0.268	0.045*	0.112	0.038*	0.080
Pz	0.119	0.416	0.152	0.064	0.058
P4	0.050*	0.294	0.119	0.047*	0.022*
T6	0.457	0.916	0.858	0.012*	0.005*
O1	0.322	0.966	0.399	0.042*	0.074
O2	0.697	0.174	0.801	0.122	0.042*

*p-value < 0.05

progression from mild cognitive impairment to dementia in post-stroke patients. Therefore, this result is expected to be used as an early warning for abnormalities in brain function. Thus, early treatment can be taken to avoid further deterioration of brain function. We know that it may be too early to conclude the results of this study, since the number of samples still a little bit, especially in post-stroke patients. Another limitation is that the normal group of post-stroke patients has not been included in this study which can be used as a baseline. However, at least, this study can provide knowledge that each group has discriminant characteristics. With the automatic classification algorithm, the proposed method can simplify the detection process as additional validation in clinical diagnoses.

4 Conclusion

This preliminary study focuses on analyzing EEG's use, especially quantitative EEG as a biosignal for the detection of post-stroke dementia. Visual observations on EEG are prone to errors due to visual limitations and the subjectivity of medical experts. With analysis through signal processing methods is expected to simplify the process and provide objective results. The quantitative EEG method is considered to have excellent performance for analyzing EEG signals in normal subjects and dementia, as explained in Sect. 3.

In this research phase, we have performed spectral analysis as a feature to characterize resting EEG signals in three groups of subjects, namely normal control (10), stroke-MCI patients (5), and stroke patients with dementia (4). A total of 19 EEG signals from the three groups have been analyzed. Relative power analysis is performed on frontal, temporal, parietal, and occipital electrodes. From this analysis, it was found that compared to the normal group, in dementia patients, there was an increase in delta activity and simultaneously a decrease in alpha, beta, and gamma activity. Statistically significant differences (p-value < 0.05) in these bands were most often found in the frontal area. In post-stroke patients, no dementia or MCI tends to have characteristics between the normal and dementia groups, with the significant differences in the relative power of beta and gamma bands. This study is expected to be used as a marker of progression from the stage of mild cognitive impairment to dementia in post-stroke patients.

Acknowledgements The authors would like to thank the Directorate General of Higher Education, Ministry of Research, Technology, and Higher Education of the Republic of Indonesia for supporting funding through the Research Grant "Penelitian Disertasi Doktor" No. 2/AMD/E1/KP.PTNBH/2020. The authors would also like to thank Hasan Sadikin Hospital, Bandung in particular the Department of Neurology for supporting EEG recording. Acknowledgments are also given to Telkom University for providing the scholarships.

References

1. Mellon L et al (2015) Cognitive impairment six months after ischaemic stroke: a profile from the ASPIRE-S study. BMC Neurol. 15(1):1–9
2. Barker-Collo SL et al (2009) Reducing attention deficits after stroke using attention process training: a randomized controlled trial. Stroke 40(10):3293–3298
3. Mohd Zulkifly MF et al (2016) A review of risk factors for cognitive impairment in stroke survivors. Sci World J
4. Mijajlović MD et al (2017) Post-stroke dementia—a comprehensive review. BMC Med 15(1): 1–12
5. O'Brien JT (2014) Vascular dementia. Pet Spect Neurol 386:417–435
6. Kementerian Kesehatan (2018) Hasil Utama RISKESDAS 2018
7. Van Der Flier WM, Scheltens P (2005) Epidemiology and risk factors of dementia. Neurol Pract 76(5)
8. Henderson G et al (2006) Development and assessment of methods for detecting dementia using the human electroencephalogram. IEEE Trans Biomed Eng 53(8):1557–1568
9. Sanei S, Chambers JA (2007) EEG signal processing. Wiley (2007)
10. Nguyen T (2013) Total number of synapses in the adult human neocortex. Undergrad J Math Model One+Two 3(1):1–13
11. Guermazi A et al (2007) Neuroradiological findings in vascular dementia. Neuroradiology 49(1):1–22
12. Kanekar S, Poot JD (2014) Neuroimaging of Vascular Dementia. Radiol Clin North Am 52(2):383–401
13. Heiss WD et al (2016) Neuroimaging in vascular cognitive impairment: a state-of-the-art review. BMC Medicin 14(1):1–8
14. Petrovic J et al (2017) Slower EEG alpha generation, synchronization and "flow"—possible biomarkers of cognitive impairment and neuropathology of minor stroke. Peer J 5:3839
15. Klimesch W (2012) Alpha-band oscillations, attention, and controlled access to stored information. Trends Cognit Sci 16(12):606–617
16. Szelies B et al (1994) Quantitative topographical EEG compared to FDG PET for classification of vascular and degenerative dementia. Electroencephalogr Clin Neurophysiol 91(2):131–139
17. Al-qazzaz NK, Ali SH (2018) Technique in discriminating vascular dementia EEGs. In: 2nd international conference on biosignal analysis, processing and systems (ICBAPS), pp 109–112
18. Al-Qazzaz NK et al (2016) EEG markers for early detection and characterization of vascular dementia during working memory tasks. In: IECBES 2016—IEEE-EMBS conference on biomedical engineering and sciences, pp 347–351
19. Al-Qazzaz NK et al (2017) Stroke-related mild cognitive impairment detection during working memory tasks using EEG signal processing. International Conference on Advances in Biomedical Engineering, ICABME
20. Sheng H, Xu J, Zheng C (2010) Time-frequency analysis of vascular dementia EEG signals using generalized S-transform. 2010 4th international conference on bioinformatics and biomedical engineering, iCBBE, pp 3–6
21. Tuffner FK, Pierre JW, Kubichek RF (2008) Computationally efficient updating of a weighted welch periodogram for nonstationary signals. In: Midwest symposium on circuits and systems, pp 799–802
22. McBride JC et al (2014) Spectral and complexity analysis of scalp EEG characteristics for mild cognitive impairment and early Alzheimer's disease. Comput Methods Programs Biomed 114(2):153–163
23. Cassani R et al (2018) Systematic review on resting-state EEG for Alzheimer's disease diagnosis and progression assessment. Dis Mark 1–26 (2018)

24. Houmani N et al (2018) Diagnosis of Alzheimer's disease with Electroencephalography in a differential framework. PLoS ONE 13(3):1–19
25. Al-Qazzaz NK et al (2014) Role of EEG as biomarker in the early detection and classification of dementia. Sci World J 1–16
26. Fraga FJ et al (2013) Characterizing Alzheimer's disease severity via resting-awake eeg amplitude modulation analysis. PLoS ONE 8(8):1–7
27. Neto E et al (2015) EEG spectral features discriminate between Alzheimer' s and vascular dementia. Front Neurol 6(February):1–9
28. Soni S et al (2017) Neourodynamics in patient with Alzheimer's disease during working memory task. Sch J Appl Med Sci 5(8D):3257–3263
29. Oakes TR et al (2004) Functional coupling of simultaneous electrical and metabolic activity in the human brain. Hum Brain Mapp 21(4):257–270
30. Handayani N et al (2016) Preliminary study of Alzheimer's Disease diagnosis based on brain electrical signals using wireless EEG. J Phys Conf Ser 694(1)

Comparative Analysis of the Phonocardiogram Denoising System Based-on Empirical Mode Decomposition (EMD) and Double-Density Discrete Wavelet Transform (DDDWT)

T. Y. Fatmawati, A. Yuliani, M. A. Afandi, and D. Zulherman

Abstract Phonocardiogram (PCG), one of the auscultation-based technique used as a diagnostic method of the heart condition, is a patient's heart sound recording. The simplicity, non-invasive, and passive brings an advantage to implement this method as a diagnosis system. Nevertheless, PCG recordings are often interrupted by various sources, for instance, noise from the surrounding environment, respiratory or lung sounds, power disturbances, and movement of the surrounding skin, so inhibit the PCG implementation as a diagnosis method. Therefore, it requires an appropriate method to eliminate the noise that exists in the PCG signals. To get an appropriate method in the PCG system, we compare the Empirical Mode Decomposition (EMD) and Double-Density Discrete Wavelet Transform (DD-DWT) method as a denoising system to minimize the noise effect in the PCG signal. Observation of the system performance used thirty data from the normal heart sound added by the additive white Gaussian noise (AWGN), and the performance parameter used signal-to-noise ratio (SNR) and mean square error (MSE). Based on the result, we obtained the best SNR value of 25.55 dB for the EMD method and SNR value of 18.19 dB for DD-DWT. Also, we perceived the best MSE value of 0.01% for the EMD method, and 0.42% for the DD-DWT. The results obtained show that the denoising process using the EMD method is better than the DD-DWT to implement in the PCG signal.

Keywords Phonocardiography · Denoising · EMD · DDDWT

T. Y. Fatmawati · A. Yuliani · M. A. Afandi · D. Zulherman (✉)
Faculty of Telecommunication and Electrical Engineering, Institut Teknologi Telkom Purwokerto, Jl. D.I. Panjaitan no. 128, Purwokerto, Indonesia
e-mail: zulherman.dodi@ittelkom-pwt.ac.id

H. Triwiyanto et al. (eds.), *Proceedings of the 1st International Conference on Electronics, Biomedical Engineering, and Health Informatics*, Lecture Notes in Electrical Engineering 746, https://doi.org/10.1007/978-981-33-6926-9_52

1 Introduction

The cardiovascular system circulating the blood into the part of the human body consists of the heart as the main organ that pumps it. Cardiovascular disorders (CVDs) is the term referring to diseases affecting the human heart [1] or the blood vessels [2]. CVDs was the primary cause of global mortality, about 17.5 million, and more death around the world in 2016 [1]. The early observation could drive the CVDs mortality impact to the lowest rate. There are several non-invasive methods to diagnose CVDs that based on electric, mechanic, or magnetic heart activities [3]. The electrocardiogram (ECG) based on electrical heart activities and tomography scans that are based on magnetic heart activities were commonly used to diagnose CVDs, but the expertise dependent and the high cost bring disadvantages to use these methods [4]. The auscultation, the method developed since the eighteenth century only requiring a stethoscope as a diagnostic device, is an alternative to diagnose heart disease and is recently named as a phonocardiogram (PCG). Since it was defined by Laennec [1], the auscultation method was commonly used as a primary diagnosis for human physiology, including heart activities, but is highly dependent on the medical doctor's experience [5] to listen and interpret sound produced by the heart. In the last decade, digital stethoscopes used to record heart sounds recorded it into digital signals so that it can be processed further [6] and reduce the clinical expertise dependent.

PCG is a signal obtained from the heart activities using a microphone attached to the chest and connected to a recording device [1]. PCG signal contains essential information about heart activities, which provides a quantitative and graphical representation of the acoustic waves generated by the mechanical activity of the heart. PCG provides one of the best graphical representations of heart sounds and murmurs (abnormal heart sounds). The PCG recording consists of four components of the heart sound (S1, S2, S3, and S4). S1 and S2 heart sounds can be heard from a healthy heart, produced by standard valve closing and opening, whereas in an abnormal heart, S3 and S4 may be present in addition to S1 and S2. S3 occurs just after S2 and S4 occur just before S1 [7]. PCG signals are used in heart rate monitoring and murmurs or detection of normal heart sounds [8].

PCG signal has a problem in the form of noise that damages the signal. Recording of heart sounds is often disturbed by various factors and noise, including electromagnetic interference from the surrounding environment, power frequency disturbances, interference with electrical signals from the human body, respiratory and digestive sounds [1, 7]. Therefore, it requires an appropriate method to remove noise in PCG signals such as the Empirical Mode Decomposition (EMD) method or wavelet-based method. The EMD method can be used for denoising PCG signals, which can be used as data analysis, especially for non-stationary and nonlinear signals. In the process of denoising the PCG signal using the EMD method, which can decompose the signal into an oscillation component called the Intrinsic Mode Function (IMF) with a filtering process [9]. Also, a wavelet-based denoising system, such as a double density discrete wavelet transform (DD-DWT), used a decomposition method to separate the information signal and the noise.

Mohguen and Bekka [10] used the EMD method to denoising ECG signal with signal-to-noise (SNR) and mean square error (MSE) as a performance parameter. Based on Mohguen and Bekka [10], our work used SNR and MSE features to analyze the denoising system performance for the PCG signal. Boudraa et al. [11] also implemented the EMD method to denoise a signal from the various noise signal. Boudraa compares them results with a wavelet-based denoising system. Based on [1, 10, 11], our work used adaptive white Gaussian noise and compared the EMD result with the wavelet-based system. The wavelet-based denoising system can be implemented in the PCG signal. Viranda et al. [12] used a wavelet packet transform to get feature extraction and identify the S1 and S2 from the phonocardiogram, and Ali et al. [1] employed a discrete wavelet transform for denoising the heart sound signal. Abdullah et al. [13] implemented a double density discrete wavelet transform (DD-DWT) to denoise the EEG signal. They said DD-DWT could be used to denoise the other biosignal forms, such as ECG or PCG. Vimala and Priya [14] showed the DD-DWT could be used to denoise the signal and image, so our work used DD-DWT to denoise the PCG signal and compared the result with the EMD method.

Based on previous work, we compared the EMD and DD-DWT method in the denoising system to remove noise contained in the PCG signal. So, we got an appropriate method to denoise the PCG signal. We used SNR and MSE value from thirty PCG signals [15, 16], the Computing in Cardiology Challenge 2016 datasets, to compare the effectiveness of the method used in the denoising process. There are two types of thresholds used in denoising PCG signals, namely soft and hard thresholds. We organized this paper into several sections, as follows: Sect. 1 showed the overview and the literature review about the denoising system. Section 2 presented the method used in this research. Section 3 discussed the experimental results, and Sect. 4 presented the conclusion of this research.

2 Method

Denoising is an extracting process from the noisy signal that separates the information with the noise. Regarding the frequency information content, the other part considered noise would be eliminated, so a new signal is obtained with the required features (such as S1 and S2 in PCG). Unlike the filter based in specific frequencies that will be discarded or maintained, the denoising process was used to decompose the signal from their noise. The PCGs' analysis system needs a denoising process to provide a high accuracy S1 and S2 nodes in raw PCG signals that are contained by other sounds from the lung, digestive system, or ambient sound from the environment. In this study, we used the PCG signal taken from the Physionet.org website [15, 16], which provided datasets that are quite complete and freely accessible. Heart sound recording was collected at either a clinical or non-clinical environment, both healthy subjects and pathological patients. We employed thirty heart sound recordings in *.wav format that consists of 23 normal and seven abnormal heart sound with duration 33,37 ± 5,81 s. There is no information about the gender and age of the subjects. All recordings have been sampled by frequency sample 2000 Hz.

This research carried out the denoising process using empirical mode decomposition (EMD) and double density discrete wavelet transform (DD-DWT) with a variation of the thresholding method. The denoising method used both EMD and DD-DWT and the system performance calculated by SNR and MSE for both methods. The study was limited to signals corrupted by additive white Gaussian noise (AWGN). AWGN contains all frequencies with equal amplitudes that means dependency of the power density from the frequency. Given a measured signal $x(t)$ with white Gaussian noise $N(0, 1)$, then,

$$x(t) = f(t) + \sigma n(t) \tag{1}$$

$f(t)$ is the original signal, $n(t)$ is the noise, σ is the noise strength (standard deviation) in this study used $\sigma = 1$ and SNR 10 dB. The denoising process objective is to eliminate the noise of the signal to recover $f(t)$. Figure 1 shows the procedure used in this work. The PCG signal extraction, this work, had several steps started by loading the PCG dataset, then preprocessing using normalized and centering process. The next step chose the EMD or the DD-DWT as a denoising method and used it to denoise the PCG signal. After the denoising process, our work calculated the SNR and MSE value as the last step to describe system performance. The EMD and DD-DWT implementation to analyze non-stationary signals such as PCG signals decompose the signal into a set of base signals. In contrast to DD-DWT, EMD uses essential functions (intrinsic mode function) derived from the signal itself, whereas DD-DWT uses a specific base signal (mother wavelet).

The EMD decomposes PCG signal $x(t)$ into a series of intrinsic mode functions (IMFs). Identifying the IMF by its time-scale characteristics, which can be determined locally by the time interval between two extrema [11]. The EMD selects the highest frequency oscillation remaining in the signal. Thus, locally, each IMF contains lower frequency oscillation than the one extracted earlier. Furthermore, the EMD does not use any pre-determined filter or wavelet function. Since EMD decomposition is based on the local characteristics time scale of the data, it applies to both nonlinear and non-stationary processes. The EMD decomposes into a sum of IMFs that must satisfy the following conditions: (1) They have the same numbers of zero crossings and extrema; and (2) they are symmetric to the local mean. The EMD method to decompose $x(t)$ into a sum of the IMFs employ several steps that describe in this the following steps [10]:

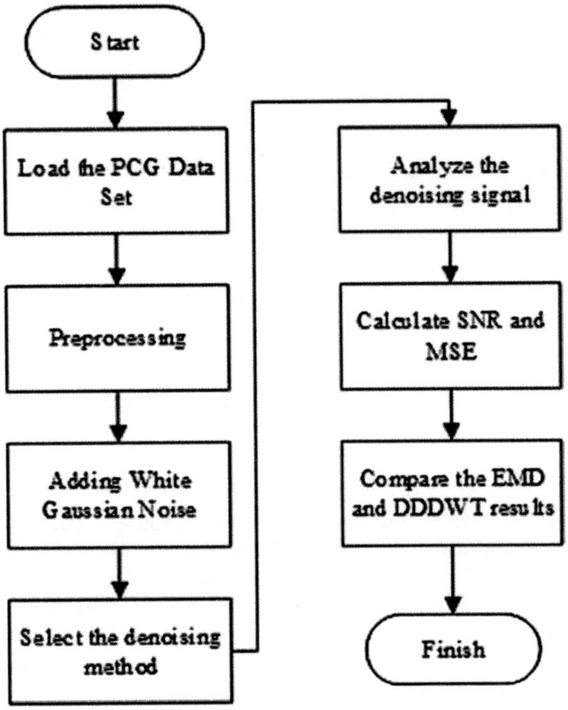

Fig. 1 PCG signal denoising flowchart

1. Find local maxima and minima in $x(t)$ to get the upper and lower envelopes respectively using cubic spline interpolation;
2. Calculate the mean envelope $m(t)$ by averaging the upper and lower envelopes;
3. Calculate the temporary local oscillation $h(t) = x(t) - m(t)$;
4. Calculate the average of $h(t)$, if average $h(t)$ is close to zero, then $h(t)$ is considered as the first IMF, named $c_i(t)$ otherwise, repeat steps (1) – (3) while using $h(t)$ for $x(t)$;
5. Calculate the residue $r(t) = x(t) - c_i(t)$;
6. Repeat steps from (1) to (5) using $r(t)$ for $x(t)$ to obtain the next IMF and residue.

The decomposition process stops when the residue $r(t)$ becomes a monotonic function or a constant that no longer satisfies the condition of an IMF.

$$\mathrm{x}(t) = \sum_{i=1}^{N} c_i(t) + r(t) \tag{2}$$

The IMF based denoising method using EMD requires thresholding and statistical classifications. The IMF, a set of functions, must meet the conditions that a

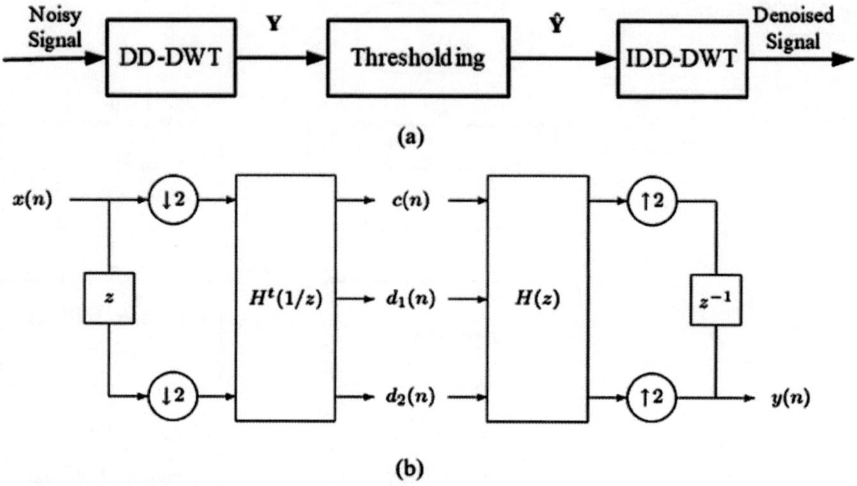

Fig. 2 Double Density-Discrete Wavelet Transform (DD-DWT) design, **a** standard scheme in using DD-DWT coefficient thresholding for denoising, **b** filter bank structure of DD-DWT

total of maximum and minimum (total of extrema) must be equal to the total number of zero-cross or not more than one.

Double density discrete wavelet transform is a type of wavelet transform that has a single scaling function and two wavelets; this wavelet is proven to be smoother than traditional DWT [17]. Like the dual-tree DWT, the overcomplete DWT described above is less shift-sensitive than an orthonormal wavelet basis. Since Discrete Wavelet Transform (DWT) techniques have been used broadly for heart sound analysis, the other form DWT like DD-DWT can be implemented to analyze heart sound. Figure 2 shows the denoising steps based on DD-DWT.

Thresholding is on the most efficient signal denoising techniques, which helps reduce the possibility of mixing the high-frequency signal with noise. In this study, two types of thresholding are used, namely hard thresholding and soft thresholding. Figure 3 shows the characteristics of the two types of thresholding used in this study [18].

$x_j(k)$ is a decomposition signal, ρ is a thresholding value, the hard-thresholding process describe in Eq. (3)

$$\tilde{x}_j = \begin{cases} x_j(k) & , |x_j(k)| > \rho \\ 0 & , |x_j(k)| \leq \rho \end{cases}. \tag{3}$$

The soft-thresholding process describe in Eqs. (4) and (5),

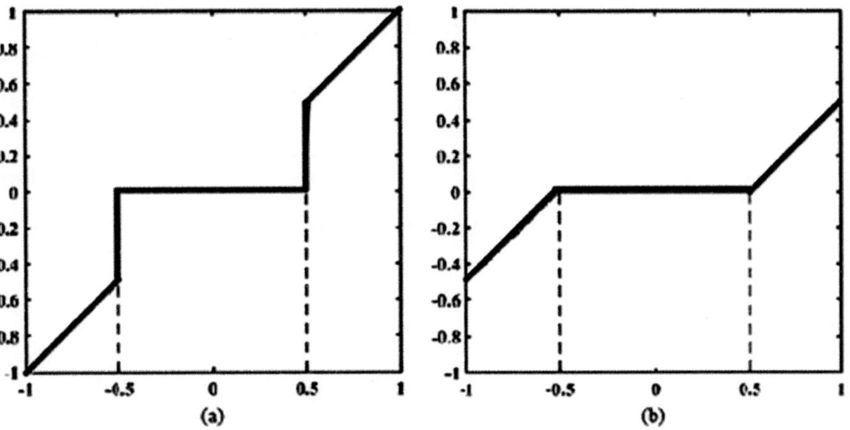

Fig. 3 Thresholding method comparison, **a** hard thresholding, **b** soft thresholding

$$signx_j = \begin{cases} 1 & ,x_j(k) > 0 \\ 0 & ,x_j(k) = 0 \\ -1 & ,x_j(k) < 0 \end{cases} \quad (4)$$

$$\tilde{x}_j(k) = sign\{x_j(k)\} \times |x_j(k) - \rho_j| \quad (5)$$

3 Results and Discussion

Analyzing the system performance in this paper used Computing in Cardiology Physionet [15] with thirty PCG signal in *.wav format. To analyze the denoising process, we used a single input that describes in Fig. 4. The signal duration shown in this paper is one point fifteen-second for easy observation. The input signal form shown in Fig. 4 consists of an S1 and S2 sequence. This picture shows that the signal used is PCG from a normal heart condition.

The DD-DWT method in this work used the 4th level filter bank and Coiflet as mother wavelet. Based on the denoising result, we got the denoised signal, like in Fig. 5. Based on the result, the DD-DWT method can remove the noise artifact from the PCG signal. Figure 6 shows the decomposition signal in the EMD method that describes the shape of the signal after the denoising process using fourth level decomposition. The EMD implementation decomposes the PCG signal into several IMF signals. From this illustration, we can get information on the 4th level that has the lowest frequency component. In this work, we used the 4th level decomposition to get denoised PCG.

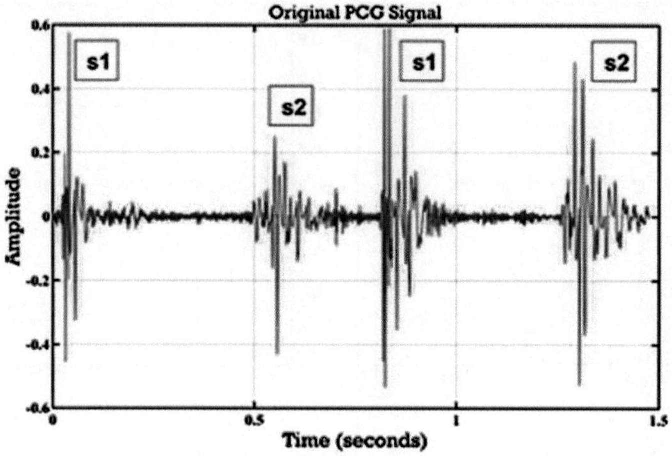

Fig. 4 PCG signal used in this design

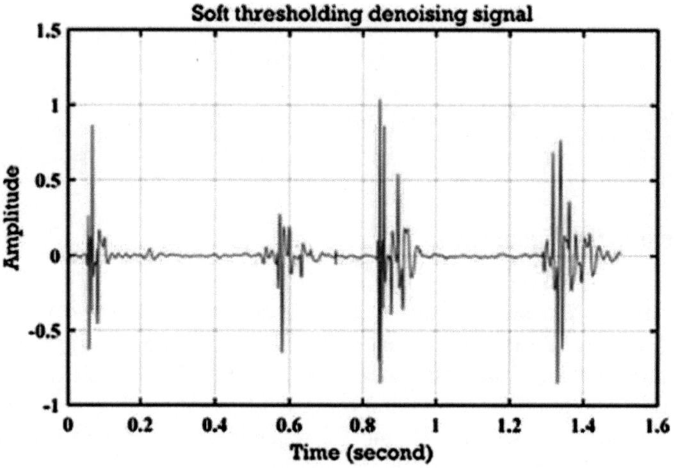

Fig. 5 Denoised PCG signal using DD-DWT method

The comparison of the SNR values of the two methods used is shown in Fig. 7. The distribution of SNR values with the soft thresholding technique is better than the hard type thresholding technique. Furthermore, the use of the EMD method for denoising PCG signal systems also shows a higher SNR value compared to the DD-DWT method. Based on the result, the best SNR value is 25.55 dB for a soft threshold-based EMD system and 18.19 dB for the soft threshold-based DD-DWT system. Based on the SNR value, the EMD gave a better performance than the DD-DWT system.

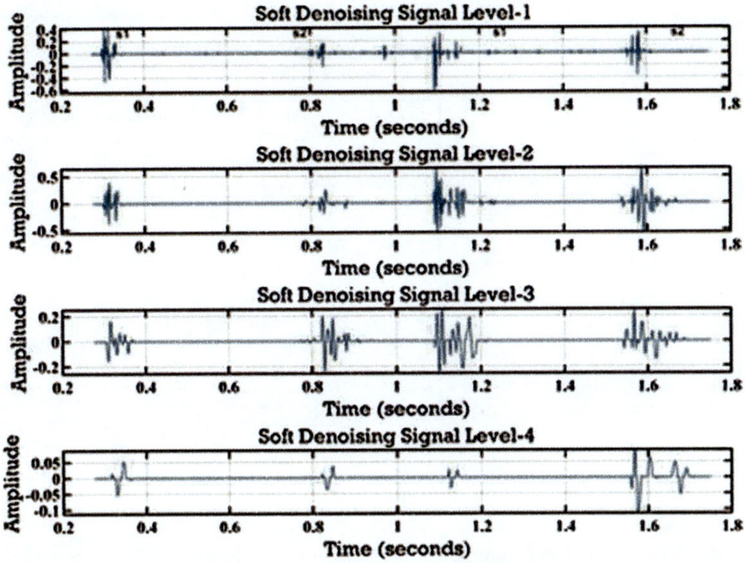

Fig. 6 Decomposition process in EMD to get denoised PCG signal

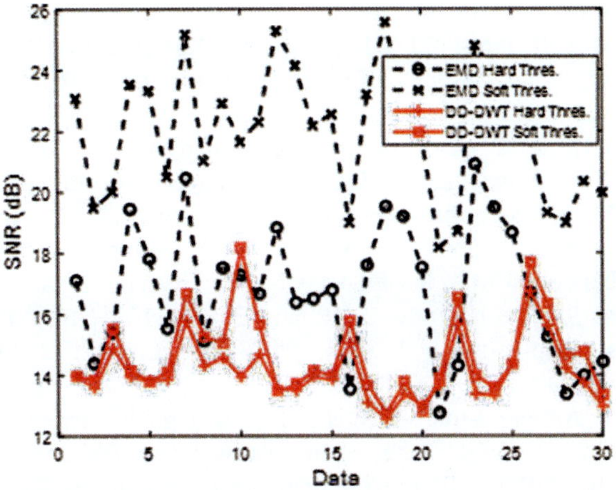

Fig. 7 SNR value of the EMD based denoising system and the DD-DWT based denoising system

The comparison of the MSE values of the two methods used is shown in Fig. 8. The distribution of MSE values with the soft thresholding technique is better than the hard type thresholding technique. Also, the use of the EMD method for denoising PCG signal systems also shows a lower MSE value compared to the DD-DWT method. Based on the result, the best MSE value is 0.00344 for the soft threshold-based EMD system and 0.14695 for the soft threshold-based DD-DWT

Fig. 8 Decomposition process in EMD to get denoised PCG signal

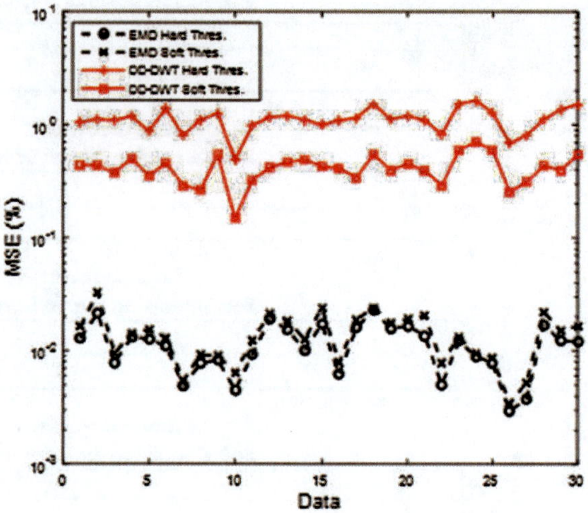

system. Based on the MSE value, the EMD gave a better performance than the DD-DWT system.

Based on statistic analysis, the SNR value is 16.75 ± 2.17 dB for hard threshold EMD and 21.99 ± 2.1 dB for soft thresholding EMD. Furthermore, the SNR value of the hard threshold DD-DWT is 14.09 ± 0.93 dB. The SNR value of soft threshold DD-DWT is 14.64 ± 1.35 dB. Based on MSE value, the denoising system performances were 0.01 ± 0.005 and 0.01 ± 0.007 for EMD hard and soft threshold, respectively. For DD-DWT, the MSE value is 1.13 ± 0.25 and 0.42 ± 0.12 for hard and soft threshold, respectively. Based on the average values, EMD has a superior result than DD-DWT, both SNR and MSE. To confirm the performance comparison between EMD and DD-DWT, we used an analysis of variance (ANOVA). Figure 9 shows the box plot comparison between EMD and DD-DWT soft-threshold. Based on ANOVA, we got p-value as 9.43×10^{-23} for SNR and 3.05×10^{-26} for MSE. Based on ANOVA, the small p-values both SNR and MSE indicates that differences between EMD and DD-DWT are significant.

Although this study is limited to signals corrupted by additive white Gaussian noise (AWGN), the results showed that EMD brings better performance than DD-DWT similarly with the report in Ismail [19]. Based on the report, research that was conducted by Salman [20] argued that EMD outperforms wavelet transform (WT) and total variation (TV) method.

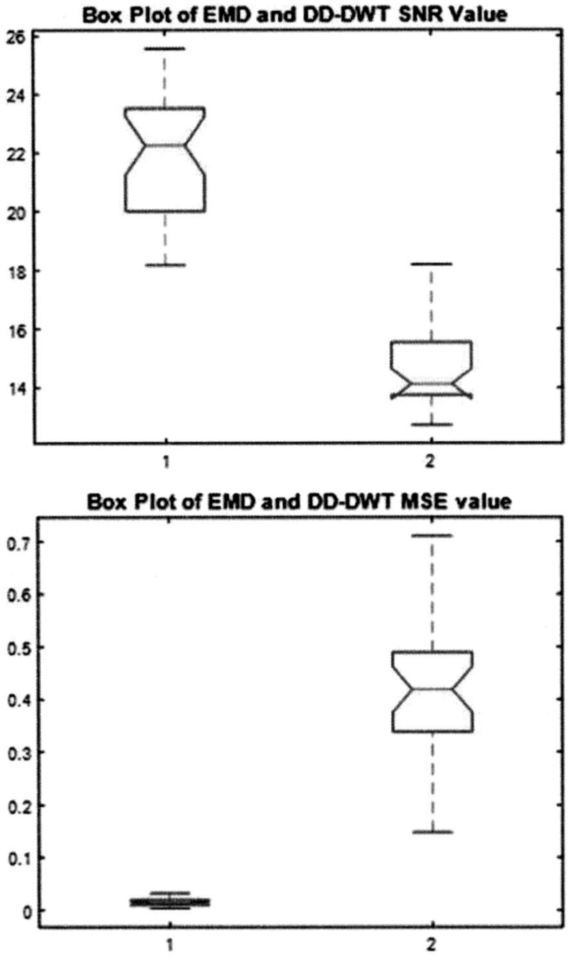

Fig. 9 Box plot of the EMD and DD-DWT comparison, (top) SNR value, (below) MSE value

4 Conclusion

To get an appropriate method in the PCG system, we compare the Empirical Mode Decomposition (EMD) and Double-Density Discrete Wavelet Transform (DD-DWT) method as a denoising system to minimize the noise effect in the PCG signal. Denoising method to suppress noise in the signal were compared with the SNR and MSE parameter. Based on results, the EMD based denoising method gave a better SNR and MSE value than DD-DWT based denoising method. Based on ANOVA, the small p-values both SNR and MSE indicates that differences between EMD and DD-DWT are significant. We argued that the EMD method is a better choice for removing noise in the PCG signals. Furthermore, these results will be highly useful for researchers in automatic the heart sound localization and classification system.

Acknowledgements Thank you to Lembaga Penelitian dan Pengabdian Masyarakat (LPPM) Institut Teknologi Telkom Purwokerto and Biomedical Engineering Program for funding this research.

References

1. Ali MN, El-Dahsan EA, Yahia AH (2017) Denoising of heart sound signals using discrete wavelet transform. J Circuits Syst Signal Process 36:4482
2. Dewangan N, Potdar RM (2014) Noise cancellation using adaptive filter for PCG signal. J Emerg Trend Tech Comput Sci 3:38
3. Low JX, Choo KW (2018) IoT-enabled heart monitoring device with signal denoising and segmentation using discrete wavelet transform. International conference on control, automation, robotic and vision, vol 15, p 119
4. Sahoo PK, Thakkar HK, Lee MY (2017) A cardiac early warning system with multi channel SCG and ECG monitoring for mobile health. J Sensors 17:1
5. Ri O et al (2015) Classification of heart sound signal using multi-modal features. J Eng Sci Tech 58:165
6. Swarup S, Makaryus AN (2018) Digital stethoscope: technology update. J Med Devices 18:29
7. Kumar P, Kumar A (2017) An adaptive thresholding method for the wavelet based denoising of phonocardiogram signal. J Biomed Signal Process Control 38:388
8. Soman KP, Ramachandran KI, Resmi NG (2010) Insight into wavelet from theory to practice, 3rd edn. Phi Learning Private Limited, New Delhi
9. Hahn SL (1996) Hilbert transforms in signal processing. Artech House, London
10. Mohguen W, Bekka RE (2017) New denoising method based on empirical mode decomposition and improved thresholding function. J Phys Conf Ser 787:012014
11. Boudaraa AO, Cexus JC, Saidi Z (2005) EMD-based signal noise reduction. J Inf Commun Eng 1:96
12. Viranda RS, Jusak J, Puspasari I (2017) Ektraksi ciri dan identifikasi sinyal suara jantung S1 dan S2 phonocardigram (PCG) menggunakan metode wavlet packet transform. J Control Netw Syst 6:187
13. Abdullah H, Cvetkovic D (2013) Double density wavelet for EEG signal denoising. International conference on machine learning and computer science, vol 2, p 51
14. Vimala C, Priya PA (2014) Noise reduction based on double density discrete wavelet transform. IEEE international conference on smart structure and systems, p 15
15. Liu C et al (2016) An open access database for the evaluation of heart sound algorithms. J Physiol Meas 12:2181
16. Goldberger A, Amaral L, Glass L, Hausdorff J, Ivanov PC, Mark R, Mietus JE, Moody B, Peng CK, Stanley HE (2001) PhysioBank, PhysioToolkit, and PhysioNet: components of a new research resource for complex physiologic signals, Circulation 101:215
17. Selesnick IW (2001) The double density DWT. J Wavelet Signal Image Anal 39
18. Zulherman D, Hendry J, Adam IF (2020) Perbandingan real valued dan complex wavelet transform pada denoising sinyal fetal-phonocardiograms. J Nas Tek Elektro dan Teknol Inf 9:63
19. Ismail S, Siddiqi I, Akram U (2018) Localization and classification of heart beats in phonocardiography signals-a comprehensive review. EURASIP J Adv Sign Process 26:1
20. Salman AH, Ahmadi N, Mengko R, Langi AZR, Mengko TLR (2015) Performance comparison of denoising methods for heart sound signal. International symposium on intelligent signals processing and communication

Time Domain Features for EEG Signal Classification of Four Class Motor Imagery Using Artificial Neural Network

Rahmat Widadi, Dodi Zulherman, and S. Rama Febriyan Ari

Abstract Brain-Computer Interface (BCI) is a system that measures and processes the activity of the human brain to improve or replace the function of the human body. In the future, this system can be a solution for people with disabilities, especially in locomotor organs such as hands and feet. The purpose of this research is to classify four classes of electroencephalogram (EEG) signals that represent four human motor imagery. The four motor imageries are left-hand, right-hand, left-foot, and right-foot that originated from motor imagery dataset. The proposed method in this research consists of filtering, feature extraction, and classification. The proposed method employed the Finite Impulse Response (FIR) in the filtering process to pass the required EEG signals such as delta, theta, alpha, beta, and gamma channels. The features are the Root Mean Square (RMS) values from the time domain filtered signal. Our system design used these features as input classification method that used the Artificial Neural Network (ANN). The training and testing data separation used 10-fold cross-validation. To analyze the testing performance used a confusion matrix. Based on the results, the proposed method brings the highest system accuracy as 61.2% on the beta channel.

Keywords EEG · MI · ANN

1 Introduction

The brain's natural intelligent computing ability to control all activities, such as human behavior, mind and motor movements, is driving the development of research in the field of signal processing and control. The main purpose is to emulate the capabilities of the human brain. One of them is the Brain-Computer Interface (BCI), which gives the ability for the human brain to interact with a

R. Widadi (✉) · D. Zulherman · S. Rama Febriyan Ari
Faculty of Telecommunication and Electrical Engineering, Institut Teknologi Telkom Purwokerto, Purwokerto, Indonesia
e-mail: rahmat@ittelkom-pwt.ac.id

H. Triwiyanto et al. (eds.), *Proceedings of the 1st International Conference on Electronics, Biomedical Engineering, and Health Informatics*, Lecture Notes in Electrical Engineering 746, https://doi.org/10.1007/978-981-33-6926-9_53

computer device [1]. It enables the user to command a computer or other peripheral device by brain activities independent of sensory nerves and muscles [1, 2]. The Electroencephalogram (EEG), the human brain activity recording, is an interpretation of potential changes in the cerebral cortex due to the interaction of various interconnected neurons [3]. The EEG signals are divided based on the delta, theta, alpha, beta and gamma channel frequencies. The features extraction of random time-varying EEG signals and accurate signals classification is the main challenge in current BCI research [1]. The use of appropriate feature extraction can produce features that represent data classes. The BCI aims to interpret the EEG signal in digital form, which performs as a command for a computer [1].

The BCI system used can be considered as a helpful method to support patients with compromised motor functions, such as 'locked-in' and 'completely-locked-in' patients [4]. Motor imagery (MI) is the process of the subject imagining the movement of one or more of his bodies. Motor-Imagery Brain-Computer Interface (MI-BCI) allows users with disabilities in the body to interact with the environment [5]. MI-BCI offers communication between people suffering from neural disorders with various devices such as robotic prostheses and wheelchairs [5]. In this work, we utilize the Root Mean Square (RMS) value as a time-domain feature. The RMS value of the signal provides the same average power with constant signals at the same load [6]. The RMS feature has low complexity in EEG signal processing [7]. The RMS feature itself has been widely used in previous EEG signal classification studies [8–10], and the resulting classification accuracy is above 70%. The choice of classification method is also important in BCI. Artificial Neural Network (ANN) is inspired by the ability of the human brain by computing network patterns to make decisions [11]. ANN is proven to be robust in multiclass classification [5]. Research on EEG based MI classification was conducted in [12] but there are only two classes, namely left and right foot. Whereas in [13] using hands and feet MI with a classification accuracy of 57%. The level of accuracy in this research needs to be improved. Based on previous work, we worked with the ANN method in the EEG classification. We organized this paper into several sections, as follows: Sect. 1 showed the overview and the literature review about EEG classification in MI-BCI. Section 2 presented the method used in this work. Section 3 discussed the experimental results, and Sect. 4 presented the conclusion of this research.

2 Method

2.1 Data

The right and left hands, legs, and tongue movements have been widely used as a paradigm for BCI interactions. In this study, we used the EEG signal obtained from thirteen subjects divided into 75 BCI EEG recording sessions with the imagery right and left hands, and legs movement. The electrode placement is based on the 10/20

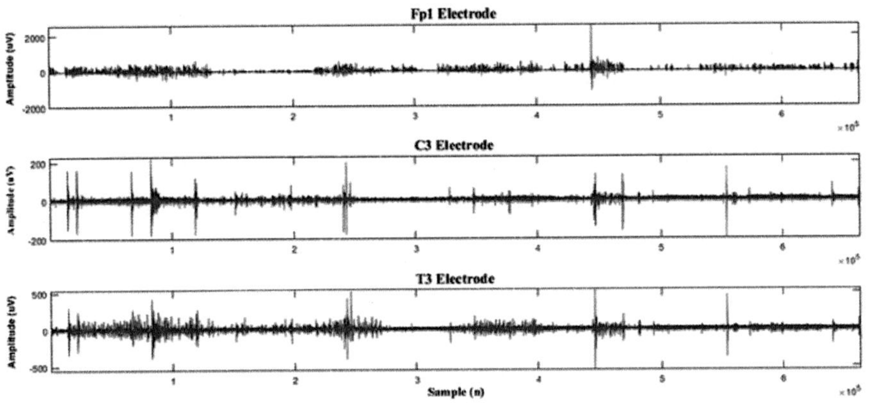

Fig. 1 Example of The Raw EEG Signal

international system. EEG signal data acquisition using the EEG-1200 JE-921A EEG device from Nihon Kohden, Japan [13]. Participants imagine the body moves according to the instructions displayed on the screen. This recorded EEG signal is called the Motor Imagery (MI) EEG signal. In this research, we use only ten subjects labelled with HaLT (Hand Leg and Tongue). Data with this label contains four classes used in this research, which are left hand, right hand, left leg, and right leg movement. The dataset has a sampling frequency of 200 Hz with 22 electrodes including 3 ground electrodes. We removed the EEG signal from the ground electrode so that only 19 electrodes were used in this research. Figure 1 shows an example of an EEG signal at the electrodes Fp1, C3, and T3 from a subject. The signal has a length of 664,400 samples.

The dataset marked several codes to define the movements. The code markers used to mark signals in a dataset divided into classes. Table 1 shows the codes that are used in the dataset that divided into nine classes. This marker data is obtained based on the instructions that appear on the screen at the time of recording.

Table 1 Code Marker in The HaLT Dataset

Code marker	Explanation
99	Relaxation
92	Experiment Finish
91	Rest
6	Right Foot
5	Tongue
4	Left Foot
3	Neutral
2	Right Hand
1	Left Hand

2.2 System Design

EEG based motor imagery classification system in this research conducted into three main stages: filtering, feature extraction, and classification. Figure 2 shows the classification system in this research to describe each stage's correlations. The preliminary stage was the filtering, which purposed to obtain EEG signals in the delta (1–4 Hz), theta (4–8 Hz), alpha (8–12 Hz), beta (12–30 Hz), and gamma (>30 Hz) channel. The type of filter used in this research was the Finite Impulse Response (FIR) filter, a non-recursive filter that has a finite number of impulse responses. The FIR is always stable, easy to realize, and provides a linear phase response. The FIR is always stable because it is implemented using an all-zero transfer function [14]. In this research, the FIR filter was designed using the windowing method that employed the Hamming window in Eq. (1).

$$W_{hamming}(n) = 0.54 - 0.46\left(1 - cos\left(\frac{2\pi n}{N-1}\right)\right); \quad 0 \leq n \leq N-1 \tag{1}$$

The filtered EEG signals were used to feature extraction process in the second stage. This stage calculated the Root Mean Square (RMS) value of the signal for each channel using Eq. (2). The feature extracted in this step for each channel consisted of the four EEG-based motor imagery classes: left hand, right hand, left foot, and right foot. These features were used as input for the Artificial Neural Network (ANN) process.

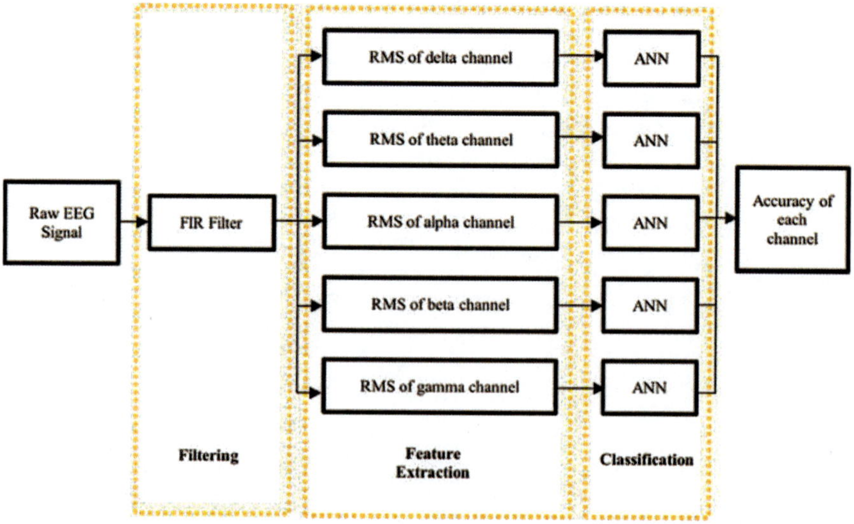

Fig. 2 The Classification System of Motor Imagery EEG Signal

$$X_{RMS} = \left(\frac{1}{n}\sum_{i=1}^{n} x_i^2\right)^{1/2} \quad (2)$$

This work employed a Multilayer Perceptron (MLP) with a backpropagation learning algorithm, one of the ANN method. The proposed methods used a simple ANN that consisted of a single input layer, hidden layer, output layer. ANN performed a cycle process that processed information to produce an optimum result for any datasets and backward algorithm to complete a network cycle. Backpropagation is an algorithm that returns the error value from the output layer to the hidden layer. Our ANN model consisted of 19 nodes in the input layer, 8 nodes in the hidden layer, and 4 nodes in the output layer. The training and testing process used 10-fold cross-validation. The system performance was analyzed by using the confusion matrix with the accuracy as the main parameter.

3 Result and Discussion

In the initial step, the proposed method filtered the EEG signal into five channels using an FIR filter. Figure 3 shows the filtered EEG signal from the Fp1 electrode signal. As we know, the delta waves have the lowest frequency, and gamma waves have the highest frequency, so it confirms in Fig. 3. Another process in pre-processing steps was giving a code marker. The filtered signal parsed based on the code maker. The classification system for motor imagery used signals with code markers 1, 2, 4 and 6 due to represent the motor imagery signals of the left hand, right hand, left foot, and right foot, respectively. The parsing signal for each subject amounted to 163 × 4 classes. So that the overall becomes 163 × 4 × 10 parsed signals. The filtered and parsed signal is then calculated its RMS value based on Eq. (2). This value is then used as an ANN input. In this research, no scenario was carried out on ANN because this research focused on the effect of channel use on the accuracy value. In addition, a classification process was carried out on each subject.

Figure 4 shows the confusion matrix of the third subject using the beta channel. Based on the confusion matrix, the ratio between the correctly classified with the total data for each marker shows the accuracy value. For example, the use of beta channels in subject 3. The system recognized 97 signals as the correct right-hand movement, 163 signals as the correct left-hand movement, 148 signals as the correct right-leg movement, and 93 signals as the correct left-leg movement. The accuracy calculated by the correct signals was 14.8% for the right hand, 24.8% for the left hand, 22.5% for the right leg, and 14.2% for the left leg. The system accuracy summarized the accuracy of each marker.

Table 2 shows the accuracy of the ten subjects used in this work. Based on the accuracy result in Table 2, we conclude that the beta or theta channel should be

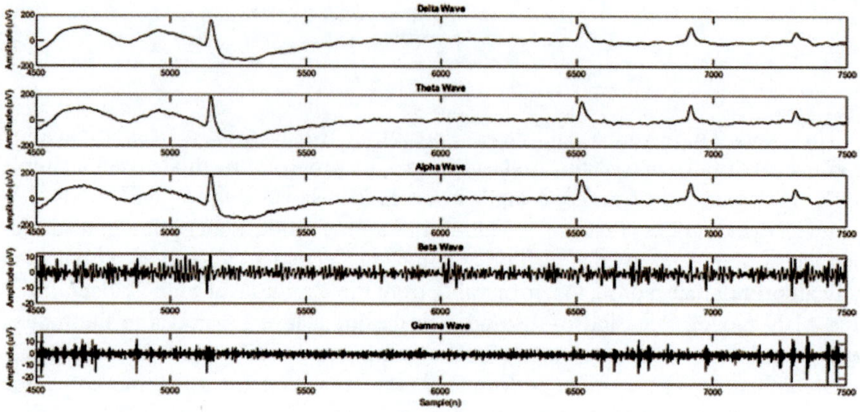

Fig. 3 Example of Filtered Signal of Fp1 Electrode

Fig. 4 Confusion Matrix of Subject 3 Beta Channel

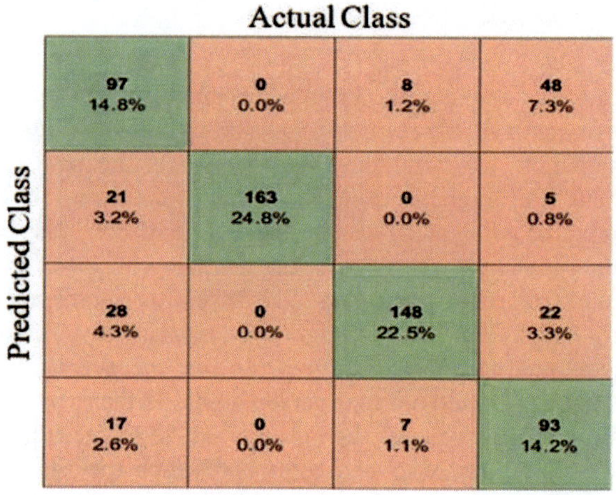

used for EEG based classification due to average accuracy for these channels superior to other channels. Several subjects show exception results like the alpha channel in subject two, seven, and ten that brings the best accuracy result for each subject. Furthermore, the gamma channel should not be used for EEG based motor-imagery classification. As a comparison, the results obtained from this study were higher than [13]. The accuracy obtained in [13] is 57% for the HaLT dataset. Meanwhile, research [12] only used 2 classes of MI, namely left and right foot. The accuracy obtained is 86.26% using linear SVM.

Table 2 Accuracy on Each Subject

Channel	Subject										Average accuracy (%)
	1	2	3	4	5	6	7	8	9	10	
Delta	36.8	39.4	76.5	80.6	55.8	61.4	79.2	60.6	58.9	58.5	60.8
Theta	35.7	39.8	81.3	81.9	54.9	60.9	77.7	59.4	60.5	58.1	61.02
Alpha	38.9	40.1	77	76.1	54.3	62.2	79.8	62.7	60	58.9	61
Beta	38.9	39.5	76.3	80.3	55.9	62.2	78.5	63.7	58.8	57.9	**61.2**
Gamma	22.7	22.8	49.2	32.7	29.2	44.5	46	48	27.2	25.2	34.75

4 Conclusion

This research discusses the classification of the four-class EEG based imagery motor. The system extracted the time-domain feature from ten subject EEG signals, which were extracted in the form of the RMS value. The channel variation employed to determine the accuracy system for each channel. ANN is used to map these features into four imagery motor classes. The highest average accuracy is 61.2% for the beta channel. Further research plans are focused on the variation of hidden layer nodes and changes in classification methods. Based on the research results, it is recommended to use the beta channel in the classification of the imagery motor EEG signal, due to the highest average accuracy.

Acknowledgements We would like heartfelt thanks to Lembaga Penelitian dan Pengabdian kepada Masyarakat, Institut Teknologi Telkom Purwokerto for funding this research.

References

1. Vaid S, Singh P, Kaur C (2015) EEG signal analysis for BCI interface: a review. In: 2015 fifth international conference on advanced computing communication technologies, pp 143–147
2. Mak JN, Wolpaw JR (2009) Clinical applications of brain-computer interfaces: current state and future prospects. IEEE Rev Biomed Eng 2:187–199
3. MacDonald DB (2015) Electroencephalography: basic principles and applications. In: Wright JD (ed) International encyclopedia of the social & behavioral sciences, Second edn. Elsevier, Oxford, pp 353–363
4. Chaudhari R, Galiyawala HJ (2017) A review on motor imagery signal classification for BCI. Signal Process An Int J 11:16–34
5. Aggarwal S, Chugh N (2019) Signal processing techniques for motor imagery brain computer interface: a review. Array 1–2:100003
6. Beranek LL, Mellow TJ (2012) Chapter 1—Introduction and terminology. In: Beranek LL, Mellow TJ (eds) Acoustics: sound fields and transducers. Academic Press, pp 1–19
7. Boonyakitanont P, Lek-Uthai A, Chomtho K, Songsiri J (2020) A review of feature extraction and performance evaluation in epileptic seizure detection using EEG. Biomed Signal Process Control 57:101702

8. Hamedi M, Salleh S, Noor AM, Mohammad-Rezazadeh I (2014) Neural network-based three-class motor imagery classification using time-domain features for BCI applications. In: 2014 IEEE region 10 symposium, pp 204–207
9. Tavakolan M, Frehlick Z, Yong X, Menon C (2017) Classifying three imaginary states of the same upper extremity using time-domain features. PLoS ONE 12:e0174161–e0174161
10. Bhuvaneswari P, Kumar JS (2015) Influence of linear features in nonlinear electroencephalography (EEG) signals. Procedia Comput Sci 47:229–236
11. Farizawani AG, Puteh M, Marina Y, Rivaie A (2020) A review of artificial neural network learning rule based on multiple variant of conjugate gradient approaches. J Phys: Conf Ser 1529:22040
12. Phang C, Ko L (2020) Global cortical network distinguishes motor imagination of the left and right foot. IEEE Access 8:103734–103745
13. Kaya M, Binli MK, Ozbay E, Yanar H, Mishchenko Y (2018) A large electroencephalographic motor imagery dataset for electroencephalographic brain computer interfaces. Sci Data 5:180211
14. Oshana R (2006) 4—Overview of digital signal processing algorithms. In: Oshana R (ed) DSP software development techniques for embedded and real-time systems. Newnes, Burlington, pp 59–121

Simple Visible Light Spectrophotometer Design Using 620 Nm Optical Filter

Meilia Safitri, Farahdiba Rahmadani, Erika Loniza, and Sotya Anggoro

Abstract The main problem of conventional spectrophotometer is its large form and complex system. This study aims to design and develop a compact and portable visible light spectrophotometer. The main contribution of this study is to simplicity the spectrophotometer design. The designed device uses a halogen lamp as the light source, and a colored lens 620 nm optical glass filters that serve to narrow the wavelength becomes monochromatic. A phototransistor sensor is utilized to convert the monochromatic light into a voltage. A differential filter is employed to reduce 15.9 Hz noise that occurred when the phototransistor detected the light. Furthermore, all processes in the developed system are automatically controlled using ATMega328. The verification of the designed spectrophotometer is carried out using cholesterol serum with various concentrations. The conducted test result shows that the designed system has more than 90% accuracy, with the highest error percentage is 5.52%, and the mean of error percentage is 2.8%. The developed spectrophotometer demonstrated high performance, portable, and cost-effective in analyzing cholesterol serum concentrations. The proposed design of the spectrophotometer was useful in the development of simple and compact devices for chemical sample analysis.

Keywords Spectrophotometer · Optical filter · Differential filter

M. Safitri (✉) · F. Rahmadani · E. Loniza
Department of Medical Electronics Technology, Universitas Muhammadiyah Yogyakarta, Jalan Brawijaya, Bantul, Indonesia
e-mail: meilia.safitri@vokasi.umy.ac.id

S. Anggoro
Department of Mechanical Technology, Universitas Muhammadiyah Yogyakarta, Jalan Brawijaya, Bantul, Indonesia

H. Triwiyanto et al. (eds.), *Proceedings of the 1st International Conference on Electronics, Biomedical Engineering, and Health Informatics*, Lecture Notes in Electrical Engineering 746, https://doi.org/10.1007/978-981-33-6926-9_54

1 Introduction

Cholesterol ($C_{27}H_{46}O$) is a substance that resembles fat in the human body and has a vital role. Cholesterol is responsible for controlling substances' movement into and out of cells [1, 2]. Furthermore, the human body requires cholesterol to make certain hormones [3], making vitamin D, forming bile, as well as the necessary substances of the body in digesting food. In order to provide cholesterol needs, the human body can create its substances. The human body also gets cholesterol intake from foods originating from animals such as eggs, meat, milk, cheese, and others. Although cholesterol is indispensable for the human body, the presence of excessive cholesterol in the blood can lead to severe illnesses. Cholesterol excess in the blood can mix with other substances in the blood and form plaque inside the artery vessels. Furthermore, some studies indicated that there is a relationship between the high concentration of cholesterol in the blood with depression [4, 5].

One of the methods can be implemented to determine blood cholesterol levels, is the spectroscopy method. Spectroscopy is a method of analyzing and interpreting the spectrum in the modern chemical field [6]. Spectrophotometry is a spectroscopic technique using *visible* rays as a light source, while the tool used in this technique is called a spectrophotometer. Spectrophotometers are used to determine a sample's composition by measuring the transmission and absorption of a solution by skipping light of a particular wavelength in a glass or quartz object called a cuvette [7]. Some light is absorbed when passing the Cuvette, and the rest will be missed. The absorbance value of the passing light will be in line with the solution concentration of the Cuvette. The use of this Spectrophotometer in analyzing a substance is determined effective since it can provide accurate results [8, 9]. Tungsten or deuterium lamp is a light source widely used in spectrophotometers [10, 11]. However, this type of Spectrophotometer has a large form and complex system that is not suitable for portable use. Moreover, equipment units and accessories' prices are high, as well as the maintenance process that must be done by professional technicians. The use of UV as a light source in a spectrophotometer has been carried out in [12, 13]; however, the method of UV spectrophotometry analysis is susceptible to the disruptors' influence, especially the colored compounds contained in samples, in which can cause analysis results to be less accurate. For the sake of overcoming this problem, an effort to improve sampling selectivity to be free from the influence of colored compounds must be carried out. It makes the sample analysis process with the UV-vis method spends a long time, in addition to the large form of UV-vis spectrophotometer that makes use of this type of Spectrophotometer less effective, mainly if it requires portable use.

The purpose of this research is to develop a compact and portable size Spectrophotometer using halogen lamps light source. Halogen lamps are chosen as visible light sources since besides their small size, they only require a voltage of 12 V. Previously, compact and portable spectrophotometers using LED light sources have been developed [8, 14, 15]. The use of LED lighting in spectrophotometer design indeed makes the tool compact and portable. However, the use of

LED lamps requires a more complex particular circuit, so it requires a somewhat complicated process in case of damage to the lamp. Also, when compared to halogen, LED lamps are more prone to heat; thus, they required unique cooling systems so that they are not easily damaged. In this study, the 620 nm optical filter is used to alter the broad spectrums wavelength polychromatic light of the halogen lamps to be monochromatic. A Phototransistor sensor is used to detect light encountering the Cuvette. Besides, a differential filter [16, 17] is used to reduce the noise detected by sensors; thus, the Spectrophotometer can produce more accurate reading results.

2 Materials and Method

2.1 Spectrophotometer

A spectrophotometer is a tool consisting of a spectrometer and a photometer. Spectrometer utilized to analyze a compound both qualitatively and quantitatively by measuring the transmittance or absorptance of a solution by skipping a particular wavelength light in a glass or quartz object called a cuvette. Some light is absorbed when passing the cuvettes, and the rest will be missed. The absorbance value of the passing light will be in line with the solution concentration of the Cuvette. The working principle of the tool was invented by Beer and Lambert, who found the law on the interaction of chemicals with light waves (electromagnetic), which in this law Beer-Lambert led to the development of chemical analysis by using the instrumentation tool that is Spectrophotometer. In the law of Beer-Lambert explained "that a transparent media as the increase rate in the intensity of the transmitted light is directly proportional to the thickness and sensitivity of the media used". The main components of a light spectrophotometer appear to generally consist of light sources (Polychromator), Monochromator, cuvettes, samples, detectors, boosters, and readers. Figure 1 is the principle of spectrophotometer work.

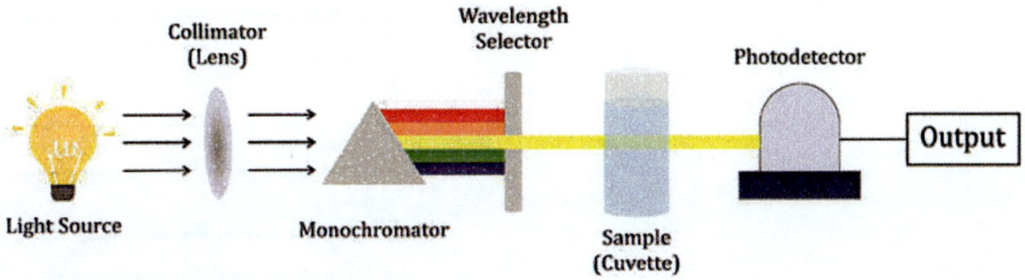

Fig. 1 Principle work of spectrophotometer

2.2 System Design

The working principle of the designed visible light spectrophotometer as shown in Fig. 2, starting from a halogen lamp, which is a polychromatic light source where light propagation consists of various wavelengths. The light enters into Monochromator (optical filter 620 nm) then exits into the sample cell (Cuvette), in the sample cell (Cuvette) there will be a process of light absorption by the substance in the sample (where the light in is brighter than the light out of the Cuvette). Furthermore, light is captured by the sensor and converts it into electrical voltage. The electrical voltage produced by the phototransistor will then be conditioned and filtered using the differential filter, then a noise-free analog signal resulted. The differential filter circuit used in the design of this Spectrophotometer is a series of different amplifiers combined with a low pass filter. On this circuit, the signal that has a frequency above 15.9 Hz will undergo filtering. The ATMega328 will then process the analog signal as output from the differential filter. Microprocessor. Signal processing results in ATMega328 microprocessors will be displayed by 2 × 14 LCD in the form of concentrations of the sample cholesterol used. A power supply supplies the entire process of this spectrophotometer circuit. The power supply set is used to obtain 220 V voltage inputs, which are then lowered and directed to generate 12 VDC and 5 VDC output.

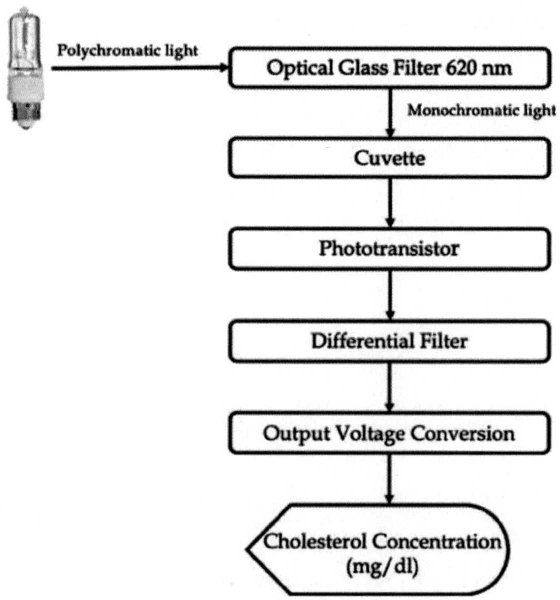

Fig. 2 Block diagram of the designed spectrophotometer

2.3 *Differential Design*

To get the output voltage that really represents the cholesterol concentration value, the input signal from the phototransistor sensor will experience three levels of gain in the buffer circuit, the differential filter circuit, and the inverting amplifier circuit as shown in Fig. 3.

The very first circuit serve as a buffer so that the input voltage value from the light sensor does not drop. Basically, this circuit aims to stabilize the light sensor voltage value. The gain in this buffer circuit is equal to 1, so the output voltage of this circuit is written as,

$$V_{in} = v_1 \tag{1}$$

with,

V_{in} = phototransistor sensor voltage
v_1 = buffer voltage.

The second circuit is a differential filter circuit. This circuit is a differential amplifier circuit combined with a filter. This circuit serves to amplify the voltage difference between the input voltage (v_1) and the reference voltage (v_{reff}). Besides, this circuit also aims to reduce existing noise. The last circuit is an inverting amplifier that aims to reverse the differential amplifier output voltage's polarity so that it is not in a negative value. In addition, this circuit is also used to widen the output voltage range.

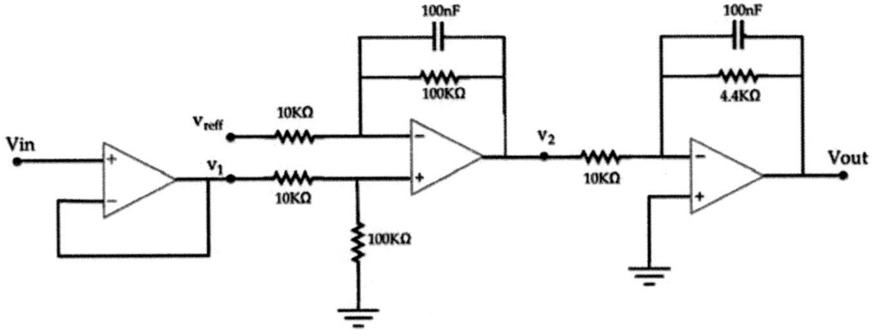

Fig. 3 Differential filter circuit

2.4 Linear Regression

Linear regression is a statistical model used in determining the relationship between two variables in a functional form. The two variables are the dependent variable (y) or also called the response variable and the independent variable (x) which is also called the predictor variable. In this paper, the linear regression method was used to determine the functional relationship between the serum cholesterol concentration value (y) and the output voltage value of the spectrophotometer. The relationship between the cholesterol concentration value and the spectrophotometer output voltage is given by the equation [18],

$$y = \beta_1 x + \beta_0 \tag{2}$$

with,

β_1 = slope of the line
β_0 = intercept of the line.

The data on the value of spectrometer voltage and cholesterol concentration can be written as $(x_1, y_1), \ldots, (x_n, y_n)$, the linear equation that best represents the relationship between the value of cholesterol concentration and the output voltage of the spectrophotometer is obtained by solving the following optimization equation.

$$\min_{\beta_0,\beta_1} = \sum_{i=1}^{n} [y_i - (\beta_0 + \beta_1 x_i)]^2 \tag{3}$$

with $\min_{\beta_0,\beta_1}$ is the minimum value β_0, β_1 so that the values of β_0 dan β_1 are given by,

$$\widehat{\beta_1} = \frac{\sum_{i=1}^{n} x_i y_i - \frac{1}{n}\sum_{i=1}^{n} x_i \sum_{i=1}^{n} y_i}{\sum_{i=1}^{n} x_i^2 - \frac{1}{n}\left(\sum_{i=1}^{n} x_i\right)^2} \tag{4}$$

$$\widehat{\beta_0} = \bar{y} - \widehat{\beta_1}\bar{x} \tag{5}$$

2.5 Testing and Analysis Method

In this research, samples serum used in designed Spectrophotometer testing are blood cholesterol serum in various concentrations, which are purchased and provided by the Asri Medical Centre Hospital. All samples of these cholesterol serums are analytical grade chemical samples. Concentrations of these serums have been prescribed and validated using chemical analyzers. The differential filter circuit testing is performed by measuring the voltage of a phototransistor sensor and the output voltage of the differential filter in the Spectrophotometer that has been given samples of cholesterol serum in various concentrations. Voltage measurements are performed using the FLUXE117 True RMS Multimeter. Determination of linear equations between the output voltage of the Spectrophotometer and the cholesterol concentration is carried out using the linear regression method—the cholesterol concentration testing target aimed to see the performance of the designed Spectrophotometer. The test is done using cholesterol samples in various concentrations. The measurement result of the cholesterol sample concentrations produced by the Spectrophotometer will be compared with the cholesterol sample actual concentration.

3 Results

Figure 4 display visible light spectrophotometer designed. The spectrophotometer has dimensions of 20 cm × 23 cm × 7.55 cm. Compact Spectrophotometer dimensions make this instrument flexible to carry and moveable.

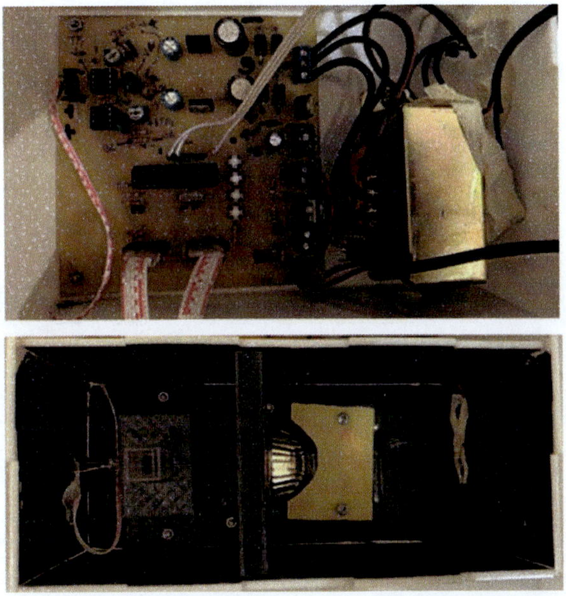

Fig. 4 The designed spectrophotometer

3.1 Differential Output

To see the effectiveness of the differential filter circuit designed in filtering noises mixed during detection by the phototransistor sensor, a comparison between the voltage values before entering the differential filter circuit (sensor voltage) and after filtered is carried out. Figure 5 is the result of a comparison of the voltage before and after the filtering.

Based on Fig. 5, it appears that the voltage value on the Phototransistor sensor shows almost the same value of about 4.8 volts. Moreover, when compared to the output voltage of the differential filter, it shows different values. It indicates that the differential filter circuit designed has succeeded in reducing the noise mixed at the time of detection by the sensor. Although the voltage value entering into the differential filter circuit is almost the same as about 4.8 volts, the output voltage value resulted varies based on the variation of the cholesterol concentration given.

3.2 Linear Analysis of Voltage and Cholesterol Concentration

To determine the equation of voltage with cholesterol concentration, Regression linear method is used. This equation will then be used by the system to determine the cholesterol concentration of the given sample. This test uses ten samples of

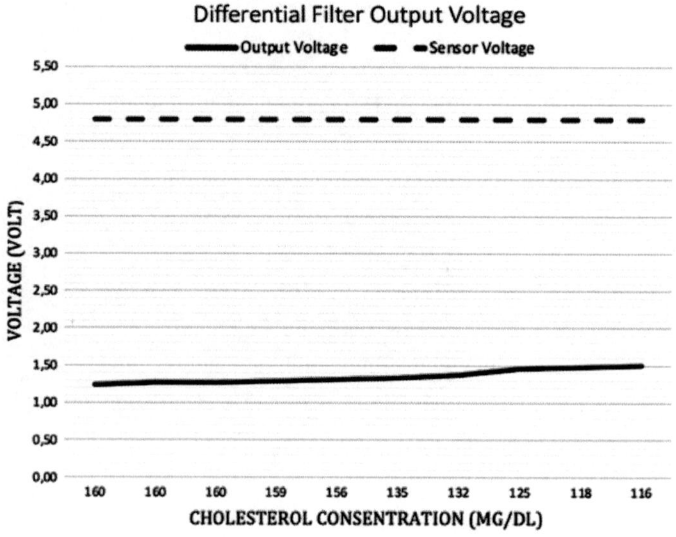

Fig. 5 Differential filter output voltage

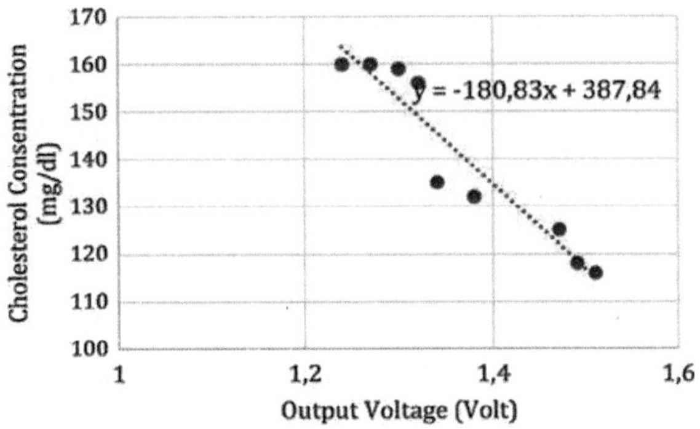

Fig. 6 Linear equations of the output voltage and cholesterol concentration

cholesterol serum in various concentration values. The concentration value of the sample cholesterol used is determined and validated using the chemical analyzer. All these samples are then used in the Spectrophotometer to determine the output voltage of the differential filter in each sample. Figure 6 is an equation graph that connects the output voltage of the spectrophotometer system designed with the value of cholesterol concentrations.

Based on Fig. 6, it appears that the concentration of cholesterol samples related inversely proportional to the output voltage spectrophotometer. The higher the value of cholesterol concentration, then the lower voltage will decrease.

3.3 The Performance and Statistical Analysis

Subsequent testing aimed to see if the designed Spectrophotometer provides accurate results in determining the concentration of cholesterol samples. This test is done using cholesterol samples in various concentrations, which has been validated previously. Table 1 shows the test results of cholesterol concentrations by using a spectrophotometer designed.

According to Table 1, it appears that the designed Spectrophotometer has provided excellent performance. The value of cholesterol concentrations provided by the Spectrophotometer is not much different from the value of actual cholesterol concentrations. The most significant error percentage given by the measurement using the Designed Spectrophotometer is 5.52%, which means that the Spectrophotometer has an accuracy value above 90%. For standard deviation (SD) and coefficient of variations (CV) result show that the designed spectrophotometer has the highest SD and CV value is about 3.99 and 2.88%, respectively. This result indicated that the designed device has high precision in measuring data.

Table 1 Measurement result sensor voltage and differential filter output voltage (based on ten times measurement)

Serum	Chemistry analyzer (mg/dl)	The designed spectrophometer (mg/dl)	Error (%)	SD	CV (%)
1	116	116.30	0.45	2.03	1.74
2	118	119.79	1.46	0.77	0.64
3	125	120.88	3.29	1.33	1.10
4	132	136.09	3.09	0.78	0.56
5	135	138.81	2.82	3.99	2.88
6	156	152.93	1.96	3.74	2.46
7	159	150.22	5.52	1.33	0.89
8	160	151.85	5.09	3.52	2.30
9	160	153.48	4.07	1.33	0.87
10	160	159.69	0.1	1.39	0.87

4 Discussion

Spectrophotometry is a quantitative measurement method in chemical analysis of a material's reflection and light transmission properties as a function of wavelength. This study demonstrates the effectiveness of using halogen lamps as light sources in the application of spectrophotometric principles in measuring cholesterol concentrations. Compared to the use of LED lamps [14, 15] as a light source on a spectrophotometer, halogen lamps have several advantages including not requiring a complex circuit in application, making it easier to maintain and repair in case of damage. In addition, compared to LEDs, halogen lamps are more resistant to heat so they do not require a special cooling system.

To convert polychromatic light produced by halogen lamps into monochromatic light, a monochromator in the form of a 620 nm optical glass filter is used. The main function of this optical glass filter is to provide light energy with a certain wavelength and spectral bandwidth. When this light energy is passed to certain media, which in this study is a serum cholesterol sample, the light intensity will decrease in proportion to the serum sample (cholesterol) concentration value. In this process, the light polarization is absorbed by the serum sample to produce a certain color (absorbance). The light produced will be detected by the phototransistor light sensor.

In principle, the phototransistor sensor produces an output voltage proportional to the wavelength of the detected light. Table 1 shows that the sensor voltage, when given cholesterol samples with various cholesterol concentrations, produces an almost identical voltage, around 4.8 volts. It is because the difference in voltage between cholesterol concentrations is very small to be detected by measuring instruments. Furthermore, the noise measured when detected by the phototransistor sensor also affects the resulting voltage value. In this study, the phototransistor sensor's voltage signal will be conditioned using amplifiers and filters so that the obtained spectrophotometer voltage truly represents the serum cholesterol concentration measured. The filter used to reduce mixed noise is a differential filter. The spectrophotometer voltage shown in Table 1 shows that the differential filter has succeeded in reducing the mixed noise during the sensor's reading. It can be seen that the output voltage value of the spectrophotometer is proportional to the value of cholesterol concentration.

The linear regression method was used to determine the functional relationship between the cholesterol concentration value and the spectrophotometer voltage value. This method has been proven for its effectiveness in determining the relationship between two variables in the spectrophotometer by Chaianantakul et al. [8]. By using the linear regression method, it is generated an equation:

$$y = -180.83x + 387.84 \tag{6}$$

The negative value at $\boldsymbol{\beta}_1$ shows the cholesterol concentration and the spectrophotometer voltage have an inversely proportional relationship. The equation obtained using the linear regression is used in microcontroller process to convert the spectrophotometer voltage into cholesterol concentration value. The test results shown in Table 1 indicate that the designed spectrophotometer has demonstrated excellent performance. The average error value obtained is below 5%. Besides that, the CV range between 0.56 and 2.88% indicated the designed device has high precision in measuring data.

The results of this study were also compared with the results of previous studies. Chaianantakul et al. proposed a spectrophotometer using LEDs as a light source and a fabricated polymer-based as a cuvette. In that study, the designed spectrophotometer was validated using a plasma glucose sample. The designed spectrophotometer has a CV range of 3.9 and 8.4% [8]. Oh and Kim developed a spectrophotometer using UV-vis as a light source. The design results were validated using dsDNA samples, and they found that the CV of the designed spectrophotometer had a range between 0.73 and 5.85% [7]. However, in these previous studies, no data was found regarding the accuracy of the designed devices.

This study has proven that a spectrophotometer's design using a halogen lamp as a light source and a 620 nm optical filter as a monochromator effectively analyzed the given chemical sample. However, this proposed device's limitation is that it only measures serum cholesterol samples and has not been tried to measure other chemical samples.

5 Conclusions

This study designed a visible light spectrophotometer that has a compact and portable size using a light source of halogen lamps. The 620 nm optical Filter is used to narrow the polychromatic light to monochromatic light. A differential filter is used to filter out mixed noise during detection by the phototransistor sensor.

Based on the test results, the differential filter circuit was designed to reduce the mixed noise during detection. Moreover, the 20 cm × 23 cm × 7.5 cm spectrophotometer performed excellently in testing the target of cholesterol concentrations. The most significant error percentage given by the measurement using the Designed Spectrophotometer is 5.52%, which means that the Spectrophotometer has an accuracy value above 90%. In the future study, this visible light spectrophotometer will aim to can be used not only for cholesterol concentration analysis, but also for other chemical samples like glucose, DHA, and the others.

References

1. Ray AG et al (2020) Novel mechanism of cholesterol transport by ABCA5 in macrophages and Its role in dyslipidemia. J Mol Biol 432(17):4922–4941
2. Pastukhov A, Krisanova N, Pyrshev K, Borisova V (2020) Dual benefit of combined neuroprotection: cholesterol depletion restores membrane microviscosity but not lipid order and enhances neuroprotective action of hypothermia in rat cortex nerve terminals. Biochim Biophys Acta Biomembr 1862(9):183362
3. Xu H, Zhou S, Tang Q, Xia H, Bi F (2020) Cholesterol metabolism: new functions and therapeutic approaches in cancer. Biochim Biophys Acta Rev Cancer 1874(1):188394
4. Cepeda MS, Kern DM, Blacketer C, Drevets WC (2020) Low levels of cholesterol and the cholesterol type are not associated with depression: results of a cross-sectional NHANES study. J Clin Lipidol
5. Shin JY, Suls J, Martin R (2008) Are cholesterol and depression inversely related? A meta-analysis of the association between two cardiac risk factors. Ann Behav Med 36(1): 33–43
6. Matinrad F, Kompany-Zareh M, Omidikia N, Dadashi M (2020) Systematic investigation of the measurement error structure in a smartphone-based spectrophotometer. Anal Chim Acta 1129:98–107
7. Oh SR, Kim S (2021) Micro-volume spectrophotometer with a slope spectroscopy technique. Measurement 167
8. Chaianantakul N et al (2018) Development of mini-spectrophotometer for determination of plasma glucose. Spectrochim Acta A Mol Biomol Spectrosc 204:670–676
9. Hespanhol MC, Souza JC, Pasquini C (2020) Feasibility of a portable, low-cost near-infrared spectrophotometer for the quality screening of omega-3 dietary supplements. J Pharm Biomed Anal 189:113436
10. Zinchenko T, Pecherskaya E, Golubkov P, Artamonov D, Kozlov G, Shepeleva Y (2020) Automated spectrophotometer control system. Procedia Comput Sci 167:477–486
11. Abdullah K, Jamil L, Saleem P (2017) Building a visible light spectrophotometer from NaI detector. Asian J Chem Sci 2(2):1–7
12. Ashfaque-E-Alam M, Islam MR, Faria IJ (2017) Development and validation of a low-cost visible light spectrophotometer. In: Presented at the 2017 4th International conference on advances in electrical engineering (ICAEE)
13. Bills MV et al (2020) Handheld UV fluorescence spectrophotometer device for the classification and analysis of petroleum oil samples. Biosens Bioelectron 159:112193
14. Veras G, Silva EC, Silva Lyra W, Soares SF, Guerreiro TB, Santos SR (2009) A portable, inexpensive and microcontrolled spectrophotometer based on white LED as light source and CD media as diffraction grid. Talanta 77(3):1155–1159

15. Zhao L, Wu D, Wu LF, Song T (2007) A simple and accurate method for quantification of magnetosomes in magnetotactic bacteria by common spectrophotometer. J Biochem Biophys Methods 70(3):377–383
16. Senthil Rajan V, Sanjay R, Kumaravel S, Venkataramani B (2019) Area and power efficient flipped voltage follower based symmetrical floating impedance scaler with improved accuracy for fully differential filters. AEU—Int J Electron Commun 106:116–125
17. Najafi-Yazdi A, Najafi-Yazdi M, Mongeau L (2015) A high resolution differential filter for large eddy simulation: toward explicit filtering on unstructured grids. J Comput Phys 292:272–286
18. Chilko SDSWD (2004) Statistics for research (Wiley Series in Probability and Statistics). Wiley, Canada (in English), p 634

Plasmodium Parasite Detection Using Combination of Image Processing and Deep Learning Approach

Alifia Revan Prananda, Hanung Adi Nugroho, and Eka Legya Frannita

Abstract The development of an intelligent system for automated malaria detection became the one of challenges since its application supported the examination process which was conducted manually by the doctor or medical personnel. Some previous studies have been done to overcome those problems. However, most of them still have problem in detecting parasite candidates. Hence, their proposed methods did not successfully detect all parasite candidates and remains a large number of false-negative. Actually, the misdetection problem occurred since the characteristic of parasites seems unclear. To overcome these problems, we applied image processing technique and deep learning architecture to detect and to ensure whether the detected candidate is a parasite or not. Our proposed method was applied to 46 digital microscopic images provided by the Department of Parasitology, Universitas Gadjah Mada and Eijkman Institute for Molecular Biology. The proposed method comprised of four steps which are normalization process using GGB (green, green, blue) color transformation, segmentation process using Otsu followed by some morphological operations, object labelling using BLOB analysis, and classification using deep learning. Our detection process successfully detected all parasites and the classification process achieved an accuracy, sensitivity, specificity, PPV and NPV of 98.97, 100, 98.08, 97.85, and 100% respectively. This result shows that our proposed method achieved outstanding performance in both detection and classification process which indicates that our proposed method had the potential to be implemented as an intelligent system for supporting the parasitologist in conducting rapid assessment of plasmodium parasite infection.

Keywords Plasmodium · Malaria · Detection · Deep learning · Image processing

A. R. Prananda · H. A. Nugroho (✉) · E. L. Frannita
Department of Electrical and Information Engineering, Faculty of Engineering, Universitas Gadjah Mada, Yogyakarta, Indonesia
e-mail: adinugroho@ugm.ac.id

H. Triwiyanto et al. (eds.), *Proceedings of the 1st International Conference on Electronics, Biomedical Engineering, and Health Informatics*, Lecture Notes in Electrical Engineering 746, https://doi.org/10.1007/978-981-33-6926-9_55

1 Introduction

Intelligent system in Plasmodium parasite detection became a necessary thing to assist the doctor to produce the diagnosis. Computer aided diagnosis (CADx) and computer aided detection (CADe) became an alternative that was recently developed by several researchers [1]. The image processing technique is one of the solutions to develop a method for detecting Plasmodium candidates even identify the species or stage of Plasmodium. Some previous research has been accomplished by applying image processing technique and successfully achieved incredible performance [2–8]. Despite the powerful results that have been accomplished, the development of detection method for Plasmodium parasite still had some hurdles. One of the hurdles is the variations of data. This problem occurs since a large number of variations not only in species variations but also in the stage of Plasmodium parasite. The amount of data variations made the automated detection system was difficult to develop [1]. In the other hand, some previous research also did not successfully detect all parasite in their experiment. This problem occurred since the digital microscopic images have low density level and show unclear parasite characteristics. Thus, most of researchers still remain a lot of false-negative rate in their studies.

Recently, deep learning approach became a model that obtained suitable result in Plasmodium parasite detection. Several studies about Plasmodium parasite detection have been done before. Research conducted by Bibin et al., proposed a detection of Malaria parasite from peripheral blood smear images by using deep belief network [9]. This study used 4100 peripheral blood smear images as a dataset consisting of parasite and non-parasite class. The DBN model used 484 visible layers and the output layer had two nodes with four hidden layers consisting of 600 hidden nodes in each layer. The proposed method successfully obtained F-score of 89.66%, sensitivity of 97.60% and specificity of 95.92%.

Study conducted by Soner et al., proposed a deep learning model for classifying Malaria [10]. This study used convolutional neural network (CNN) in the classification process, then the system selected from the incoming images using the convolution process, which is the most efficient features for training by revealing the separating properties from that images. The feature that selected, then pass through the artificial neural network and then the estimations were compared with the actual values, after that the network was updated and optimized. The dataset that used for this study consists of 27,558 cell images taken from the U.S National Library of Medicine. The result of this study reached the training accuracy rate of 0.97 and the testing accuracy of 0.95. Besides, the training and test accuracy values were 0.07 and 0.16 respectively. Research conducted by Esra et al., proposed deep transfer learning for detection Malaria parasite [11]. This study applied transfer learning method to detect and classify the malaria parasites. The pre-trained process used CNN Model VGG19 for 20 epochs on 1428 samples of Plasmodium Vivax, 1425 samples of Plasmodium Ovale, 1446 samples of Plasmodium Falciparum, 1450 samples of Plasmodium Malariae, and 1440 of non-parasite samples.

This cstudy achieved 80, 83, 86, 75% of precision, and 83, 86, 86, 79% of F-measure test from the 19 test images.

Research conducted by Yuhang et al., proposed a deep convolutional neural network for classifying Malaria [12]. This study classified Malaria infected cells using deep convolutional neural network. The research used LeNet-5 for training and testing. This study achieved 95% of accuracy. Research conducted by Yuhang et al., proposed an evaluation method of deep convolutional neural network for automatic identification of Malaria [13]. This study used three types of well-known convolutional neural network, which is LeNet, AlexNet, and GoogLeNet. All of those three types that used for this study, achieved classification accuracy over 95%.

Regarding the outperforming performance of deep learning, we decided to adopt this approach for detecting the plasmodium parasite especially to distinguish Plasmodium parasites and other objects. We combined the image processing approach and deep learning to find the location of parasite candidate and to analyze whether the detected object is a parasite or artifact. To address the research gap, we presented the contributions including of:

1. Several previous studies in both image processing and machine learning or deep learning have been done to detect the Plasmodium parasites. However, most of them still have problem in the detection process in which occurred by the unclear characteristic of parasite. Thus, we performed GGB color combination to sharpen those characteristics since it worked nicely for reducing unnecessary red color in the images like digital microscopic images.
2. After performing GGB color combination, we applied image processing process to detect all parasite candidates.
3. In the last step, we performed deep learning approach to validate our detection result and to distinguish whether the detected candidate is a parasite or not.

All steps of this paper were organized as follow: dataset was described in Sect. 2, deep learning approach was drawn in Sect. 3, plasmodium detection process was stated in Sect. 4, experimental result was described in Sect. 5 and finally the conclusion was stated in Sect. 5.

2 Methodology

Our proposed method was developed by conducting several processes which are pre-processing for sharpening the characteristic of Plasmodium parasites, segmentation, detection, and classification as depicted in Fig. 1.

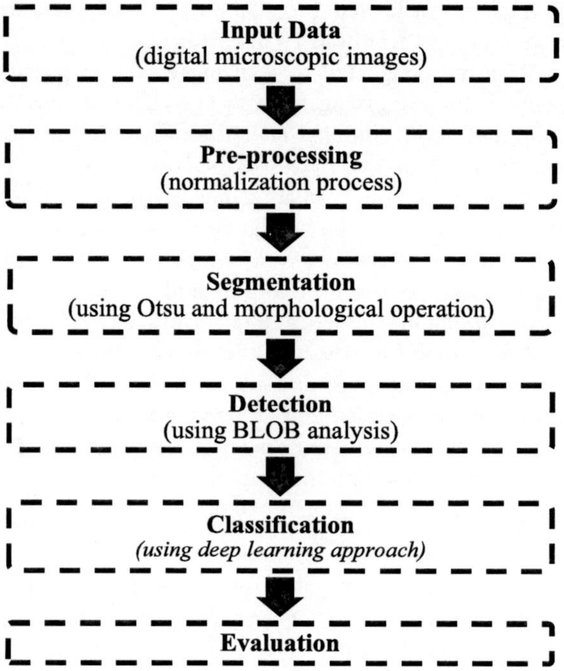

Fig. 1 Steps of development of Plasmodium detection method

2.1 Dataset and Hardware Specification

Development of plasmodium detection method required the digital microscopic images. We performed 46 thin blood smear digital microscopic images provided by Department of Parasitology, Faculty of Medicine, Public Health and Nursing, Universitas Gadjah Mada and Eijkman Institute for Molecular Biology. The dataset was the raw data with a size of 1280 × 960 captured by the OptiLab camera. The dataset was also completed with the ground truth marked by the parasitologist and processed to be a binary image. An example of dataset is illustrated in Fig. 2. For the development process, we used a personal computer with specification as follow: processor—Intel(R) Core(TM) i5-4210U, CPU—1.7 GHz (Turbo Boost up to 2.40 GHz), RAM—8 GB.

2.2 Pre-processing

Pre-processing step was used to enhance the quality of images since our dataset contained of some unwanted objects like artifact and noise. In this study we used GGB color transformation as the normalization process proposed by [14]. The objective of this normalization process is to sharpen the image. The improvement of

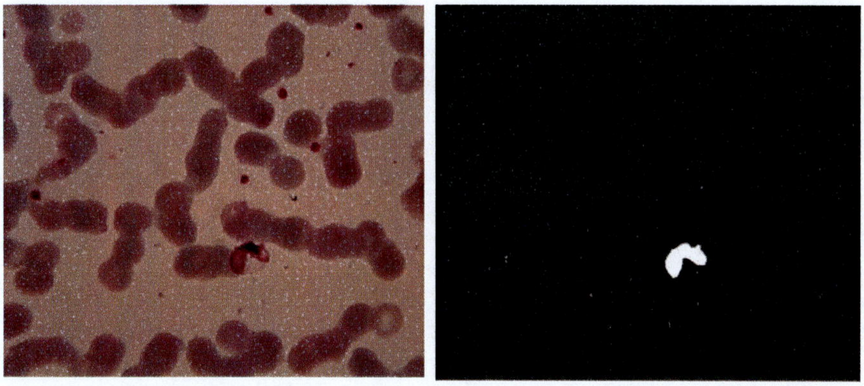

(a) (b)

Fig. 2 An example of dataset: **a** raw data and **b** ground truth of images (**a**)

image quality was very useful for segmentation process since it performed to strengthen objects with unique characteristic.

The GGB color transformation was performed by several steps. Firstly, it separated each channel of RGB followed by calculating G_n using (1).

$$G_n = \frac{G}{G_{mean}} \tag{1}$$

with G is pixel value of green channel and G_{mean} is mean value of green channel image. The result of Eq. (1) was then enhanced by applying contrast adjustment. The result of this process was defined as G′. Then, pre-processing step was continued by calculate B_n using (2).

$$B_n = \frac{B}{B_{mean}} \tag{2}$$

with B is pixel value of blue channel and B_{mean} is mean value of blue channel. In the last step, it was created a new image combination by combining G′, G′ and B_n which was called GGB. The result of GGB color transformation was then used in the segmentation process.

2.3 *Segmentation Process*

In the next step, we performed Otsu thresholding [15] to segment the parasite candidates by using B_n as input image and calculate the threshold value from G′. We chose B_n as input image since it contained object with strengthened characteristic and low pixel value of background. Then, we calculated threshold value from G′ because image G′ provided homogeny pixel value which close to parasite characteristic in image B_n. We also performed the morphological operation [16] to flesh out the imperfection object of segmentation result.

2.4 Detection Process

Result of segmentation process was then analyzed to detect the location parasite candidates. We stored the location of Plasmodium candidates by using result of segmentation process. This process was conducted by using BLOB analysis [17]. After finding the location of parasite candidates, we labelled those objects as parasite candidate and cropped it in size of 251 × 251 pixel.

2.5 Classification Process

Result of detection process was a cropped image that represent the Plasmodium parasite. However, we need to ensure whether those objects were correctly parasite or not. To validate the detection result, we performed the classification process by using deep learning approach. We used LeNet architecture with the following configuration. We used size of 100 × 100 of input image with the number mini batch size of 6 and batch size of 8. We also used number of channels of 3 since our dataset comprised of 3 channels (RGB). LeNet architecture had 6 layers which are input layer, convolution layer 1, subsampling layer 1 (max pooling), convolution layer 2, subsampling layer 2 (max pooling), dense layer and output layer.

2.6 Evaluation

In the last step, we calculated accuracy, sensitivity, specificity, positive predictive value (PPV) and negative predictive value (NPV) using Eqs. (3, 4, 5, 6, 7).

$$accuracy = \frac{TP + TN}{TP + TN + FP + FN} \tag{3}$$

$$sensitivity = \frac{TP}{TP + FN} \tag{4}$$

$$specificity = \frac{TN}{TN + FP} \tag{5}$$

$$PPV = \frac{TP}{TP + FP} \quad (6)$$

$$NPV = \frac{TN}{TN + FN} \quad (7)$$

3 Experimental Result

After conducting all processes, our experiment in pre-processing step using GGB color transformation and Otsu followed by morphological operation achieved good results as illustrated in Fig. 3.

Result of normalization process is illustrated in Fig. 3b. This result illustrates that parasite candidate was more clearly than image in Fig. 3a. This result was then used in segmentation process by separating G′ and B_n in Fig. 3b. Image B_n is illustrated in Fig. 3d and image G′ is illustrated in Fig. 3c. Since parasite in Fig. 3d seems more clearly, this image was used as an input image in segmentation process. While image G′ was used to calculate the threshold value since it contained homogeny pixel value that close to the parasite characteristic as delineated in

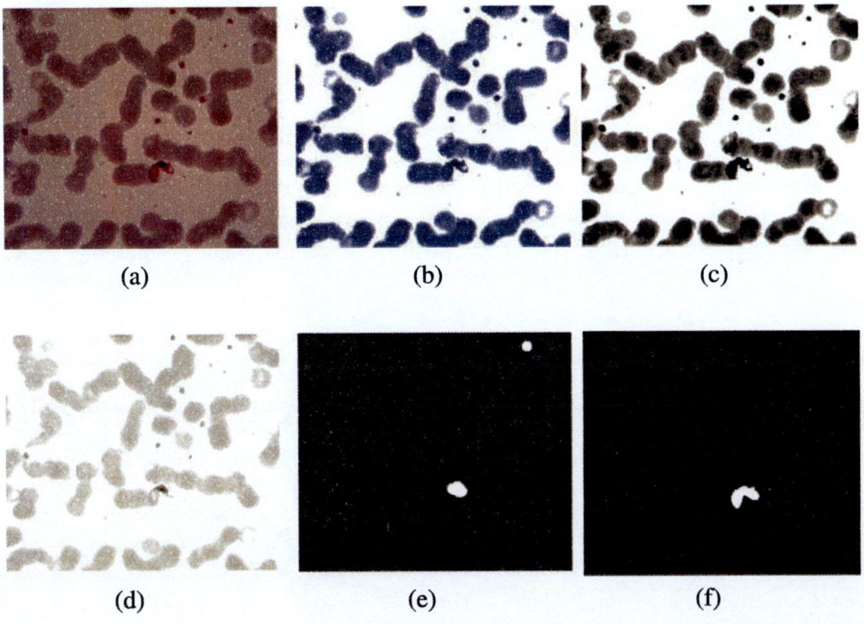

Fig. 3 Result of pre-processing step and segmentation step: **a** raw data, **b** result of GGB, **c** image G', **d** image B_n, **e** final result of segmentation process and **f** ground truth of image **(a)**

Fig. 3c. After applying threshold value from Fig. 3c to image in Fig. 3d, we achieved segmentation result as depicted in Fig. 3e. As illustrated in Fig. 3e, our proposed method successfully segmented the parasite although it produced 2 unwanted objects that call false positive.

After conducting segmentation process, we stored the location of all detected objects and gave the label on them as illustrated in Fig. 4b. The labelled object was then evaluated with the ground truth. If the detected object was match with the ground truth, so it labelled as true positive (TP). If we found an unwanted object that does not match with the ground truth, so it labelled as false positive (FP). Figure 4 illustrates the result of labelling process.

As illustrated in Fig. 4, location of detected objects in Fig. 4a was stored and validated in the ground truth as presented in Fig. 4b. The location of detected object is drawn by yellow rectangle. In this figure we successfully detect the parasite, but we also produce 2 false positive as illustrated in Fig. 4c. All detected object was the cropped in size of 251 × 251.

Our proposed method successfully detected all parasite candidates, however it also produced a large number of false positive. Due to this problem, we conducted the data augmentation using flip and rotation function using 90° on the detected parasite. This data augmentation process achieved 487 images of parasite and 488 images of non-parasite. This data was then used as an input data in the classification model with the proportion data of 80% for training data and 20% for testing data. Our classification process successfully achieved good result as follow (Table 1).

4 Discussion

In the experimental result, our proposed method successfully achieved outstanding performance in both detection and classification of Plasmodium parasite. In the detection process, we successfully detected all parasites. In the classification process, we achieved accuracy, specificity, positive predictive value, F-measure, ROC

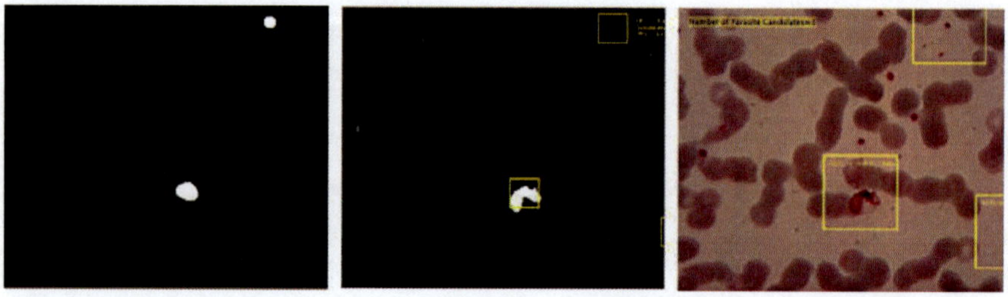

(a) (b) (c)

Fig. 4 Result of detection step: **a** segmentation result, **b** validation on the ground truth, **c** detection result

Table 1 Experimental result using deep learning

Parameters	Performance
Accuracy	98.97%
Sensitivity	100%
Specificity	98.08%
Positive predictive value	97.85%
Negative predictive value	100%
F-measure	0.990
ROC area	0.996
Computational time	952.05 s

Fig. 5 Confusion Matrix

Predicted Class \ Actual Class	Non-parasite	Parasite
Non-parasite	91	2
Parasite	0	102

area of 98.97%, 98.08%, 97.85%, 0.990, 0.006, respectively, while sensitivity and negative predictive value achieved a perfect score. As illustrate in the confusion matrix depicted in Fig. 5, there were only 2 objects that were misclassified which indicates that our classification process can distinguish the parasite characteristic perfectly. Despite those outstanding performance, our proposed still need more improvement to overcome some problem such as high computational time and a lot of false positive rate.

5 Conclusion

The development of detection system to assist the parasitologist in analyzing digital microscopic images is necessary to conduct early detection of Plasmodium parasites. In this work, we present a combination of image processing technique for detecting the parasite candidates and deep learning approach for distinguishing that the detected object is parasite or not. Our proposed method comprised of four processes which are pre-processing for sharpening the characteristic of Plasmodium parasites, segmentation, detection, and classification. This model achieved accuracy, sensitivity, specificity, PPV and NPV of 98.97, 100, 98.08, 97.85, and 100% respectively. It indicates that our proposed method provides powerful performance in detecting and classifying Plasmodium parasites.

Acknowledgements This study is funded by Directorate General of Higher Education, Ministry of Research, Technology and Higher Education through the Research Grant of "Penelitian Dasar Unggulan Perguruan Tinggi". The authors would also like to thank Intelligent System research group in Department of Electrical and Information Engineering for inspiring discussion and motivation.

References

1. Preedanan W, Phothisonothai M, Senavongse W, Tantisatirapong S (2016) Automated detection of plasmodium falciparum from Giemsa-stained thin blood films. In: 2016 8th international conference on knowledge and smart technology (KST), pp 215–218
2. Nugroho HA, Nurfauzi R, Frannita EL (2019) Plasmodium candidate detection on thin blood smear images with luminance noise reduction. In: 2019 5th international conference on science in information technology (ICSITech), pp 146–149
3. Haryanto SEV, Mashor MY, Nasir ASA, Jaafar H (2017) A fast and accurate detection of Schizont plasmodium falciparum using channel color space segmentation method. In: 2017 5th international conference on cyber and IT service management (CITSM), pp 1–4
4. Gatc J, Maspiyanti F (2018) Plasmodium parasite detection on thin blood smear image using double thresholding and BLOB analysis. In: 2018 international conference on applied engineering (ICAE), pp 1–6
5. Peñas KED, Rivera PT, Naval PC (2017) Malaria parasite detection and species identification on thin blood smears using a convolutional neural network. In: 2017 IEEE/ACM international conference on connected health: applications, systems and engineering technologies (CHASE), pp 1–6
6. Nugroho HA, Imaroh K, Ardiyanto I, Frannita EL (2020) Automated detection of plasmodium ovale and malariae species on microscopic thin blood smear images. Int J Adv Soft Compu Appl 12
7. Mohammed HA, Abdelrahman IAM (2017) Detection and classification of Malaria in thin blood slide images. In: 2017 international conference on communication, control, computing and electronics engineering (ICCCCEE), pp 1–5
8. Prananda AR, Nugroho HA, Ardiyanto I (2019) Enumeration of plasmodium parasites on thin blood smear digital microscopic images. In: 2019 5th international conference on science in information technology (ICSITech), pp 223–228
9. Bibin D, Nair MS, Punitha P (2017) Malaria parasite detection from peripheral blood smear images using deep belief networks. IEEE Access 5:9099–9108
10. Kalkan SC, Sahingoz OK (2019) Deep learning based classification of malaria from slide images. In: 2019 scientific meeting on electrical-electronics & biomedical engineering and computer science (EBBT), pp 1–4
11. Var E, Tek FB (2018) Malaria parasite detection with deep transfer learning. In: 2018 3rd international conference on computer science and engineering (UBMK), pp 298–302. https://doi.org/10.1109/ubmk.2018.8566549
12. Dong Y, Jiang Z, Shen H, Pan WD (2017) Classification accuracies of malaria infected cells using deep convolutional neural networks based on decompressed images. In: SoutheastCon 2017, pp 1–6
13. Dong Y et al (2017) Evaluations of deep convolutional neural networks for automatic identification of malaria infected cells. In: 2017 IEEE EMBS international conference on biomedical & health informatics (BHI), pp 101–104
14. Hegde R, Prasad K, Hebbar H, Singh BM (2018) Development of a robust algorithm for detection of nuclei and classification of white blood cells in peripheral blood smear images. J Med Syst 42

15. Otsu N (1979) A threshold selection method from gray-level histograms. IEEE Trans Syst Man Cybern 9:62–66
16. Davies ERBT-CV (ed) (2018) Chapter 3—Image filtering and morphology (Fifth ed). Academic Press, pp 39–92
17. Nugroho HA, Saputra WA, Permanasari AE, Murhandarwati EEH (2017) Automated determination of plasmodium region of interest on thin blood smear images. In: 2017 international seminar on intelligent technology and its applications (ISITIA), pp 352–355

Rapid Assessment of Breast Cancer Malignancy Using Deep Neural Network

Alifia Revan Prananda, Hanung Adi Nugroho, and Eka Legya Frannita

Abstract Breast cancer is one of the deadly diseases that have high morbidity and mortality rate. Traditionally, doctors or radiologists should delineate the malignancy suspicious in a manual procedure such as manual segmentation or making diagnosis decisions. This medical examination may occur some problems such as time-consuming, tedious, and possible to produce subjective results. An alternative way to overcome this problem is that implementing technology to support this examination process. Hence, we propose a deep neural network model to reach the development of a rapid classification system for breast cancer. Our model was performed in the Breast Cancer Wisconsin (Diagnostic) dataset consisting of 569 instances and 30 attributes. Our proposed model was started by balancing the data in the preparation step. After conducting the preparation step, we performed a deep neural network model with three hidden layers and two dropout layers. Our experiment achieved the best performance compared to the previous study with accuracy, sensitivity, specificity, positive predictive value, and negative predictive value of 98.536, 98.466, 98.765, 99.689, 94.118, and 98.500% respectively which indicates that our proposed method has suitable performance for assessing cancerous of breast cancer.

Keywords Breast cancer · Deep neural network · Cancer malignancy · Classification

1 Introduction

Breast cancer is one of dangerous disease that has high morbidity and mortality. In 2017, United States Breast Cancer Statistics estimated that there were 252,710 new malignancy cases that should be analyzed [1]. In the same year, Health Institution

A. R. Prananda · H. A. Nugroho (✉) · E. L. Frannita
Department of Electrical and Information Engineering, Faculty of Engineering, Universitas Gadjah Mada, Yogyakarta, Indonesia
e-mail: adinugroho@ugm.ac.id

H. Triwiyanto et al. (eds.), *Proceedings of the 1st International Conference on Electronics, Biomedical Engineering, and Health Informatics*, Lecture Notes in Electrical Engineering 746, https://doi.org/10.1007/978-981-33-6926-9_56

of Malaysia also analyzed and assumed that Malaysian woman has one of 20 chances to be diagnosed as a patient with malignancy cases [1]. Other country such as China also reported that mortality rate caused by breast cancer has been increased particularly in both urban and rural area with the increasing number of 38.9 and 39.7% respectively [2].

Traditionally, for assessing the cancerous of breast cancer, doctor or radiologist should delineate the malignancy suspicious in a manual procedure such as manual segmentation or making diagnosis decision. Nevertheless, this manual procedure needed more time and depended on the operator or radiologist. Recently, computer aided diagnosis which is well-known as CAD became an effective system to overcome this manual problem and operator dependency. CAD related with the technology used to analyzed medical problem regarding to make a diagnosis decision. CAD was developed to decrease the subjectivity and error affected by manual examination procedure [1, 3, 4].

Currently, numerous researchers have been accomplishing studies regarding to CAD development and concluding that machine learning was one of powerful methods to be implemented in the development of CAD. In the breast cancer problem, machine learning approach also performed a powerful performance. For example, in classification process conducted by Bayrak et al. [5] in the Wisconsin Breast Cancer (original) dataset achieved accuracy of 96.9957% using support vector machine classifier. This classification process aimed to distinguish 699 instances into two classes which are benign and malignant. Classification process was performed based on 11 integer-valued attributes provided by the dataset without any pre-treatment. Despite the performance of classification model was high enough, this classification process was conducted without any pre-treatment before. Hence, if the pre-treatment was conducted before, it might increase the performance of classification model.

Other same cases in the breast cancer classification using Wisconsin Breast Cancer has been conducted by Amrane et al. [6]. This classification process was started by conducting data acquisition. Since the dataset contained of missing data for 16 observations, this classification process only used 683 instances from 699 instances provided by dataset. For the classification process, nearest neighbor algorithm with k value of 3 and Naïve Bayes were used as classifier and achieved accuracy of 97.5109 and 96.1932% respectively. These results show that pre-processing affects the classification result. The same pre-processing step also conducted in other research with same dataset and obtained accuracy of 96.85% by using C-SVM classifier [7]. Other cases with the same scenario obtained accuracy of 97.9% by using support vector machine classifier [8]. All accomplished studies were conducted in the same dataset and used machine learning for classifying breast cancer in the malignant and benign classes.

Regardless of machine learning performance in breast cancer classification cases, implementation of machine learning for classifying breast cancer still leaves a few problems and still has some efforts to achieve high performance such as preprocessing and feature selection process. In the other hand, recently, deep neural network approach became a powerful method to overcome the limitation of machine learning approach. In the same case, deep neural network also successfully classified breast cancer into two classes (benign and malignant) with accuracy of 97.4468% by using Wisconsin Breast Cancer (original) dataset consisting of 699 instances [9]. Another research conducting in this field, Darapurredy et al. [10] also proposed a deep neural network for classifying breast cancer using Wisconsin Breast Cancer (diagnostic) dataset and achieved accuracy of 97%. In the other hand, Shajib et al. [11] conducted convolutional neural network for classifying breast cancer and obtained accuracy of 98%. Those studies successfully achieve high performance for classifying breast cancer in the case of Wisconsin dataset in which mostly accuracy was more than 97%. According to this result, it can be assumed that deep learning approach had a potential to be implemented in breast cancer classification problem.

In this study, we presented a deep neural network model to classify breast cancer into two classes (benign and malignant). We used Wisconsin Breast Cancer (diagnostic) dataset that was updated from Wisconsin Breast Cancer (original) and consisted of 569 instances. This dataset also consisted of 30 attribute that had high variation. Hence, we assumed that machine learning might be difficult to resolve this classification problem since the data was complex enough. To address these research gap, we performed a deep neural network architecture regarding to increase the performance of classification and overcome the limitation of machine learning approach since deep neural network was estimated to be a powerful method that had better performance than machine learning approach. We adopted and modified the deep neural network proposed by Yuefeng [9] by applying the different configuration in both activation function and optimizer. We also conducted the data balancing process before inputting our data to the deep neural model. We also analyzed and compared the performance of classification obtained from deep neural network with some machine learning approaches.

2 Materials and Method

This research work is conducted in the Breast Cancer Wisconsin (Diagnostic) dataset by performing three processes as delineated in Fig. 1. These all processes were data preparation, development deep neural network architecture and evaluation. The detail explanation of dataset and each step were described in the following subsection.

2.1 Dataset

In this study, we used Breast Cancer Wisconsin (Diagnostic) dataset provided in the UCI Machine Learning website [12, 13]. Breast Cancer Wisconsin (Diagnostic) dataset was updated dataset from Wisconsin Breast Cancer (original) and consisted

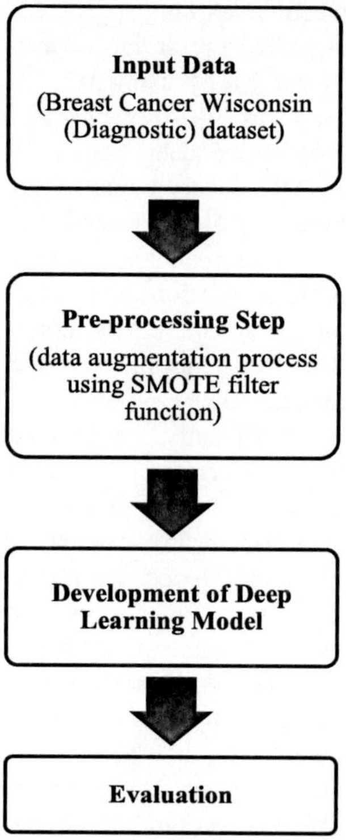

Fig. 1 Block diagram of the proposed method

of 569 instances and 30 attributes. The 30 attributes are shown in Table 1 and the example of data are shown in Table 2. Notation M in Table 2 indicates the malignant cancer, while notation B in Table 2 indicates the benign cancer. Hence, there are two classes which are malignant and benign that will be classified in the study.

Table 1 Attributes of Breast Cancer Wisconsin (Diagnostic) dataset

Attributes of data		
1. Radius mean	11. Radius se	21. Radius worst
2. Texture mean	12. Texture se	22. Texture worst
3. Perimeter mean	13. Perimeter se	23. Perimeter worst
4. Area mean	14. Area se	24. Area worst
5. Smoothness mean	15. Smoothness se	25. Smoothness worst
6. Compactness mean	16. Compactness se	26. Compactness worst
7. Concavity mean	17. Concavity se	27. Concavity worst
8. Concave points mean	18. Concave points se	28. Concave points worst
9. Symmetry mean	19. Symmetry se	29. Symmetry worst
10. Fractal dimension mean	20. Fractal dimension se	30. Fractal dimension worst

Table 2 Example of attributes value

No	Radius mean	Texture mean	Perimeter mean	…	Diagnosis
1	17.99	10.38	122.8	…	M
2	20.57	17.77	132.9	…	M
3	19.69	21.25	130	…	M
4	11.42	20.38	77.58	…	M
5	20.29	14.34	135.1	…	M
6	12.45	15.7	82.57	…	M
7	18.25	19.98	119.6	…	M
8	13.54	14.36	87.46	…	B
…	…	…	…	…	…
569	9.504	12.44	60.34	…	B

2.2 *Data Preparation*

Since our proposed method was performed in the imbalance and insufficient dataset, we should have conducted data balancing and increased the amount of data. In this research work, we performed SMOTE (Synthetic Minority Oversampling Technique) filter function to overcome this problem. This filter function was work by balancing the amount of data. This filter function was also powerful to be implemented as a data augmentation process. Hence, we used this filter function to conduct these purposes.

SMOTE filter function is a kind of over-sampling methods proposed by Chawla et al. [14–16] which was used to alleviate the risk of overfitting caused by random sampling process. SMOTE filter function was also powerful to overcome imbalance data problem. SMOTE filter function worked by the three following steps:

- Select a random minority observation $\vec{a}$.
- Select instance $\vec{b}$ amidst its k nearest minority class neighbors.
- Create a new sample $\vec{x}$ by applying (1) as a randomly interpolating formula of two samples with w defines a random weight. See Fig. 2.

Fig. 2 An illustration of SMOTE filter function with k = 4 [14]

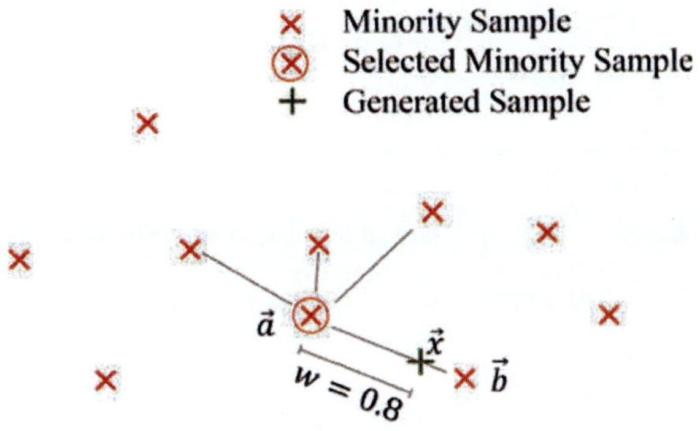

$$\vec{x} = \vec{a} + w * \left(\vec{b} - \vec{a}\right) \quad (1)$$

In this process, we set up some parameter such as nearest neighbors and percentage of data augmentation. For nearest neighbor parameter, it was suggested that 5 was the best value. However, to validate this value, we tried some number between 1 and 5 and found that 3 was the best number to increase the performance of accuracy. For the percentage of data augmentation process, we filled 500% since deep neural network needed a lot of data.

2.3 Development of Deep Neural Network Model

Since deep neural network offered the powerful performance, we adopted it in this research work to resolve our classification problem. In the development of deep neural network model step, we adopted and modified a deep neural network architecture proposed by [9]. This architecture is delineated in Fig. 3 and all parameters that is used in this work is described in Table 3.

As depicted in Fig. 3, we put three hidden layers and two dropout layers. The two dropouts' layer were used for eliminating the lowest weight to avoid the overfitting. In the first hidden layer, we used dense layer with number of outputs of 9 and took ReLU as an activation function. In the second hidden layer, we used dense layer with number of outputs of 5 and took ReLU as an activation function. In the last hidden layer, we used dense layer with number of outputs of 1 and took ReLU as an activation function. The previous work [9] used sigmoid function in

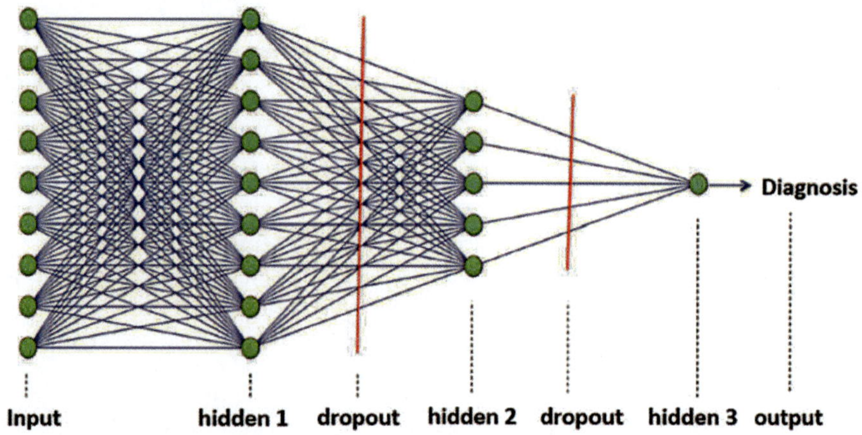

Fig. 3 The proposed deep neural network architecture [9]

Table 3 Parameter of the deep neural network architecture

Layer	Number of outputs
Hidden layer 1	9
Dropout layer 1	9
Hidden layer 2	5
Dropout layer 2	5
Hidden layer 3	1

this layer, however we modified and changed into ReLU. ReLU was chosen since it worked effectively. ReLU worked by eliminating an unnecessary value for example if the value was lower than 0, then it replaced to 0. This process was very useful to reduce the used memory. This fact is that causing ReLU works better than another activation function. Hence, we considered to use ReLU with assumption that ReLU has better performance than sigmoid. We also used Adam optimizer function to increase the accuracy. Our model was run in 50 epoch and batch size of 16 in training step.

In this study, we chose this architecture since it successfully worked in previous research conducted by Yuefeng [9]. However, we conducted some additional process because the number of data and the number of attributes were very different. Yuefeng [9] only used small attributes for classification process, while we used 30 attributes that may increase the accuracy. Thus, we still use that architecture, but we modified it and performed additional process to keep the performance.

2.4 Evaluation

Performance evaluation was step to analysis how the proposed model or method resolve the main problem. In this study, we used five parameters to evaluate the performance proposed model. The five parameters were accuracy, sensitivity, specificity, positive predictive value (PPV) and negative predictive value (NPV). These five parameters are described in the following equations with TP defines as the true positive rate, TN defines as the true negative rate, FP defines as the false positive rate and FN defines as the false negative rate.

$$accuracy = \frac{TP + TN}{TP + TN + FP + FN} \tag{2}$$

$$sensitivity = \frac{TP}{TP + FN} \tag{3}$$

$$specificity = \frac{TN}{TN + FP} \tag{4}$$

$$PPV = \frac{TP}{TP + FP} \quad (5)$$

$$NPV = \frac{TN}{TN + FN} \quad (6)$$

3 Experimental Result

In our experiment, we conducted pre-processing step by using SMOTE filter function. Our experiment successfully increased and balanced the data with an increasing number of 1629 of instances. This data was then inputted in the deep neural network model with proportion of 75% for training data and 25% for testing data. By using architecture that is described in the subsection before, we get an evaluation result as delineated in Fig. 4 and Table 4.

To point out the difference performance of our proposed method with the previous study proposed by Yuefeng [9], we illustrate a result when the dataset is performed in the architecture proposed by Yuefeng [9] without any additional process or modification (Table 5).

Since the Breast Cancer Wisconsin (Diagnostic) dataset has been used in numerous research such as Ashraf et al. [17] that used k-NN classifier to classify the breast cancer, Singh et al. [18] that applied several classifiers in their experiment, Darapureddy et al. [10] that used deep neural network to classify the malignancy of

Fig. 4 Confusion Matrix

Predicted Class \ Actual Class	Malignant	Benign
Malignant	321	5
Benign	1	80

Table 4 Experimental result for the testing process using deep neural network

Parameters	Proposed method
Accuracy	98.536%
Sensitivity	98.466%
Specificity	98.765%
Positive predictive value	99.689%
Negative predictive value	94.118%
F-measure	98.500%
ROC area	0.999
Computational time	267.64 s

Table 5 Experimental result for the testing process using Yuefeng's method [9] without any additional process or modification

Parameters	Proposed method
Accuracy	63.83%
Sensitivity	85.71%
Specificity	24%
Positive predictive value	67.24%
Negative predictive value	48%
F-measure	60%
ROC area	0.578
Computational time	155.35 s

Table 6 Comparison results

Methods	Performance evaluation							
	Accuracy (%)	Sensitivity (%)	Specificity (%)	PPV (%)	NPV (%)	F-measure (%)	ROC area	Time (s)
SVM [18]	80	100	0	80	NaN	NaN	0.50	0.72
MLP [18]	98.53	98.16	100	100	93.10	98.5	0.99	5.34
Naive Bayes [17, 18]	95.33	95.09	96.29	99.04	82.98	95.5	0.99	0.01
Random Forest [18]	98.03	98.77	95.06	98.77	95.06	98	0.99	0.35
Deep Neural Network [10]	97	–	–	–	–	–	–	–
Deep Neural Network [9]	63.83	85.71	24	67.24	48	60	0.58	155.35
RBF	98.28	98.47	97.53	99.38	94.05	98.3	0.99	0.32
Proposed method	**98.54**	**98.47**	**98.77**	**99.69**	**94.12**	**98.5**	**0.99**	**267.64**

breast cancer, and Shahnaz et al. [11] that used several classifiers to evaluate the classification process. Thus, we compared our experimental result with those previous studies. Table 6 shows the comparison result with some previous studies. We also conducted experiment in another classifier such as RBF.

4 Discussion

Table 6 shows the comparison result between the proposed method and other methods such as SVM, Naive Bayes, Random Forest, and another deep neural network. SVM seems achieve the lowest performance with accuracy of 80% and zero value in some evaluation parameter such as PPV, NPV and F-measure. These zero values are occurred since the classifier did not success to classify the data into two classes, however the classifier only can identify the data as a malignant class. In the other hand, MLP, Naive Bayes, Random Forest, and RBF provided good performance with accuracy of 98.526, 95.332, 98.034, 98.280%, respectively. Those results show that the classifiers are successfully in distinguish the benign and malignant data. We also compared our proposed method with another deep neural network conducted by Darapureddy et al. [10] which achieves accuracy of 97%. This study did not conduct another measurement of parameter evaluation. Our proposed method also outperformed the previous study conducted by Yuefeng [9] which achieves accuracy of 63.83%. Finally, our proposed method is successfully outperformed another classifier with accuracy of 98.536%. It indicates that our proposed method provides an outstanding performance since the dataset was complex enough and consisted of many features. Our proposed method also achieves high performance in sensitivity, specificity, positive predictive value, negative predictive value and F-measure with the value of them are 98.466%, 98.765%, 99.689%, 94.118%, and 98.500% respectively. Despite this successful achievement, our proposed method needs more time to execute the data. Hence, in future work, some optimization was needed to decrease the computational time and to keep the performance high.

5 Conclusion

The development of a classification model to assist the doctor and radiologist in diagnosing breast cancer was necessary to reduce subjectivity problem. In this work, we present a deep neural network model to classify breast cancer into two classes (benign and malignant) by using Breast Cancer Wisconsin (Diagnostic) dataset provided in the UCI Machine Learning website. Our experiment comprised of three major processes which are pre-processing data, development of deep neural network model and evaluation. Our deep neural network model consisted of three hidden layers and two dropout layers. This model achieved accuracy, sensitivity, specificity, PPV and NPV of 98.536, 98.466, 98.765, 99.689, 94.118 and 98.500% respectively. However, our deep neural network model needed more computational time compared with machine learning classifier.

Acknowledgements This study is funded by Directorate General of Higher Education, Ministry of Research, Technology and Higher Education and Department of Electrical and Information Engineering, Faculty of Engineering, Universitas Gadjah Mada through research grant of "Hibah Departemen". The authors would also like to thank Intelligent System research group in Department of Electrical and Information Engineering for inspiring discussion and motivation.

References

1. Ting FF, Tan YJ, Sim KS (2019) Convolutional neural network improvement for breast cancer classification. Expert Syst Appl 120:103–115
2. Fang Y et al (2019) Image classification toward breast cancer using deeply-learned quality features. J Vis Commun Image Represent 64:102609
3. Ekici S, Jawzal H (2020) Breast cancer diagnosis using thermography and convolutional neural networks. Med Hypotheses 137:109542
4. Jarosik P, Klimonda Z, Lewandowski M, Byra M (2020) Breast lesion classification based on ultrasonic radio-frequency signals using convolutional neural networks. Biocybern Biomed Eng 40:977–986
5. Bayrak EA, Kırcı P, Ensari T (2019) Comparison of machine learning methods for breast cancer diagnosis. In: 2019 Scientific meeting on electrical-electronics & biomedical engineering and computer science (EBBT), pp 1–3
6. Amrane M, Oukid S, Gagaoua I, Ensarİ T (2018) Breast cancer classification using machine learning. In: 2018 Electric electronics, computer science, biomedical engineerings' meeting (EBBT), pp 1–4
7. Akbugday B (2019) Classification of breast cancer data using machine learning algorithms. In: 2019 Medical technologies congress (TIPTEKNO), pp 1–4
8. Khourdifi Y, Bahaj M (2018) Applying best machine learning algorithms for breast cancer prediction and classification. In: 2018 International conference on electronics, control, optimization and computer science (ICECOCS), pp 1–5
9. Zhang Y (2019) Deep learning breast cancer diagnosis. https://towardsdatascience.com/deep-learning-in-winonsin-breast-cancer-diagnosis-6bab13838abd
10. Darapureddy N, Karatapu N, Battula TK (2019) Implementation of optimization algorithms on Wisconsin breast cancer dataset using deep neural network. In: 2019 4th International conference on recent trends on electronics, information, communication & technology (RTEICT), pp 351–355
11. Ghosh S et al (2017) Efficient approaches for accuracy improvement of breast cancer classification using Wisconsin database. In: 2017 IEEE region 10 humanitarian technology conference (R10-HTC), pp 792–797
12. Sarmento R (2019) Breast cancer Wisconsin (diagnostic) data set
13. Learning UM. Breast cancer Wisconsin (diagnostic) data set. https://archive.ics.uci.edu/ml/datasets/Breast+Cancer+Wisconsin+(Diagnostic)
14. Chawla NV (2005) Data mining for imbalanced datasets: an overview BT. In: Maimon O, Rokach L (eds) Data mining and knowledge discovery handbook. Springer, US, pp 853–867
15. Guo C, Ma Y, Xu Z, Cao M, Yao Q (2019) An improved oversampling method for imbalanced data–SMOTE based on Canopy and K-means. In: 2019 Chinese automation congress (CAC), pp 1467–1469
16. Tallo TE, Musdholifah A (2018) The implementation of genetic algorithm in smote (synthetic minority oversampling technique) for handling imbalanced dataset problem. In: 2018 4th international conference on science and technology (ICST), pp 1–4
17. Ashraf M, Le K, Huang X (2011) Iterative weighted k-NN for constructing missing feature values in Wisconsin breast cancer dataset. In: The 3rd international conference on data mining and intelligent information technology applications, pp 23–27
18. Singh SN, Thakral S (2018) Using data mining tools for breast cancer prediction and analysis. In: 2018 4th international conference on computing communication and automation (ICCCA), pp 1–4

Investigation on Natural Frequency of Different Thicknesses of Cartilage in Myringoplasty

Hidayat Hidayat, Sudarsono Sudarsono, Sarwo Pranoto, and Rozaini Othman

Abstract A human middle ear system which includes tympanic membrane and ossicles (three tiny bones) has a function as a mechanical system transmitted sound and vibration from outer through to the inner ear section. Myringoplasty is an operation performed to repair a hole (perforation) in the tympanic membrane (TM). Sliced cartilage is generally used by an otolaryngologist to repair tympanic membrane perforation. The natural frequency for different thicknesses of cartilage in myringoplasty was compared to the normal tympanic membrane to find proper thickness in order to get the best hearing of the human ear system. The purpose of this work is to show the effect of different thicknesses of cartilage in myringoplasty using the Finite Element Method (FEM). The geometrical model of the human middle ear system was generated by the CAD Software using the physical properties of the human middle ear system reported by the previous researcher. Then, Hypermesh was used to create the Finite Element (FE) model. The eigen-value analysis is performed to obtain the mode shape and natural frequency of the human middle ear system with varied thicknesses of cartilage from 0.1 to 10 mm. Thus, by comparing the first natural frequencies of each cartilage thicknesses, we found that the maximum natural frequency of the human ear system when the cartilage's thickness is 0.13 mm. This disorder is the effect of the human middle ear system's mass and stiffness.

Keywords Tympanic membrane · Myringoplasty · Cartilage

H. Hidayat (✉)
Department of Mechanical Engineering, Politeknik Negeri Samarinda, Samarinda, Indonesia
e-mail: hidayat@polnes.ac.id

S. Sudarsono
Department of Mechanical Engineering, Universitas Halu Oleo, Kendari, Indonesia

S. Pranoto
Department of Electrical Engineering, Politeknik Negeri Ujung Pandang, Makassar, Indonesia

R. Othman
Faculty of Mechanical Engineering, Universiti Teknologi MARA, Pematang Sauh, Malaysia

H. Triwiyanto et al. (eds.), *Proceedings of the 1st International Conference on Electronics, Biomedical Engineering, and Health Informatics*, Lecture Notes in Electrical Engineering 746, https://doi.org/10.1007/978-981-33-6926-9_57

1 Introduction

The human ear was divided into three parts, namely the outer, middle and inner ears. The TM, three tiny bones called ossicles, some ligaments, and tendons comprise the human middle ear. As a mechanical device, it has a purpose to convey vibration and sound through the inner ear. The condition when the sound and vibration are unable to reach the human inner ear called conductive hearing loss. A hole in the tympanic membrane can cause this type of hearing loss. The tympanic membrane has a hole, also known as tympanic membrane perforation. In this case, the TM having a hole can be closed by a surgery called myringoplasty. The cartilage graft is generally used in myringoplasty. Due to the different material properties between cartilage and tympanic membrane, then the proper thickness of sliced cartilage is necessary to define. Increasing or reducing the thickness of sliced cartilage will affect the mass and stiffness of TM.

Several researchers on the tympanic membrane perforation repaired by sliced cartilage in myringoplasty had been reported. It has been reported an experimental data and model analysis to predict conductive hearing loss using tympanic membrane perforation [1]. Another researcher reported a quantitive model of the human middle ear with the tympanic membrane perforation constrained by several types of acoustic measurement [2]. The three dimensional model of human middle ear and an application for clinics tympanoplasty had been carried out by finite element analysis [3]. The optimal graft thickness for cartilage in myringoplasty was determined by using finite element analysis. Three different size types of tympanic membrane were generated in part tensa [4]. Performing frequency response analysis of the human middle ear system with tympanic membrane perforation had been carried out by researchers [5]. Our previous study performing eigen-value analysis to find out the dynamic behavior of human eardrum which has a hole using FEM [6]. Acoustic transfer characteristic was investigated by varying thickness of sliced cartilage and its mechanical deformation [7]. However, there is no study performing the effect of different thicknesses of sliced cartilage in myringoplasty.

In this study, the effect of thickness of sliced cartilage on natural frequencies in myringoplasty was investigated. The thickness of cartilage was varieted from 0.01 to 10 mm. The geometrial shapes of human ear was considered from our previous published [8]. Then, Hypermesh was used to generate the finite element model. Finally, the eigen-value analysis was carried out to obtain mode shape and the natural frequency in this study.

2 Method

2.1 FE Model of Human TM in Myringoplasty

The FE model of the human TM in myringoplasty was divided into 2245 pieces of six-node triangular elements. The Solidworks (CAD Software) was used to create the geometrical shape of the human TM. Then, the Hypermesh software was used to generate the finite element model of human middle ear system. The material properties of the human tympanic membrane are shown in Table 1. In this work, our previous study [9] were considered as the material properties of the human tympanic membrane. The geometrical of the tympanic membrane is a concave elliptic shape. The human tympanic membrane with sliced cartilage in myringoplasty is shown in Fig. 1.

The Young's Modulus, mass density and Poisson's ratio of sliced cartilage were 2.8×10^6 N/mm^2, 1.3×10^3 kg/m^3 and 0.3, respectively. As for the boundary condition of the human TM, the shell elements which adjusted 45° to the horizontal were used. The mass density and Poisson's ratio of boundary condition were the same as the human tympanic membrane. Then, value of E (Young's modulus) = 319.3×10^6 N/m^2 was found using trial and error by performing eigenvalue analysis.

2.2 FE Model of Human Middle Ear System

The FE model of the human middle ear with sliced cartilage in myringoplasty is shown in Fig. 2. The human middle ear system consists of the thin membrane called tympanic membrane and three tiny bones called ossicles, ligaments and

Table 1 Material Properties of Human Middle Ear System

Human Ear Components	Young's Modulus (MPa)	Mass Density × 10^3 (kg/m^3)	Poisson's ratio
Tympanic Membrane	32	1.2	0.3
Malleus	14,000	2.55	0.3
Incus	14,000	2.36	0.3
Stapes	14,000	2.20	0.3
Superior Malleal Ligament	0.048	2.50	0.3
Lateral Malleal Ligament	0.067	2.50	0.3
Anterior Malleal Ligament	0.021	2.50	0.3
Superior Incudal Ligament	0.049	2.50	0.3
Posterior Incudal Ligament	0.65	2.50	0.3
Tensor Tympanic Tendon	2.60	2.50	0.3
Stapedius Annular Ligament	0.06	1.20	0.3

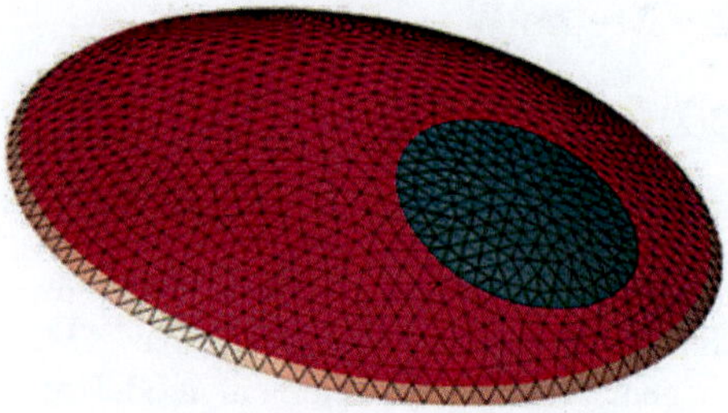

Fig. 1 Human tympanic membrane with cartilage in myringoplasty

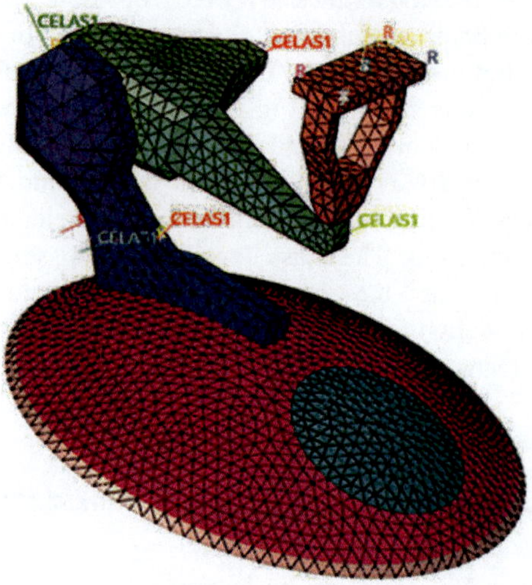

Fig. 2 Human middle ear system with cartilage in myringoplasty

tendons. The ligaments, tendon and tensor tympanic membrane were considered as springs element in x-, y- and z-directions. The value of springs constant was defined considering the previous published [8]. The spring element in x-direction was defined in the perpendicular direction of the ossicles's surface. As for the human middle ear system, the previous published was considered as geometrical shape. In the FE model of the human middle ear system, the tympanic membrane and the three tiny bones called ossicles were divided by using ten-node tetrahedron element and six-node triangular element, respectively.

2.3 Eigen-Value Analysis of Human Middle Ear

In this study, eigen-value analysis was carried out to obtain natural frequency and mode shape of the human middle ear system. The thicknesses of graft cartilage used in myringoplasty were varied from 0.01 to 10 mm. Then, the first natural frequency of the human tympanic membrane was compared to find out the effect of thicknesses of sliced cartilage in myringoplasty. The solver Optistruct was used to perform an eigen-value analysis of the human middle ear system. The natural frequency formula is shown Eq. 1 below [10].

$$f_i = \frac{1}{2\pi}\frac{K}{M} \tag{1}$$

where f_i, K and M are i-th natural frequencies, stiffness and mass, respectively.

3 Result

Table 1 shows The material properties of the human middle ear, which consist of the tympanic membrane, three tiny bones, namely malleus, incus and stapes, ligaments and tendons. The physical properties of the human ear components were considered our previous published [8].

Figure 3 shows the effect of thicknesses of graft cartilage on natural frequencies. The first natural frequencies of each thickness of sliced cartilage were compared. The natural frequencies of the human middle ear system were increased until the thickness of sliced cartilage 0.13 mm. The natural frequency of the system is determined by mass and stiffness. The stiffness effect is higher than the mass effect before 0.13 mm so that the natural frequencies increased. Then, the effect of mass is higher than stiffness after 0.13 mm. Thus, the first natural frequencies of each thickness of graft cartilage were decreased from 0.13 to 10 mm.

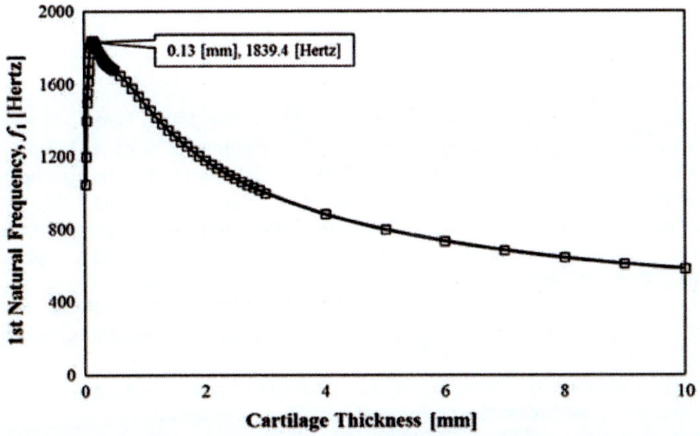

Fig. 3 Effect of thicknesses of sliced cartilage on natural frequencies

4 Discussion

This study only performs eigenvalue analysis to obtain the natural frequency of the human ear system with the repaired tympanic membrane in myringoplasty using different thicknesses of cartilage. The first natural frequencies for each thickness of cartilage were compared. The proper thickness of cartilage in myringoplasty was determined by the researcher using frequency response analysis but the dynamic behavior, which is natural frequency and mode shape, was not considered. In order to clarify the result, so that the mode shapes of each natural frequency need to be considered in the future work to define the optimal thickness of sliced cartilage used in myringoplasty.

5 Conclusion

In this study, the effect of different thicknesses on natural frequency of human middle ear system in myringoplasty had been investigated. Eigen-value analysis of the human middle ear system consisting of tympanic membrane, ossicles, ligaments and tendon had been carried out to obtain natural frequencies. The natural frequencies of the human middle ear increased from 0.01 mm until 0.13 mm then, decreased when cartilage thickness becomes larger. The maximum natural frequency is 1839.4 Hz when the thickness of sliced cartilage 0.13 mm. The natural frequencies for different thicknesses of cartilage need to be clarified by using vibration mode for each frequency in the future work.

References

1. Mehta RP, Rosowski JJ, Voss SE, O'Neil E, Merchant SN (2006) Determinants of hearing loss in perforations of the tympanic membrane. Otol Neurotol 27(2):136–143
2. Voss SE, Rosowski JJ, Merchant SN, Peake WT (2001) Middle-ear function with tympanic-membrane perforations. II. A simple model. J Acoust Soc Am 110(3):1445–1452
3. Higashimachi T, Shiratake Y, Maeda T, Sug K, Toriya R (2013) Three-dimensional finite element analysis of the human middle ear and an application for clinics for tympanoplasty. WIT Trans Eng Sci 78:61–72
4. Lee CF, Chen JH, Chou YF, Hsu LP, Chen PR, Liu TC (2007) Optimal graft thickness for different sizes of tympanic membrane perforation in cartilage myringoplasty: a finite element analysis. Laryngoscope 117(4):725–730
5. Hidayat H, Sudarsono S, Aviva D, Othman R (2019) Frequency response of the human middle ear system with eardrum perforation. Int J Sci Tech Res 8(4)
6. Hidayat H, Sudarsono S, Othman R (2020) Dynamic behavior of human tympanic membrane perforation using finite element method. In: IOP conference series: materials science and engineering, vol 797, no 1, p 012025
7. Zahnert T, Hüttenbrink KB, Mürbe D, Bornitz M (2000) Experimental investigations of the use of cartilage in tympanic membrane reconstruction. Am J Otol 21(3):322–328

8. Hidayat H, Okamoto S, Lee JH, Hato N, Yamada H, Takagi D (2016) Finite element dynamics of human ear system comprising middle ear and cochlea in inner ear. J Biomed Sci Eng 09(13):597–610
9. Hidayat H, Okamoto S, Lee JH, Matsuura K, Hato N, Yamada H (2016) Dynamics analyses of human middle ear system using finite element method. In: International conference on engineering & technology, computer, basic & applied science, ECBA-2016, vol 127, no 5
10. Lalanne M, Berthier P, Der Hagopian J (1984) Mechanical vibrations for engineers

Detection of Diabetic Macular Edema in Optical Coherence Tomography Image Using Convolutional Neural Network

Sarwo Pranoto, H. Hidayat, S. Sudarsono, and M. P. Lukman

Abstract Diabetic macular edema (DME) is known as the main cause of patients with Diabetic Retinopathy loss their vision. The vision loss can be prevented if DME could be detected and diagnosed in the early stage. The purpose of this research is to detect DME from retinal-Optical Coherence Tomography (OCT) images using Convolutional Neural Network (CNN). In this research, 2 pre-trained models using Transfer Learning namely MobileNet and VGG-16 and 1 custom CNN models were used to classify the retinal-OCT images. The dataset of the retinal-OCT images used in this research has been obtained from Kaggle website. The dataset is organized into 3 folders (train, validation, and test) and contains subfolders for DME image category and normal image category. There are 37,663 retinal-OCT images used in the training dataset, 484 images in the validation dataset, and 16 images in the testing dataset. In this research, the custom 5 layer CNN model was compared with the 2 pre-trained models to estimate the performance of DME detection. The results show both the 2 pre-trained models using Transfer Learning and the custom 5 layer CNN model could detect DME from retinal-OCT images. Compared with the 2 pre-trained models, the custom 5 layer CNN model distinguishing DME images from normal images achieved the highest accuracy of 96%.

Keywords Diabetic macular edema · Optical coherence tomography · Convolutional neural network

S. Pranoto (✉) · M. P. Lukman
Department of Electrical Engineering, Politeknik Negeri Ujung Pandang, Makassar, Indonesia
e-mail: sarwo.pranoto@poliupg.ac.id

H. Hidayat
Department of Mechanical Engineering, Politeknik Negeri Samarinda, Samarinda, Indonesia

S. Sudarsono
Department of Mechanical Engineering, Faculty of Engineering, Universitas Halu Oleo, Kendari, Indonesia

H. Triwiyanto et al. (eds.), *Proceedings of the 1st International Conference on Electronics, Biomedical Engineering, and Health Informatics*, Lecture Notes in Electrical Engineering 746, https://doi.org/10.1007/978-981-33-6926-9_58

1 Introduction

Diabetic macular edema (DME) is one of the causes that patients with Diabetic Retinopathy loss their vision [1]. DME is caused by the fluid which accumulated in the macula as a result of the disrupted blood-retinal barrier [2]. Although DME could be cured if it is detected in the early stage, many people especially in rural areas are suffering from DME due to their ignorance and unawareness [3]. Therefore, early detection and treatment of DME play an important role in preventing patients with Diabetic Retinopathy loss their vision. Many researchers have used retinal-OCT images for guiding the diagnosis and treatment of DME [4]. By using retinal-OCT images, the information about retinal internal structures can be obtained. Moreover, retinal-OCT images can be used to identify early symptoms of retinal disease [5]. However, it is a tedious task and time-consuming for ophthalmologists to diagnose the DME by using the retinal-OCT image due to the high similarity between DME image and healthy image [6]. Then various algorithms such as segmentation [7, 8], and classification [9–15] have been developed to analyze automatically the retinal-OCT image. However, the developments of the algorithms are still in early stage as only academic works and still open for improvements [16].

This research focuses on the implementation of pre-trained models using Transfer Learning and custom convolutional neural network (CNN) model to detect DME from the retinal-OCT images. The pre-trained models that widely used and reimplemented in this research are MobileNet [17] and VGG-16 [18].

2 Methodology

2.1 Dataset Description

In this research, a dataset of retinal-OCT images from [19] was used to evaluate the models. The dataset contains four categories (normal, CNV, DME, DRUSEN). However, only retinal-OCT images of normal and DME categories were used to evaluate the models. The dataset consists of 38,163 retinal-OCT images (11,598 DME and 26,565 normal categories). Each category contains retinal-OCT images with different resolutions. The dataset was divided into three parts, namely training data (37,663 images), validation data (484 images), and testing data (16 images).

2.2 OCT Image Classification

The implementation of pre-trained and custom models for detecting DME from retinal-OCT images can be shown as a block diagram in Fig. 1.

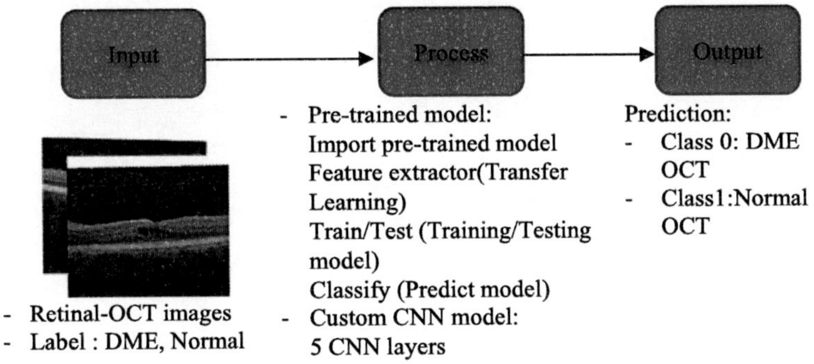

Fig. 1 Block diagram of the implementation of pre-trained and custom models

As can be seen from Fig. 1, the retinal-OCT images were used as the input for the pre-trained and custom models. As the retinal-OCT images have various resolutions, all retinal-OCT images used in this research were resized to $224 \times 224 \times 3$. The two pre-trained models using Transfer Learning and one custom CNN models were used to classify the OCT-retinal images. The two pre-trained models, namely MobileNet and VGG-16 were implemented by loading the models with Imagenet weights and replacing the top layer with new fully connected layers. As all the convolutional layers are pre-trained, the last four layers were frozen during the training of the full connected layer preventing their weights from being updated during training.

While the custom CNN model consists of five convolution layers with 3×3 kernel and max poll layer in the first, second, and third layers. The dropout layer was also added in all convolutional layers in order to avoid overfitting problems. During the training process, the batch size was set to 16 for the MobileNet and VGG-16 models. While the batch size for the custom CNN model was set to 8.

The experiment was implemented by using Keras Framework with NVDIA Compute Unified Device Architecture (CUDA) v10.1 and CUDA Deep Neural Network v7.6.4 accelerated library. All experiments were implemented under Windows 10 Home operating system with CPU Intel Core i7-4750HQ 2.00 GHz, GPU NVDIA GeForce GTX 950 M, and RAM 8 GB.

3 Result and Discussion

Two different numbers of training samples were used to evaluate the performances of the models. In the first experiment, the number of training samples was set to 10% which contains of 1135 DME images and 2632 normal images. While in the second experiment, the number of training samples was set to 100%. The validation dataset for both experiments was kept the same using 484 images (242 DME images and 242 normal images).

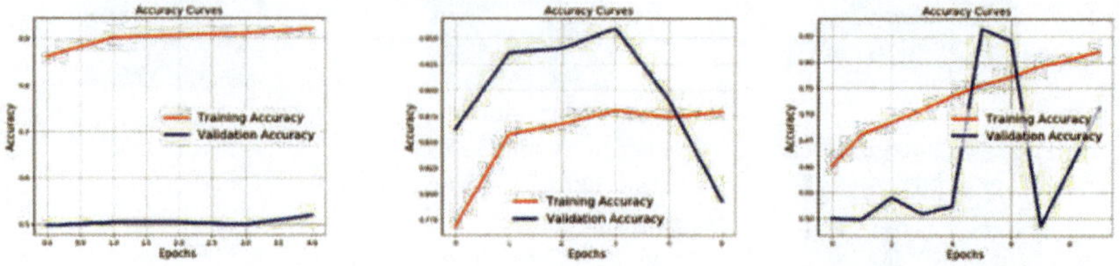

MobileNet VGG-16 Custom 5 layer CNN

(a) Accuracy values of the three CNN models with the number of training samples set to 10%

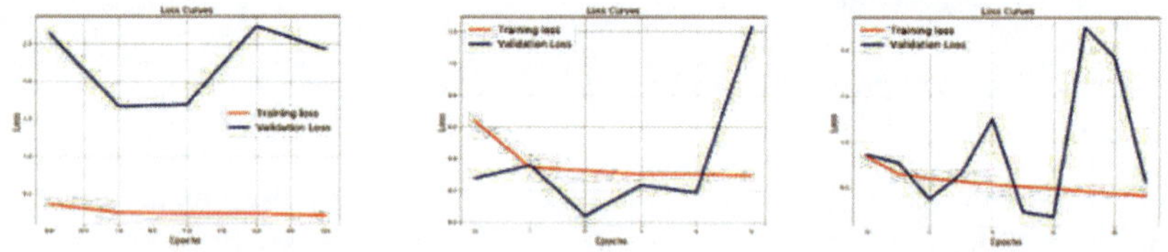

MobileNet VGG-16 Custom 5 layer CNN

(b) Loss values of the three CNN models with the number of training samples set to 10%

Fig. 2 Performances in the training and validation dataset of the three CNN models with the number of training samples set to 10%

Figure 2 shows the performances in the training and validation dataset of the three CNN models with the number of training samples set to 10%. As can be seen from Fig. 2a the training accuracy of MobileNet is increasing gradually over time and achieves a maximum of 93%. Although the validation accuracy also increases, it stalls around 64% in the training process. The difference in accuracy between training and validation accuracy is around 29% which indicates overfitting. The training accuracy of the VGG-16 reaches about 88% at the maximum, while the validation accuracy achieves about 79% at the end of the epoch. In addition, the training accuracy of the custom 5 layer CNN reaches about 82% at the maximum and the validation accuracy of the custom one reaches 71% at the end of the epoch. The training accuracies and validation accuracies of the three models are off by large margin and the models achieved only around 64, 79, and 71% accuracies on the validation dataset for MobileNet, VGG-16, and the custom one respectively. In this experiment, the training was stopped due to the validation loss has not decreased for 3 number of epochs as shown in Fig. 2b.

Figure 3 shows the performances in the training and validation dataset of the three CNN models with the number of training samples set to 100%. The performance of the three models generally improves as the number of training samples increase. As can be seen from Fig. 3a, the training accuracy of MobileNet is increasing over time. It reaches a maximum of 93%, while the validation accuracy reaches a maximum of 64%. The training and validation accuracies of the VGG-16

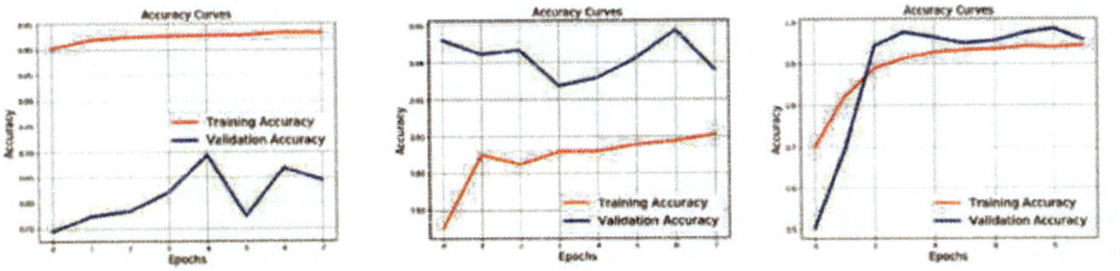

MobileNet VGG16 Custom 5 layer CNN

(a) Accuracy values of the three CNN models with the number of training samples set to 100%

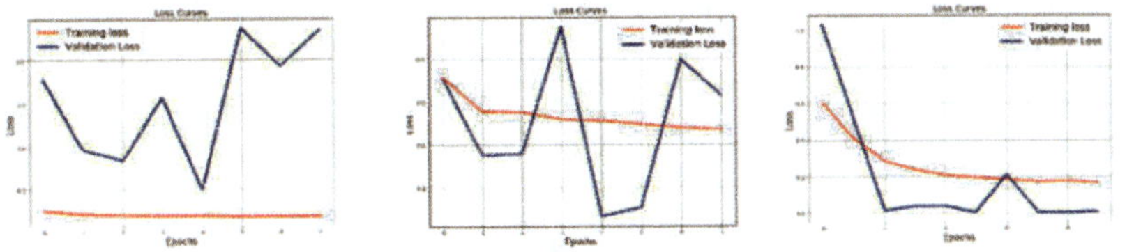

MobileNet VGG16 Custom 5 layer CNN

(b) Loss values of the three CNN models with the number of training samples set to 100%

Fig. 3 Performances in the training and validation dataset of the three CNN models with the number of training samples set to 100%

reach about 90 and 93% at the end of the epoch respectively. The training and validation accuracies of the custom 5 layer CNN model reach about 94 and 96% at the maximum respectively. In this experiment, the training was stopped due to the validation loss has not decreased for 3 number of epochs as shown in Fig. 3b. Both the pre-trained models still have large gaps of training and validations accuracies means that the models have a difficult time generalizing on a new dataset. On the other hand, the custom 5 layer CNN model has training accuracy and validation accuracy by 1% gap means that the model could make generalizing on a new dataset.

Figure 4 shows the confusion matrixes of those classification models of the validation image dataset with the number of training samples set to 100%. The validation image dataset consists of 242 DME images and 242 normal images. Using the MobileNet model, 90 of DME images and all normal images are correctly predicted. Oppositely, 152 of normal images are incorrectly predicted as DME images. Using the VGG-16 model, 202 of DME images and 242 normal images are correctly predicted. Oppositely, 34 of normal images are incorrectly predicted as DME images. While using the custom 5 CNN model, 222 of DME images and all normal images are correctly predicted. Oppositely, 20 of normal images are incorrectly predicted as DME images.

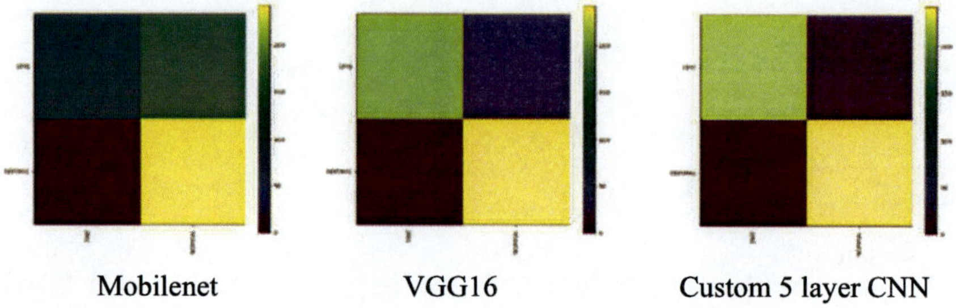

Fig. 4 Confusion matrixes of those classification models of the validation image dataset with the number of training samples set to 100%

Labels	DME	Normal
OCT Images	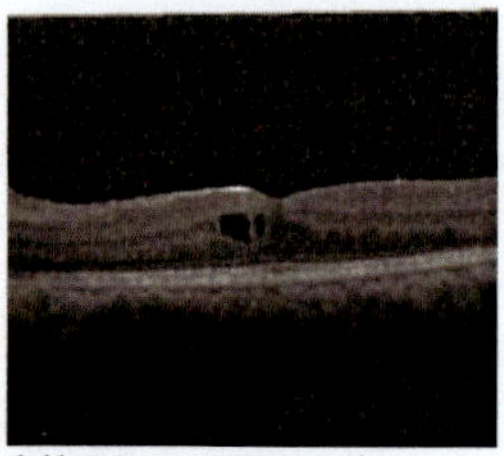	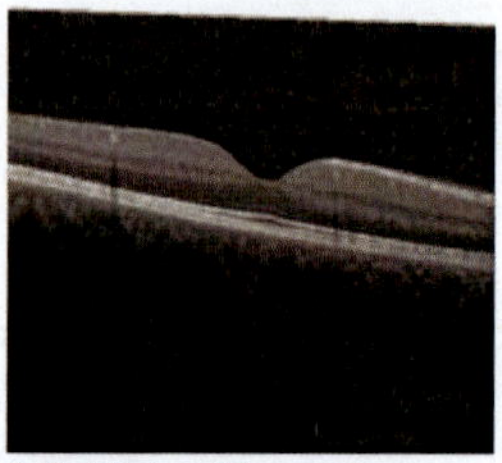
Prediction Results	MobileNet = Normal VGG-16 = DME Custom 5 Layer CNN = DME	MobileNet = Normal VGG-16 = Normal Custom 5 Layer CNN = Normal

Fig. 5 Examples of prediction results of the three classification models

In this research, the test dataset was used for testing the models with new data. The test dataset consists of 16 images (8 DME images and 8 normal images). The 10 out of 16 images were randomly selected to test the models. Figure 5 shows examples of the prediction results of the three classification models used in this research. As can be observed from Fig. 5, the DME can confuse the MobileNet. Some DME images in the test dataset are treated as normal ones by MobileNet.

Table 1 shows the classification reports of the three models using validation image dataset with the number of training samples set to 100%. The best performance of the models was obtained by the custom 5 layer CNN with an accuracy 96%.

Table 1 Classification reports of the three models

Models	Classes	Precision	Recall	F1-Score
MobileNet	DME	1.00	0.37	0.54
	Normal	0.61	1.00	0.76
	Accuracy			0.69
	Macro average	0.81	0.69	0.65
	Weighted average	0.81	0.69	0.65
VGG-16	DME	1.00	0.86	0.92
	Normal	0.88	1.00	0.93
	Accuracy			0.93
	Macro average	0.94	0.93	0.93
	Weighted average	0.94	0.93	0.93
Custom 5 layer CNN	DME	1.00	0.92	0.96
	Normal	0.92	1.00	0.96
	Accuracy			**0.96**
	Macro average	0.96	0.96	0.96
	Weighted average	0.96	0.96	0.96

4 Conclusion

This research aims to detect diabetic macular edema (DME) from retinal-OCT images using CNN. Two pre-trained models using Transfer Learning techniques namely MobileNet and VGG-16 and one custom 5 layer CNN models are implemented to classify the retinal-OCT images. The results of this research show that using the small number of training samples, the three models suffer from overfitting problems. However, by increasing the number of training samples, the performances of the three models increase. Comparing the performances of the models, VGG-16 model and 5 layer CNN model performed better than MobileNet model. The 5 layer CNN model is best-performed model out of 3 models. The 5 layer CNN model has the highest accuracy value which reaches 95%. In future works, it is expected that the pre-trained and custom models can be implemented to detect Drusen and Choroidal Neovascularization (CNV) from retinal-OCT images automatically.

References

1. Das A, McGuire PG, Rangasamy S (2015) Diabetic macular edema: pathophysiology and novel therapeutic targets. Ophthalmology 122(7):1375–1394
2. de Sisternes L, Jonna G, Moss J, Marmor MF, Leng T, Rubin DL (2017) Automated intraretinal segmentation of SD-OCT images in normal and age-related macular degeneration eyes. Biomed Opt Express 8(3):1926

3. Gargeya R, Leng T (2017) Automated identification of diabetic retinopathy using deep learning. Ophthalmology 124(7):962–969
4. van Velthoven MEJ, Faber DJ, Verbraak FD, van Leeuwen TG, de Smet MD (2007) Recent developments in optical coherence tomography for imaging the retina. Prog Retin Eye Res 26(1):57–77
5. Brezinski ME et al (1996) Optical coherence tomography for optical biopsy: properties and demonstration of vascular pathology. Circulation 93(6):1206–1213
6. Liu YY et al (2011) Computerized macular pathology diagnosis in spectral domain optical coherence tomography scans based on multiscale texture and shape features. Investig Ophthalmol Vis Sci 52(11):8316–8322
7. Hassan T, Akram MU, Masood MF, Yasin U (2019) Deep structure tensor graph search framework for automated extraction and characterization of retinal layers and fluid pathology in retinal SD-OCT scans. Comput Biol Med 105(July 2018):112–124
8. Xu R, Niu S, Chen Q, Ji Z, Rubin D, Chen Y (2019) Automated geographic atrophy segmentation for SD-OCT images based on two-stage learning model. Comput Biol Med 105(September 2018):102–111
9. Otani T, Kishi S, Maruyama Y, Otani T, Kishi S, Maruyama Y (1999) Patterns of diabetic macular edema with optical coherence tomography. Am J Ophthalmol 127(6):688–693
10. Farsiu S et al (2014) Quantitative classification of eyes with and without intermediate age-related macular degeneration using optical coherence tomography. Ophthalmology 121(1):162–172
11. Srinivasan PP et al (2014) Fully automated detection of diabetic macular edema and dry age-related macular degeneration from optical coherence tomography images. Biomed Opt Express 5(10):3568
12. Venhuizen FG et al (2017) Automated staging of age-related macular degeneration using optical coherence tomography. Investig Ophthalmol Vis Sci 58(4):2318–2328
13. Lemaître G et al (2016) Classification of SD-OCT volumes using local binary patterns: experimental validation for DME detection. J Ophthalmol 2016
14. Albarrak A, Coenen F, Zheng Y (2013) Age-related macular degeneration identification in volumetric optical coherence tomography using decomposition and local feature extraction. In: Proceedings of 2013 international conference on medical image, understanding and analysis, pp 59–64
15. Alsaih K et al (2016) Classification of SD-OCT volumes with multi pyramids, LBP and HOG descriptors: application to DME detections. Proc Annu Int Conf IEEE Eng Med Biol Soc EMBS 2016(Octob):1344–1347
16. Alsaih K, Lemaitre G, Rastgoo M, Massich J, Sidibé D, Meriaudeau F (2017) Machine learning techniques for diabetic macular edema (DME) classification on SD-OCT images. Biomed Eng Online 16(1)
17. Howard AG et al (2017) MobileNets: efficient convolutional neural networks for mobile vision applications. Available [online] http://arxiv.org/abs/1704.04861
18. Simonyan K, Zisserman A (2015) Very deep convolutional networks for large-scale image recognition. In: 3rd International conference on learning representations ICLR 2015—conference track proceedings, pp 1–14
19. Kaggle Homepage. https://www.kaggle.com/paultimothymooney/kermany2018. Accessed Jun 15, 2020

Graphical User Interface for Heartbeat and Body Temperature Monitoring System Using Internet of Things (IOT)

Raja Siti Nur Adiimah Raja Aris, Amri Mohd Azhari, Lia Safiyah Syafie, Farah Hanan Azimi, and Suzanna Ridzuan Aw

Abstract Nowadays, the zvariation of the diseases revolution had become a major thread to the human kind population. The repercussion of this uncontrolled situation had led to the increasing trend regarding to the number of the patient those visited the hospital in order to obtain a treatment from the professional in the medical sector. As the number of the patient is keep increasing by the day, the number of hospital staff still not able to meet the requirement in providing the optimum service to all of their patients. The development of this project is to reduce the burden bear by the hospital staff especially the doctor by the implementation of the IOT technology. The purpose of this study is to develop a system based on the ESP8266 microcontroller that internally installed a WIFI shield provide internet connectivity easily for the user to measure the heart rate and the body temperature. By the help of Arduino environment platform, the IOT based project can be developed. This project will focus in capturing and measure the two parameters from the human body which are the heart rate and the body temperature. The sensor used are heart rate sensor, MAX30100 and the body temperature sensor, MLX90614. As the results, this system will process the raw data from the two sensors into a desire value and display the data on the OLED display and the application display. The implementation of IOT technology to this system will provide a continuous data streaming through thinger.io website and showing a live development of patients for the user who is has the permission access by only using their own smart devices. Based on the finding, its shows that the comparison percentage deviation between heartbeat sensor and blood pressure monitor is 3.37% and the comparison percentage deviation between body temperature sensor and digital thermometer is 0.54%. The Graphical User Interface through Internet of Things (IOT) application system is proven to monitor accurately for heartbeat sensor measurement and body temperature sensor measurement.

Keywords IoT · Heart rate sensor · Body temperature sensor · Monitoring system · Microcontroller

R. S. N. A. Raja Aris (✉) · A. Mohd Azhari · L. S. Syafie · F. H. Azimi · S. Ridzuan Aw
University College TATI, Kemaman, Terengganu, Malaysia
e-mail: rsnara95@gmail.com

H. Triwiyanto et al. (eds.), *Proceedings of the 1st International Conference on Electronics, Biomedical Engineering, and Health Informatics*, Lecture Notes in Electrical Engineering 746, https://doi.org/10.1007/978-981-33-6926-9_59

1 Introduction

1.1 Background

Nowadays, the development of the technology in medical sector had rapidly increased in providing the best solution to the patients who is needed a treatment. Despite of the conventional method in obtaining the patient heart rate and body temperature, an automatic technology method with a low cost are mostly prefer by the user in improving their health monitoring method. There are a few factor influence that give a chance to propose the system. First factor is inclusively the increasing of the patient number. The numbers of patients seem to be keeping increasing from day by day. This situation happened when the diversity of the diseases revolution such as influenza H1N1 and dengue had frequently attack the human kind resulted to the uncontrolled situation at the medical institutions. At the critical time which is when the emergence of the new epidemics attacked human, most of the clinic and hospital facing a hard time in providing the optimum service to their patients due to the lack of staff to support their daily treatment duty. Second problem is the time managements of a doctor in monitoring all of their patients at one single time. Every single patient that is in charged into the patient ward is not experience a same illness. Most of them are critically need to be monitor by the professional staff. Even the diseases is different experience by difference patients, the overall treatment process always considered to monitor the heart rate of the patient in order to make sure that the patient is the normal human condition. The body temperature of patient will be monitored according to the specific cases such dengue fever that need to consistently monitor the body temperature of the patient. As for the solution, the proposed system able to reduce the time lag in between actual treatment service requirement and improve the efficiency of this organization working procedure.

Internet of thing is an intelligent system that has a capability to interpret the variety of sensors and driver and directly read their context by using the network capabilities so that a new communication way will be developed. This kind of communication allow the project system accessing the open source internet services and provide a platform for the project system to be interacting with the human world. One of the implementation of the Internet of thing in the healthcare sector able to ease the doctor responsibility and tasks that need to be performed by the doctors in providing the optimum treatment to their patient.

Measurement a consistent patient heart rate and the body temperature of all the patients by a single on duty doctor will be easier by taking the advantages of the IOT technology. In order to realize the system, the specific intelligent sensor name MAX30100 is applied to measure the heart rate by sensing the changes in blood volume in the a human finger artery when every single time the heart keep pumping the blood to the whole human body system. Heart rate is the number of heart beats per unit of time and usually expressed in beats per minute (bpm). This type of heart rate sensor also capable to calculate the oxygen level (Spo2) in the human blood by using the specific algorithm provided. Body temperature may seem like not a vital parameter to be measure on the normal patients but it was really important parameter that always monitor by the doctor if the patients is critically experience a dangerous diseases. In order to ensure measurement method more efficient and practically, the monitoring system for body temperature sensor is presenting for this paper. The temperature sensor which is the MLX90614 has been used to measure the human body temperature.

Vikramsingh et al. presented a wireless heartbeat and temperature monitoring system based on a microcontroller ATmega328 (arduino uno). The system consists of sensors to measure heartbeat and body temperature and display on LCD monitor. The ATmega328 (arduino uno) microcontroller will process all the data measurement and display it in LCD as well as sends it to the receiving end for displaying at the remote place [1]. Nur Hudha et al. designed a system that provide information on the user's health condition by measuring of heart rate and body temperature using a heart rate sensor (finger-tip sensor). The sensor heat changes converted into electricity, through digital form with 10-bit ADC by using ATMega 16 as a controller and will displayed on the LCD [2]. Uysal developed a wireless sensor network system for a heart rate monitoring application using Matlab GUI as interface. The wireless sensor networks (WSN) used as based for design heart rate monitoring system using Bluetooth. Pulse-Oximeter (SPO2) data, which is received from the patients, forwarded wirelessly through Arduino to the personal computer (PC) using HC-05 Bluetooth module also processed on PC. The MATLAB program used to design Graphical User Interface (GUI) as interface to observe the measurements of the pulse of the heart rate, simultaneously [3].

In the other application, Huang et al. developed an embedded automatic body temperature estimation system which could continuously and unconsciously measure the human temperature in real-time. By implementation with face tracking and fuzzy-control of Pan-tilt unit, the system ensures that human face is focused during measuring process [4]. Similar to this study, Daniel et al. presented electronic monitoring system for measuring heart rate and skin temperature in small ruminants [5]. The system be able to measure the heart rate and skin temperature in small ruminants. There are two components which are a mobile base unit, mounted on the animal under study, and a fixed base unit. The communication between the mobile and fixed units through wireless concept using a Xbee Series 2 radio frequency transceiver. All the data were recorded and transferred to a secure digital card in the mobile unit. The reference equipment is used as a device to mount in Santa Inês crossbred sheep while the animals were restrained in steel cages.

Hashim et al. studied on the system that can minimize the costing at hospital. Hence, a prototype involve software and hardware are developed. The completed system are combination of design for graphical user interface (GUI) based on Visual Basic Net 2010 software and the hardware interface is Peripheral Interface Controller (PIC) 16F877A microcontroller [6]. Based on Kazi et al., a development of heart disease monitoring system in a real time measurement is presented. This system is using Raspberry Pi as controller, pulse rate sensor to measure the heart rate, Arduino UNO and Thing Speak cloud [7].

Some other researchers, Hassanalieragh et al. have conducted research on Internet-of-Things (IoT) Sensing with Cloud-based for Health Monitoring and Management system [8]. Patel et al. presented the application of IoT based for heart rate monitoring dan heart attack recognition system. The heart beat reading is measured by sensor will send the data through the internet. The limitation of heartbeat for high level and low level can be set by user. Once heart beat readings goes above or below the limit set, the system will response for risks of heart attack [9]. Mallick et al. designed a monitoring system for heart rate using a principal of photophelthysmography (PPG) technique through a fingertip and Arduino. The sensor applied for this system is an infrared light-emitting-diode (IR LED) and a photo diode [10]. Regarding Koshti et al., presented a novel easy-to-use system intended for the fast and noninvasive monitoring of the Lead I electrocardiogram (ECG) signal by using a wireless steering wheel. The system is developed using Raspberry Pi as interface and ECG Signal as heart rate detection. The signal detect will convert through Analog-to-Digital Convertor (ADC) of Arduino and the data will be stored in the EEPROM of Arduino. All the data will display on GUI interface by using XBEE module [11].

This paper proposes a heart rate and body temperature based on the IOT monitoring system where the development progress of the patients can be easily access on the data stored in the cloud system by the doctor at any times and anywhere by using their smart devices. Monitoring activity will be more advance when the doctor is able to monitor the real-time of the patient development through the application designed. The MAX30100 sensor is applied to measure the heart rate and the MLX90614 sensor has been used to measure the human body temperature. The data from the sensor will convert into web hosting and the databased server through NodeMcu ESP8266 Lolin microcontroller board. The Thinger.io IOT platform is used to send data from the ESP8266 Lolin microcontroller that obtained from the sensor by using Wi-Fi communication. It had a digital dashboard where the graphical user interface for this project can be generated. The value stored in database will be sent to PC or hand phone via serial (RS232) wired interface and a serial port will be opened on processing 3 graphical user interface (GUI). The application is develop based on the both computer and Smartphone user and all the data such as the heart rate, the blood oxygen saturated level (SPo2) and the body temperature are display in the animation graphic (GUI). Thus, the doctor daily treatment activity was improved by the help of the project system and the implementation of the Internet of Thing.

2 Materials and Method

This research can be divided into two important parts. The first part is automatically capturing and measuring the importance parameter from the sensors which is the human heart rate and the human body temperature. The data form sensor is able to transfer directly to the cloud web-based system through the IOT technology. The second part of the system is development of IOT entitled the Thinger.io IOT platform. With the special features of NodeMcu ESP8266 Lolin microcontroller board, the data from both sensors can always be transfer into web hosting and the databased server. As long as the internet connectivity is available, user can always monitor the development of patient in easily through internet.

2.1 *System Design Development*

This research is focused in automatically monitoring the heart rate and body temperature measurement in the system. An Internet platform is very helpful in this system as an interface to replace the conventional method with the automatic monitoring system. The users be able to monitor the measurement in any place using the internet support. The general project design of this research is shown (see Fig. 1). The system consists of Lolin ESP8266 microcontroller, heart rate sensor, temperature sensor, LCD display, web hosting and data base server. The MAX30100 sensor is applied to measure the heart rate by sensing the changes in blood volume in the human finger artery when every single time the heart keep pumping the blood to the whole human body system. Heart rate is the number of heart beats per unit of time and usually expressed in beats per minute (bpm). The heart rate sensor was able to provide a measurement value within the desire value which is in between 60 and 100 bpm for rest position. The MLX90614 sensor has been used to measure the human body temperature. The normal reading for body temperature which in between 36.0 °C and 37.5 °C while for the fever range is between 37.6 °C and 41.0 °C. In order to evidence the reliability of the sensor

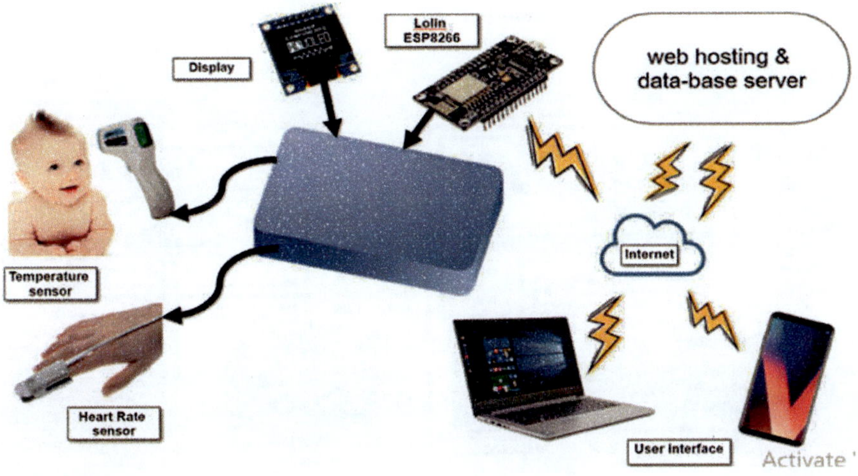

Fig. 1 Sketch for system setup

result as the one of the medical measurement instrumentation, an analysis had been perform in comparing the heart rate and body temperature measurement for 10 person in rest state condition measure by sensor with the blood pressure monitor and digital thermometer method.

The raw data capturing by the both sensors will be transfer to the process segment. This segment involving the Lolin Esp8266 microcontroller board to calculate the raw data into a desired value based on the algorithm set in the project system coding. Once the desired value is successfully calculated, the data on Esp8266 microcontroller board will transfer to Output segment. The output segment is web-based hosting and data-base server via Wi-Fi. The output will displayed on oled LCD display. On the same time, the data can be monitored by IOT monitoring system. All the data measurement such as the heart rate, the blood oxygen saturated level (SPo2) and the body temperature can be monitored continuously and are displayed in the animation graphic.

2.2 Electrical Circuit Schematic Design

The electrical circuit system (see Fig. 2) was design as separately in between two sensors in order two established the sensor reading and thinger.io IOT monitoring running simultaneously. The monitoring system is equipped with two sensor where is each sensor had their own ESP8266 microcontroller. The mlx90614 temperature sensor is connected to I2C communication in order to maintain output value. Meanwhile the Max30100 sensor need a strict timing in collecting data continuously. The data will sent to the each ESP8266 microcontroller. The heart rate sensor raw data will be converted into two parameters where the heart rate in beat per minute (bpm) and the oxygen level in blood (Spo2) in the percentage unit. While temperature sensor data is converted into the temperature value with the both

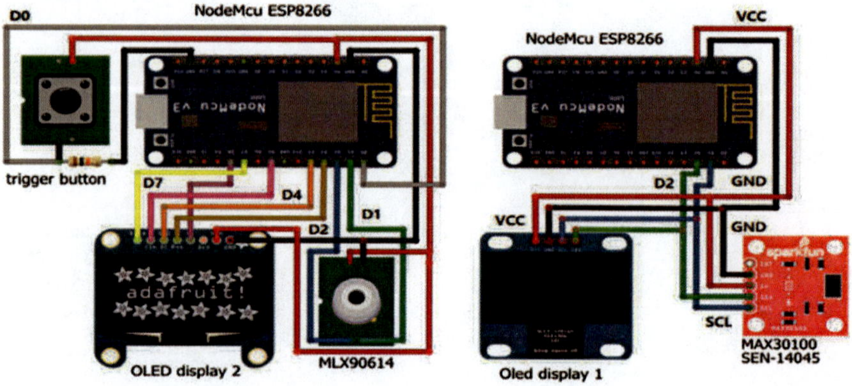

Fig. 2 Electrical schematic diagram

Celsius and Fahrenheit unit. The output result for heart rate and body temperature measurement will displayed on the OLED LCD display.

3 Results and Discussions

3.1 Data Recording

The developed system will monitor the required parameter by using the processing 3.0 Sketches software and the thinger.io IOT application. It had a digital dashboard where the graphical user interface for this project can be created by simple setup in the website. The processing 3 graphical user interface (see Figs. 3 and 4) for heart rate and body temperature display on the IoT monitoring system. With the implementation of this IoT application, all the data from sensors can be obtained continuously by using Wi-Fi communication. The heart rate of a healthy adult at rest is around 72 beats per minute (bpm). Athletes normally have lower heart rates than less active people. The heart rate rises gradually during exercises and returns slowly to the rest value after exercise. Thus, the normal range for heart rate varies with age, however it is generally accepted that the average resting pulse rate in a healthy person is approximately 60–100 beats per minute. Meanwhile, the normal reading for body temperature which in between 36.0 °C and 37.5 °C while for the fever range is between 37.6 °C and 41.0 °C. The heart rate raw data will be obtained from the human fingertip by attaching the sensor together on the fingertip surface. While for the body temperature raw data is collected by detecting the IR rays to quantize the temperature range.

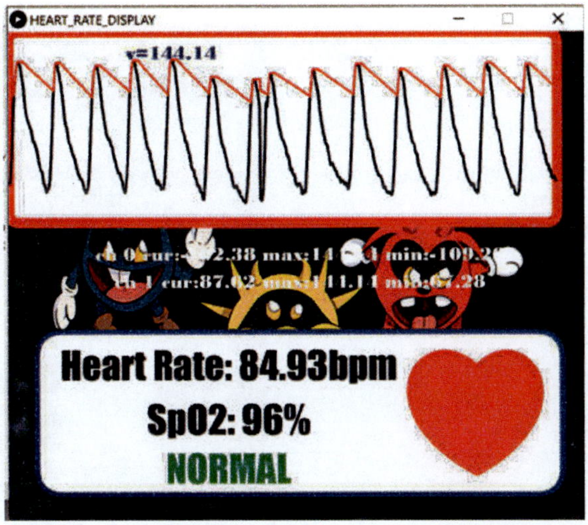

Fig. 3 The processing 3 graphical user interface (heart rate)

All data acquired were graphically transformed into table and line charts. An analysis on consistency of the sensor have been done in real time monitoring. An experimental had been perform in comparing the heart rate and body temperature of the 10 person in rest state condition measure by sensor and by the manual method.

3.2 The Heart Rate Sensor Measurement Result

A max30100 pulse oximeter sensor or known as heart rate sensor is a sensor that had a capability to measure the heart rate (bpm) and the blood oxygen saturation level (spo2) from the human fingertip. The results obtained (see Fig. 5) for human heart rate and blood oxygen saturation level measurement. Results show that the sensor competent consistently measure and capture the human heart rate continuously. The normal heart rate for human is between 60 and 100 bpm during the rest condition. Meanwhile for the blood oxygen saturation level result for human, the Spo2 value above than 95% to keep alive.

3.3 The Temperature Sensor Measurement Result

The measurement result obtain (see Fig. 6) from the mlx90614 temperature sensor for a normal condition human. A normal body temperature range for human is in

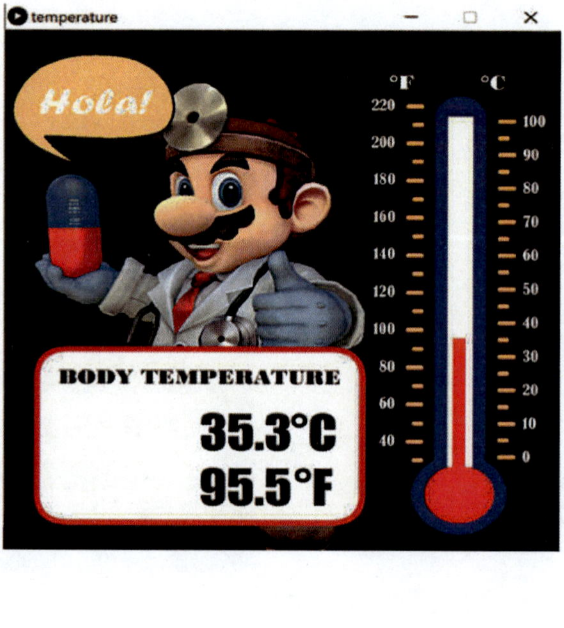

Fig. 4 The processing 3 graphical user interface (body temperature)

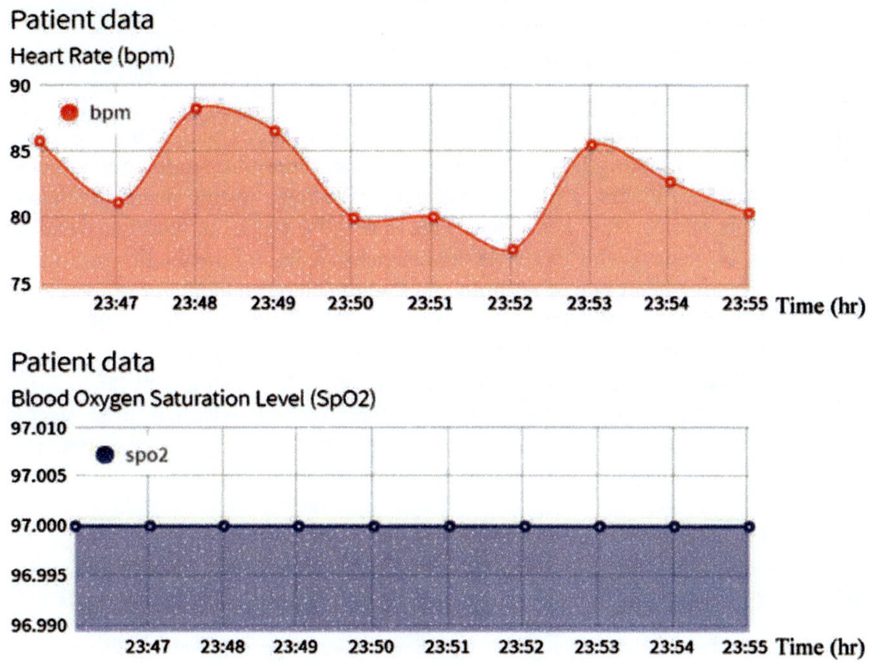

Fig. 5 The max30100 sensor measurement data

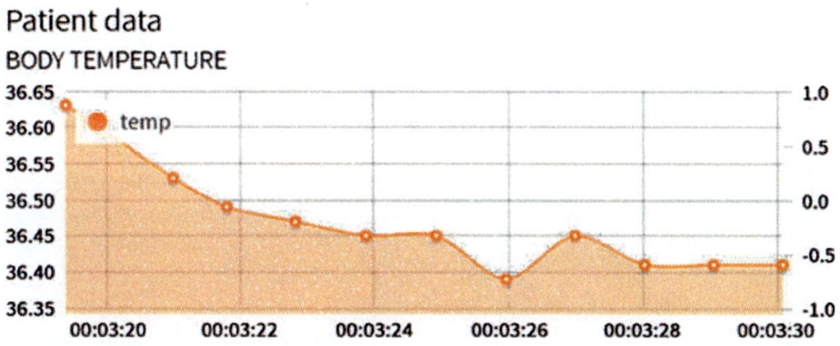

Fig. 6 The max90614 sensor measurement data

between 36.0 °C until 37.5 °C. Result show that the measurement reading from the sensor was consistently provided for every second for normal human body temperature.

3.4 The Comparison Between Heart Rate Sensor and Blood Pressure Monitor Measurement

A healthy resting heart rate for adults is 60–80 bpm. Adults with a high level of fitness may have a resting heart rate below 60 and some elite endurance athletes (such as marathon runners or professional cyclists) have a resting heart rate below 40. An average adult resting heart rate range is 60–100 bpm, but the higher end of this range is associated with increased health risks including metabolic syndrome. An elevated resting heart rate of 80 bpm and higher can be an indicator of increased cardiovascular risk and all-cause mortality risk, according to studies. The risk is most pronounced when the resting heart rate goes above 90 bpm.

Table 1 show the result of the heart rate (see Fig. 7) measurement taken from randomly 10 adult people by using two different methods which is from sensor measurement and manually calculated from the wrist point. From the experimental,

Table 1 The comparison heart rate measurement between Heart Rate Sensor and Blood Pressure Monitor

Individual	Heart rate (bpm)		Percentage Deviation (%)
	Sensor	Blood Pressure Monitor	
A	85.7	84.0	2.02
B	72.7	72.0	0.97
C	80.4	82.0	1.95
D	67.6	66.0	1.55
E	70.8	72.0	1.67
F	82.1	80.0	2.63
G	96.6	96.0	0.63
H	64.2	64.0	0.31
I	72.1	70.0	3.00
J	88.9	86.0	3.37

Fig. 7 The comparison heart rate measurement by using sensor and manual method max90614 sensor measurement data

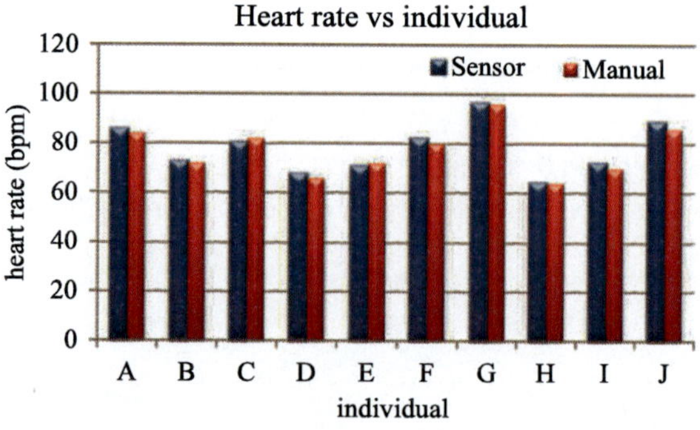

measuring the heart rate by using sensor was easier and effective compare to the conventional method. From the data collection, the measurement value of the heart rate achieved from the sensor was similar compared to the blood pressure monitor measurement value. Based on the result reached, its shows that the comparison percentage deviation maximum between heartbeat sensor and blood pressure monitor is 3.37%.

3.5 The Comparison Between Body Temperature Sensor and Digital Thermometer Measurement

The accuracy of temperature sensor is one of the analysis have been investigated under this research. The two body temperature condition which is during fever and after fever was taken from five different individual. The normal body temperature of adult people should be lie in between 36.0 °C until 37.5 °C and the fever temperature will be indicated from 37.6 °C to 41.0 °C according to the level of the fever. Table 2 show that the body temperature measurement (see Fig. 8) result of five individual under fever and after fever condition.

Result shows that the reading from the temperature sensor is similar compared with the measurement value by using digital thermometer. Using ESP8266 as the microcontroller, the data from both sensors is transferred into web hosting and database server. User is able to monitor the patient situation through online with permissible buffer changing time. Based on the findings, its show that the comparison percentage deviation between body temperature sensor and digital thermometer is 0.54%. There are a few limitation found from this research. First, the measurement result for heart rate only show in average value with unit beat per minute (bpm) for every patient. In the meantime for the heart rate sensor clip it is required only for suitable finger size to accurately measure the heart rate. The measurement result of heart rate is only valid for an adult age range.

Table 2 The comparison body temperature measurement between body temperature sensor and digital thermometer (during fever and after fever)

Individual	Body temperature condition					
	Fever (°C)			After fever (°C)		
	Sensor	Digital Thermometer	Percentage Deviation (%)	Sensor	Digital Thermometer	Percentage Deviation (%)
A	37.6	37.7	0.27	36.0	36.1	0.28
B	38.1	38.3	0.52	36.8	36.9	0.27
C	40.7	40.8	0.25	36.6	36.8	0.54
D	36.6	36.8	0.54	36.9	37.1	0.54
E	37.7	37.9	0.53	36.2	36.3	0.28

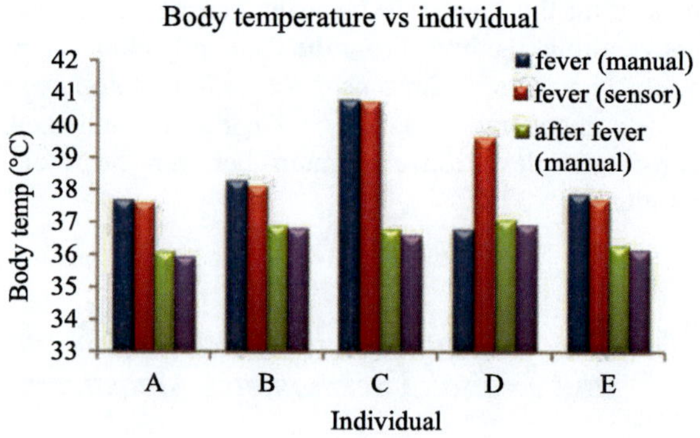

Fig. 8 The comparison body temperature measurement by using sensor and manual method (during fever and after fever)

4 Conclusion

The limitations of conventional technique for measuring and monitoring heart rate and body temperature has led to a successful development of monitoring system that can be monitored automatically. The monitoring system for heartbeat and body temperature project was successfully measuring the human heart rate and body temperature by using low cost microcontroller with internal build-in Wi-Fi configuration which the NodeMcu ESP8266. There are two main sensors involved which MAX30100 heart rate sensor and MLX90614 temperature sensor. A few experimental had successfully performed for analyzed the sensor measurement with the blood pressure monitor and digital thermometer measurement. The data collected using Iot platform which is Thinger.io is displayed on Graphical User Interface (GUI). The characteristics in the developed Thinger.io application for the system includes monitoring the details information of heart rate and body temperature. The user able to monitor the system either through desktop or smartphones method where the hardware system can be controlled via finger touch. This method will give another benefit to user without the need to be at the particular area. Referring to the outcome presented, its shows that the comparison percentage deviation between heartbeat sensor and blood pressure monitor is 3.37% and the comparison percentage deviation between body temperature sensor and digital thermometer is 0.54%. There are a few enhancement can be implement in the future. The human blood pressure is one of the most frequent parameter that will be consider as important to checked by the doctor. For Future development, a sensor that had a capability to measure the human blood pressure should be integrate with this system to ensure the monitoring system can be more versatile in monitoring the human health parameter.

References

1. Parihar VR, Tonge AY, Ganorkar PD (2017) Heartbeat and temperature monitoring system for remote patients using arduino. Int J Adv Eng Res Sci 4(5):55–58
2. Wijaya NH, Fauzi FA, Helmy ET, Nguyen PT, Atmoko RA (2020) The design of heart rate detector and body temperature measurement device using ATMega16. J Robot Control 1 (2):40–43
3. Uysal Z, Kalkancı G, İmren T, Değ A, Karal Ö, Çankaya İ (2016) A heart rate monitoring application using wireless sensor network system based on Bluetooth with Matlab GUI. IJESC, vol 6, no 8, pp 2862–2866
4. Huang PW, Chang TH, Lee MJ, Lin TM, Chung ML, Wu BF (2017) An embedded non-contact body temperature measurement system with automatic face tracking and neural network regression. In: 2016 International automatic control conference (CACS 2016), pp 161–166
5. Costa DS, Turco SHN, Ramos RP, Silva FMFM, Freire MS (2018) Electronic monitoring system for measuring heart rate and skin temperature in small ruminants. J Brazilian Assoc Agric Eng 38(2):166–172
6. Hashim NMZ, Anuar MR, Jaafar A, Aziz MZAA, Salleh A, Ja'afar AS (2014) Graphical user interface for wireless patient monitoring system using Zigbee communication. ARPN J Eng Appl Sci 9(9):1554–1558
7. Kazi SS, Bajantri G, Thite T (2018) Remote heart rate monitoring system using IoT. Int Res J Eng Technol 05(04):2956–2963
8. Hassanalieragh M et al (2015) Health monitoring and management using internet-of-things (IoT) sensing with cloud-based processing: opportunities and challenges. In: Proceedings—2015 IEEE International conference on services computing (SCC 2015), pp 285–292
9. Patel N, Patel P, Patel N (2018) Heart attack detection and heart rate monitoring using IoT. Int J Innov Adv Comput Sci IJIACS 7(4):611–615
10. Mallick B, Patro AK (2016) Heart rate monitoring system using finger tip through arduino and processing software. Int J Sci Eng Technol Res 5(1):84–89
11. Koshti M, Ganorkar S, M.E. Student (2016) IoT based health monitoring system by using Raspberry Pi and ECG signal. Int J Innov Res Sci Eng Technol (An ISO Certif Organ) 5 (5):8977–8985
12. Punit Gupta PKD, Agrawal D, Chhabra J (2016) IoT based Smart HealthCare Kit. ICCTICT, 237–242
13. Gómez J, Oviedo B, Zhuma E (2016) Patient monitoring system based on internet of things. Procedia Comput Sci 83(Ant):90–97

Investigation on the Effect of Varying Bubble Size and Location in Electrical Resistance Tomography Using Conducting Boundary Strategy

Suzanna Ridzuan Aw, Farah Hanan Azimi, Lia Safiyah Syafie, Ruzairi Abdul Rahim, Yasmin Abd Wahab, Nurain Izzati Shuhaimi, Raja Siti Nur Adiimah Raja Aris, and Ida Laila Ahmad

Abstract This paper demonstrates a Linear Back Projection (LBP) algorithm based reconstruction of conductivity distributions to investigate the effect of varying different size and location of the bubble phantom in a vertical metallic column. Sixteen electrodes were placed evenly along the circumference of the column. Simulation and experimental studies applying conducting boundary strategy were conducted to investigate the performance of the system. The reconstructed images of the phantom under test are presented. All LBP images obtained by simulation and experiment then be presented and analysed using the Mean Structural Similarity Index (MSSIM) and Area Error (AE) analysis. The number and spatial distribution of the bubble phantom can be clearly distinguished wherever they are located in the pipeline. Bubbles with a greater size than 6 mm and especially the one that is located near the wall boundary are much easier to detect. This research has successfully been applied to a metallic column and contribute the knowledge on the effect of varying both the size and location of the bubble in the column.

S. R. Aw (✉) · F. H. Azimi · L. S. Syafie · R. S. N. A. R. Aris
Faculty of Engineering Technology, University College TATI (UC TATI), Jalan Panchor, Telok Kalong, 24000 Kemaman, Terengganu, Malaysia
e-mail: suzanna_aw@uctati.edu.my

R. A. Rahim
Process Tomography and Instrumentation Engineering Research Group (PROTOM-I), Innovative Engineering Research Alliance, Faculty of Electrical Engineering, Universiti Teknologi Malaysia, UTM Skudai, 81310 Skudai, Johor, Malaysia

Y. A. Wahab
Department of Instrumentation & Control Engineering (ICE), Faculty of Electrical & Electronics Engineering, Universiti Malaysia Pahang, 26600 Pekan, Pahang, Malaysia

N. I. Shuhaimi
Faculty of Electrical Engineering, UiTM Shah Alam, Shah Alam, Malaysia

I. L. Ahmad
Department of Mechatronics and Robotics, Faculty of Electrical and Electronic Engineering, Universiti Tun Hussein Onn Malaysia, 86400 Batu Pahat, Johor, Malaysia

H. Triwiyanto et al. (eds.), *Proceedings of the 1st International Conference on Electronics, Biomedical Engineering, and Health Informatics*, Lecture Notes in Electrical Engineering 746, https://doi.org/10.1007/978-981-33-6926-9_60

Keywords Electrical resistance tomography · Linear back projection · Bubble · MSSIM · AE

1 Introduction

1.1 Background

Tomography is now of paramount interest to researchers as it can provide ample information about the internal structure of an object without the need to interrupt the process. One of the most extensive tomography modalities is Electrical Resistance Tomography (ERT). ERT is an accepted diagnostic technique for imaging the interior of opaque systems. It is relatively safe and inexpensive to operate and is relatively fast, thus enabling the real-time monitoring of processes. This technique has been applied in numerous areas, including medical imaging, environmental monitoring, and industrial processes. Knowing the process flow conditions can help in managing the downstream processes. It would be highly beneficial to measure the flow of each phase in the pipe; ideally the mass, volume, and degree of mixing within the pipe. By adapting ERT, early monitoring of the existence of gas can be facilitated, resulting in an ability to monitor or assess the effect of process changes on process quality and efficiency.

There are numerous examples of ERT being employed to qualitatively image the material distribution of multiphase processes within electrically insulated (non-conducting) walls. Among them are the research by Low et al. [1] which demonstrated the great potential of ERT in measuring active volume in a mixing column for multiphase flow, Sardeshpande et al. [2, 3] published papers on the use of ERT in visualising the gas liquid flows in a stirred tank reactor and Hashemi et al. [4] investigated bubble behaviour in an aerated mixing vessel of a viscous corn syrup solution. Babaei et al. [5] used ERT to analyse gas phase behaviour in an activated sludge bubble column. Bubble size and conductivity of the boundary of bubbles in flotation froth were estimated by Nissinen et al. [6].

However, only a few studies deploying ERT within electrically conducting columns have been reported, and these have primarily provided qualitative results for the purpose of process monitoring. These are as published by Wang et al. [7, 8], Yuen et al. [9], Grieve [10], Liter et al. [11], and Davidson [12]. In this research, a measurement system using ERT techniques to monitor the two phase (liquid/gas) flow for the application of a conducting bubble column wall is proposed.

This paper focused on a number of simulations and experiments done in reconstructing the image of bubble phantoms in a metal wall using conducting strategy in ERT. The aim of this research is to investigate the effect of varying bubble phantom size and location in a vertical metal pipe applying conducting boundary strategy in ERT to obtain the images.

2 ERT Image Reconstruction

LBP algorithm is one of the types from back projection algorithm and is essentially based on the linearization of a normalized form of the original problem. The projection data from each sensor with its sensitivity maps is combined to generate the concentration profile in LBP. Theoretically, providing by the corresponding sensitivity map, LBP can be viewed as a weighted back projected or "smearing" of each one of the normalized measurements along its sensing zone [13].

The principle of this back-projection in ERT is that a relative change of the boundary measurement, $\Delta V_{i,j}/V_{i,j}$ with its sensitivity at each pixel as its weight factor is back-projected to the whole domain as relative changes of the conductivity at each pixel in the i, j projection. Because of its linear approach and fixed weight factors, LBP could not provide an accurate image. Nonetheless, it provides a fast online view or a preview for initial visualization [14].

For the LBP implementation in this research, the calibration for the homogeneous system needs to be done first. The homogeneous flow for this research is a full flow of tap water with conductivity of 8.33×10^{-3} S/m. Later, the system can then be used to reconstruct the cross-sectional image of the region of interest based on Eq. 1 that represents the LBP algorithm.

$$\mathrm{LBP}\ (\mathrm{x},\mathrm{y}) = \sum_{\mathrm{Tx}=0}^{n} \sum_{\mathrm{Rx}=0}^{n} A_{\mathrm{Tx,Rx}} \times \bar{S}_{\mathrm{Tx,Rx}}(x,y) \tag{1}$$

where LBP (x, y), is the profile showing the concentration image obtained using LBP algorithm in n × n (128 × 128) matrix where n equals to the dimension of the sensitivity matrix; $\bar{S}_{\mathrm{Tx,Rx}}(x,y)$ is the normalized sensitivity map for the view of transmitter Tx to receiver Rx, and $A_{\mathrm{Tx,Rx}}$ is the sensor loss value which refers to the difference of the homogeneous and non-homogeneous flow for the projection of transmitter Tx to receiver Rx. Non-homogeneous flow refers to the flow condition when there is a phantom or object exists inside the pipe. $A_{\mathrm{Tx,Rx}}$ is represented in Eq. 2 below:

$$A_{Tx,Rx} = \frac{V_{homo}(Tx,Rx) - V_{non-homo}(Tx,Rx)}{V_{homo}(Tx,Rx)} \tag{2}$$

where $V_{homo}(Tx,Rx)$ is the electric potential measured when Tx act as source electrode and Rx act as the receiver electrode in the condition of full water flow; while $V_{non-homo}(Tx,Rx)$ is the electric potential measured when Tx act as source electrode and Rx act as the receiver electrode in the condition of non-homogeneous flow.

The algorithm is then applied in a programming environment along with the sensor loss data and sensitivity maps to be computed and programmed to generate the image. Authors use the MATLAB programming environment to reconstruct the image.

3 Methodology

3.1 Proposed System

For this research, the proposed system is first simulated and being verified experimentally. The modelling and simulation of the system in 2D was performed using COMSOL. This simulation aimed to investigate and analyse the effect of varying bubble size and location on the potential distribution which are represented by the reconstructed images of ERT, applying conducting columns. Sixteen rectangular electrodes denoted as e in Fig. 1 were implemented. The electrodes were attached evenly along the circumference of a stainless-steel pipe wall. It was important to ensure these were insulated from the metal wall. Adopting the conducting boundary strategy, a constant current was applied at source electrode es, and the output voltages from 15 pairs of electrodes from e1 to e15 were measured. The column itself was grounded and acted as the current sink. The model under investigation and the clearer view of electrode fabrication using flexible circuit board are presented in Figs. 1 and 2 respectively.

3.2 Experimental Setup

Sixteen electrodes were placed equidistantly around the inner periphery of the column so that it contacted the fluid inside the pipe but did not disturb the flow inside. The conducting boundary approach was adopted in the experiment whereby

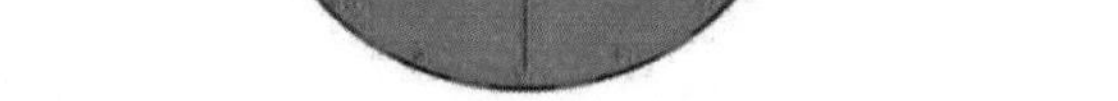

Fig. 1 2D View of Model Under Investigation

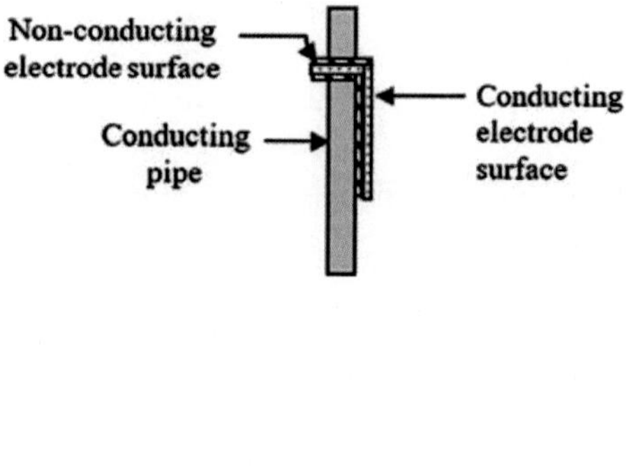

Fig. 2 Electrode fabrication using flexible circuit board

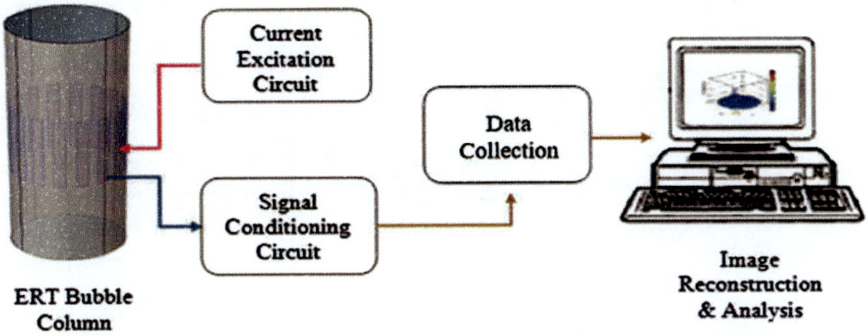

Fig. 3 ERT experimental setup

a 5 mA bidirectional pulse current was injected into the system and the output voltages were gathered. The output voltage from the receiving electrode was then amplified in the signal conditioning part. The pipe itself acted as a ground. Cross-sectional images of the bubbles were reconstructed using LBP after the data collection process was completed. The experimental setup for this system is illustrated in Fig. 3.

3.3 Test Profile for Simulation and Experiment

In validating the measurement system, a number of known test profiles (gas bubble model) were implemented. The test profiles were placed in the investigation column in a pre-defined position as shown in Table 1. Phantoms A, to E were of 20 mm diameter whilst phantoms F to H were of 10 mm diameter. Phantoms I and J were of 6 and 3 mm diameter respectively.

The output potentials of the system were obtained from COMSOL simulation and the tomogram was reconstructed using the LBP technique. The simulations were then verified through the experiment. The tomogram for both simulation and experiment means were then reconstructed using the LBP techniques.

3.4 LBP Routine

For each phantom under investigation, the sensor loss data were loaded into the software before performing the LBP algorithm for image reconstruction. Subsequently, the LBP routine in Fig. 4 was applied towards the selected phantom. For the routine, the output potential at receiver 1 was recorded first when transmitter 1 transmitted the current source. All possible independent measurements for that

Table 1 Test profile information

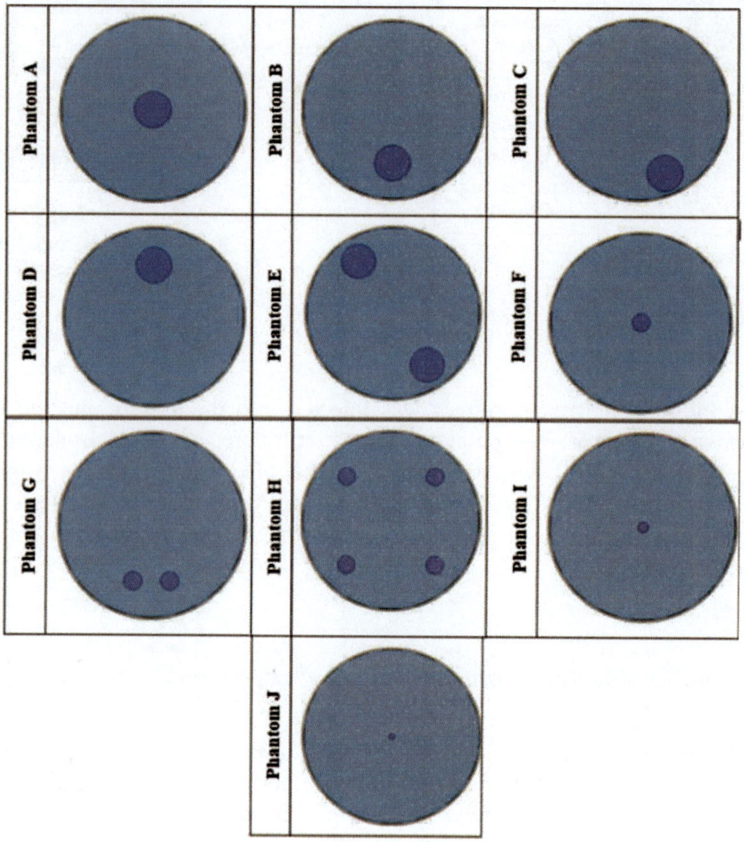

particular phantom were then taken to obtain the sensor loss. Once the sixteen scans were completed, the tomogram was reconstructed by performing the LBP algorithm.

4 Results and Discussions

The results of varying bubble size were first presented. This will be followed by the reconstructed ERT images of other bubble phantoms.

Fig. 4 LBP routine

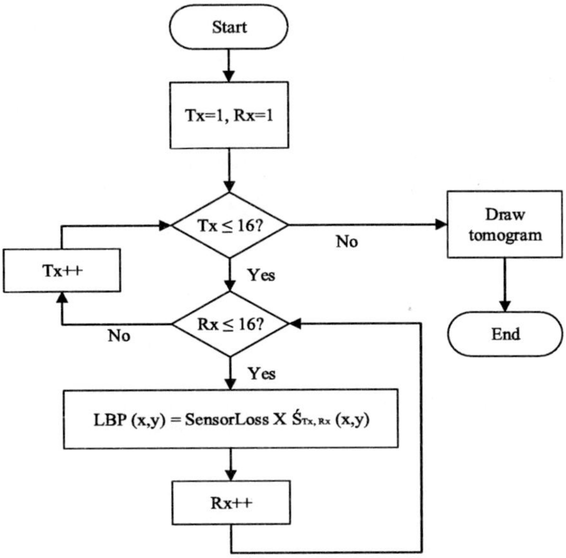

4.1 *Limitation of Bubble Phantom Size*

Three bubble phantom sizes of 10, 6 and 3 mm diameter were placed at the central region of the pipe. The output potential from the COMSOL simulation was gathered to obtain the sensor loss. The sensor loss data were then implemented, using the LBP algorithm in MATLAB, to generate the image shown in Table 2. The same procedures were completed in the experiment to confirm the simulation. A cylinder rod was used in the experiment to resemble the 2D cross section of the bubble phantom, as modelled in COMSOL.

The first investigation in COMSOL involved a 10 mm diameter bubble phantom which was shown to be detected for the ERT system. The image was reconstructed correctly and a bubble phantom was clearly shown at the centre of the pipe. The experimental results agreed with the simulation. The phantom size was then reduced to 6 mm diameter and was detected correctly. Finally, the phantom size was reduced to 3 mm diameter; however, this could not be detected correctly. These results agreed with the simulation presented in [15], where bubble phantoms of 6 mm diameter and above were said to be more sensitive towards the injected current and yielded higher differences in the sensor loss data.

Table 2 LBP Image for centred bubble phantom of Difference Phantom Size

Phantom Position	**COMSOL Results**	**Experimental Results**
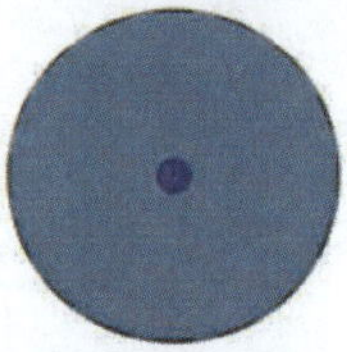 Phantom F	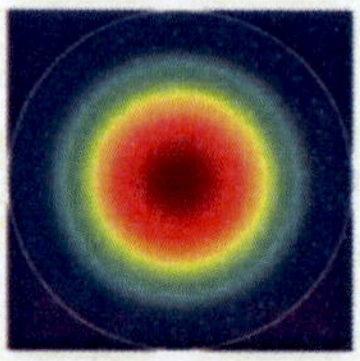	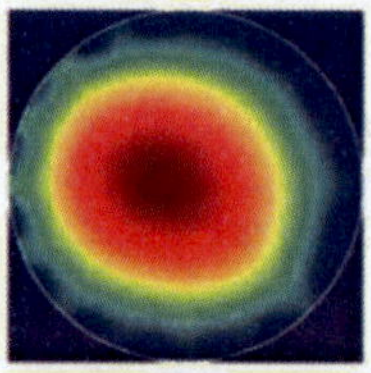
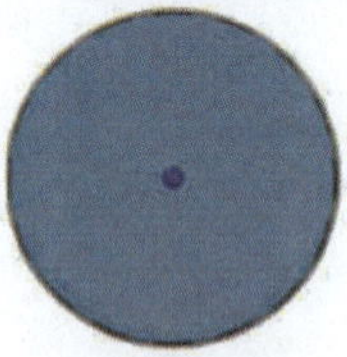 Phantom I	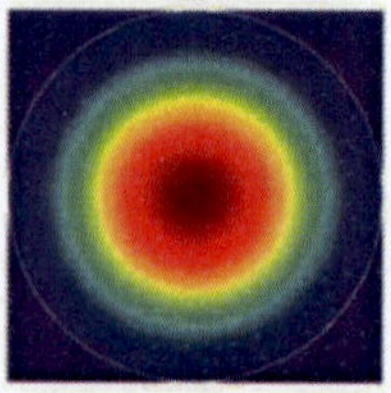	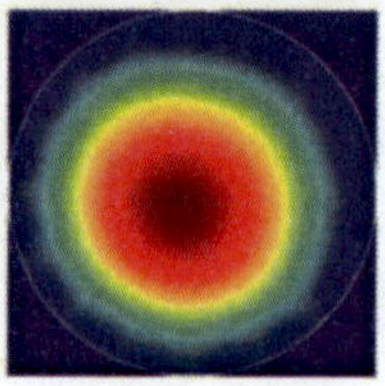
 Phantom J	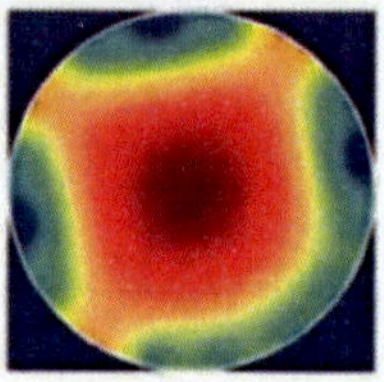	No available 3mm diameter rod for test

4.2 *Reconstructed Image Using LBP (Non-Threshold Technique)*

The reconstructed tomogram for the simulation and experiment for each phantom is tabulated in Table 3. The darkest red region shows the most concentrated region which denotes the existence of the bubble phantom. The images from the experimental results agree with the simulation, where only a slight difference in the 2D view was observed. When two phantoms are located near each other, as in Phantom E, the image is not able to show the solid existence of two bubbles using LBP because of the very dense conductivity distribution at this location.

MSSIM Analysis for Test Profile

MSSIM compares the reconstructed image to a reference image that closely matches the cross section of the model. The reference image was generated on the computer, using MATLAB. To represent the cross section of the flow conveying

Table 3 2D view of LBP tomograms for simulation versus experiment

	Simulation	Experiment
Phantom B	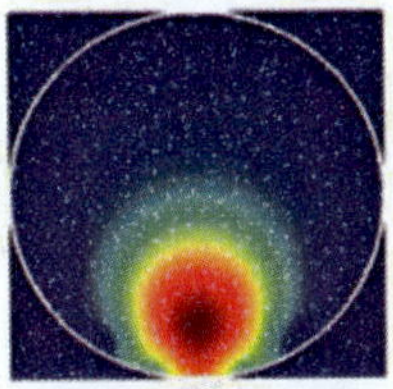	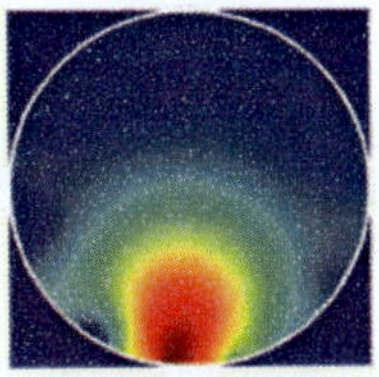
Phantom C	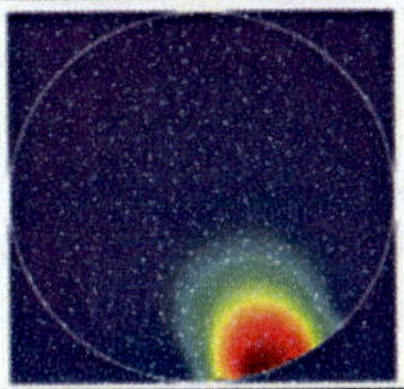	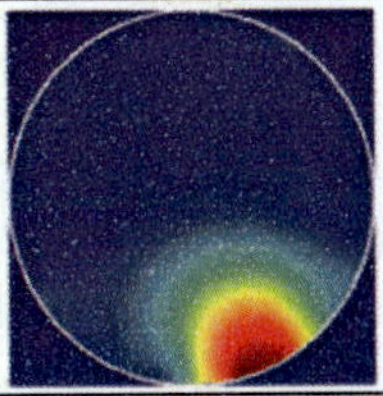
Phantom D	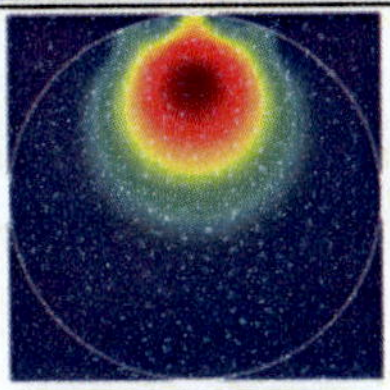	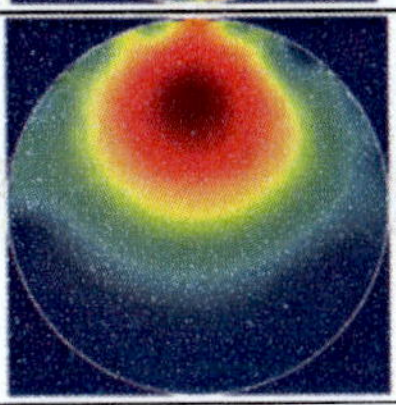
Phantom E	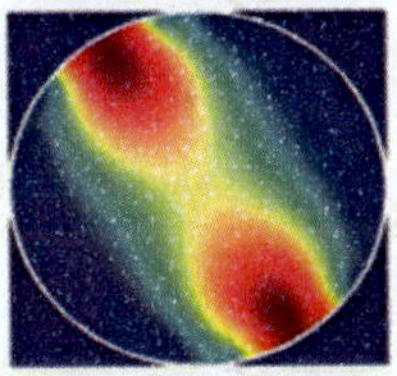	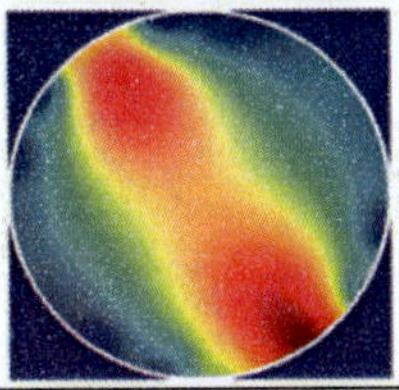
Phantom G	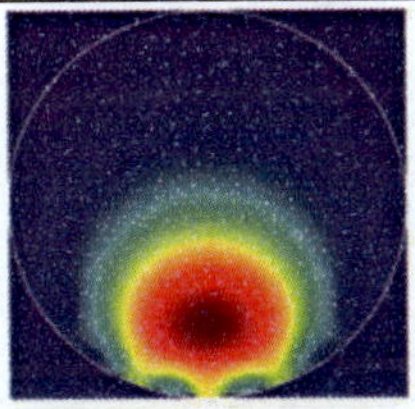	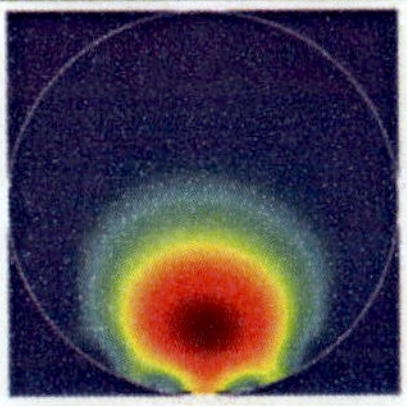
Phantom H	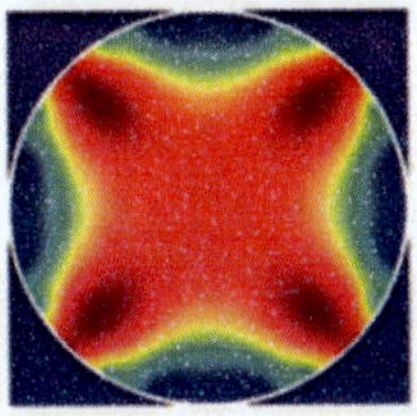	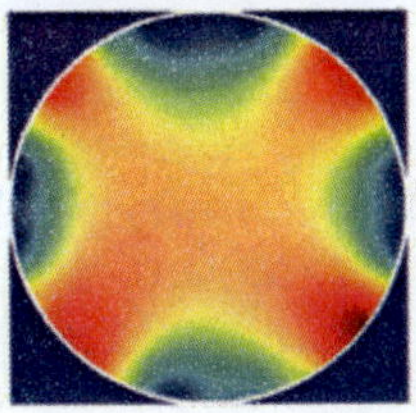

pipe, the image plane was divided into P square (128 × 128) image pixels. The effective area that represents the cross section of the full liquid medium for the system under investigation equalled to 12,851 pixels. To produce the image of a two-phase flow (liquid and gas phantom), a circle was drawn with an appropriate radius that resembles the gas phantom used.

The MSSIM index measured for each phantom investigated in the simulation and experiment is presented in Table 4. The corresponding graph is shown in Fig. 5.

The plot shows that the MSSIM gives a higher value for the simulation results than the experimental results. This is because of accurate readings in the simulation, compared with the error introduced in the experiment that made the results fluctuate from theoretical readings. Phantom C and Phantom G give the highest indexes in the simulation and experiment, respectively. A higher MSSIM index indicates a better reconstructed image. When there are four sparse bubble phantoms located in the conducting column, as in Phantom H, the MSSIM index yields a low value due to the high difference in conductivity distribution, compared with the homogeneous

Table 4 MSSIM Indexes measured on reconstructed test profiles

Phantom	Simulation	Experiment
A	0.2588	0.1334
B	0.2032	0.1066
C	0.3028	0.1055
D	0.1763	0.1055
E	0.1338	0.1099
F	0.1176	0.0931
G	0.169	0.1524
H	0.0791	0.0759
I	0.1164	0.0986
J	0.0769	Null

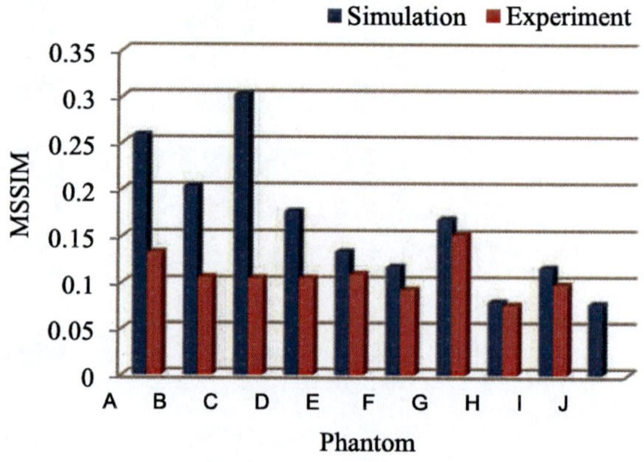

Fig. 5 MSSIM Indexes measured on reconstructed test profiles

medium. Phantom J in the simulation has the smallest value of MSSIM. This accords with the low accuracy of the smallest bubble image reconstructed previously.

Area Error (AE) Analysis for Non-Threshold Test Profile.

Area error (AE), which measures the error of the cross-sectional area between the reference image and the reconstructed image, was also analysed. Table 5 tabulates the AE measured on every phantom in the simulation and experiment, the corresponding plot for which is depicted in Fig. 6.

The error in the cross-sectional area of the 20 mm gas phantom under investigation is smaller than the 10, 6, and 3 mm diameter gas bubble phantoms. The value of the AE in the simulation and experiment produced the same reading. Comparing the AE between the phantoms shows that the gas phantom located in the deepest region of the conductivity distribution yields a very high value of the AE with values of 282.6222 and 1417.11 for 6 and 3 mm centre bubble phantoms,

Table 5 AE measured on reconstructed test profiles

Phantom	Simulation	Experiment
A	23.1267	23.1267
B	23.1267	23.1267
C	24.0747	24.0747
D	24.0747	24.0747
E	11.5373	11.5373
F	97.938	97.938
G	48.469	48.469
H	23.7345	23.7345
I	282.6222	282.6222
J	1417.11	Null

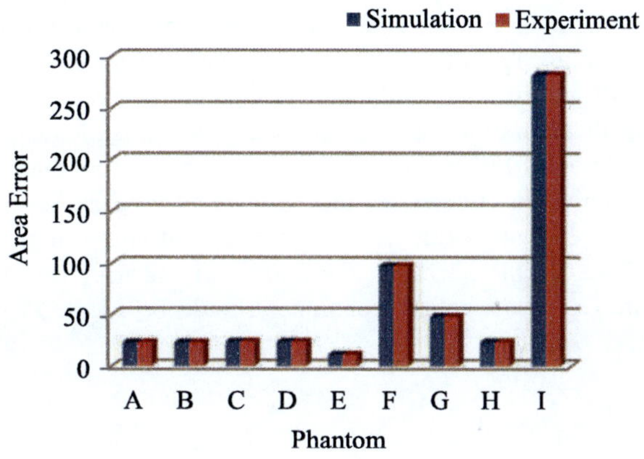

Fig. 6 AE measured on reconstructed test profiles

respectively. This is due to the central region problem in ERT. For a phantom of 10 mm diameter that is not located at the centre, such as in G and H, the AE provides smaller error.

4.3 Discussions

In the simulation of the two-phase flow model using COMSOL, the properties for each material under investigation were based on their real properties in the experiment. Based on the sensor loss and sensitivity maps obtained, MATLAB was used to reconstruct the image using an LBP algorithm. A number of bubble phantoms were tested to justify the research. To verify the efficiency and feasibility of the research as well as the sensitivity-based image reconstruction algorithm, the reconstructed images of ten phantoms for the two-phase flow (water and gas) are presented.

The constructed LBP images obtained from COMSOL simulation data were analysed using the MSSIM and the AE. These were then compared with the images obtained from experimental data. The results show that the reconstructed images successfully displayed the location of the phantom of interest correctly using the LBP algorithm. The sensitivity values decrease when the excitation electrode is located farther from the measurement electrode. Furthermore, the sensor loss value is higher when there is an object between the source electrode and receiver electrode. This causes the concentration profile to become higher and denser at the located object.

For a single phantom, the location of the bubble image resembles the real location of the phantom. For images where more than one phantom exists, such as those illustrated in Phantom E, G, and H, LBP is still sufficient to produce the correct location of the image even though the shape of phantom is not 100% accurate. This is caused by the smearing effect in LBP because of its linear approach and fixed weight factor. When the bubble is located at the centre of the pipe, an artefact in the image occurs. When the bubble phantom is located near to the boundary of the pipe, the grounded wall will introduce a much greater artefact and blurring to the boundary, or even distort the reconstructed image. However, LBP is still sufficiently adequate to be implemented for initial visualisation and verification of the study. Conversely, it is not adequate enough to obtain the images of bubbles located near to one another. The conductivity distribution changes too much when bubbles are too close to each other, as in Phantom G.

Even though LBP provides a sufficient image to give information on the location of the bubble phantom, the noise and smearing effect remained high. Thus, other image reconstruction techniques should be adopted to improve the image MSSIM and AE.

5 Conclusion

The effect of varying bubble phantom size and location in a vertical metal pipe applying conducting boundary strategy in ERT to obtain the images has successfully being investigated. The LBP remains a widespread choice in ERT image reconstruction since it can provide sufficient images. Although it cannot provide an accurate image, it does provide an acceptable view for initial visualisation. Simulation results for ten bubble phantoms demonstrated that the invasive ERT sensor in a metal pipe applying a conductivity boundary strategy, together with the sensitivity-based reconstruction algorithm, can feasibly provide cross-sectional images of the water and gas two-phase flow. The locations of the bubble can be clearly distinguished. However, the exact shape of the conductivity distribution was not obtained because of the aforementioned imperfections of the linear method approximations in the algorithm used. To improve the image quality, a thresholding technique or other advance image reconstruction techniques can be implemented.

Acknowledgements The authors fully acknowledge University College TATI (UC TATI) for giving financial support for this conference and grateful to the PROTOM Research Group UTM for the facilities and instrumentations that makes this important research viable and effective.

References

1. Low SC, Allitt D, Eshtiaghi N, Parthasarathy R (2018) Measuring active volume using electrical resistance tomography in a gas-sparged model anaerobic digester. Chem Eng Res Des
2. Sardeshpande MV, Gupta S, Ranade VV (2017) Electrical resistance tomography for gas holdup in a gas-liquid stirred tank reactor. Chem Eng Sci 2017(170):476–490
3. Sardeshpande MV, Kumar G, Aditya T, Ranade VV (2016) Mixing studies in unbaffled stirred tank reactor using electrical resistance tomography. Flow Meas Instrum
4. Hashemi N, Ein-Mozaffari F, Upreti SR, Hwang DK (2016) Experimental investigation of the bubble behavior in an aerated coaxial mixing vessel through electrical resistance tomography (ERT). Chem Eng J
5. Babaei R, Bonakdarpour B, Ein-Mozaffari F (2015) Analysis of gas phase characteristics and mixing performance in an activated sludge bioreactor using electrical resistance tomography. Chem Eng J
6. Nissinen A, Lehikoinen A, Mononen M, Lähteenmäki S, Vauhkonen M (2014) Estimation of the bubble size and bubble loading in a flotation froth using electrical resistance tomography. Miner Eng
7. Wang M, Dickin FJ, Williams RA (1994) Electrical resistance tomography of metal walled vessels and pipelines. Electron Lett
8. Wang M, Dickin FJ, Williams RA (1995) Modelling and analysis of electrically conducting vessels and pipelines in electrical resistance process tomography. IEE Proc Sci Meas Technol
9. Yuen EL, Mann R, York TA, Grieve BD (2001) Electrical resistance tomography imaging of a metal-walled solid-liquid filter. In: 2nd World Congress on Industrial Process Tomography. Hannover, Germany

10. Grieve BD (2002) On-line electrical impedance tomography for industrial batch processing [Internet]. Department of Chemical Engineering [Manchester, UK]: UMIST, 2002. Available from https://www.escholar.manchester.ac.uk/api/datastream?publicationPid=uk-ac-man-scw:10776&datastreamId=FULL-TEXT.PDF
11. Liter SG, Shollenberger KA, Torczynski JR, Ceccio SL (2002) Measuring material distributions of multiphase flows in electrically conducting vessels using electrical-impedance tomography. Am Soc Mech Eng Fluids Eng Div FED
12. Davidson JL (2004) Three-dimensional electrical impedance tomography applied to a metal-walled filtration test platform. Meas Sci Technol 2004(15):2263–2274
13. Rahiman MHF, Zakaria Z, Rahim RA, Ng WN (2009) Ultrasonic tomography imaging simulation of two-phase homogeneous flow. Sens Rev
14. Wang M, Mann R, Dickin FJ (1999) Electrical resistance tomographic sensing systems for industrial applications. Chem Eng Commun
15. Ridzuan Aw S, Abdul Rahim R, Fazalul Rahiman MH, Mohamad EJ, Mohd Yunus FR, Wahab YA et al (2015) Simulation study on electrical resistance tomography using metal wall for bubble detection. J Teknol 2015(73):31–35

Initial-to-Point of Motion Planning on Exoskeleton Arm for Post Stroke Rehabilitation

W. T. Wan Faizura, M. Z. Muhammad Luqman, O. Mohd Hafiz, M. Safuan Naim, and M. S. Muhamad Habiibullah

Abstract There were several statements of problem that initially rise and cause the invention. Currently, there are some problems that are still the main cause of adult disability in Malaysia and various countries. Although stroke can cause deficiencies in some neurological domains, the most normally affected is the motor system. Furthermore, given the central role normally played by hand movements in human existence, much focus is placed on remedial research focused on understanding and restoring the function of hand motor after stroke. In this study is to design arm exoskeleton for use in the field of hand rehabilitation based on the application of therapy and closely related movement training. Although the system already exists, past exoskeleton efforts involve large, expensive, invasive, and moored products and costs. Therefore, this study is m to build a cheap, smooth and effective exoskeleton system. To overcome this problem, the rehabilitation for human therapy will be a low-cost, ergonomic device actuated through sensors measuring the user's motion. The study of exoskeleton arm is particularly interest to the researchers. Various methods have been proposed by past researchers to improve motion planning for the exoskeleton arm. However, some are still limited because the techniques are not appropriate for therapeutic applications. Motion planning is very important for the patients need to do movement as a therapist. The purpose of this study is to develop motion planning on exoskeleton arm for post-stroke rehabilitation. The motion planning from the initial to the target point. By using third order polynomial system, the trajectory planning is carried out. The starting point is known as the initial point and final point is known as target achieved. By taking the number of degrees of freedom and time, motion planning has been produced. The motion planning of exoskeleton arm is depending on the angle joint and the time to achieve the target movement.

W. T. Wan Faizura · M. Z. Muhammad Luqman (✉) · O. Mohd Hafiz ·
M. Safuan Naim · M. S. Muhamad Habiibullah
Faculty of Engineering Technology, University College TATI,
Kemaman, Terengganu, Malaysia
e-mail: m_luqman@uctati.edu.my

H. Triwiyanto et al. (eds.), *Proceedings of the 1st International Conference on Electronics, Biomedical Engineering, and Health Informatics*, Lecture Notes in Electrical Engineering 746, https://doi.org/10.1007/978-981-33-6926-9_61

Keywords Motion planning · Trajectory planning · Exoskeleton arm and rehabilitation

1 Introduction

Stroke is one of the leading causes of disability worldwide. Lack of motor function due to stroke affects the mobility of patients, their limitations in the activities of daily life, their participation in society and the possibility of them returning to professional activities [1]. Most hands rehabilitation in Malaysia are a manual exercise or conventional therapy. Conventional therapy is usually performed by professional medical therapists, who require labor and, therefore, are expensive. To overcome this lack of manually assisted arm training, many upper limb exoskeleton systems are investigated and designed to help patients. Therefore, this stroke hand needs a more practical and modern therapy like hand device or hand tool that can assist and help human hand movement. The main human focus organ is the brain. Where the brain functions to send and receive all information. The ability of the human hand to move is through stimuli and signals sent by the brain. In some studies, it shows that the use of sensors is important for the construction of robot hands. According to Li et al. [2] through the use of onboard sensing, the framework can provide rich data i.e. distance used in physical therapy. Where such data can be used by physicians and patients to track improvement more accurately over time. At low cost, hospitals can use many tools and help a larger patient population. In addition, it can also be used at home for physical therapy, which will dramatically improve the patient's quality of life. With this, the therapist to monitor the exercise remotely. This solution is unique in that it will be a low-cost ergonomic device powered by a sensor that measures user movement. Previously, stroke was the most common neurological disease and often caused disability. Stroke can cause the patient to be affected by daily life as its characteristic feature is a decrease in the patient's limbs. To reduce the sports injuries of stroke patients, the best method is to perform specific rehabilitation exercises [3]. The exoskeleton arm is an external structural mechanism with joints and connections that correspond to those on the human limb. The exoskeleton sends torque from the proximal mover through the rigid exoskeleton link to the human joint. Exoskeleton is designed to be used for wrist and forearm movements. It currently consists of a seven-degree exoskeleton of freedom (DOF), designed to overcome the full range of motion of the main movement of the arm, which is at shoulder, elbow and wrist levels, combined or individually. Thus, the work has expanded to the level of passive recovery, which means that the exoskeleton performs movements along a predetermined crossing that moves the subject's arm with its own movement to help increase range of motion [4]. Most exoskeleton systems have been designed and operated to assist or inhibit human movement depending on the type of application in which the system includes larger parts of the human body or just individual joints. A large number of control methods here focus on increasing the effectiveness of the user in terms of joint motion or joint torque. To enable safe interaction between the exoskeleton and the user, a common approach is to use an impedance or entry operator by the researcher [5]. Some researchers focus on planning the movement of hand exoskeletons for rehabilitation. To improve hand movement techniques, parameters have been performed. Mehmet el al. proposed [6] exoskeleton design recommendations for wrist and forearm recovery. The contribution of this study is to offer a methodology that shows how to adapt a serial manipulator that reduces the number of actuators used in exoskeleton design for rehabilitation. The system presented is a combination of end-effector and exoskeleton-based devices. The passive exoskeleton is attached to the effector manipulator, which provides movement for the purpose of the recovery process. The Denso VP 6-Axis Articulation Robot is used to control the movement of the exoskeleton throughout the rehabilitation process. Clemetree et al. [7] also proposed a motion planning system based on Learning by Demonstration (LBD) for upper-limb exoskeletons that allow successfully supporting patients during Activities of Daily Living (ADLs) in unstructured environment, while ensuring that anthropomorphic criteria are satisfied in the whole human-robot workspace. Motion planning systems combine LDB Dynamic Motion Primitives calculations and machine learning techniques to build task-specific and patient-specific joint trajectories based on learned trajectories. Verification of this system has been done simulated and also in real condition with limb exoskeleton which is 4 DOF, wrist exoskeleton is 5 DOF and four patients with Limb Girdle Muscular dystrophy.

1.1 Conventional Therapist for Arm Post-stroke Rehabilitation

Conventional therapy is a training manual used for stroke patients to recover part of the hand and arm. There are various methods of therapy used such as inner arm stretch, wrist and hand stretch, elbow strength, crawling strength, wrist motion, end elbow weight training, finger walk and seated push up [8] (Fig. 1).

1.2 Modern Therapist

Hemiparetic Arm for post-stroke rehabilitation

The hemiparetic arm is designed based on the application of gyro sensors and accelerometers. The purpose of the research for post-processing and progressive status processing Subjects should wear a set of sensors on the wrist while performing some basic arm movements. The data will be converted into a network of data that can be read and stored on a microSD card and then taken to a computer for

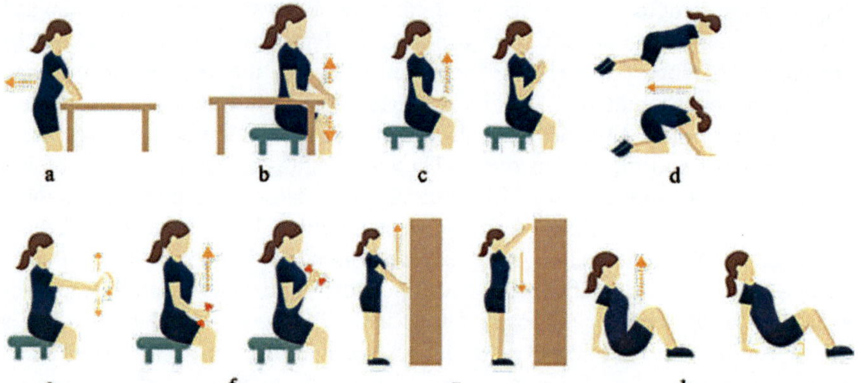

Fig. 1 Conventional Therapist **a** inner arm stretch **b** wrist and hand stretch **c** elbow stretch **d** crawling strength **e** wrist motion **f** end elbow weight training **g** finger walk and **h** seated push up [8]

pattern analysis. These experiments demonstrate the ability of sensors to produce extensive information on arm movement activities. It is believed that this system offers more information than conventional methods as well as the ability to improve the quality of training, outcomes, and patient progress. For initial conceptual evidence, the system will be tested for healthy normal subjects. It is understood that studies have been conducted in the rehabilitation of stroke patients using gyroscopes and accelerometers [9] (Fig. 2).

RECUPERA Exoskeleton for Stroke Rehabilitation

Robot-assisted therapy is more popular and useful in post-stroke rehabilitation. The research is to design and control the two-arm RECUPERA exoskeleton to provide strong therapy and self-training for sensory motor rehabilitation in the upper body. Exoskeleton has a lightweight design, high modularity level, decentralized computing, and various levels of security implementation. Due to its modularity, the

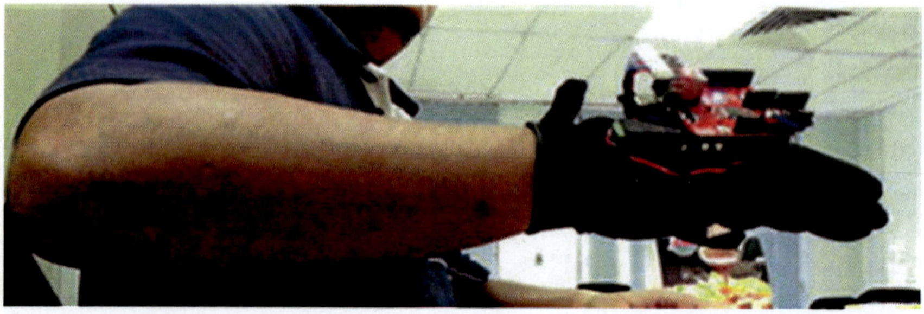

Fig. 2 Hemiparetic Arm for post-stroke rehabilitation [9]

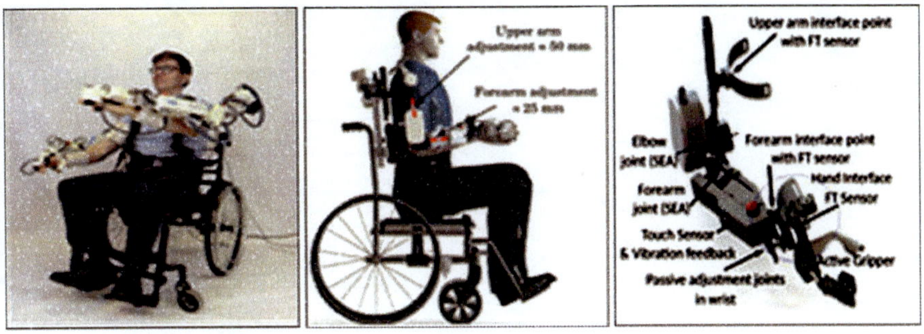

Fig. 3 RECUPERA Exoskeleton for Stroke Rehabilitation [10]

system can be used as a system mounted in a wheelchair or as a full body system. Both of these systems enable different types of therapy while placing system weight effectively and without compromising patient mobility. Further, two rehabilitation therapies implemented on the exoskeleton system, namely teaching and repetition therapy and mirror therapy, are presented along with the experimental outcomes. The main goal behind the second mechatronic design of the RECUPERA exoskeleton configuration is to obtain a lightweight modular system that provides high support capabilities and safety assurance without compromising patient mobility. This is achieved by using highly modular architecture in the mechanical and electronic domains [10] (Fig. 3).

From previous studies, various methods have been proposed by researchers. This study is to improve conventional therapy to become automatic training. Based on the conventional therapy of wrist motion and finger walk as shown in Fig. 1, the arm will move from one point to another. The purpose of this study is to develop motion planning of exoskeleton arm for post-stroke rehabilitation. By using the exoskeleton arm as a therapeutic tool, the arm can move from one point to another using trajectory planning. The starting point is known as "initial point" and the end point is known as "target point". The research also uses third order polynomial trajectory planning to determine the position, velocity and acceleration.

2 Methodology

In order to implementation of exoskeleton arm movement planning, ideas for planning and exoskeleton arm movement techniques refer to previous studies. Figure 4 shows the research flow. The first step, research is focused on mathematical modeling using third order polynomial of trajectory of planning. Mathematical modeling is an important part of finding exoskeleton arm movements. The second step, the research is to plan the exoskeleton arm for trajectory planning.

Fig. 4 Research flow

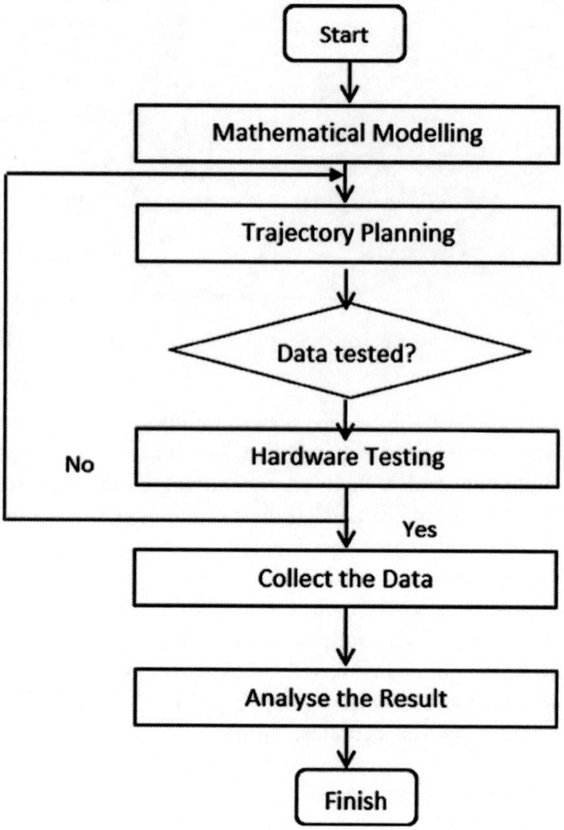

The movement of the exoskeleton arm will be tested using point to point as shown in Fig. 6. Then, data will be collected and finally the results will be analyzed.

2.1 *Mechanical Design of Exoskeleton Arm*

There are two main parts in the designing of this exoskeleton arm, the first part is exoskeleton arm controller and the second part are the point to reach the target. The movement of the exoskeleton arm is controlled by two motors, where that motors are joint 1 and joint 2 which is to control the movement from top to bottom and movement from left to right. The component used in designing of exoskeleton arm such as aluminum, force sensor, motor, laser sensor and Arduino microcontroller. The place to achieved the target point is called as therapy training board. This research is primarily concerned with the design of hands therapeutics devices with suitable material and mechanical structure idea. Therapy training board is the path

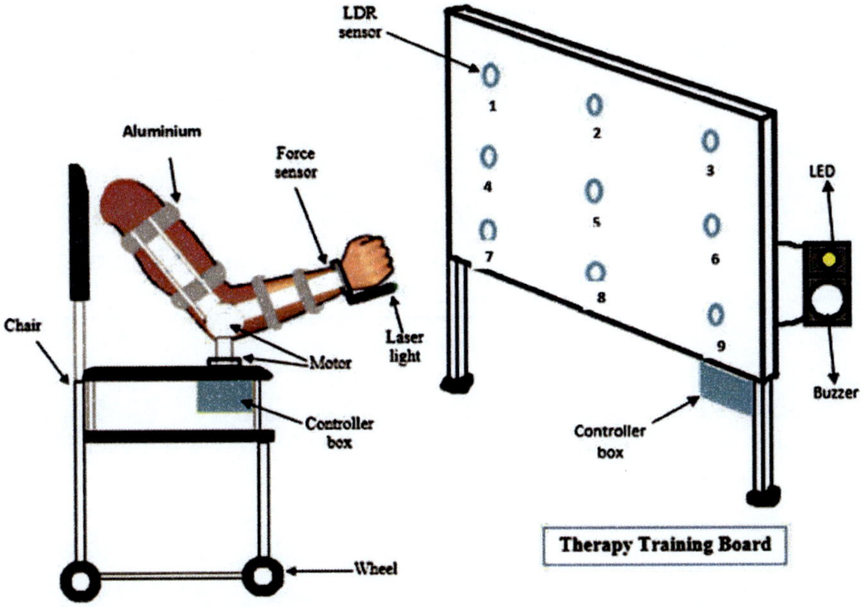

Fig. 5 Motion Planning of exoskeleton arm

or trajectory or tracking for movement of exoskeleton arm. Therapy training board $3' \times 3'$, which is the height and wide of the board and the maximum load (hand) less than 8 kg when operation. There are consisted of LDR sensor, LED, buzzer and Arduino microcontroller. The mathematical model and details of motion planning on therapy training board is discussed in Sects. 2.2 and 2.3 (Fig. 5).

2.2 Motion Planning of Exoskeleton Arm

Motion Planning or trajectory planning is concerned about when each part of the path must be attained, thus specifying timing. It is depending on the position, velocities and accelerations, where the target points will be reached at different times. The motions of the exoskeleton arm can be planned in joint space using different schemes. Using third-order polynomial cross-sectional planning, research will consider the problem of moving the exoskeleton arm from its initial position to the goal position in a given period of time. The initial location and orientation of the exoskeleton arm tool is known, and using the inverse kinematic equations is to find the final joint angles for the desired (goal) position and orientation. Now consider one of the joints, which at the beginning of the motion segment at time t_i is at θ_i. The joint move to a new value of θ_f (final joint) at time t_f (final time) as shown in Fig. 6 [11].

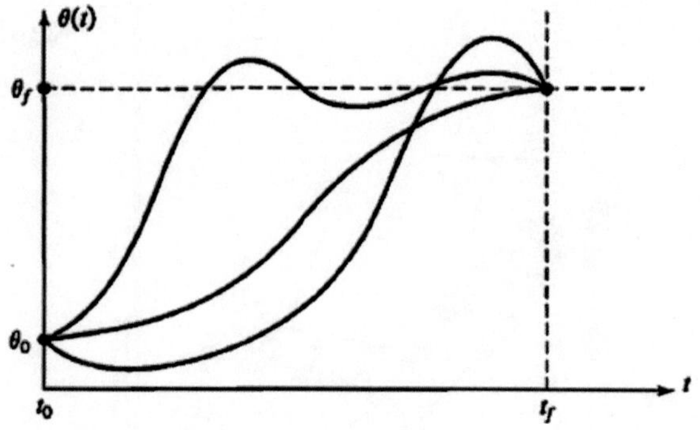

Fig. 6 Several path shape for a single joint [11]

To plan the trajectory in making a single smooth motion, we use polynomial such that at least four constraints on θ(t) are evident [11]. Two constraints come from the selection of initial and final values:

$$\theta(0) = \theta_0 \tag{1}$$

$$\theta(\mathrm{tf}) = \theta_\mathrm{f} \tag{2}$$

An additional two constraints are the velocity, which the initial and final velocity are zero:

$$\dot{\theta}(0) = 0 \tag{3}$$

$$\dot{\theta}(\mathrm{tf}) = 0 \tag{4}$$

These four constraints can be met by a polynomial at least third degree. The cubic polynomial has four coefficients, so it can be made to meet the four constraints. A cubic has the form:

$$\theta(t) = a_0 + a_1 t + a_2 t^2 + a_3 t^3 \tag{5}$$

The first equation is determining the position of exoskeleton arm for a single joint. Then, taking the first derivative of θ(t), then get equation of velocity is:

$$\dot{\theta}(t) = a_1 + 2a_2 t + 3a_3 t^2 \tag{6}$$

For the second derivative, the joint acceleration has been shown:

$$\ddot{\theta}(t) = 2a_2 + 6a_3 t \tag{7}$$

2.3 *Initial Point to Target Points*

In the research there are two joint angles to control movement of exoskeleton arm. The motion planning of exoskeleton arm using polynomial third order system to movement point to point as shown in Fig. 6. For first join is to control movement from up and down, the second joint to control left and right. There are 9 points used for motion planning of exoskeleton arm which are point 1 (P1), point 2 (P2), point 3 (P3), point 4 (P4), point 5 (P5), point 6 (P6), point 7 (P7), point 8 (P8), point 9 (P9). The main point is initial point (PO) where the starting point before achieved the target point. Figures 7 and 8 shows the motion planning of exoskeleton arm from initial to target points. There are similar joint angles of movement of exoskeleton arm from initial point (down) goes to targets point (up) for points (P1, P2, P3), (P4, P5, P6) and (P7, P8, P9) which are parallel line. The angle joint 1 for point 1 are point 1 (P1), point 2 (P2) and point 3 (P3) is 130°, point 4 (P4), point 5 (P5) and point 6 (P6) is 110° and point 7 (P7), point 8 (P8) and point 9(P9) is 90°. In order to movement of exoskeleton arm for joint 2, the points (P1, P4, P7), (P2, P5, P8) and (P3, P6, P9) are parallel line from left to right. The joint angle for points (P1, P4, P7 = 30°), (P2, P5, P8 = 45°) and (P3, P6, P9 = 60°).

3 Results and Discussion

In the research, there are two joints to control the movement of exoskeleton arm for rehabilitation. The first joint is controlling the movement up and down and the second joint is to control the left and right of exoskeleton arm. By using third order

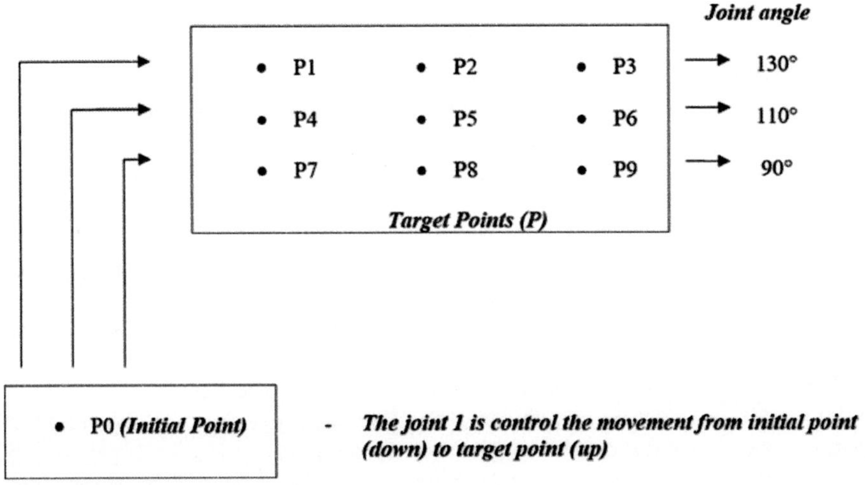

Fig. 7 Motion Planning for Joint 1 From initial to Points

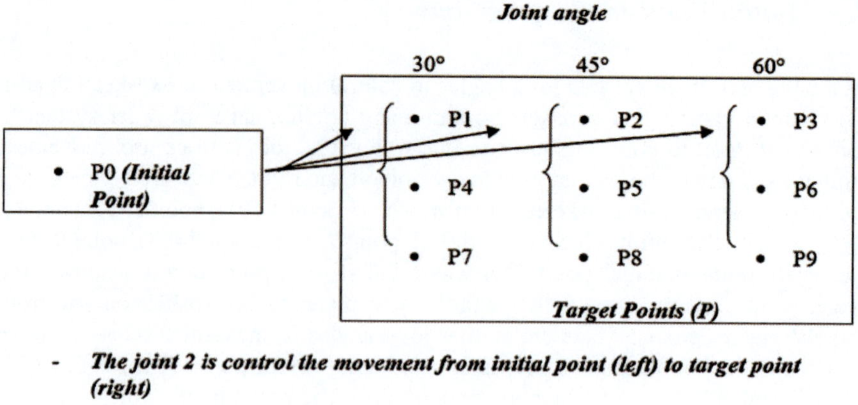

Fig. 8 Motion Planning for Joint 2 From initial to Points

Fig. 9 Graph of Motion Planning of Joint 1 from initial to P1, P2 and P3

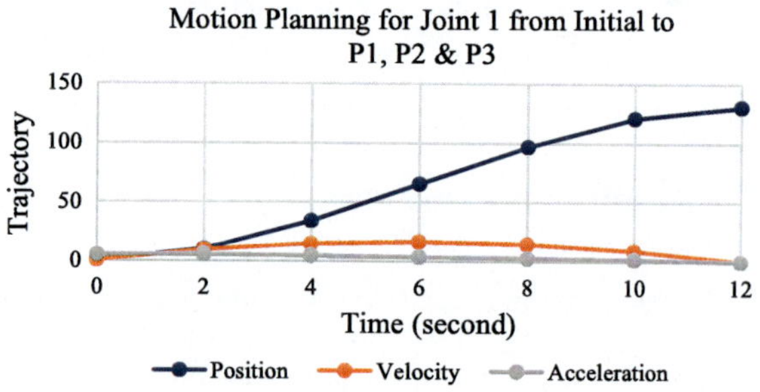

polynomial trajectory planning, the motion planning of exoskeleton arm will be shown in Fig. 9 until Fig. 14.

Figure 9 shows the results of motion planning of joint 1 from initial (P0) to point 1 (P1), point 2 (P2) and point 3 (P3). The results are based on the values of position, velocity and acceleration. The time duration to achieved the target point is 12 s. The starting position is 0 and the higher degree is 130 degree/sec, at the same time the values of velocity and acceleration are 0 (Table 1).

Figure 10 shows the results of motion planning of joint 1 from initial (P0) to point 4 (P4), point 5 (P5) and point 6 (P6). The results are based on the values of position, velocity and acceleration. The time duration to achieved the target point is 10 s. The starting position is 0 and the higher degree is 110 degree/sec, at the same time the values of velocity and acceleration are 0 (Table 2).

Figure 11 shows the results of motion planning of joint 1 from initial (P0) to point 7 (P7), point 8 (P8) and point 9 (P9). The results are based on the values of position, velocity and acceleration. The time duration to achieved the target point is 8 s. The starting position is 0 and the higher degree is 90 degree/sec, at the same time the values of velocity and acceleration are 0 (Table 3).

Table 1 Results of Motion Planning of Joint 1 from initial to P1, P2 and P3

Time (second)	Position (degree)	Velocity (degree)	Acceleration (degree)
0	0	0	5
2	9.63	9.03	5.42
4	33.7	14.44	4.51
6	64.99	16.24	3.61
8	96.27	14.44	2.71
10	120.33	9.02	1.8
12	129.93	0	0

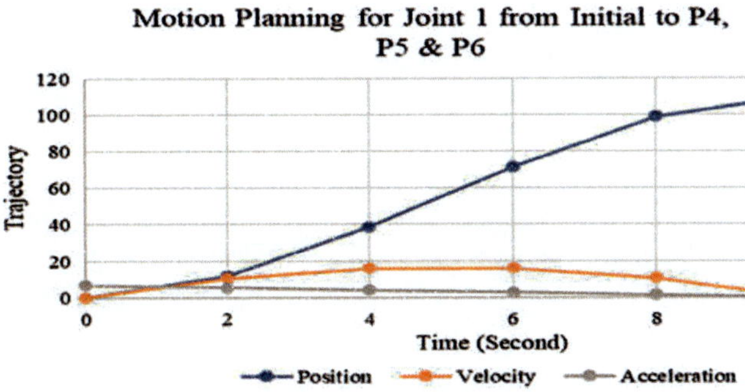

Fig. 10 Graph of Motion Planning of Joint 1 from initial to P4, P5 and P6

Table 2 Results of Motion Planning of Joint 1 from initial to P4, P5 and P6

Time (second)	Position (degree)	Velocity (degree)	Acceleration (degree)
0	0	0	6.6
2	11.44	10.56	5.28
4	38.72	15.84	3.96
6	71.28	15.84	2.64
8	98.56	10.56	1.32
10	110	0	0

Fig. 11 Graph of Motion Planning of Joint 1 from initial to P7, P8 and P9

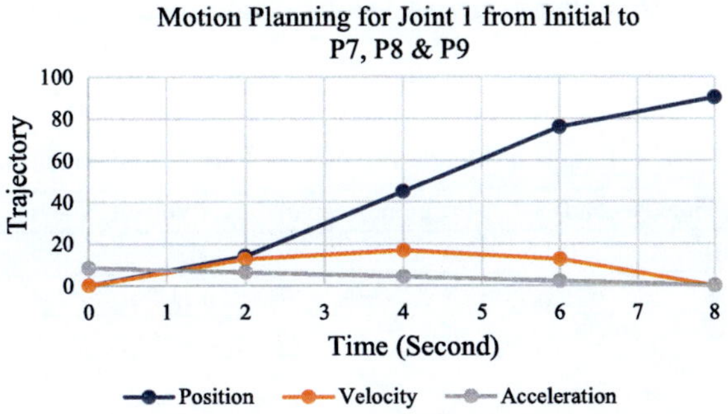

Table 3 Results of Motion Planning of Joint 1 from initial to P7, P8 and P9

Time (second)	Position (degree)	Velocity (degree)	Acceleration (degree)
0	0	0	8.44
2	14.06	12.65	6.32
4	44.99	16.87	4.22
6	75.93	12.65	2.11
8	89.98	0	0

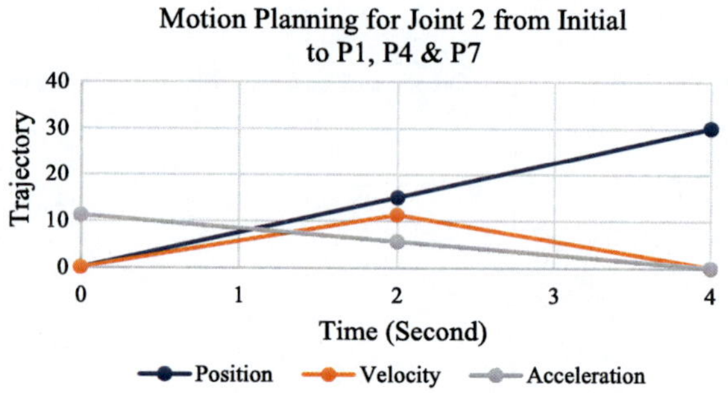

Fig. 12 Graph of Motion Planning of Joint 2 from initial to P1, P4 and P7

Figure 12 shows the results of motion planning of joint 2 from initial (P0) to point 1 (P1), point 4 (P4) and point 7 (P7). The results are based on the values of position, velocity and acceleration. The time duration to achieved the target point is 4 s. The starting position is 0 and the higher degree is 30 degree/sec, at the same time the values of velocity and acceleration are 0 (Table 4).

Figure 13 shows the results of motion planning of joint 2 from initial (P0) to point 2 (P2), point 5 (P5) and point 8 (P8). The results are based on the values of position, velocity and acceleration. The time duration to achieved the target point is 6 s. The starting position is 0 and the higher degree is 44.993 degree/sec, at the same time the values of velocity and acceleration are 0 (Table 5).

Figure 14 shows the results of motion planning of joint 2 from initial (P0) to point 3 (P3), point 6 (P6) and point 9 (P9). The results are based on the values of position, velocity and acceleration. The time duration to achieved the target point is 8 s. The starting position is 0 and the higher degree is 59.987 degree/sec at the same time the values of velocity and acceleration are 0 (Table 6).

Table 4 Results of Motion Planning of Joint 2 from initial to P1, P4 and P7

Time (second)	Position (degree)	Velocity (degree)	Acceleration (degree)
0	0	0	11.25
2	15	11.25	5.625
4	30	0	0

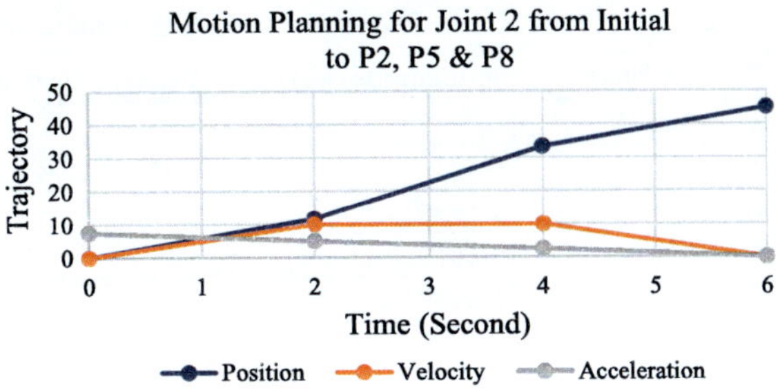

Fig. 13 Graph of Motion Planning of Joint 2 from initial to P2, P5 and P8

Table 5 Results of Motion Planning of Joint 2 from initial to P2, P5 and P8

Time (second)	Position (degree)	Velocity (degree)	Acceleration (degree)
0	0	0	7.5
2	11.664	9.999	4.999
4	33.331	9.999	2.499
6	44.993	0	0

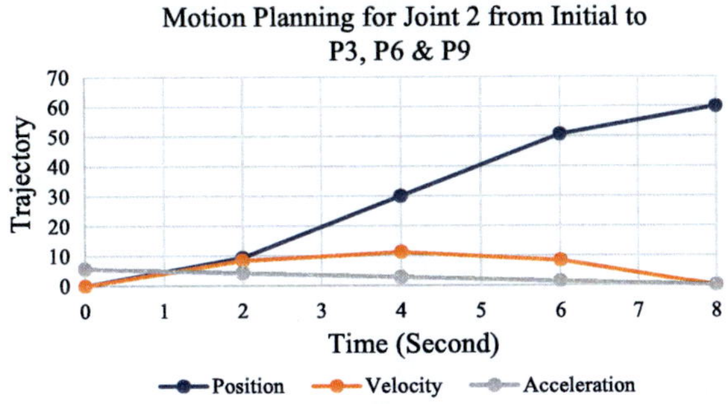

Fig. 14 Graph of Motion Planning of Joint 2 from initial to P3, P6 and P9

Overall, the motion planning of exoskeleton arm is depending on time to achieve the target movement. Figures 9, 10, 11, 12, 13, 14 show the movement of joint 1 and joint 2 movement where the starting point is at the initial point to the target point with different angles. The terms of Pos, Vel and Acc are referred to as Position, Velocity and Acceleration. The angle of movements from initial to points are referred to the point 1 (P1), point 2 (P2), point 3 (P3), point 4 (P4), point 5 (P5), point 6 (P6), point 7 (P7), point 8 (P8) and point 9 (P9) and the angle of the joint 1 are 130°, 110° and 90° and the angle of joint 2 are 30°, 45° and 60°. There are two movements of exoskeleton arm are “from down to up” and “from left to right” as be discussed in Figs. 7 and 8. The first movement of joint 1 that is from the initial point to other points (P1, P2 and P3) at 130° with 12 s. Second movement, the initial point to point 1, point 2 and point 3 (P1, P2 and P3) at 110° with 10 s. Third movement, the angle joint at 90° with 8 s. For movement of joint 2, the angle is 30°

Table 6 Results of Motion Planning of Joint 2 from initial to P3, P6 and P9

Time (second)	Position (degree)	Velocity (degree)	Acceleration (degree)
0	0	0	5.625
2	9.375	8.437	4.218
4	29.998	11.248	2.812
6	50.619	8.435	1.405
8	59.987	0	0

Table 7 Comparison of angle movement of Joint 1 (from down to up)

Time (seconds)	130 degree (P1, P2 and P3)			110 degree (P4, P5 and P6)			90 degree (P7, P8 and P9)		
	Pos	Vel	Acc	Pos	Vel	Acc	Pos	Vel	Acc
0	0	0	5	0	0	6.6	0	0	8.44
2	9.63	9.03	5.42	11.44	10.56	5.28	14.06	12.65	6.32
4	33.7	14.44	4.51	38.72	15.84	3.96	44.99	16.87	4.22
6	64.99	16.24	3.61	71.28	15.84	2.64	75.93	12.65	2.11
8	96.27	14.44	2.71	98.56	10.56	1.32	89.98		
10	120.33	9.02	1.8	110					
12	129.93								

Table 8 Comparison of angle movement of Joint 2 (from left to right)

Time (seconds)	30 degree (P1, P4 and P7)			45 degree (P2, P5 and P8)			60 degree (P3, P6 and P9)		
	Pos	Vel	Acc	Pos	Vel	Acc	Pos	Vel	Acc
0	0	0	11.25	0	0	7.5	0	0	5.625
2	15	11.25	5.625	11.664	9.999	4.999	9.375	8.437	4.218
4	30	0	0	33.331	9.999	2.499	29.998	11.248	2.812
6				44.993	0	0	50.619	8.435	1.405
8							59.987	0	0

with 4 s. The next movement of joint 2 are 45° with 6 s and 60° with 8 s. As a result, the value position, velocity and acceleration are depending on time. When the position is higher, the time will be longer and when the position is lower, the time will be shorter. Also, when the position reaches the target, the velocity and acceleration will be 0 and stop (Tables 7 and 8).

4 Conclusion

Motion planning is very important for the patients need to do movement as a therapist. The purpose of this study was to develop motion planning on exoskeleton arm for post-stroke rehabilitation. Basically, motion planning is needed to determine movement in more detail than just by stating the desired final configuration. One way to include more detail in a road description is to provide the desired point sequence (intermediate between initial to final positions). Therefore, in completing the motion, the tool frame must go through a set of intermediate positions and orientations as described by the passing point. Each point through this is actually a frame that determines the position and orientation of the tool relative to the station. Name path points include all endpoints plus starting and ending points Along with the constraints of space on movement, this study is to determine the temporal nature of movement. For example, the time elapsed between points can be determined in the description of the path. In this study, the motion planning of exoskeleton arm for post-stroke rehabilitation will be carried out. The third order polynomial trajectory planning is determining the motion of exoskeleton arm. The motion planning of exoskeleton arm for rehabilitation is considering the motion using point to point. The angle movement and time period are important to determine point to point of motion planning of exoskeleton arm of post-stroke rehabilitation. The study also improved the conventional therapy as discussed in literature review section. Future work, the new methods or techniques of motion planning can be explored for post-stroke rehabilitation.

Acknowledgements We thank all the reviewers for the suggestions and comments to improve the paper. This research is completely supported by University College TATI Short Term Grant, 9001-1804. The author fully acknowledged University College TATI (UCTATI) for the facilities and instrumentations that makes this important research viable and effective.

References

1. Hatem SM, Saussez G, Faille MD et al (2016) Rehabilitation of motor function after stroke: a multiple systematic review focused on techniques to stimulate upper extremity recovery. Front Hum Neurosci 10:1–22
2. Li G, Fang Q, Xu T, Zhao J, Cai H, Zhu Y (2019) Inverse kinematic analysis and trajectory planning of a modular upper limb rehabilitation exoskeleton. Tech Health Care 27:123–132
3. Ochoa-Luna C, Rahman MH, Saad M, Archambault PS (2018) Hand exoskeleton for rehabilitation therapies with integrated optical force sensor. Adv Mech Eng 10(2):1–11
4. Fitle KD, Pehlivan AU, O'Malley MK, 2015 A robotic exoskeleton for rehabilitation and assessment of the upper limb following incomplete spinal cord injury, Int. Conf. on Robot Autom 215:4960–4966
5. Petric T, Peternel L, Morimoto J, Babic J (2019) Assistive arm-exoskeleton control based on human muskular manipulability. Front Neurorobot 30
6. Kütük ME, Dülger LC, Das MT (2019) Design of a robot-assisted exoskeleton for passive wrist and forearm rehabilitation. Mech Sci 10:107–118

7. Lauretti C, Cordella F, Ciancio AL et al (2018) Learning by demonstration for motion planning of upper—limb exoskeleton. Front Neurorobot 12:30
8. Hoffman H. Reclaim your strength with these 8 arm exercises for stroke patients information page. https://www.saebo.com/blog/reclaim-your-strength-with-arm-exercises-for-stroke-recovery/. Accessed 2020/07/29
9. Salim S, Jamil MMA (2014) Monitoring of rehabilitation process via gyro and accelerometer sensor. In: Proceedings of the international colloquium on sports science, exercise, engineering and technology
10. Kumar S, Wöhrle H, Trampler M, Simnofske M, Peters H, Mallwitz M, Kirchner EA, Kirchner F (2019) Modular design and decentralized control of the RECUPERA exoskeleton for stroke rehabilitation. J Appl Sci 9:2–23
11. Craigh JJ (2018) Introduction to robotics: mechanics and control, 4th edn. Pearson, pp 203–204

Fabrication of Porous Mg–Ca–Zn Alloy by High Energy Milling for Bone Implants

Ika Kartika, Doty Dewi Risanti, Hardhian Restu P. Laksana, Franciska Pramuji Lestari, Fendy Rokhmanto, and Aprilia Erryani

Abstract Biodegradable porous magnesium-based alloys are essential in hard tissue engineering, such as mechanical support during healing process, and disappear after completion of the healing process, avoiding the secondary surgery. The present study aims to fabricate Mg–Ca–Zn degradable metallic foam implant for domestically made bone replacement. The foam was introduced through the variation of TiH_2 addition as blowing agent that will create a large volume fraction of gas-filled pores during heating. A High-Energy-Milling (HEM) was performed by a horizontal rotating cylinder ball mill with a rotation speed of 130 rpm for 48 h, with the ratio of metallic powders: balls are 3:7 followed by a compacting process. Some samples were subjected to preheating at 450 °C for 2 h before sintering process to observe its effect on pore formation of the green compact, followed by sintering at the temperature of 550 and 650 °C for 3 h. Samples sintered at 650 °C showed profuse micro-cracks, due to uncontrollable release of H_2 gas in the liquid film creating pore rupture and MgO formation that detected from XRD analysis, that impedes the sintering process. While sintering at a lower temperature showed a dependence on preheating process. The preheated samples containing MgO suffered from micro-cracking, except for sample with 3 wt% of TiH_2, where TiH_2 can act as oxygen scavenger that hinders the formation of MgO. In contrast, all samples without preheating remained intact without obvious micro-cracks. Those samples have a comparable hardness value to that of the bone. The pores in the materials measured according to Archimedes procedure behave as gypsum. Thus concerning mechanical properties, the samples can be regarded as bone implants.

I. Kartika · F. P. Lestari · F. Rokhmanto · A. Erryani
Research Center for Metallurgy and Material–Indonesian Institute of Sciences,
Gedung 470, Kawasan PUSPIPTEK Serpong, Tangerang Selatan 15343, Indonesia

D. D. Risanti (✉) · H. R. P. Laksana
Department of Engineering Physics, Institut Teknologi Sepuluh Nopember Kampus ITS,
Keputih Sukolilo, Surabaya 60111, Indonesia
e-mail: risanti@ep.its.ac.id

H. R. P. Laksana
PT. Eforel Citra Utama, Rungkut Megah Raya Blok H-30 Jl. Raya Rungkut no. 5,
Surabaya 60293, Indonesia

H. Triwiyanto et al. (eds.), *Proceedings of the 1st International Conference on Electronics, Biomedical Engineering, and Health Informatics*, Lecture Notes in Electrical Engineering 746, https://doi.org/10.1007/978-981-33-6926-9_62

Keywords Mg–Ca–Zn alloy · Metal foam · Blowing agent

1 Introduction

Magnesium and its alloys are widely studied as materials for orthopaedic applications due to its mechanical properties of interest, such as lower Young's modulus (41–45 GPa) [1, 2] and strength (160–230 MPa) [3] compared with other metallic implants, close mechanical properties to that of natural bone and low density (1.74–2.0 g/cm^3) [1, 2] as well as biocompatibility and biodegradability [4]. As an important factor in many metabolic processes, Mg in the human body is mainly contained in bone tissue. Mg plays an essential role in preservation of healthy bones, it is taken into the body everyday in large quantities, promotes the development of osteoblasts and osteoclasts cells, assuring the bone growth and repair. Another important phenomenon that occurs during bone recovery is stress shielding as a result of the excessive stiffness of the implant material which is unfavorable to the healing bone [4]. This problem can be tackled through the introduction of pores in Mg/Mg alloys in the form of metallic foams which later will significantly reduce Young's modulus and the yield strength compared to dense counterparts.

To date, the development of processing technologies, especially for the manufacture of implant using metallic foam is increasing rapidly. Among these, the powder metallurgy (PM) remains one of the most appropriate routes for the production of Mg foam because of its nature that easily burns in air. PM leaves benefits such as low segregations, grain refinement, homogeneous microstructure, an extension of solubility, formation of different phases, low preparation temperatures avoiding oxidation of particles, and finally, manufacture of the complex shape with high-precision of the dimensions [5–7]. Mechanical milling, as a part of PM process, has been considered one of the successful techniques for obtaining nanocrystalline metal alloys, achieving size in the range of 30–50 nm [8]. One should carefully control the ball/powder ratio, time, and speed in mechanical milling, as they can affect the properties of the resulting materials [9].

To mimic the structure of the human bone, the bioresorbable metallic implant must be porous instead of solid one. Apart from reducing the stiffness and strength, the pores will allow bone regeneration and vascularization [10, 11]. However, the mechanical strength of the implant still has to be kept sufficiently comparable to that of the bone itself, since it is necessary especially in surgical handling and bearing osteogenic loads during healing. To sustain such load, Mg has to be alloyed with other elements, such as Al, Zn, Ca, Ag, Ce, and Th that will produce different microstructures and the mechanical properties of the resulting Mg alloy are thus improved [12–15]. Among them, Ca is the major bone constituent, has a function as a grain-refining agent in Mg alloys for up to 0.5% of the Ca content [16]. Ca, that abundantly available in human bone, is important for bone cell signaling and beneficial for bone healing. Earlier findings have reported that Mg-1Ca alloy pins implanted in rabbit femoral shafts keeps osteocytes remain active around the pins, indicating good biocompatibility and bioactivity [17]. Another element, zinc (Zn) is one of the most available basic nutrients in the human body and is non-toxic for biomedical use [18]. The presence of Zn in Mg allows strengthening of the mechanical properties in Mg alloys via solid solution hardening, it has been reported to be beneficial in reducing corrosion rate, too [19]. Porous scaffolds can be obtained using a pore-forming agent, such as TiH_2 through PM method. Porosity is produced in this phase by trapping gas that is released into the Mg powder from the hydride foaming agent as reported in [20]. Therefore, in this study, we report the fabrication of Mg–Ca–Zn alloy metallic with the TiH_2 as a foaming agent. The objective of the present study is to analyze the effect of TiH_2 preheating and non-preheat, as well as the amount of TiH_2 on the pore formation of the Mg–Ca–Zn alloys. In addition, the Vicker's hardness of the implant was quantified and analyzed.

2 Material and Method

Materials used in this study are 99.9% Magnesium powder, Calcium granular with the particle size of less than 2.6 mm, 99.8% Zinc powder with the particle size 45 μm, and 98% TiH_2 powder. All the metal powders are made by Merck. The weight per alloy compositions before the high energy milling (HEM) is 70 g, as can be seen in Table 1.

The mechanical milling was done using a horizontal rotating cylinder ball mill with a rotation speed of 130 rpm for 48 h. The ball mills used are made of steel with a diameter of 8 and 10 mm and each of them weighs 3.5 and 5.6 g, respectively. The metallic powders and balls were put in a jar mill with the ratio of small balls:large balls inside the jar was 4:1, while the ratio of metals powder:balls was 3:7. The compacting process was carried out by the compression machine with a pressure of 3750 psi (~26 MPa) for 3 min at room temperature. The die for making a green compact has the cylinder shape with a diameter of 25 mm. The sintering process used a vacuum tube furnace with a flow rate of 0.1 l/min and increases every 5 °C/min. Prior to sintering process, the samples were subjected to preheating at 450 °C for 2 h, and the sintering was undertaken at 550 and 650 °C for 3 h. Some samples were subjected to directly sintering the green compact at 550 °C for 3 h without preheating.

Table 1 Composition of the Mg alloys (wt%)

Studied Alloys	wt%			
	Ca	Zn	TiH_2	Mg
Mg–Ca–Zn	1	3	0	96
Mg–Ca–Zn–0,5TiH_2	1	3	0.5	95.5
Mg–Ca–Zn–1,5TiH_2	1	3	1.5	94.5
Mg–Ca–Zn–3TiH_2	1	3	3	93

The XRD was carried out using Philips X'pert MPD (30 kV, 40 mA) using Cu–Kα source to characterize the phase that formed after sintering in studied Mg alloys. Also, the mapping elements carried out by scanning electron microscopy (SEM) JEOL JSM-6390A equipped with energy-dispersive X-ray spectroscopy (EDX) JED-2300 and SEM-FEI-Inspect S50 to observe the homogeneity of the distribution elements after the mechanical milling and morphology of the pore after sintering. The mechanical properties of the Mg alloys after heat treatment was measured using Vickers hardness test using Leitz Microhardness Tester under the load of 50 kgf and holding time of 30 s according to ASTM E92 standard. The density and porosity of the alloys were performed by the Archimedes method according to ASTM B311-93 standards. The sample density is calculated using Eq. (1).

$$\rho_b = \frac{m_1}{m_3 - m_2} \times \rho_{water} \tag{1}$$

ρ_b is the theoretical density (gr/cm^3), m_1 = sample dry weight (gram), m_2 = sample weight in water (gram), m_3 = sample wet weight (gram), ρ_{water} is water density (gr/cm^3).

The porosity is calculated using Eq. (2) after the density obtained.

$$\mu = 1 - \frac{\rho_t}{\rho_b} \times 100\% \tag{2}$$

where μ = porosity, ρ_b = wet density (gr/cm^3), ρ_t = dry density (gr/cm^3).

3 Result and Discussion

3.1 *High Energy Milling Result*

During mechanical milling process, severe plastic deformations occur due to continuous collision among powders, balls, and vial along with the rotation of the ball, resulting in particles breaking up into small fragments and agglomeration as indicated in Table 2. Moreover, consecutive fracturing, cold welding, and folding of Mg, Ca, Zn and TiH_2 particles during collision, result in layered structures in the particles or a flatter form particles as seen in Fig. 1 which is in accord with [21]. Agglomeration in this case is due to cold welding stage during the milling process [22]. It is likely that even after 48 h of milling, the fracture process of milling has not fully achieved. All elements are distributed evenly (Fig. 2), where some Ca, Zn and TiH_2 particles are located between Mg layers and likely cold-welded to Mg powders. Although, some Ca, Zn, and TiH_2 particles cannot be completely incorporated into Mg layers or they can be separated from Mg powders by subsequent

Table 2 Particle Size After Milling

Element	Powder Original Size (mm)	Alloys Composition	As-Milled Size (μm)
Mg	0.06–0.3	Mg–Ca–Zn	456.29
Ca	<2.6	Mg–Ca–Zn–0.5TiH_2	415.38
Zn	<0.045	Mg–Ca–Zn–1.5TiH_2	208.75
TiH_2	0.045	Mg–Ca–Zn–3TiH_2	246.53

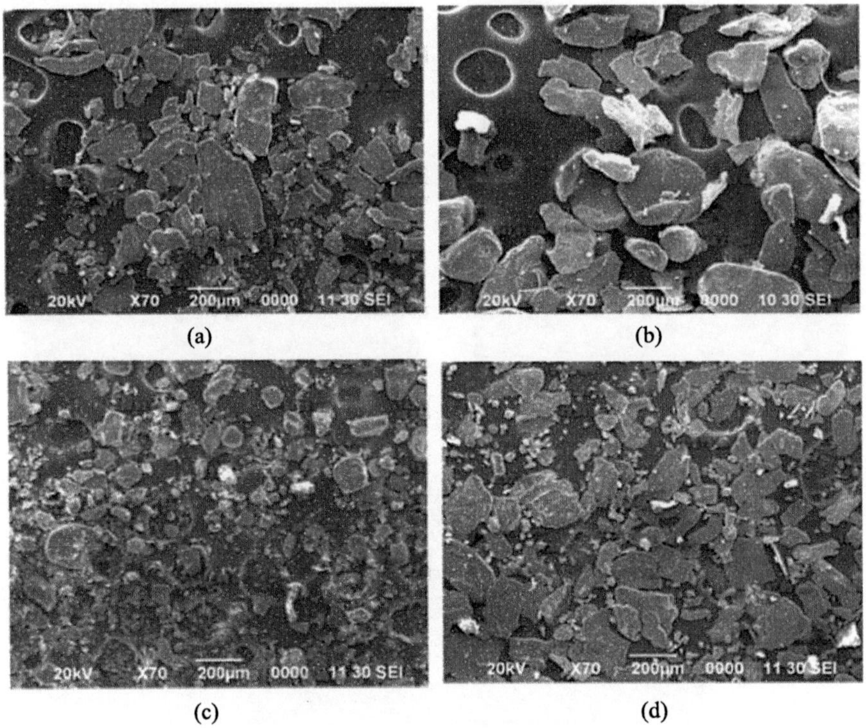

Fig. 1 Secondary electron images of Mg–Ca–Zn powders after 48 h of milling **a** 0 wt%, **b** 0.5 wt %, **c** 1.5 wt% and **d** 3 wt% of TiH_2

fracturing. Thus, during pressing the powders into green compact, these particles form and adhere to the outer surface of Mg powders.

3.2 Microstructure After Sintering

Figure 2 illustrates the secondary electron images of un-/preheated samples underwent sintering at 550 and 650 °C. It is seen that the unpreheated samples

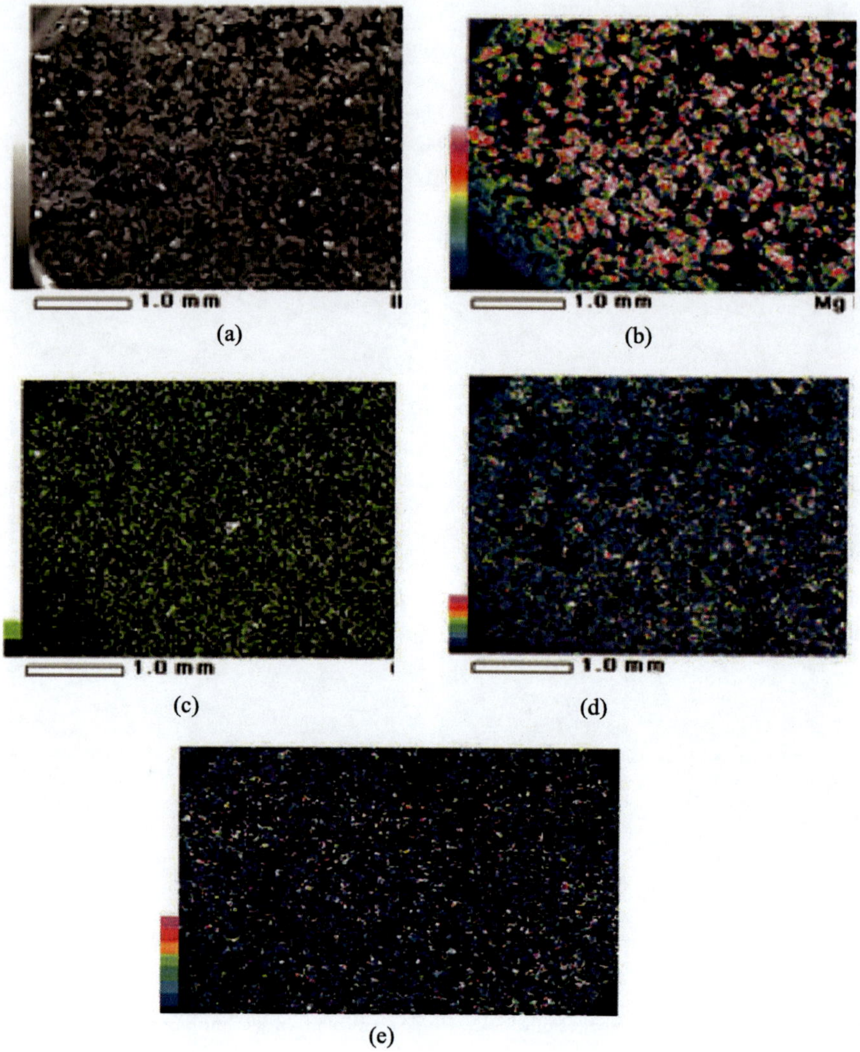

Fig. 2 Elemental mapping of Mg–Ca–Zn–3TiH_2 powder after 48 h of milling indicating distribution of **a** Mg, **b** Ca, **c** Zn, and **d** Ti

show pore formation which raises with the increase in TiH_2. On the other hand, all preheated samples show marked micro-cracks and surface detachment except for sample containing 3% TiH_2 and sintered at 550 °C (Fig. 3 (b_3)).

To address the effect of TiH_2 preheating on the pore formation, the XRD analysis results were shown in Fig. 4. It is seen that the unpreheated samples only show the presence of α-Mg and Mg_2Ca phases, while the preheated samples at

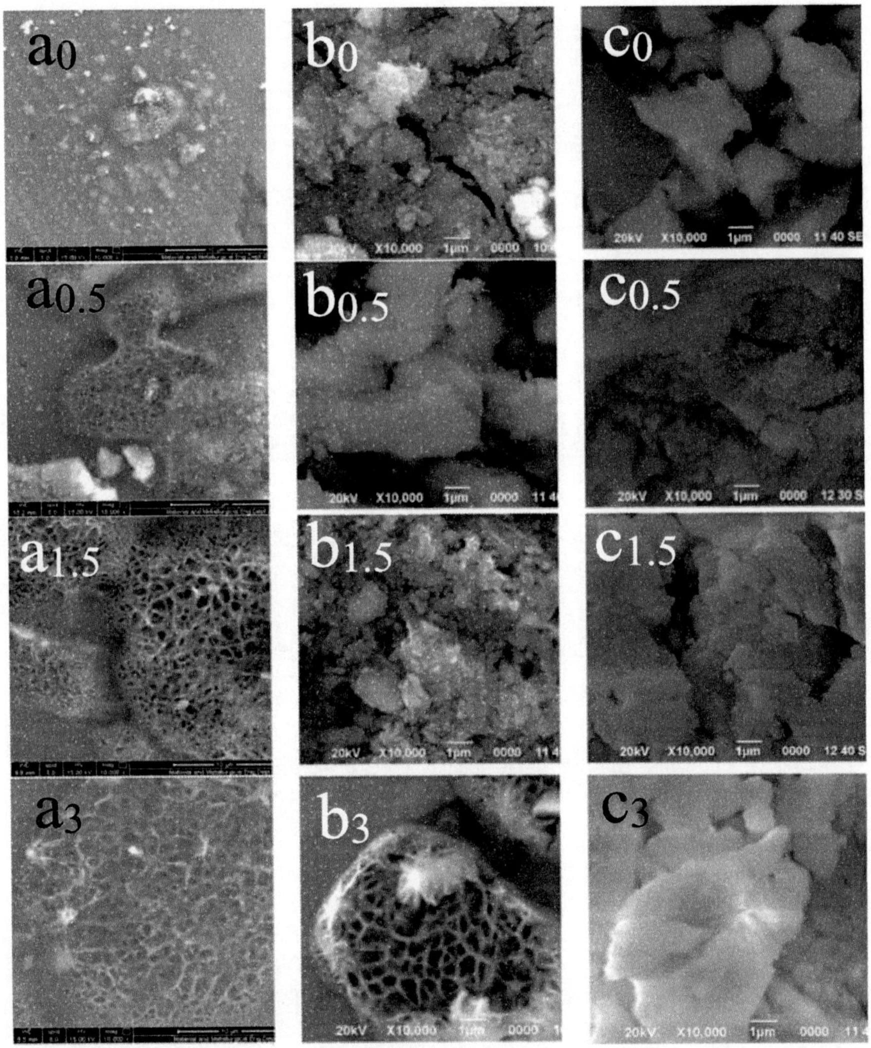

Fig. 3 Secondary electron images of **a** unpreheated samples and preheated samples: **b** sintered at 550 °C and **c** sintered at 650 °C. The amount of TiH_2 is indicated in figure

550 °C indicate the presence of MgO particularly on samples containing TiH_2 of less than 3 wt%. It is clear MgO may form easily due to the high affinity of Mg with oxygen and its existence causes the micro cracks to take place as indicative of the sintering process being hindered [23]. Similar alloys containing MgO sintered at a similar condition were reported to experience the same problem [24]. Given the effect of TiH_2, the MgO formation acts as a barrier for hydrogen being release in the green compact, thus it requires a higher temperature for foam formation [25].

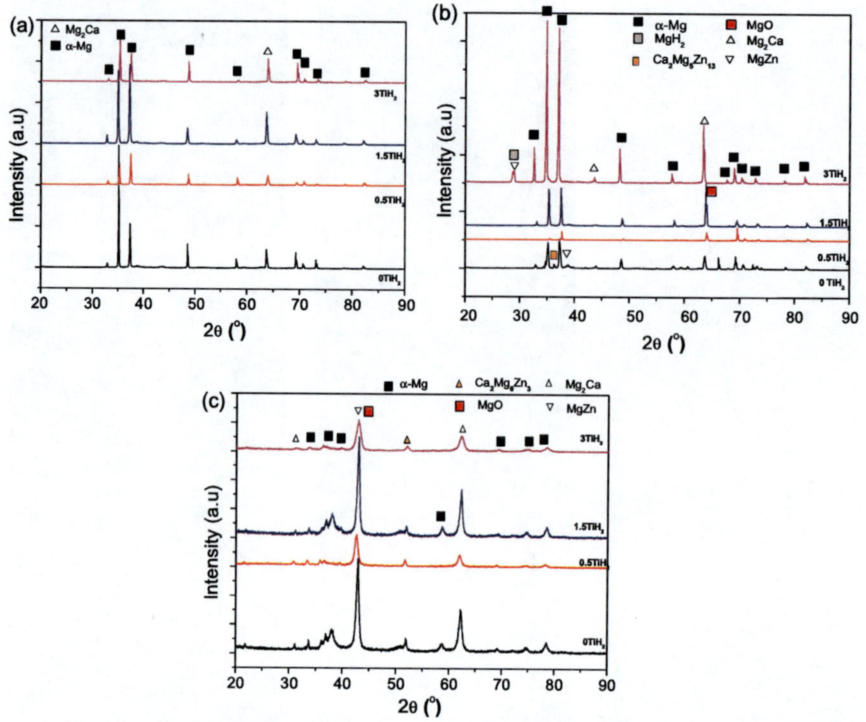

Fig. 4 X-Ray diffraction spectra of **a** unpreheated, **b** preheated/sintered at 550 °C and **c** preheated/sintered at 650 °C. The amount of TiH_2 and phases present are indicated in figure

Except for sample with 3 wt% of TiH_2 does not reveal the occurrence of MgO, nevertheless, it shows the abundance of α-Mg and Mg_2Ca with some traces of MgZn and MgH_2. The surface cleaning effects of TiH_2 during the dehydrogenation process permit the hydrogen atoms in TiH_2 powder at sufficient amount allowing the oxygen removal from metastable Ti_2O_3 and partly TiO_2, thus, TiH_2 may act as an oxygen scavenger to improve the sintering of Mg–Ca–Zn alloys [26].

As for samples sintered at 650 °C, the strong peak of MgZn/MgO is obvious, while the presence of α-Mg is significantly reduced. At this temperature, Mg is completely melted. As reported earlier, the formation of liquid phase allows a fast expansion of TiH_2 [27, 28] which blows the liquid foam films but it cannot preserve its structure due to poor sintering quality, thus resulting in micro-cracks formation [29]. The poor quality sintering of Mg powders is affected by the evidence of MgO, since it is known that stable MgO leads to Mg particles cannot be bonded completely and remain separated in the vicinity of powder covered by MgO [30]. The presence of MgZn can be explained that liquid Zn in the product already reacts with the residual Mg to form the molten Mg–Zn. Besides, high mobility of Mg atoms markedly at high temperatures may help in Mg migration within the Mg grain to react with Zn and further forms MgZn [31].

3.3 Mechanical Properties

Mechanical properties of the alloys were studied through hardness measurement. However, the hardness of samples suffered from profuse microcracks cannot be carried out. In general, the obtained hardness values are close to that of human bone, i.e. 33.30–43.82 HV [32], which is good for avoiding stress shielding. Porosity and density were estimated using the Archimedes principle (Eqs. 1 and 2), data are tabulated in Table 3. The analysis involves the relation between hardness and porosity using an empirical approach in the form of exponential expression [33], as well as Gibson-Ashby model [34]. The results are displayed in Fig. 5. Figure 5a represents the hardness and porosity behavior similar to that of porous polycrystalline solid such as gypsum, where intergrowth and interlocking of crystals or the connectivity of the dense part of the foam significantly may affect the mechanical properties. Also, Fig. 5b shows the dependence of hardness of a metallic foam and the relative density according to the formula:

$$H = \sigma_c\left(1 + 2\frac{\rho}{\rho_s}\right) \quad (3)$$

where H is hardness, σ_c is collapse strength, ρ is density, and ρ_s is the density of the cell wall material (alloy without TiH_2). Thus, the x-axis of the plot is referred to as the parameter in the bracket of Eq. (3), the obtained slope is the collapse strength, i.e. the strength at which the foam inside the material is collapsing. According to Gibson-Ashby model, since the relative density ρ/ρ_s is more than 0.3, i.e. our results indicate the value ~0.8, there should be a strong dependence of mechanical strength on the relative density. Further investigations should be made to optimize the selective foaming agent and milling process.

Table 3 Hardness and Porosity Data

Alloy Composition	Heat Treatment	Hardness (HV)	Porosity (%)	Density
Mg–Ca–Zn	550 °C	30.78	19.87	0.62
Mg–Ca–Zn–0.5TiH_2		50.96	9.75	0.54
Mg–Ca–Zn–1.5TiH_2		44.13	10.37	0.46
Mg–Ca–Zn–3TiH_2		49.25	9.82	0.53
Mg–Ca–Zn–3TiH_2	450°C/550 °C	40.13	10.97	0.47

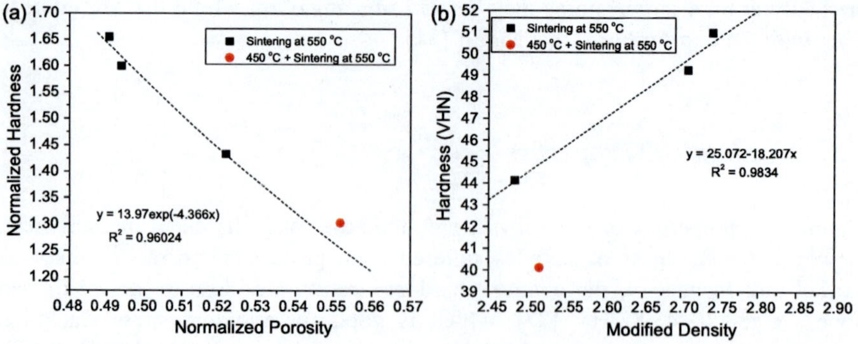

Fig. 5 Dependence of **a** porosity and **b** density of studied alloys on mechanical properties

4 Conclusion

Mg–Ca–Zn porous implants were fabricated using high energy milling, compaction, and sintering process. Different concentrations of TiH_2 were applied for foam fabrication. Most of the preheated samples studied suffered from microcracks due to the presence of MgO. TiH_2 of 3 wt% can act as an oxygen scavenger that inhibits the MgO formation. Sintering at the melting temperature of Mg resulted in a profuse cracking due to the uncontrollable foaming process. With the hardness value being comparable to that of bone, the pores produced in the materials behave as gypsum, where the connectivity of the dense part of the foam is crucial, hence the present metallic foam can be considered for being used as bone implant.

Acknowledgements This research was financially supported by The Research Center for Metallurgy and Materials, Indonesian Institute of Sciences. The main contributor to this manuscript is Ika Kartika and Doty Dewi Risanti.

References

1. Staiger MP, Pietak AM, Huadmai J, Dias G (2006) Magnesium and its alloys as orthopedic biomaterials: a review. Biomaterials 27:1728–1734
2. Wolf FI, Cittadini A (2003) Chemistry and biochemistry of magnesium. Mol Aspects Med 24:3–9
3. Manakari V, Parande G, Doddamani M, Gupta M (2017) Enhancing the ignition, hardness and compressive response of magnesium by reinforcing with hollow glass microballoons
4. Chagnon M, Guy L-G, Jackson N (2019) Evaluation of magnesium-based medical devices in preclinical studies: challenges and points to consider. Toxicol Pathol 47:390–400
5. Matsuzaki K, Hatsukano K, Hanada K, Takahashi M, Shimizu T (2006) Mechanical properties and formability of PM Mg-Al based alloys. In: Kainer KU (ed) Magnesium: proceedings of the 6th international conference magnesium alloys and their applications 2003. Wiley, United States, pp 170–175

6. Zhou YJ, Jiang AY, Liu JX (2013) The effect of sintering temperature to the microstructure and properties of AZ91 magnesium alloy by powder metallurgy. Appl Mech Mater 377:250–254
7. Fogagnolo JB, Velasco F, Robert MH, Torralba JM (2003) Effect of mechanical alloying on the morphology, microstructure and properties of aluminium matrix composite powders. Mater Sci Eng A 342:131–143
8. Galindez Y, Correa E, Zuleta AA, Valencia-Escobar A, Calderon D, Toro L, Chacón P, Echeverría EF (2019) Improved Mg–Al–Zn magnesium alloys produced by high energy milling and hot sintering. Met Mater Int
9. Varol T (2018) The effect of milling time, milling speed and ball to powder weight ratio on the physical properties of submicron Al_2O_3 ceramic particles fabricated by mechanical milling method. Pamukkale Univ J Eng Sci 24:635–642
10. Götz HE, Müller M, Emmel A, Holzwarth U, Erben RG, Stangl R (2004) Effect of surface finish on the osseointegration of laser-treated titanium alloy implants. Biomaterials 25:4057–4064
11. Kuboki Y, Jin Q, Takita H (2001) Geometry of carriers controlling phenotypic expression in BMP-induced osteogenesis and chondrogenesis. JBJS, 83
12. Yang H, Liu C, Wan P, Tan L, Yang K (2013) Study of second phase in bioabsorbable magnesium alloys: phase stability evaluation via Dmol3 calculation. APL Mater 1:52104
13. Tie D, Feyerabend F, Hort N, Hoeche D, Kainer KU, Willumeit R, Mueller WD (2014) In vitro mechanical and corrosion properties of biodegradable Mg–Ag alloys. Mater Corros 65:569–576
14. Hirvinen LJM, Litsky AS, Samii VF, Weisbrode SE, Bertone AL (2009) Influence of bone cements on bone-screw interfaces in the third metacarpal and third metatarsal bones of horses. Am J Vet Res 70:964–972
15. Zheng Y, Gu X (2011) Research activities of biomedical magnesium alloys in China. JOM 63:105–108
16. Li YC, Li MH, Hu WY, Hodgson PD, Wen CE (2010) Biodegradable Mg-Ca and Mg-Ca-Y alloys for regenerative medicine. Mater Sci Forum 654–656:2192–2195
17. Li Z, Gu X, Lou S, Zheng Y (2008) The development of binary Mg–Ca alloys for use as biodegradable materials within bone. Biomaterials 29:1329–1344
18. Li J, Song Y, Zhang S, Zhao C, Zhang F, Zhang X, Cao L, Fan Q, Tang T (2010) In vitro responses of human bone marrow stromal cells to a fluoridated hydroxyapatite coated biodegradable Mg–Zn alloy. Biomaterials 31:5782–5788
19. Zhang S, Zhang X, Zhao C, Li J, Song Y, Xie C, Tao H, Zhang Y, He Y, Jiang Y, Bian Y (2010) Research on an Mg–Zn alloy as a degradable biomaterial. Acta Biomater 6:626–640
20. Lestari FP, Laksana HR, Annur D, Amal MI, Sriyono B, Kartika I (2014) Development of magnesium alloy foam with TiH_2 as foaming agent. In: Proceeding, the Indonesian biomaterials conference 2014 in conjunction with the 2nd regional biomaterials scientific meeting 2014, Surabaya
21. Vahid A, Hodgson P, Li Y (2018) Effect of high-energy ball milling on mechanical properties of the Mg–Nb composites fabricated through powder metallurgy process. Adv Eng Mater 20:1700759
22. Sezer N, Evis Z, Kayhan SM, Tahmasebifar A, Koç M (2018) Review of magnesium-based biomaterials and their applications. J Magnes Alloy 6:23–43
23. Wolff M, Ebel T, Dahms M (2010) Sintering of magnesium. Adv Eng Mater 12:829–836
24. Amal MI, Annur D, Lestari FP, Sutowo C, Kartika I (2016) Processing of porous Mg-Zn-Ca alloy via powder metallurgy. AIP Conf Proc 1778:030010
25. Kadoi K, Babscan N, Nakae H (2009) Heat treatment of TiH_2 powder to control decomposition phenomenon for aluminum foam fabrication by melt route. Mater Trans 50:727–733
26. Hao H, Wang Y, Jafari Nodooshan HR, Zhang Y, Ye S, Lv Y, Yu P (2019) The effects of sintering temperature and addition of TiH_2 on the sintering process of Cu. Mater (Basel, Switzerland), 12

27. Neu T, Mukherjee M, Moreno FG, Banhart J (2011) Magnesium and magnesium alloy foams. In: Hur B-Y, Kim B-K, Kim S-E, Hyun S-K (eds) 7th International conference on porous metals and metallic foams (MetFoam2011). Busan, pp 139–146
28. Jiménez C, Garcia-Moreno F, Pfretzschner B, Kamm PH, Neu TR, Klaus M, Genzel C, Hilger A, Manke I, Banhart J (2013) Metal foaming studied in situ by energy dispersive X-ray diffraction of synchrotron radiation, X-ray radioscopy, and optical expandometry. Adv Eng Mater 15:141–148
29. Hao GL, Han FS, Li WD (2009) Processing and mechanical properties of magnesium foams. J Porous Mater 16:251–256
30. Vahid A, Hodgson P, Li Y (2017) New porous Mg composites for bone implants. J Alloys Compd 724:176–186
31. Deng C-J, Wong ML, Ho MW, Yu P, Ng DHL (2005) Formation of MgO and Mg–Zn intermetallics in an Mg-based composite by in situ reactions. Compos Part A Appl Sci Manuf 36:551–557
32. Wu W-W, Zhu Y-B, Chen W, Li S, Yin B, Wang J-Z, Zhang X-J, Liu G-B, Hu Z-S, Zhang Y-Z (2019) Bone hardness of different anatomical regions of human radius and its impact on the pullout strength of screws. Orthop Surg 11:270–276
33. Soroka I, Sereda PJ (1968) Interrelation of hardness, modulus of elasticity, and porosity in various gypsum systems. J Am Ceram Soc 51:337–340
34. Ashby MF, Evans AG, Fleck NA, Gibson LJ, Hutchinson HNG, Wadley JW (2000) Metal foams: a design guide. Butterworth-Heinemann, Woburn, MA

Performance Comparison of Strain Sensors for Wearable Device in Respiratory Rate Monitoring

Ahmad Akbar Khatami, Husneni Mukhtar, and Dien Rahmawati

Abstract Respiratory rate (RR), a clinical sign of ventilation, should be measured and recorded periodically for patients on acute care. Among the other common vital signs, a change in RR can be used as the first sign of deterioration and can avoid the possibility of missing the trends' identification as occurs in intermittent monitoring. Meanwhile some devices have experiences in false detection due to the different body motions. Hence, this study aims to develop a continuous RR monitoring with accuracy improvements using wearable sensors and data recording. In this RR monitoring work, we compared the performances of the flex sensor (2.2″ in size) and the force-sensing resistor (FSR402) by placing them on the abdomen of a relaxing subject using a belt for 6 h every 10 min. The monitoring data were not only displayed on a smartphone but also stored on firebase platform. The system therefore took the advantages of a web service architecture to send, retrieve, and access data from the cloud. The comparison results of the flex and the FSR402 sensors due to the average RR differences (and the mean average error) compared to the breath manual count are 0.30 bpm (0.90 bpm) and 1.45 bpm (2.25 bpm), respectively. In this study, we show a way to improve the sensor performance by automatically adjusting the sensitivity of the strain sensors for adapting the RR measurement on abdomen of the test subject. Furthermore, this study demonstrates that the system is able to measure and fast transmit the RR data as the monitoring process using the IoT Firebase platform and that the performance of the flex sensor provides the possibility of further development and improvement in obtaining much better result.

Keywords Respiratory rate · Vital sign · Flex · Strain sensor

A. A. Khatami · H. Mukhtar (✉) · D. Rahmawati
School of Electrical Engineering, Telkom University, Bandung, Indonesia
e-mail: husnenimukhtar@telkomuniversity.ac.id

A. A. Khatami · H. Mukhtar
Biospin Laboratory, Telkom University, Bandung, Indonesia

H. Triwiyanto et al. (eds.), *Proceedings of the 1st International Conference on Electronics, Biomedical Engineering, and Health Informatics*, Lecture Notes in Electrical Engineering 746, https://doi.org/10.1007/978-981-33-6926-9_63

1 Introduction

Vital signs such as respiration rate (RR), heart rate (HR), blood pressure (BP) and body temperature should be measured and recorded periodically for patients on acute care or emergency department because it is able to overcome the problem of overcrowding in the emergency unit which can lead to the disadvantageous clinical results. The early and repeated measurement of vital signs and the assessment of early warning scores are critical in prioritizing the patients requiring the immediate attention and identifying the deteriorating clinical conditions [1, 2]. This procedure is a clinical priority as a clinical quality foundation. It has been proven to be effective in the UK [3]. However, in many countries, the monitoring of vital signs is rarely performed, especially the RR measurement, due to various reasons such as patient handling standard and difficulty in providing the continuous monitoring.

Besides, countries that have RR measurement monitoring in the acute care or emergency department still need RR monitoring in the general ward. Please note, the RR monitoring for patients in general wards is almost neglected. Medical staffs only examine the patients every few hours [4, 5]. A decrease in the patient's condition can occur between those examinations or even the in-hospital mortality rate may be triggered after the ICU-patients were transferred to the wards [4–7].

Respiratory rate, among the other common vital signs, is probably the most important one to monitor continuously [8, 9] as means of keeping the patient's safety because a change in RR can be used as the first sign of patient deterioration and avoid the possibility of missing the trends identification as occurs in intermittent monitoring [2, 8, 10]. In addition, the RR changes may cause other vital signs changes such as the heart rate and blood pressure [9]. In general, to measure a manually RR, a clinician observes the patient by counting the number of both inhale and exhale of breathing motions on the chest in half or one minute. But doing this way continuously will take a lot of time and add the workload of the clinicians. Moreover, it is not possible to perform the monitoring in overcrowded units and also it has a risk of measuring errors [3]. As a consequence, a continuous RR monitoring might not be provided. A device should be used to support the measurement.

There are several devices available for measuring and monitoring the RR that are having advantages and limitations. For instance, an impedance pneumography is used for continuous RR measurement by locating two surface electrodes on patient's chest to record the movement. False detections of this device often come from other movements of tremors and abnormal breathing due to apnea [11, 12]. To overcome those drawbacks, the acoustic transducers have been developed with high accuracy but several motions such as cough and sneeze affect the performance [11, 13]. Another device based on infrared thermal camera may also counted on the RR monitoring, but it is also sensitive to other different body motions [11, 14]. Those devices seemed to be limited to other movements originating either from the body or the outside body. Ones should continue to improve those devices or find other alternative techniques to minimize the measurement error.

In terms of finding other alternative ones, this study chooses strain sensor due to a schematic review of classification and methodological approach. Compared to other sensors and other methods, strain sensors are the best to use for clinical, occupational and sport settings in both controlled and uncontrolled environments. The unobtrusiveness and motion artifacts are its main advantage and drawback in respectively [15]. This study uses two strain sensors, flex and FSR402 as an aim to compare the performances of both sensors for continuous RR monitoring based on wearable sensor. Both sensors are placed on the abdomen of a relaxing subject using a belt for 6 h every 10 min. An automatic threshold value is introduced on device as each time the device is used by a test subject in order to minimize the error of RR measurement.

2 Material and Method

The respiratory rate monitoring proposed in this paper was carried out by comparing the performances of two types of strain sensors in measuring the RR of a relaxing subject for 6 h every 10 min. Those sensors are a 22 in. flex sensor and a force sensing resistor (FSR402) simultaneously used in measuring the RR during the monitoring period. The outline and the electronic schematic of this system are shown in Figs. 1 and 2.

Beside the selection reasons from the schematic review mentioned in the last part of the introduction section, there are other considerations of choosing the strain sensors. First, the sensor shape is like a small, thin sheet that can be easily attached onto the abdomen as a wearable sensor, which is expected to be comfortable for the subject to wear. Second, the direct measurement of the inhalation motion of the abdomen is predicted producing the RR values closer to the true values; Third,

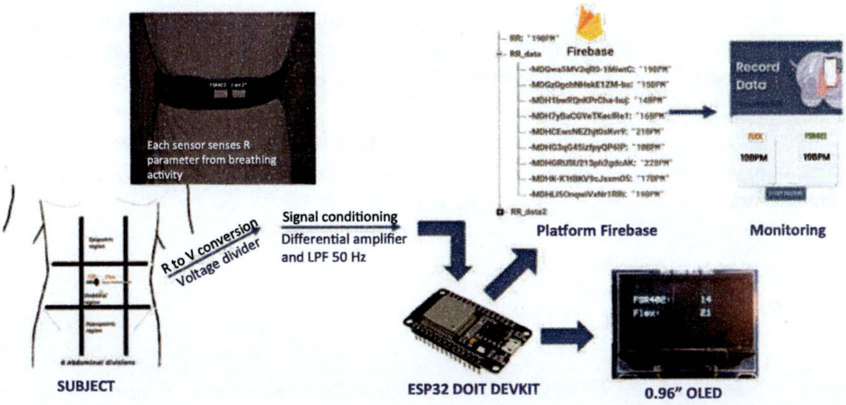

Fig. 1 The working principle of wearable sensors for continuous RR monitoring

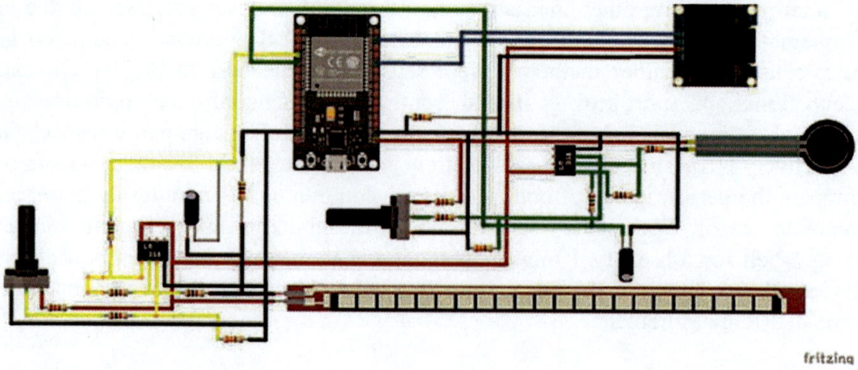

Fig. 2 The electronic schematic of RR monitoring

the obtained value is then be compared with a manual count for further analysis and study in order to reduce the measurement error. The two sensors were finally chosen to be tested because they met the criteria and were also widely available, easy to obtain, and relatively cheap.

2.1 Flex Sensor

Flex sensor, or a variable resistor, has a polymer ink with the embedded conductive particles on one side of the sensor. Flex sensor used in this study is FS-L-0055 with 2.2 in. of size, low resistance type, 0–5 V of the operating voltage, 5 W of continues power rating, 25 kΩ flat resistance, ±30% of resistance tolerance, and 45–125 kΩ of bend resistance range.

The working principle of this sensor is based on a change in resistance in response to surface linearity or mechanical deformation. The increasing change in resistance referred to the particles moves further apart from the ink when the sensor is flexed or bent away. In other words, flex sensor measures the amount of bending or deflecting. For the RR measurement purpose, this sensor detects the angle changes of abdomen movements when a subject breathes, then converts it to the resistance parameter. A typical voltage divider circuit is then used to convert the resistance parameter to voltage parameter.

2.2 Force Sensing Resistor

Force Sensing Resistor (FSR) is a kind of piezoresistive sensor technology which also functions as a variable resistor. FSR model used in this study is FSR402 with dimension 13 mm circle × 56 mm. FSR402 has 2 layers of flexible substrate films with printed semiconductor and active element dots that is separated by an adhesive spacer. The sensor resistance changes because the particles touch the conducting electrode as a force is applied to a sensing film surface. In further, the generated force sensitivity is able to be optimized for medical devices as well as RR monitoring [16]. This low-cost sensor uses a voltage divider with a 10 kΩ static resistor and has similar operating work with flex sensor, the difference is the large active area on FSR.

Both sensors are placed on a subject's abdomen using a rubber cloth belt with Velcro (see Fig. 1). The converted analogue voltage is sent to the ADC in the microcontroller after being amplified using a differential amplifier (LM384) and conditioned using a 50 Hz noise filter. The ADC conversion results are in RR data in unit of beats per minute (BPM). The arrangement of both sensors in the monitoring system is derived in Fig. 2.

2.3 RR Monitoring System

Respiratory rate monitoring in this study is performed using a microcontroller ESP32 DOIT Devkit with 4 MB flash memory, a Wi-Fi module and Firebase platform. In this study, ESP32 Devkit, as an IoT mobile device, is a board of a low power single chip from DOIT based on the ESP-WROM-32 microcontroller and provided optimal performances with peripheral set, WiFi and Bluetooth support. Wi-Fi network is used as a wireless connection between the IoT device and the internet. Instead of using GPRS/GSM network or Local Area Network (LAN) cable, Wi-Fi network is chosen due to the advantages of wireless-enabled device, mobile connection and the signal quality.

Firebase platform, an IoT-based cloud service, enables data storage with integration of software platform and operating system. Cloud replaces the use of data storage in data logger. As a platform with a real- time backend database, Firebase has several features such as cloud data storage, for examples Real-time data base and Firebase storage [17]. This study uses these features to record and show the RR measurement. The RR data from the two sensors are sent via ESP32 to the Firebase platform and also displayed on 0.96″ OLED. In addition, this OLED display can be used either in online or offline mode. Those steps will be repeated in next ten minutes (see the flowchart in Fig. 3a).

2.4 Accuracy Improvement

One of the goal parts in this study is to improve the accuracy of RR measurement to support the continuous RR monitoring in acute care or emergency units or in other conditions. As shown in Fig. 3a, RR monitoring is started with the adjustment of

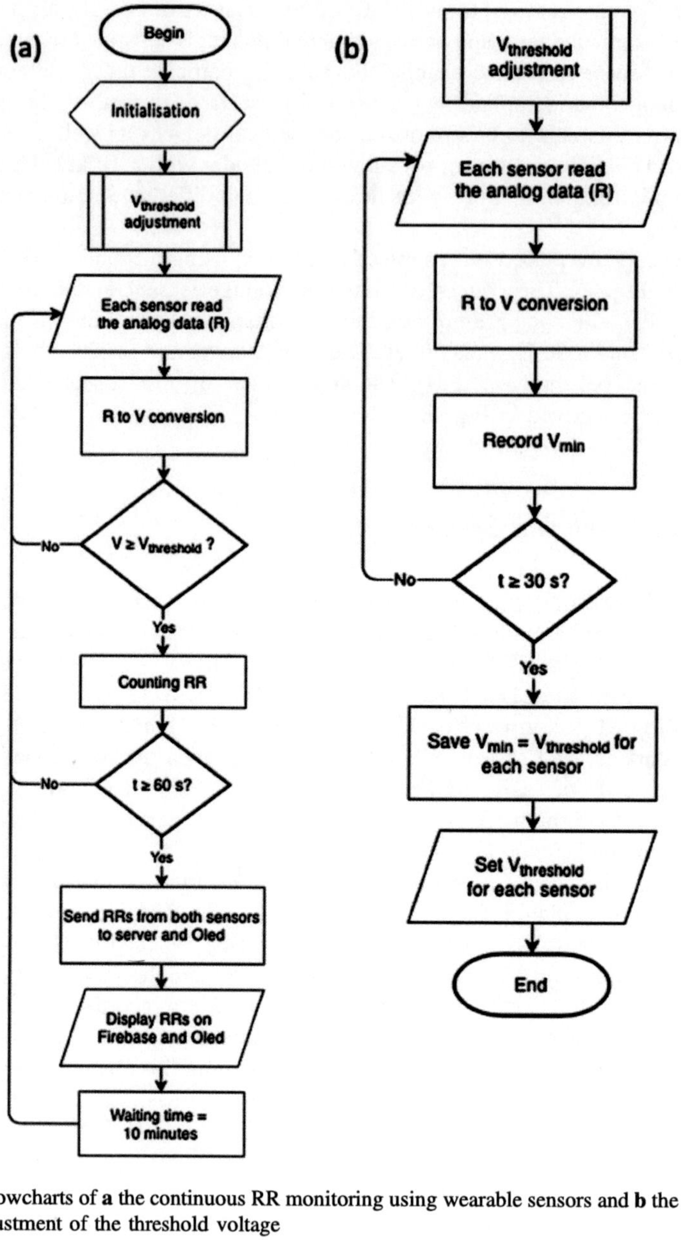

Fig. 3 Flowcharts of **a** the continuous RR monitoring using wearable sensors and **b** the procedure of the adjustment of the threshold voltage

voltage parameter obtained from sensing. Adjustments are made to improve the sensitivity of the sensor reading to abdominal motion for each test subject. The adjustment process (shown in Fig. 3b) is carried out once at the first moment of wearing the device on a test subject in the following steps:

1. Device measures the first abdomen movement. A voltage value is obtained from the conversions, then this value is saved as the threshold voltage, say $_{t}$ = 2.2 V.
2. Device measures the second abdomen movement, then a new voltage, say = 2.05 V, is produced from this measurement. is compared to the threshold voltage to determine the smaller number as the threshold value, say < $_{t}$ then $_{t}$ = 2.05 V.
3. Device continues measuring the next abdomen movement and compares the value with the threshold value for 30 s. The last $_{t}$ is saved and used as the threshold value for RR measurement.

3 Result and Discussion

In this section, we present the result continued by discussing the performance of the flex and FSR402 sensors. For the test comparison and the accuracy, this study used a method of the manual breath count because it is the common reference standard used in hospitals for one minute breath and in other reviews [18, 19]. The results of RR measurement carried out on a group of 20 males of the test subjects aged 20–25 years with different BMI (normal and overweight). The test was done in condition of relaxed test subjects by placing both sensors on their *umbirical* abdomen area.

The adjustment of the threshold voltage for determining the minimum voltage as the threshold of counted breath was automatically executed by the device system for each test subject at the first use, as explained in Subsect. 2.4. The threshold voltages are different for each subject, it depended on the abdominal motion when one breathed. In general, the threshold voltage of the test subject with an overweight BMI is bigger than the one with a normal BMI. The exhale motion is counted as one breath indicating the abdominal area enlarge and makes the sensors supressed.

Some of the RR measurement results using each sensor and the reference standard of the breath manual count are shown in Table 1. The comparisons of these strain sensors are then presented in the forms of the mean relative error (MRE) and the mean absolute error (MAE). The values of MRE, average difference and MAE are calculated using formulas in Eqs. (1) until (3). The variables of *m* and *s* respectively represent the values of the breath manual count and the sensor, i = 1, 2, 3, …, n is the data total.

$$MRE = \frac{1}{n}\left[\sum_{i=1}^{n}\frac{|m_i - s_i|}{m_i}\right] \times 100\% \quad (1)$$

$$Average\ difference = \frac{1}{n}\left(\sum_{i=1}^{n} m_i - s_i\right) \quad (2)$$

Table 1 Comparison of the RR measurements of each sensor to the manual count

Nth Subject	Respiratory Rate (RR) in unit of breaths per minute (bpm)		
	Flex sensor	FSR402	Manual count
1	22	21	23
2	21	18	22
3	22	23	21
4	22	19	23
5	25	22	24
6	21	17	20
7	21	19	23
8	21	19	20
9	21	21	21
10	22	24	22

$$MAE = \frac{1}{n}\left|\sum_{i=1}^{n} m_i - s_i\right| \quad (3)$$

The mean relative errors and the measurement error of each sensor compared to the breath manual count are 4.21% for flex sensor and 10.37% for FSR402. These errors show that the performance of accuracy of flex sensor is better than the FSR402. Meanwhile, the MAE of flex and FSR402 sensors are 0.90 and 2.25 bpm, respectively.

In order to compare and analyze the results of RR measurement, Table 2 presents the statistical analysis using the parameters of the average difference, standard deviation, and the standard error. The measurement comparisons observed are between that of the manual and flex, the manual and FSR402, and the flex and the FSR402. One can see that the average RR difference of the manual-flex methods is the smallest one than the others. It indicates that the measurement result of the flex sensor is very close to the manual count. This result is supported and validated by the smallest values of the standard deviation and the standard error. In contrary, the measurement result of FSR sensor is the poorest one compared to the manual count and the flex sensor. Hence, the performance comparison of both sensors is that the flex sensor is better than the FSR402. In addition, compared to other studies using flex sensor [20, 21], this system generates less error. The errors are not caused by the motion changing of the test subject, for instance from sitting to lying down or vice versa. It does not result in the false detection.

However, the performances of both sensors were improved by introducing the threshold voltage as the minimum input of physical parameter that led to create a detectable voltage change as the output of counting of the respiratory activity. In other words, the threshold adjustment is carried out to adjust or adapt the sensitivity of the sensor to the abdominal condition of each subject when breathing.

Table 2 Comparison of the RR measurements of each sensor to the manual count

Comparison of the methods of RR measurements	Statistical analysis for RR measurements in unit of breaths per minute (bpm)		
	Average difference	Standard deviation	Standard error
Manual—Flex	0.30	1.03	0.23
Manual—FSR402	1.45	2.16	0.48
Flex—FSR402	1.15	1.73	0.39

The performance difference between these two sensors might be caused by several factors, one of them is related to the sensitivity error of sensor responses. The dimension of the active part of the sensor compared to the pressure of the abdominal diaphragm of the test subject during breathing may have relationship affecting the sensor measurement result, where FSR402 is smaller in length than flex sensor. It is possible to find another FSR model with longer dimension, that is FSR408 with 10 × 622 mm strip. This FSR408 model has similar shape with flex sensor.

Finally, the development results of the continuous RR monitoring device using two wearable sensors on abdomen of a test subject in relaxing condition is shown in Fig. 4. This monitoring was performed every 10 min for 6 h. The RR data were displayed on Oled display and Firebase platform, then also recorded in Firebase storage.

The responses of both sensors in Fig. 4 generally show the conformity. However, in terms of qualitative analysis-based time series, it can be observed that the FSR402 sensor is more unstable than the flex sensor. For example, at 8.30, the FSR402 sensor was late in responding to the decrease in respiratory rate, moreover at 11.30 the FSR402 sensor changed ahead of time. Otherwise, the flex sensor was more stable in response to the actual measurements.

In Fig. 5, the RR data distribution is analyzed using the linearity concept applied on both sensors and the manual count. The responses of both sensors in measuring RR show a poor correlation ($r^2 = 0.40$), as shown in scatter plot of Fig. 5a. This is

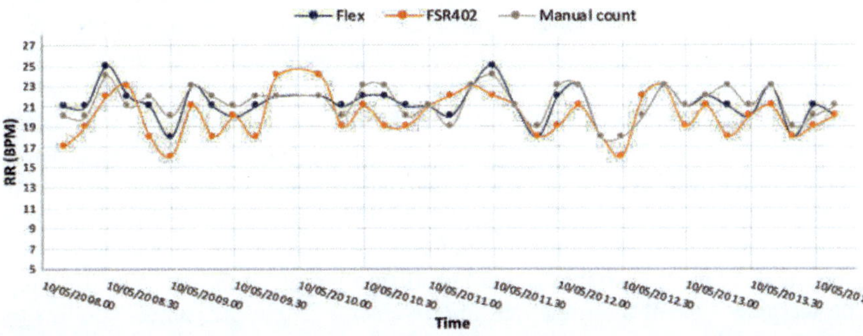

Fig. 4 The recorded data of continuous RR monitoring using flex and FSR402 sensors every 10 min for 6 h

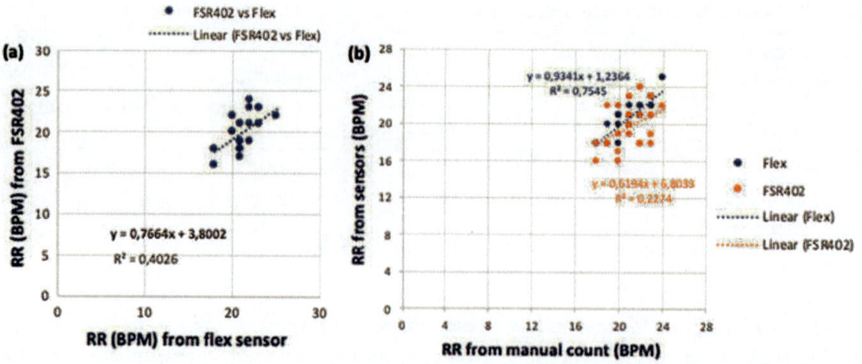

Fig. 5 Comparisons of sensor responses **a** between flex and FSR402 and **b** both sensors to the manual count, in continuous RR monitoring every 10 min for 6 h

probably due to the instability of the FSR402 sensor, inadequate abdominal sensor dimensions, etc. Furthermore, the responses of both sensors as compared to manual count also generally shows a good performance for the flex sensor ($r^2 = 0.75$) and less for the FSR sensor ($r^2 = 0.23$) based on the scatter plot in Fig. 5b.

We can underline some important things for summing up this section that in this developed device can be counted on to assist the duties of the medical staffs in either the ICU or the wards in measuring, recording and monitoring the patient's RR regularly and continuously. Besides, this device may cut off the human error for the RR counting. Last but not least, the use of this relatively inexpensive technology can be applied in most hospitals with low-resource issue [18].

4 Conclusion

This study has demonstrated the development of the continuous RR monitoring using two strain sensors for comparing the sensor performances. This system used the concept of wearable sensor to measure the respiratory rate directly. The threshold adjustment was introduced on the system for first use in each test subject to reduce the measurement limitation such as false detection, incapability to detect the abdominal motion in respiration or too sensitive. Flex sensor has much better performance than FSR402, where its average difference RR compared to manual count and MAE are 0.3 and 0.90, respectively. This result is seemed promising to be explored and improved in further studies such as adding the warning status not only on the display but also in hospital installation by integrating the sound source for the warning. One of the important improvements is that the subject comfort to the use of wearable sensor should be investigated and treated in order to be able to use in clinical condition.

References

1. Dias D, Cunha JPS (2018) Wearable health devices—vital sign monitoring, systems and technologies. Sensors 18(8):2–28
2. Gandevia SC, McKenzie DK (2008) Respiratory rate: the neglected vital sign. Med J Aust 189(9):657–659
3. TRC of Emergency Medicine (2019) Vital signs in adults national quality improvement project report. RCEM, England
4. Goldhill DR, McNarry AF, Mandersloot G (2005) A physiologically—based early warning score for ward patients: the association between score and outcome. Anaesthesia 189(9): 547–553
5. McGain F et al (2008) Documentation of clinical review and vital signs after major surgery. Med J Aust 189(7):1326–5377
6. Buist M, Bernard T, Nguyen TV, Moore G, Anderson J (2004) Association between clinically abnormal observations and subsequent in-hospital mortality: a prospective study. Resuscitation 62(2):137–141
7. Rosenberg AL, Watts C (2000) Patients readmitted to ICUs: a systematic review of risk factors and outcomes. Chest 118(2):492–502
8. Kelly C (2018) Respiratory rate 1: why measurement and recording are crucial. Nursing Times 114(4):23–24
9. Dix A (2018) Respiratory rate 6: the benefits of continuous monitoring. Nursing Times 114 (4):36–37
10. Wheatley I (2018) Respiratory rate 5: using this vital sign to detect deterioration. Nursing Times 114(4):45–46
11. Guechi Y, Pichot A, Frasca A, Rayeh-Pelardy F, Lardeur JY, Mimoz O (2015) Assessment of noninvasive acoustic respiration rate monitoring in patients admitted to an emergency department for drug or alcoholic poisoning. J Clin Monit Comput 29(6):721–726
12. Marjanovic N, Mimoz O, Guenezan J (2020) An easy and accurate respiratory rate monitor is necessary. J Clin Monit Comput 34(2):221–222
13. Eisenberg ME, Givony D, Levin R (2020) Acoustic respiration rate and pulse oximetry-derived respiration rate: a clinical comparison study. J Clin Monit Comput 34 (2):139–146
14. Liu H, Allen J, Zheng D, Chen F (2019) Recent development of respiratory rate measurement technologies. Physiol Meas 40(7):1–27
15. Massaroni C, Nicolò A, Lo Presti D, Sacchetti M, Silvestri S, Schena E (2019) Contact-based methods for measuring respiratory rate. Sensors 19(4):1–47
16. Interlink electronics Homepage. https://www.interlinkelectronics.com/fsr-400-series. Accessed 2020/09/02
17. Al-Kababji A et al (2019) IoT-based fall and ecg monitoring system: wireless communication system based firebase realtime database. In: Proceedings—2019 IEEE Smartworld, Ubiquitous intelligence & computing, advanced & trusted computing, scalable computing & communications internet people smart city innovation. IEEE Explore, Auckland University of Technology, pp 1480–1485
18. Ginsburg AS, Lenahan JL, Izadnegahdar J, Ansermino JM (2017) A systematic review of tools to measure respiratory rate in order to identify childhood pneumonia. Am J Respir Crit Care Med 197(9):1116–1126
19. Smith I, Mackay J, Fahrid N, Krucheck D (2011) Respiratory rate measurement: a comparison of methods. Br J Health Assist 5(1):18

20. Kristiani DG, Triwiyanto T, Nugraha PC et al (2019) The measuring of vital signs using internet of things technology (heart rate and respiration). In: Proceedings 2019 international seminar on application for technology of information and communication: industry 4.0: retrospect, prospect, and challenges. IEEE, Indonesia, pp 417–422
21. Miyagi SA, Mak'ruf MR, Setioningsih ED, Das T (2020) Design of respiration rate meter using flexible sensor. J Electronic Electromed Eng Med Inform 2(1):13–18